Pain Management: A Multidisciplinary Approach

Pain Management: A Multidisciplinary Approach

Edited by Sidney Gillespie

hayle medical
New York

Hayle Medical,
750 Third Avenue, 9th Floor,
New York, NY 10017, USA

Visit us on the World Wide Web at:
www.haylemedical.com

ISBN: 978-1-63241-437-3

The publisher's policy is to use permanent paper from mills that operate a sustainable forestry policy. Furthermore, the publisher ensures that the text paper and cover boards used have met acceptable environmental accreditation standards.

Printed in China.

Cataloging-in-Publication Data

Pain management : a multidisciplinary approach / edited by Sidney Gillespie.
p. cm.
Includes bibliographical references and index.
ISBN 978-1-63241-437-3
1. Pain--Treatment. 2. Pain. 3. Pain--Physiological aspects. 4. Pain medicine. I. Gillespie, Sidney.
RB127 .P35 2017
616.047 2--dc23

Table of Contents

Preface

Pain Management is defined as the treatment of chronic pain and injury. This book on pain management deals with topics related to injury and pain management, long-term and immediate treatment of pain and its diagnosis, etc. Pain management treatment has various techniques such as physiotherapy and massage, interventional injections, behaviour therapy and psychotherapy and alternative medicinal practices such as acupuncture. Chronic pain often goes misdiagnosed and misunderstood, especially among the elderly. This book discusses fundamental as well as modern approaches of pain management. It consists of contributions made by international experts. This book will be helpful for students, experts and researchers in the field of pain management.

The information shared in this book is based on empirical researches made by veterans in this field of study. The elaborative information provided in this book will help the readers further their scope of knowledge leading to advancements in this field.

Finally, I would like to thank my fellow researchers who gave constructive feedback and my family members who supported me at every step of my research.

Editor

1

Central Administration of C-X-C Chemokine Receptor Type 4 Antagonist Alleviates the Development and Maintenance of Peripheral Neuropathic Pain in Mice

Xin Luo[1,4], Wai Lydia Tai[1,4], Liting Sun[1,4], Qiu Qiu[1,4], Zhengyuan Xia[1,3], Sookja Kim Chung[2,3,4], Chi Wai Cheung[1,3,4]*

1 Department of Anaesthesiology, The University of Hong Kong, HKSAR, China, **2** Department of Anatomy, The University of Hong Kong, HKSAR, China, **3** Research Center of Heart, Brain, Hormone and Healthy Aging, The University of Hong Kong, HKSAR, China, **4** Laboratory and Clinical Research Institute for Pain, The University of Hong Kong, HKSAR, China

Abstract

Aim: To explore the roles of C-X-C chemokine receptor type 4 (CXCR4) in spinal processing of neuropathic pain at the central nervous system (CNS).

Methods: Peripheral neuropathic pain (PNP) induced by partial sciatic nerve ligation (pSNL) model was assessed in mice. Effects of a single intrathecal (central) administration of AMD3100 (intrathecal AMD3100), a CXCR4 antagonist, on pain behavior and pain-related spinal pathways and molecules in the L3-L5 spinal cord segment was studied compare to saline treatment.

Results: Rotarod test showed that intrathecal AMD3100 did not impair mice motor function. In pSNL-induced mice, intrathecal AMD3100 delayed the development of mechanical allodynia and reversed the established mechanical allodynia in a dose-dependent way. Moreover, intrathecal AMD3100 downregulated the activation of JNK1 and p38 pathways and the protein expression of p65 as assessed by western blotting. Real-time PCR test also demonstrated that substance P mRNA was decreased, while adrenomedullin and intercellular adhesion molecule mRNA was increased following AMD3100 treatment.

Conclusion: Our results suggest that central (spinal) CXCR4 is involved in the development and maintenance of PNP and the regulation of multiple spinal molecular events under pain condition, implicating that CXCR4 would potentially be a therapeutic target for chronic neuropathic pain.

Editor: Sam Eldabe, The James Cook University Hospital, United Kingdom

Funding: Funding for this study was provided by the departmental fund, Department of Anaesthesiology, The University of Hong Kong; the department fund, Department of Anaesthesiology, The University of Hong Kong had no further role in study design; in the collection, analysis and interpretation of data; in the writing of the report; and in the decision to submit the paper for publication.

Competing Interests: Co-author Professor Sookja K. Chung is a PLOS ONE Editorial Board member but this does not alter the authors' adherence to PLOS ONE Editorial policies and criteria.

* Email: cheucw@hku.hk

Introduction

Chemokine receptors have been intensively studied for their roles in nociception and considered novel targets for neuropathic pain therapy [1]. C-X-C chemokine receptor type 4 (CXCR4) is the receptor of chemokine (C-X-C motif) ligand 12 (CXCL12), which belongs to the G protein-coupled receptor (GPCR) family. CXCR4 is widely expressed in the peripheral and central nervous system (PNS and CNS) and exerts numerous important functions, such as modulation of neurotransmission, synaptic plasticity, and neuroglial interactions [2]. Increasing number of studies reported roles of CXCR4 in pain processing in the PNS, as CXCR4 is expressed on primary sensory neurons, satellite cells, Schwann cells, and endothelial cells in the peripheral nociceptive structure [3–9]. Recent immunohistochemistry studies also showed that CXCR4 would be involved in the modulation of pain signaling in the CNS. CXCL12 and CXCR4 were positive in neurons, astrocytes, microglia/macrophages, and leukocytes in the lumbar spinal cord and their spinal immunoreactivity was found to be increased in a central neuropathic pain model [10]. The activation of spinal CXCR4 by the intrathecal administration of CXCL12 has been found to induce mechanical allodynia for 3 days, which could be reversed by a CXCR4-neutralizing antibody given intrathecally [9].

Currently, systematic (intraperitoneal) administration of CXCR4 antagonist, AMD3100, was demonstrated to have analgesic effects on opioid-induced hyperalgesia [8] and neuropathic pain induced by peripheral neuropathy [3] and by anti-AIDS therapy [6,7]. These studies implicated the potential application of AMD3100 for analgesia. However, central roles of CXCR4 in pain transduction remain unclear and there has been no study evaluating the effects of pharmacological inhibition of

CXCR4 on central pain signal processing. Therefore, in this study, we aimed to explore the roles and mechanisms of central CXCR4 in pain modulation using specific CXCR4 antagonist AMD3100 and a peripheral neuropathic pain (PNP) model using partial sciatic nerve ligation (pSNL) in mice.

Materials and Methods

Animals

This research was approved by the Committee on the Use of Live Animals in Teaching and Research (CULATR) (Permit Number: 2610-11), the University of Hong Kong, and performed according to the guidelines for the care and use of laboratory animals as established by the Laboratory Animal Unit (LAU) at the University of Hong Kong. The mice were housed at 23±3°C, with humidity ranges between 25% and 45% under a 12-hour light/12-hour dark cycle (lights on at 07:00). The mice were offered free access to water and food. They were fed with Lab Diet 5012 (1.0% calcium, 0.5% phosphorus, and 3.3 IU/g of vitamin D3).

The experiments were conducted using adult male C57BL/6 wild-type mice (25–30 grams). Total number of mice used in this project was 86. In Rotarod test, 20 mice that had not received any operation or behavior test were randomly divided into four groups ($n = 5$ in each group). The mice of four groups were treated intrathecally with AMD3100 1 μg (AMD3100 1 μg group), 5 μg (AMD3100 5 μg group), 25 μg (AMD3100 25 μg group) or saline (saline group). To study the roles of CXCR4 in the development of PNP, the mice were randomly divided into four groups. Two groups received either pSNL (pSNL group, $n = 6$) or sham surgery (sham group, $n = 6$) without intrathecal drug administration. The other two groups were treated 1 hour before pSNL surgery with a single intrathecal injection of either AMD3100 (5 μg, AMD3100 + pSNL group, $n = 12$) or saline (saline + pSNL group, $n = 12$). To study the roles of CXCR4 in the maintenance of PNP, mice were randomly divided into four groups, and all received pSNL surgery. On post-operative day (POD) 7, four groups were treated with a single intrathecal injection of AMD3100 or of saline. The dosages given to the four groups were 1 μg (pSNL + AMD3100 1 μg group, $n = 5$), 5 μg (pSNL + AMD3100 5 μg group, $n = 6$), 25 μg (pSNL + AMD3100 25 μg group, $n = 6$), or saline (pSNL + saline group, $n = 5$). To study the effects of a single intrathecal injection of AMD3100 (intrathecal AMD3100) on pain pathways in the lumbar spinal cords of pSNL-injured mice, the mice were treated with a single injection of either AMD3100 25 μg (AMD3100 group) or saline (saline group) on POD 7 ($n = 8$ per group). To study the effects of intrathecal AMD3100 on pain molecules in the lumbar spinal cords of pSNL-injured mice, the mice were treated with a single injection of either AMD3100 25 μg (AMD3100 group) or saline (saline group) on POD 7 ($n = 6$ per group).

Partial sciatic nerve ligation surgery

A pSNL surgery was used as the PNP model in this study [11]. The mice were anesthetized with halothane in a 1:1 mixture of O_2 and N_2O. Under aseptic conditions, the right sciatic nerve (SN) was exposed by an incision from the right sciatic notch to the distal thigh. The location of the SN ligation was identified using the femoral head as a landmark. Approximately 1/2 of the SN was tightly ligated with a 7-0 silk suture. In the sham-operated mice that were used as controls, the right sciatic nerve was exposed, but not ligated. The incision was closed with 5–0 cotton suture and disinfected with ethanol.

Drug administration

AMD3100 (Sigma), a CXCR4 antagonist, was prepared in saline on the day of the experiment. As the dosage of AMD3100 for intrathecal administration in mice has not been determined, dosages of 1 μg, 5 μg, and 25 μg were used in this study. AMD3100 was administrated as a single dose intrathecally, according to a previous study [12]. Before the injection, the animals were anesthetized using halothane with mixture of oxygen and N_2O as described above. Using a syringe (Hamilton) with a 30-gauge needle, a spinal cord puncture was made between the L3 and L5 levels in order to deliver a total volume of 5 μl to the subarachnoid space. Successful administration was identified by tail swinging or a tail configuration of the "S" type immediately after injection.

von Frey test

Mechanical allodynia is the symptom of PNP, which is indicated by a reduction in the paw withdrawal threshold (PWT). This condition was assessed by von Frey test which was performed in our previous research [13]. For habituation before the experiment, the mice were placed in a transparent plastic dome with a metal mesh floor for 20 to 30 minutes. Their PWT was measured with a series of von Frey filaments (IITC). The filaments were applied perpendicularly to the plantar surface of both hind paws, with sufficient force to bend the filaments into an "S" shape. Quick withdrawal or licking of the paw was considered a positive response.

Rotarod test

To assess whether there would be any the potential side-effect of a single intrathecal injection of AMD3100 (intrathecal AMD3100) on motor function, a rotarod test was conducted to measure the motor coordination and balance of the mice._ENREF_18 Twenty mice that had not received any operation or behavior test were randomly divided into four groups. These animals were habituated to the rotarod apparatus (IITC) for 2 consecutive days at low-speed rotation (5 rpm) for 600 seconds each day before basal measurement. During the experiment, the animals were tested in three accelerating trials of 300 seconds, with the rotarod speed increasing from 5 to 40 rpm over 300 seconds, and with an inter-trial interval of at least 20 minutes. The animals' latency in falling from the rod was recorded for each trial, with a cutoff time at 300 seconds.

Western blotting

The sciatic nerve of C57BL/6 mice is composed from elements of L3 and L4 segments of spinal cord with a smaller contribution from L5 segment [14]. Therefore, after euthanizing each mouse with pentobarbital, the L3-L5 section of its spinal cord was quickly removed and homogenized in ice-cold RIPA lysis buffer. After concentration determination, protein samples were separated in 10% SDS-PAGE and electrotransferred onto PVDF membranes. Protein samples were then probed with antibodies for extracellular signal-regulated kinase (ERK, 4695, Cell Signaling), phosphorylated ERK (pERK, 4511, Cell Signaling), c-Jun N-terminal kinase (JNK, 9258, Cell Signaling), phosphorylated JNK (pJNK, 4668, Cell Signaling), p38 (9212, Cell Signaling), phosphorylated p38 (p-p38, 4511, Cell Signaling), AKT (9272, Cell Signaling), phosphorylated AKT (pAKT, 4060, Cell Signaling), Signal transducer and activator of transcription 3 (STAT3, 9132, Cell Signaling), phosphorylated STAT3 (pSTAT3, 9131, Cell Signaling), or p65 (4764, Cell Signaling) with alpha-tubulin (T5168, Sigma) used as a loading control. The membranes were visualized with horseradish

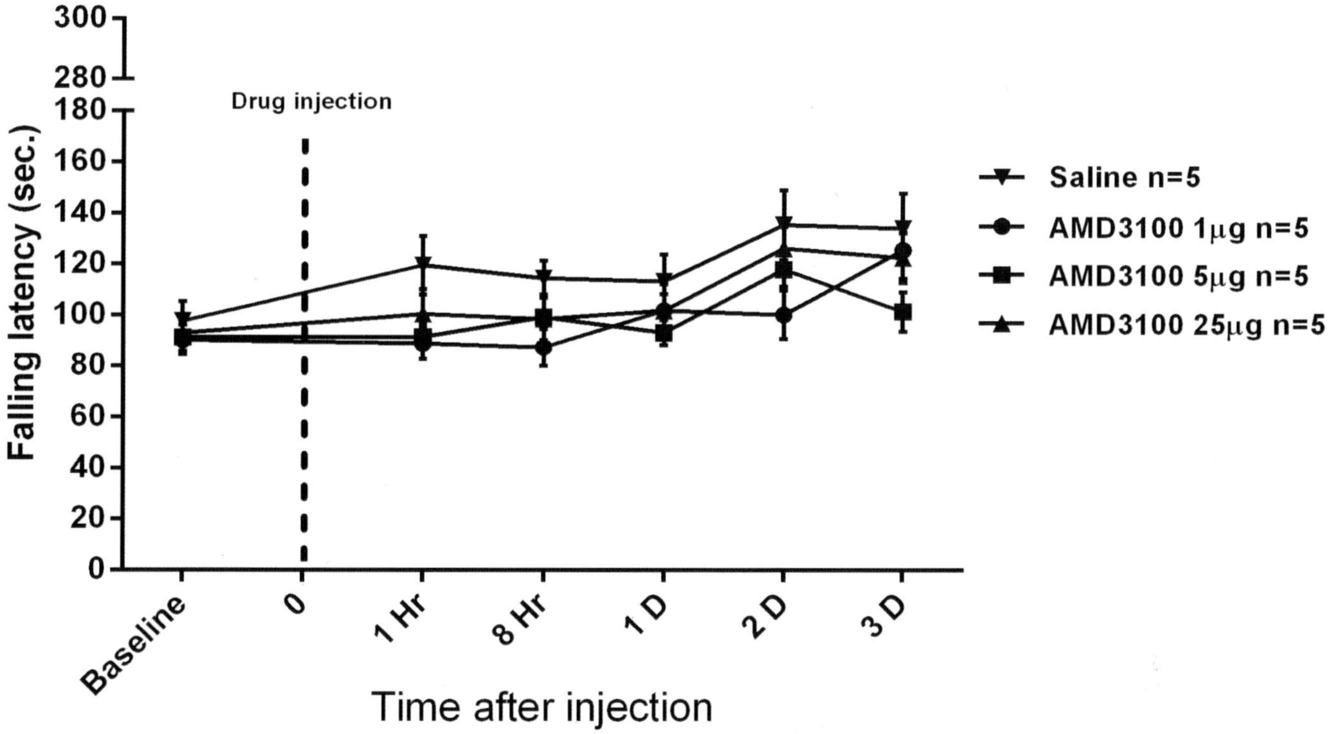

Figure 1. The effects of intrathecal AMD3100 on the motor function of normal mice. There was no significant change in falling latency among the three groups with intrathecal AMD3100, compared to the saline group from hour 1 to day 3 after the injection. Results are mean ± SEM ($n = 5$). Sec. = second, D = day, Hr = hour, 0 = time of intrathecal injection.

peroxidase (HRP)-conjugated secondary antibodies (anti-rabbit IgG and anti-mouse IgG, Sigma).

Real time PCR

After euthanizing each mouse with pentobarbital, the L3-L5 section of its spinal cord was quickly removed and stored at −80°C until RNA extraction. mRNA was extracted from homogenized spinal cord segements following the manufacturer's protocol (Takara). After the quality and quantity determination, mRNA samples were made to cDNA library with reverse transcriptase (Life Technologies). Prepared cDNA samples were diluted and stored at −20°C until further tests. Real time PCR reactions were performed with the SYBR green chemistry method or the Taqman chemistry method (Applied biosystems). The specific primers for substance P (SP), adrenomedullin (AM), calcitonin gene-related peptide (CGRP) and 18S rRNA were reported in our previous study [13], and used with Fast SYBR green master mix (Applied Biosystems). The Taqman Probes for mouse Tumor necrosis factor-α (TNF-α, Mm00443258), interleukin-1β (IL-1β, Mm00434228), interleukin-6 (IL-6, Mm00446190), intercellular adhesion molecule (ICAM, Mm00516023), vascular cell adhesion molecule (VCAM, Mm00449197), excitatory amino-acid transporter-2 (EAAT-2, Mm00441457) and actin-β (Mm01205647) were purchased from Applied Biosystems.

Statistical analysis

The data were expressed as means ± SEM. Student's t tests was used to analyze Western blot and real time PCR data. Results from von Frey test was analyzed using a student's t test or a two-way analysis of variance (ANOVA), followed by a Tukey's multiple comparison post test. Results from the rotarod test were analyzed using a two-way analysis of variance (ANOVA), followed by a Tukey's multiple comparison post test. In all cases, $p<0.05$ was considered as statistically significant.

Results

Effects of intrathecal AMD3100 on the motor function of mice

The effects of intrathecal AMD3100 on motor function had not been studied before. Any impairment in motor function might affect the assessment of pain and intrathecal AMD3100 would not be suitable for potential analgesic treatment if that was the case. Therefore, motor function after intrathecal AMD3100 was assessed by a rotarod test in this study. The falling latency of the three groups with intrathecal AMD3100 showed no significant change compared to the saline group after the injection ($p>0.05$; ANOVA; $n = 5$; Figure 1). These results indicated that intrathecal AMD3100 did not influence the motor function of mice.

Effects of intrathecal AMD3100 on the development and maintenance of mechanical allodynia in pSNL-injured mice

AMD3100 or saline was given intrathecally at one hour before pSNL surgery, and the involvement of central CXCR4 in the development of PNP was evaluated by von Frey tests. Sham surgery ($n = 6$) did not affect ipsilateral PWT, but pSNL surgery ($n = 6$) decreased ipsilateral PWT significantly on POD 1 ($p<0.001$; ANOVA). These results demonstrated that mechanical allodynia was induced immediately by pSNL, but not by sham operation. Pretreatment of a single intrathecal injection of saline (intrathecal saline) did not have any effect on ipsilateral PWT in

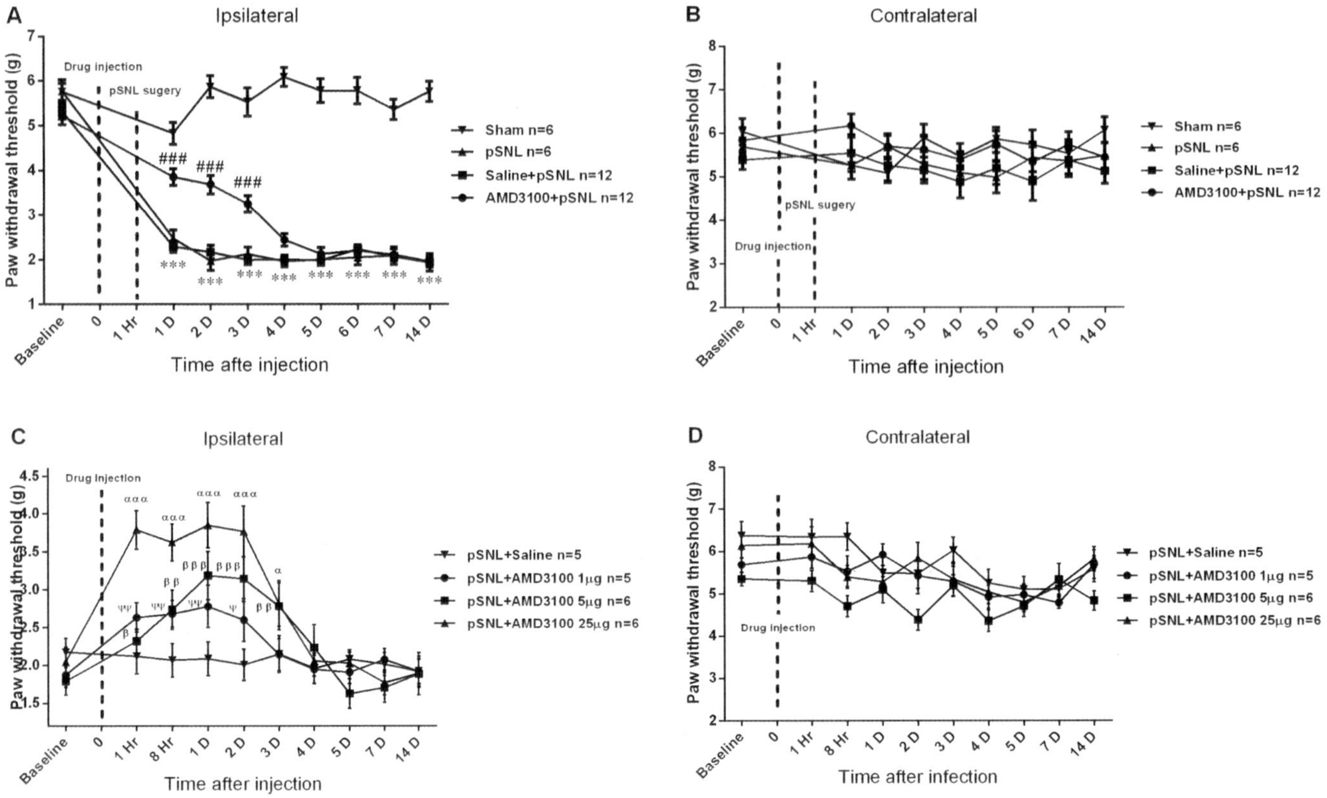

Figure 2. The effects of intrathecal AMD3100 on the development and maintenance of PNP in pSNL-injured mice. The preemptive intrathecal AMD3100, but not intrathecal saline, increased ipsilateral PWT of pSNL mice for 3 days after the surgery (A), but did not affect contralateral PWT (B). On POD 7, intrathecal AMD3100 at dosages of 1 μg, 5 μg and 25 μg increased the ipsilateral PWT of pSNL mice for 2, 3 and 3 days, respectively (C), but did not affect contralateral PWT (D). Results are mean ± SEM ($n = 5–12$). $^{***}p<0.001$ versus the pSNL group at the corresponding timepoints. $^{\#\#\#}p<0.001$ versus the Saline + pSNL group at the corresponding timepoints. $^{\alpha\alpha\alpha}p<0.001$, $^{\alpha}p<0.05$, $^{\beta\beta\beta}p<0.001$, $^{\beta\beta}p<0.01$, $^{\beta}p<0.05$, $^{\Psi\Psi}p<0.01$ and $^{\Psi}p<0.05$ versus the baseline. g = gram, D = day, Hr = hour, 0 = time of intrathecal injection.

the pSNL + saline group (n = 12), as compared with that in the pSNL group without any intrathecal medication ($p>0.05$; ANOVA). However, intrathecal AMD3100 before pSNL surgery increased ipsilateral PWT significantly from day 1 to day 3 ($p<0.001$; ANOVA; n = 12) after drug injection, as compared with the pSNL + saline group (Figure 2A). No difference in contralateral PWT was found among the four study groups ($p>0.05$; ANOVA; Figure 2B). These results suggested that intrathecal AMD3100 could delay the development of mechanical allodynia by pSNL.

To study the role of central CXCR4 in the maintenance of PNP, pSNL-injured mice received either intrathecal AMD3100 or intrathecal saline on POD 7. Mechanical allodynia from hour 1 to day 14 after the injection was assessed by von Frey test. Intrathecal AMD3100 1 μg increased ipsilateral PWT from hour 1 to day 2 ($p<0.01$ or 0.05; student's t test; n = 5; Figure 2C) after the injection. Intrathecal AMD3100 5 μg increased ipsilateral PWT from hour 1 to day 3 ($p<0.001$ or 0.01 or 0.05; student's t test; n = 6; Figure 2C) after the injection. Intrathecal AMD3100 25 μg increased ipsilateral PWT from hour 1 to day 3 ($p<0.001$ or 0.05; student's t test; n = 6; Figure 2C) after the injection. Intrathecal saline did not have any effect on ipsilateral PWT ($p>0.05$; student's t test; n = 5; Figure 2C). No significant difference was shown in contralateral PWT among any of the four groups ($p>0.05$; student's t test; Figure 2D). These results suggested that intrathecal AMD3100 could transiently reverse established mechanical allodynia by pSNL in a dose-dependent way.

Effects of intrathecal AMD3100 on the production of pain molecules in the lumbar spinal cord of pSNL-injured mice

Following the peripheral nerve injury, the central release of neuropeptides (e.g. SP, CGRP and AM), pro-inflammatory cytokines (e.g. TNF-α, IL-1β and IL-6), cellular adhesion molecules (e.g. ICAM and VCAM) and glutamate transporter (e.g. EAAT-2) contribute to neuronal central sensitization and persistent pain [15,16]. Therefore, we also investigated whether intrathecal AMD3100 could affect the spinal production of these neuropeptides and pro-inflammatory cytokines. The mRNA level of SP was decreased but the mRNA level of AM and ICAM were increased significantly on the ipsilateral side of the L3-L5 spinal cord segment in pSNL-injured mice with intrathecal AMD3100 25 μg (n = 6) compared to the saline group (n = 6) at 8 hour after the injection ($p<0.05$; student's t test; Figures 3B, C and G). However, the mRNA levels of CGRP, TNF-α, IL-1β, IL-6, VCAM and EAAT-2 in the L3-L5 spinal cords of pSNL-injured mice were not affected by intrathecal AMD3100 (all $p>0.05$; student's t test; Figures 3A, D, E, F, H and I).

Effects of intrathecal AMD3100 on pain signaling pathways in the lumbar spinal cord of pSNL-injured mice

Spinal mitogen-activated protein kinases (MAPKs), phosphoinositide 3-kinase (PI3K), STAT3 and nuclear factor kappa-light-chain-enhancer of activated B (NF-κB) pathways were shown to be significantly activated on POD 7 using PNP models [17–20]. Our

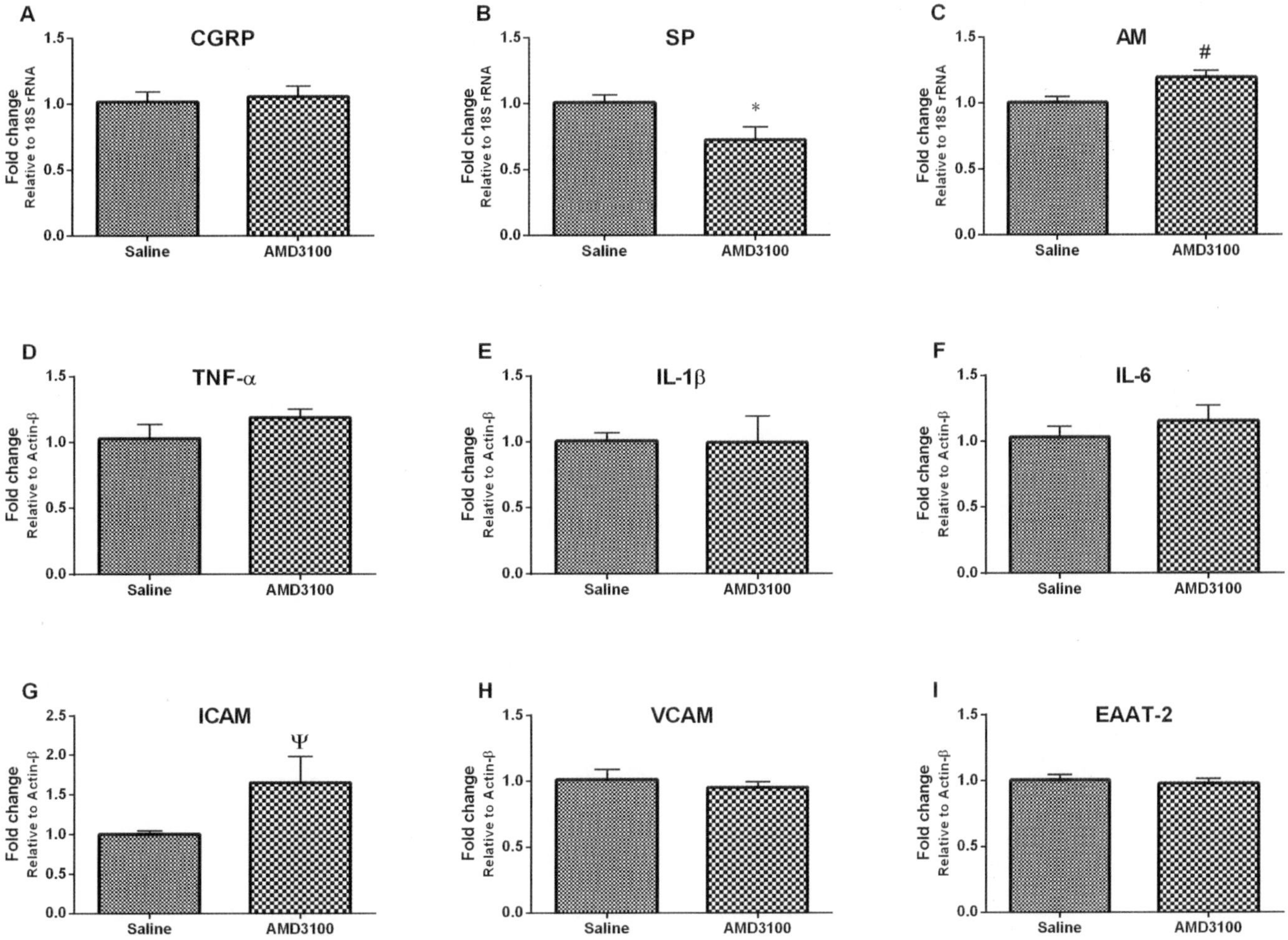

Figure 3. The effects of intrathecal AMD3100 on the production of neuropeptides and pro-inflammatory cytokines, and cellular adhesion molecules in the ipsilateral L3-L5 spinal cord segment of pSNL-injured mice. Real time PCR revealed that intrathecal AMD3100 decreased mRNA level of SP (B) and increased mRNA level of AM (C) and ICAM (G), but did not affect mRNA levels of CGRP (A), TNF-α (D) and IL-1β (E), IL-6 (F), VCAM (H) or EAAT-2 (I) at hour 8 after the injection. Results are means ± SEM (n = 6). *$p<0.01$, $^{\#}p$ and $^{\Psi}p<0.05$ versus the saline group.

result found that intrathecal AMD3100 in all used dosage produced analgesic effects on pSNL-injured mice at hour 8 after the drug injection. Therefore, we harvested lumbar spinal cord sample from this time-point and detected whether intrathecal AMD3100 could affect the activation of members of these pathways. The phosphorylation level of JNK1 ($p<0.01$; student's t test; Figure 4C) and p38 ($p<0.05$; student's t test; Figure 4E) and the expression level of p65 ($p<0.05$; student's t test; Figure 4H) was decreased significantly on the ipsilateral side of the L3-L5 spinal cord segment in pSNL-injured mice with intrathecal AMD3100 25 μg (n = 8), compared to the saline group (n = 8). However, the activation (phosphorylation) levels of ERK1, ERK2, and JNK2 in the L3-L5 spinal cords of pSNL-injured mice were not affected by intrathecal AMD3100 (all $p>0.05$; student's t test; Figures 4A, B, D, F and G).

Discussion

Although recent immunohistochemistry study has suggested the involvement of CXCR4 in pain processing in the CNS [10], central roles of CXCR4 in nociception remain unclear. Therefore, in order to explore the function of CXCR4 in pain modulation in CNS, we studied the pharmacological effects of intrathecal administration of CXCR4 antagonist (AMD3100) on PNP using a pSNL model. The pSNL model is a widely used PNP model, and long-lasted mechanical allodynia is induced following partial sciatic ligation [11]. Our present work employed a single intrathecal injection of AMD3100 before pSNL surgery or on POD 7 with similar methods used in antagonism studies of other chemokine receptors [21,22]. Evidence for the involvement of central CXCR4 in the initiation of PNP came from the observation that the pretreatment of AMD3100 led to an attenuation of pSNL-induced allodynia. Essentially, this CXCR4 antagonist was also effective in alleviating mechanical allodynia when pSNL-induce neuropathy had been established. The results indicated that CXCR4 also contribute to the early maintenance of PNP state. Moreover, the reliability of these behavioral anti-nociceptive effects was enhanced by the facts the intrathecal AMD3100 did not impair any motor function.

Previous studies reported analgesic effects of systematic administration of AMD3100 only lasted for hours [8,10], but the effects of central administration of AMD3100 as used in our current study could last for several days. As CXCR4 is widely distributed on nearly all cell types and plays important roles in the tissue development [23], systematic (intraperitoneal) administration of

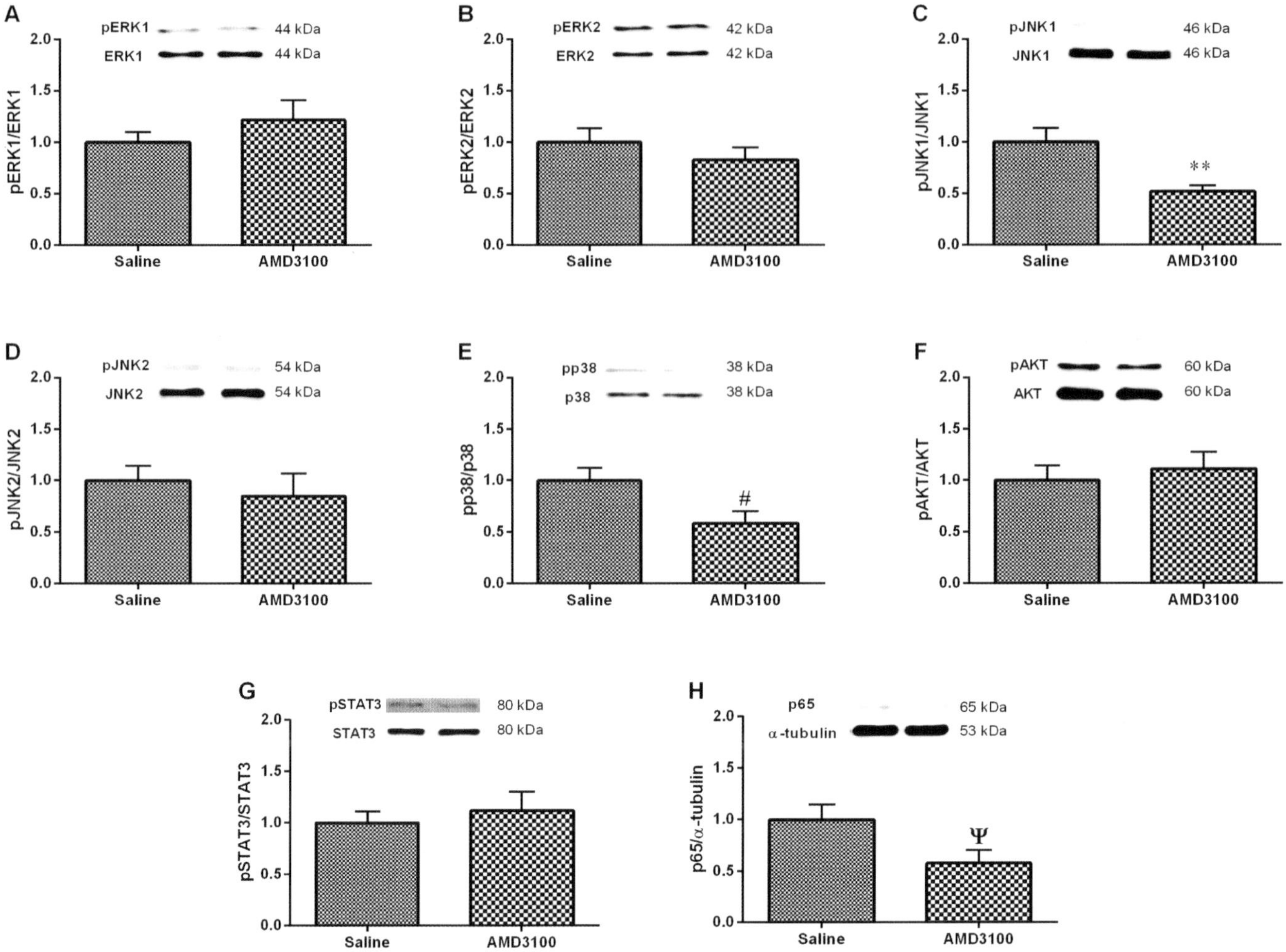

Figure 4. The effects of intrathecal AMD3100 on pain pathways in the ipsilateral L3-L5 spinal cord segment of pSNL-injured mice. Western blotting revealed that intrathecal AMD3100 decreased the phosphorylation level of the JNK1 (C), p38 (E) and p65 (H) pathway, but did not affect the phosphorylation levels of the ERK1 (A), ERK2 (B), JNK2 (D), AKT (F) or STAT3 (G) at hour 8 after the injection. Results are means ± SEM (n = 8). $^{**}p<0.01$, $^{\#}p$ and $^{\Psi}p<0.05$ versus the saline group.

CXCR4 antagonist would be of lower nociceptive structure-specificity and anti-nociceptive efficiency relative to central (intrathecal) administration of AMD3100 theoretically. Moreover, intrathecal delivery of AMD3100 is highly specific to spinal cord, implicating that central (spinal) administration of CXCR4 antagonist for analgesia would be more effective than peripheral injection. While the effects of AMD3100 on DRG have been previously reported [3,4,6–8], its spinal effects have not been studied. Multiple mechanisms would accounts for the anti-nociceptive effects of intrathecal AMD3100, as CXCR4 is expressed on neuron, glia and other cell types in the lumbar spinal cord [9,10]. Therefore, in the current study, we explored its effects on well-known pain pathways and molecules at the lumbar spinal cord.

GPCR coupled signaling, including MAPKs, PI3K, STAT3 and NF-κB pathways, are proposed to function in CXCR4 signaling, and these pathways are also activated in the lumbar spinal cord following peripheral neuropathy [17–20]. As these pathways are activated by different cell type-specific mechanisms, antagonism study of intrathecal AMD3100 on these pathways can explain how CXCR4 signaling works on PNP in the CNS. The present study found that, among MAPK pathways, intrathecal AMD3100 downregulated spinal phosphorylation level of JNK1 and p38, but did not affect ERK1, ERK2 or JNK2. Peripheral neuropathy activates ERK1/2 in neuron, astrocyte and microglia. pSNL-induced activation of JNK1/2 is restricted to spinal astrocyte, while, the activation of p38 is restricted to spinal microglia [17]. This study also uncovered that intrathecal AMD3100 reduced the spinal expression of p65. The family of NF-κB transcription factors is associated with neuropathic pain, and the activation (increase in expression) of these factors is selectively restricted in spinal glial cells (astrocyte and microglia) [18,24]. Peripheral neuropathy also activates STAT3 (restricted to spinal microglia [20]) and AKT (restricted to spinal neuron [19]); however our present study did not found any effect of intrathecal AMD3100 on STAT3 or AKT pathways. Therefore, this research found that, among pain-related CGRP pathways, some pathways activated in spinal glial cells would account for anti-nociceptive effects of intrathecal AMD3100.

This research also studied the effects of intrathecal AMD3100 on pain-related molecules. Our study showed that AMD3100 given intrathecally reduced the spinal production of SP and increased that of AM, but its effects on CGRP were not detectable. SP is locally expressed by secondary sensory neuron at the lumbar spinal cord [25], and spinal SP expression is inducible following neuropathy, implicating that SP may account for the pain signaling to higher level of nociceptive structure [26]. AM is a pain-related neuropeptide with partial homology to CGRP, and recent research with transgenic technology unveiled its central role in pain processing was more complicated than previously surmised [27]. Because the presence of pre-synaptic and post-synaptic CXCR4 receptor implicates the potential interaction of CXCR4 signaling and the release of neurotransmitters [9], our results verified this hypothesis that neuronal CXCR4 may modulate SP and AM-mediated synaptic activity in central nociception. TNF-α, IL-1β and IL-6 are mainly released by spinal glial cells and contribute to the alteration of pain processing centrally [28]. Spinal production of these cytokines was transiently increased at early stage following peripheral neuropathy, implicating that these pro-inflammatory cytokines would be important to the development, but not the maintenance, of neuropathic pain [29]. Therefore, our results indicated that effects of intrathecal AMD3100 on maintenance of PNP did not involve the regulation of these pro-inflammatory cytokines. Moreover, our study found that AMD3100 given intrathecally increased the spinal mRNA level of ICAM. The blood-spinal cord barrier (BSCB) offers a specialized microenvironment for the cellular constituents of the spinal cord, and increasing evidence shows that BSCB is involved in nociception following neuropathic injury [30]. The expression level of ICAM correlates with the permeability of BSCB and the infiltration of immune cells to the CNS [31]. Therefore, this result indicated that central CXCR4 would be involved in the regulation of the permeability of BSCB and the immune response to PNP at the spinal cord. Spinal expression of EAAT-2 is decreased with peripheral neuropahty, and the prevention of downregulated EAAT-2 expression can potentially be an analgesic target [32]. Nevertheless, this studied did not show the involvement of central CXCR4 in the regulation of EAAT-2 expression.

In conclusion, this study firstly reports that central administration of CXCR4 antagonist AMD3100 can attenuate the development and the maintenance of PNP after pSNL without any impairment in motor function. Among well-known pain related pathways and molecules, the analgesic effects of intrathecal AMD3100 involve the downregulation of JNK1, p38 and p65 pathways, with the decrease in SP and the increase in AM and ICAM in the lumbar spinal cord of pSNL-injured mice. This study is an essential step toward understanding the contribution of CXCR4-mediated pain processing in CNS, which can lead to chemokine-targeted analgesia in the future.

Acknowledgments

We would like to thank Dr. Amy Cheuk Yin Lo, who assisted with animal experiments.

Author Contributions

Conceived and designed the experiments: LX CSK CCW. Performed the experiments: LX TWL QQ. Analyzed the data: LX TWL SLT QQ XZY CSK CCW. Contributed reagents/materials/analysis tools: LX TWL SLT XZY CSK CCW. Wrote the paper: LX TLW QQ.

References

1. Rostene W, Dansereau MA, Godefroy D, Van Steenwinckel J, Goazigo ARL, et al. (2011) Neurochemokines: a menage a trois providing new insights on the functions of chemokines in the central nervous system. Journal of Neurochemistry 118: 680–694.
2. Li MZ, Ransohoff RA (2008) Multiple roles of chemokine CXCL12 in the central nervous system: A migration from immunology to neurobiology. Progress in Neurobiology 84: 116–131.
3. Dubovy P, Klusakova I, Svizenska I, Brazda V (2010) Spatio-temporal changes of SDF1 and its CXCR4 receptor in the dorsal root ganglia following unilateral sciatic nerve injury as a model of neuropathic pain. Histochemistry and Cell Biology 133: 323–337.
4. Oh SB, Tran PB, Gillard SE, Hurley RW, Hammond DL, et al. (2001) Chemokines and glycoprotein 120 produce pain hypersensitivity by directly exciting primary nociceptive neurons. Journal of Neuroscience 21: 5027–5035.
5. Bhangoo S, Ren D, Miller RJ, Henry KJ, Lineswala J, et al. (2007) Delayed functional expression of neuronal chemokine receptors following focal nerve demyelination in the rat: a mechanism for the development of chronic sensitization of peripheral nociceptors. Molecular Pain 3: 38.
6. Bhangoo SK, Ren DJ, Miller RJ, Chan DM, Ripsch MS, et al. (2007) CXCR4 chemokine receptor signaling mediates pain hypersensitivity in association with antiretroviral toxic neuropathy. Brain Behavior and Immunity 21: 581–591.
7. Bhangoo SK, Ripsch MS, Buchanan DJ, Miller RJ, White FA (2009) Increased chemokine signaling in a model of HIV1-associated peripheral neuropathy. Molecular Pain 5: 48.
8. Wilson NM, Jung HS, Ripsch MS, Miller RJ, White FA (2011) CXCR4 signaling mediates morphine-induced tactile hyperalgesia. Brain Behavior and Immunity 25: 565–573.
9. Reaux-Le Goazigo A, Rivat C, Kitabgi P, Pohl M, Parsadaniantz SM (2012) Cellular and subcellular localization of CXCL12 and CXCR4 in rat nociceptive structures: physiological relevance. European Journal of Neuroscience 36: 2619–2631.
10. Knerlich-Lukoschus F, von der Ropp-Brenner B, Lucius R, Mehdorn HM, Held-Feindt J (2011) Spatiotemporal CCR1, CCL3(MIP-1 alpha), CXCR4, CXCL12(SDF-1 alpha) expression patterns in a rat spinal cord injury model of posttraumatic neuropathic pain. Journal of Neurosurgery-Spine 14: 583–597.
11. Bennett GJ, Xie YK (1988) A peripheral mononeuropathy in rat that produces disorders of pain sensation like those seen in man. Pain 33: 87–107.
12. Fairbanks CA (2003) Spinal delivery of analgesics in experimental models of pain and analgesia. Advanced Drug Delivery Reviews 55: 1007–1041.
13. Hung VKL, Chen SMY, Tai LW, Chen AYS, Chung SK, et al. (2012) Over-expression of endothelin-1 in astrocytes, but not endothelial cells, ameliorates inflammatory pain response after formalin injection. Life Sciences 91: 618–622.
14. Rigaud M, Gemes G, Barabas ME, Chernoff DI, Abram SE, et al. (2008) Species and strain differences in rodent sciatic nerve anatomy: Implications for studies of neuropathic pain. Pain 136: 188–201.
15. Basbaum AI, Bautista DM, Scherrer G, Julius D (2009) Cellular and Molecular Mechanisms of Pain. Cell 139: 267–284.
16. Chaudhary P, Marracci GH, Bourdette DN (2006) Lipoic acid inhibits expression of ICAM-1 and VCAM-1 by CNS endothelial cells and T cell migration into the spinal cord in experimental autoimmune encephalomyelitis. Journal of Neuroimmunology 175: 87–96.
17. Ji RR, Gereau RW, Malcangio M, Strichartz GR (2009) MAP kinase and pain. Brain Research Reviews 60: 135–148.
18. Chou CW, Wong GTC, Lim G, Wang SX, Irwin MG, et al. (2011) Spatiotemporal Pattern of Concurrent Spinal and Supraspinal NF-kappa B Expression After Peripheral Nerve Injury. Journal of Pain 12: 13–21.
19. Xu JT, Tu HY, Xin WJ, Liu XG, Zhang GH, et al. (2007) Activation of phosphatidylinositol 3-kinase and protein kinase B/Akt in dorsal root ganglia and spinal cord contributes to the neuropathic pain induced by spinal nerve ligation in rats. Experimental Neurology 206: 269–279.
20. Dominguez E, Rivat C, Pommier B, Mauborgne A, Pohl M (2008) JAK/STAT3 pathway is activated in spinal cord microglia after peripheral nerve injury and contributes to neuropathic pain development in rat. Journal of Neurochemistry 107: 50–60.
21. Serrano A, Pare M, McIntosh F, Elmes SJR, Martino G, et al. (2010) Blocking spinal CCR2 with AZ889 reversed hyperalgesia in a model of neuropathic pain. Molecular Pain 6: 90.
22. Milligan ED, Zapata V, Chacur M, Schoeniger D, Biedenkapp J, et al. (2004) Evidence that exogenous and endogenous fractalkine can induce spinal nociceptive facilitation in rats. European Journal of Neuroscience 20: 2294–2302.
23. McGrath KE, Koniski AD, Maltby KM, McGann JK, Palis J (1999) Embryonic expression and function of the chemokine SDF-1 and its receptor, CXCR4. Developmental Biology 213: 442–456.
24. Meunier A, Latremoliere A, Dominguez E, Mauborgne A, Philippe S, et al. (2007) Lentiviral-mediated targeted NF-kappa B blockade in dorsal spinal cord glia attenuates sciatic nerve injury-induced neuropathic pain in the rat. Molecular Therapy 15: 687–697.
25. D'Mello R, Dickenson AH (2008) Spinal cord mechanisms of pain. British Journal of Anaesthesia 101: 8–16.
26. Malmberg AB, Basbaum AI (1998) Partial sciatic nerve injury in the mouse as a model of neuropathic pain: behavioral and neuroanatomical correlates. Pain 76: 215–222.
27. Fernandez AP, Serrano J, Martinez-Murillo R, Martinez A (2010) Lack of Adrenomedullin in the Central Nervous System Results in Apparently Paradoxical Alterations on Pain Sensitivity. Endocrinology 151: 4908–4915.

28. Watkins LR, Milligan ED, Maier SF (2001) Glial activation: a driving force for pathological pain. Trends in Neurosciences 24: 450–455.
29. Lee HL, Lee KM, Son SJ, Hwang SH, Cho HJ (2004) Temporal expression of cytokines and their receptors mRNAs in a neuropathic pain model. Neuroreport 15: 2807–2811.
30. Bartanusz V, Jezova D, Alajajian B, Digicaylioglu M (2011) The Blood-Spinal Cord Barrier: Morphology and Clinical Implications. Annals of Neurology 70: 194–206.
31. Lee SJ, Benveniste EN (1999) Adhesion molecule expression and regulation on cells of the central nervous system. Journal of Neuroimmunology 98: 77–88.
32. Nakagawa T, Kaneko S (2010) Spinal Astrocytes as Therapeutic Targets for Pathological Pain. Journal of Pharmacological Sciences 114: 347–353.

2

An Efficient, Optimized Synthesis of Fentanyl and Related Analogs

Carlos A. Valdez[1,2], Roald N. Leif[1,2], Brian P. Mayer[1,2]*

1 Physical and Life Sciences Directorate, Lawrence Livermore National Laboratory, Livermore, California, United States of America, **2** Forensic Science Center, Lawrence Livermore National Laboratory, Livermore, California, United States of America

Abstract

The alternate and optimized syntheses of the parent opioid fentanyl and its analogs are described. The routes presented exhibit high-yielding transformations leading to these powerful analgesics after optimization studies were carried out for each synthetic step. The general three-step strategy produced a panel of four fentanyls in excellent yields (73–78%) along with their more commonly encountered hydrochloride and citric acid salts. The following strategy offers the opportunity for the gram-scale, efficient production of this interesting class of opioid alkaloids.

Editor: Martina Lahmann, Bangor University, United Kingdom

Funding: The authors (CAV, BPM, and RNL) received funding from Lawrence Livermore National Laboratory (llnl.gov) under the Laboratory Directed Research and Development (LDRD) program, project number 14-ERD-048. The funders had no role in study design, data collection and analysis, decision to publish, or preparation of the manuscript.

Competing Interests: The authors have declared that no competing interests exist.

* Email: mayer22@llnl.gov

Introduction

Very few synthetic drugs generate an immediate and powerful impact in the biomedical field shortly after their inception. This has been the case particularly within the areas of pre-surgical, surgical, and post-surgical anesthesiology where the need for fast acting, effective pain relievers is a key element in the overall patient care practice. Morphine (**1**) and Tramadol (**2**) (Fig. 1) are two opioid-based compounds that are widely recognized for being the gold standard prescriptions for patients with moderate to severe pain after surgery or with certain disease states (*e.g.* cancer) [1–6]. Due to their potency, these therapeutics, however, are also well known for their ability to foster chemical dependencies in patients and other users [7].

Though it is often difficult to surpass the established therapeutic records and efficiency profiles by the aforementioned drugs, occasionally new drug candidates are identified that accomplish this seemingly difficult feat. Such is the case for a class of synthetic alkaloids whose birth and swift entrance in the medical field of anesthesiology originated with the synthesis of fentanyl (**4**, Fig. 1) by Paul Janssen in 1960 [8–11]. Since its synthesis, inspired partly by the necessity to improve the potency and bioavailability of the structurally related opiate Demerol (**3**), fentanyl analogs with superior pharmacokinetic properties, onset time, and effective dosage have been successfully produced [12,13]. Currently, a significant array of fentanyl analogs exists spanning a large range of physicochemical properties, which strictly determine their ultimate application. Some of these compounds, along with their potency relative to morphine, are given in Fig. 2 [12,14].

With drugs of this kind, propensity of their users to become physiologically dependent has been reported, and indeed there exist issues involving the use of fentanyl and its analogs [15,16]. For example, these compounds have been the epicenter of fatal incidents involving overdoses by users who self-administer quantities that are just minimally beyond the carefully prescribed doses for controlling pain in a clinical setting. Additionally, there has been documented military misuse of these compounds for their crowd controlling properties. As a particularly infamous case, the presumed use of gaseous/aerosolized fentanyl derivatives by Russian security forces to incapacitate terrorists during a Moscow theater hostage crisis in 2002 led to the death of 170 people, 127 of them hostages [17–21]. The powerful effects of these compounds at such low doses combined with the lack of medical training in cases of illicit use make these drugs extremely dangerous outside the clinical environment.

Fentanyl (prescribed more commonly by its trade name Sublimaze) is approximately 50–100 times more potent than morphine, a quality that has righteously cemented this drug and its congeners in the medical field as the primary choice for a fast acting anesthetic during perioperative procedures. Their *modus operandi* is believed to involve the binding to the transmembrane μ-opioid receptors on cell surfaces resulting in a cascade of intracellular signals that eventually results in their biological effect [22,23]. Even though to date a detailed description of this receptor binding event remains undiscovered, a suitable model can be proposed based on the known binding of similar opioids to various nociceptive/opioid receptors for which few crystallographic structures have been solved [24–27].

Due to the importance of this class of opioids in the biomedical field as well as their history of illicit use, it is not surprising that several synthetic routes have been devised for their construction since Janssen's original disclosure [28–31]. However, most of these routes focus on specific transformations along the original

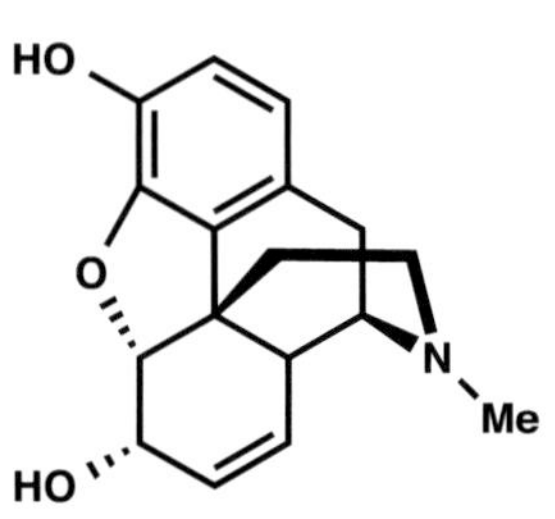

1

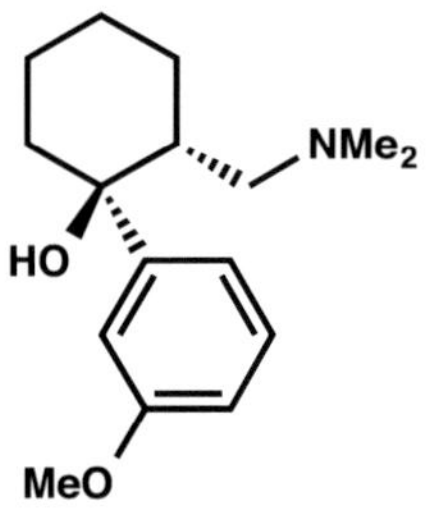

2

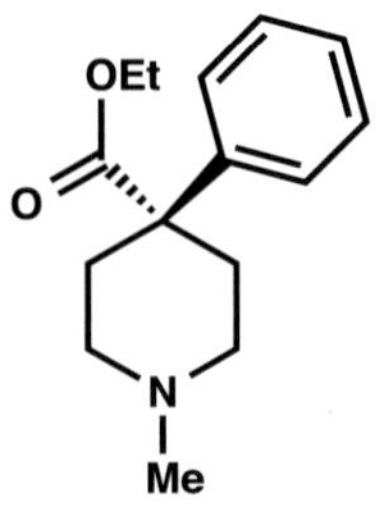

3

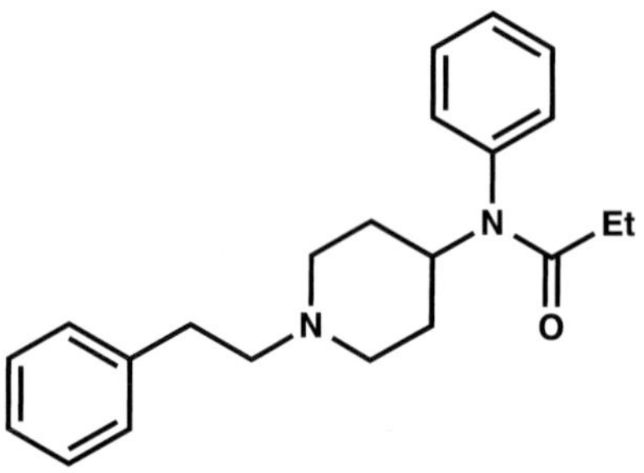

4

Figure 1. Various commonly administered opioids: (1) morphine, (2) Tramadol, (3) Demerol, and (4) fentanyl.

sequence to eventually provide fentanyl (**4**) in moderate yields. The need to understand fentanyl receptor activation and to develop potential countermeasures for illicit use coupled to the lack of established procedures for procuring high quality materials in gram quantities prompted us to revisit and optimize the synthetic route for parent fentanyl **4** along with additional analogs. The routes described herein were optimized to obtain fentanyls in high yields using an efficient, three-step synthetic strategy. The four analogs that our efforts focused on are: fentanyl (**4**), acetylfentanyl (**9**), thiofentanyl (**10**) and acetylthiofentanyl (**11**). The opioids were synthesized as the free bases as well as their more clinically relevant hydrochloride and citric acid salts (Fig. 3).

Materials and Methods

Solvents used during the syntheses were removed by using a Büchi rotary evaporator R-200 equipped with a Büchi heating bath B-490 and coupled to a KNF Laboport Neuberger UN820 vacuum pump. Analytical thin layer chromatography (TLC) was conducted on Agela Technologies silica gel glass plates coupled with detection ceric ammonium molybdate (CAM), exposure to iodine vapor and/or UV light ($\lambda = 254$ nm). ^{1}H NMR (600 MHz) and ^{13}C NMR (150 MHz) were recorded in $CDCl_3$ and D_2O. Spectra were obtained using a Bruker Avance III 600 MHz instrument equipped with a Bruker QNP 5 mm cryoprobe (Bruker Biospin, Billerica, MA) at 30.0±0.1°C. NMR data is reported as follows: chemical shift (δ) (parts per million, ppm); multiplicity: s (singlet), d (doublet), t (triplet), q (quartet) and br (broad); coupling constants (J) are given in Hertz (Hz). ^{1}H NMR chemical shifts are calibrated with respect to residual chloroform in $CDCl_3$ centered at 7.26 ppm, whereas for ^{13}C NMR, the center peak for $CDCl_3$, centered at 77.0 ppm, was used for the calibration. All NMR spectra can be found in Information S1. HRMS analyses were obtained at the Forensic Science Center at the Lawrence Livermore National Laboratory using either Chemical Ionization (CI) or Electrospray Ionization (ESI). Elemental analyses were conducted at Galbraith Laboratories (Knoxville, TN).

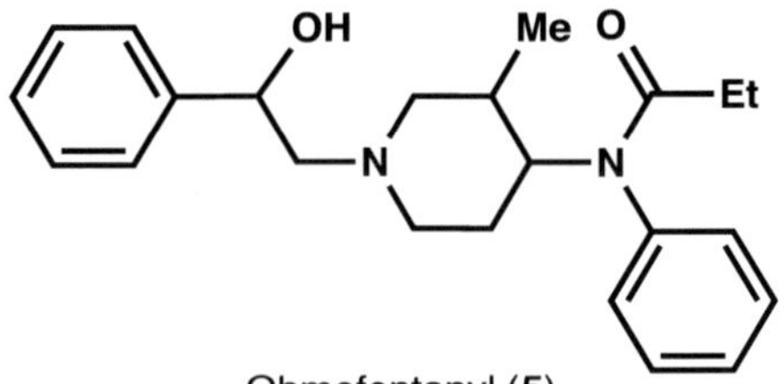

Ohmefentanyl (**5**)
[6300x]

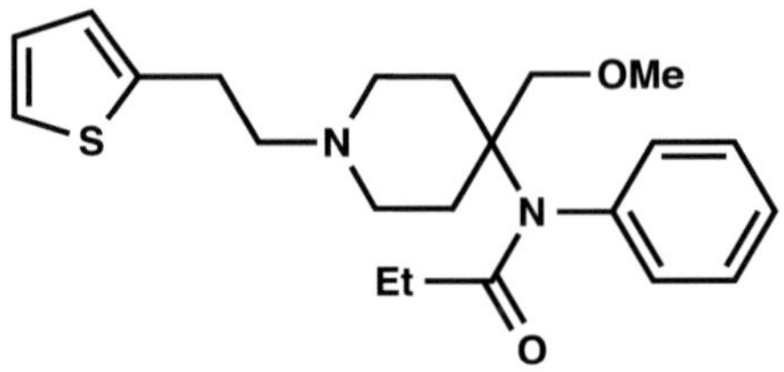

Sufentanyl (**6**)
[500x]

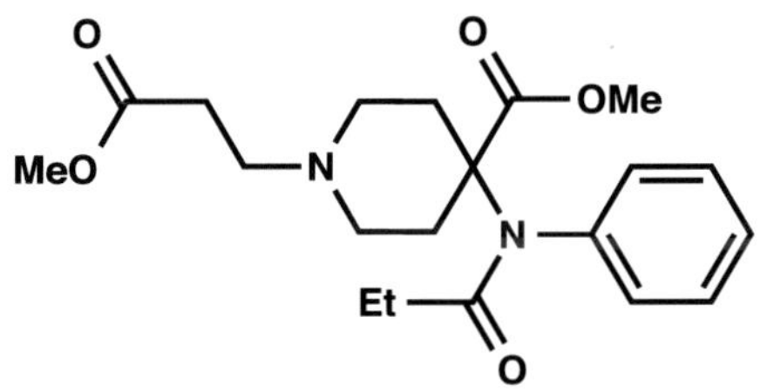

Remifentanyl (**7**)
[100-200x]

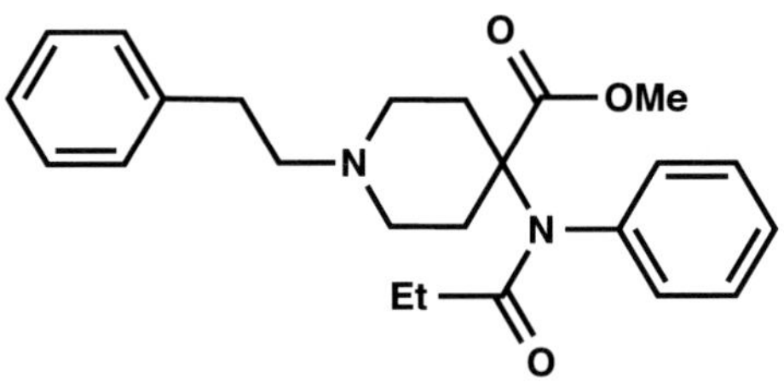

Carfentanyl (**8**)
[1000x]

Figure 2. Fentanyl analogs and their potencies relative to morphine.

Results and Discussion

Our final, optimized synthetic path to fentanyl (**4**) is outlined in Fig. 4 and it begins with the alkylation of commercially available 4-piperidone monohydrate hydrochloride **12** with 2-(bromoethyl)-benzene in the presence of cesium carbonate to furnish alkylated piperidone **13** in 88% yield. Reductive amination with aniline of **13** mediated by sodium triacetoxyborohydride in the presence of acetic acid yielded the 4-piperidineamine precursor **14** in excellent yield (91%). Lastly, piperidineamine **14** was acylated using propionyl chloride in the presence of Hunig's base to provide fentanyl (**4**) in 95% yield. Likewise, piperidineamine **14** was treated with acetic anhydride in the presence of Hunig's base to provide acetylfentanyl (**9**) in 98% yield. Conversion of **4** and **9** into their hydrochloride and citrate salts proceeded smoothly in nearly

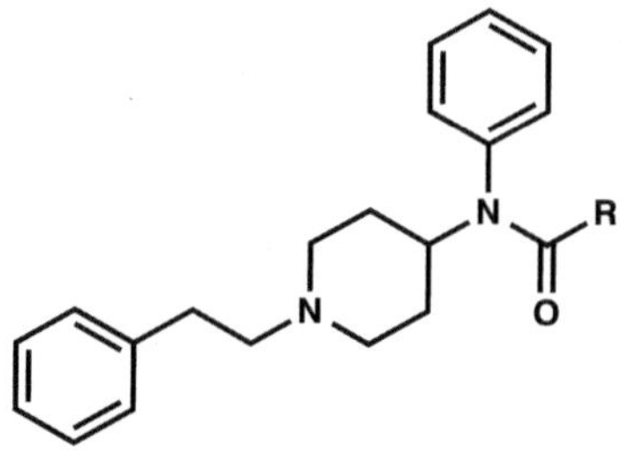

Fentanyl (R = Et, **4**)
Fentanyl HCl (R = Et, **15**)
Fentanyl citrate (R = Et, **16**)
Acetylfentanyl (R = Me, **9**)
Acetylfentanyl HCl (R = Me, **17**)
Acetylfentanyl citrate (R = Me, **18**)

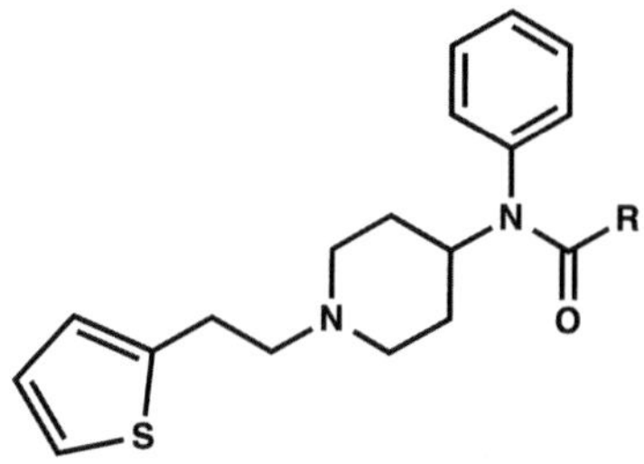

Thiofentanyl (R = Et, **10**)
Thiofentanyl HCl (R = Et, **23**)
Thiofentanyl citrate (R = Et, **24**)
Acetylthiofentanyl (R = Me, **11**)
Acetylthiofentanyl HCl (R = Me, **25**)
Acetylthiofentanyl citrate (R = Me, **26**)

Figure 3. Fentanyl analogs synthesized in this work.

quantitative yields (Fig. 3). The synthesis of the thiofentanyl analogs was accomplished in a similar fashion as shown in Fig. 5. Thus, 4-piperidone monohydrate hydrochloride **12** was alkylated with 2-(thiophen-2-yl)ethyl methanesulfonate (**19**) [32] in the presence of cesium carbonate to give *N*-[2-(2-thienyl)ethyl]-4-piperidinone (**20**) in 90% yield. Reductive amination with aniline of **20** with sodium triacetoxyborohydride and acetic acid yielded the 4-piperidineamine precursor **21** in 87% yield. Lastly, piperidineamine **21** was acylated using propionyl chloride to provide thiofentanyl (**10**) in 97% yield. Likewise, piperidineamine **21** was treated with acetic anhydride in the presence of Hunig's base to provide acetylthiofentanyl (**11**) in 94% yield. As before, conversion of **10** and **11** to their respective hydrochloride and citric acid salts was accomplished smoothly in nearly quantitative yields (Fig. 3).

Due to the low-yielding characteristics of our initial attempts, we decided to explore optimization studies for the synthesis of fentanyl (**4**) and then apply these to the syntheses of the analogs. Several conditions for each one of the steps composing the overall sequence were considered and evaluated (Table 1). We deduced that optimal conditions discovered for the synthesis of **4** could be directly translated to the syntheses of fentanyls **9–11** as they all share a common synthetic pathway. Thus, it was found that the use of acetonitrile instead of dimethylformamide increased the yields of the first alkylation step from 72 to 88% (Table 1, entries 1 and 2). This was also observed during the synthesis of the thiofentanyl precursor (**20**) that made use of the mesylate (**19**) as the alkylating species where the yield markedly increased from 62 to 83% (Table 1, entries 3 and 4). For the reductive amination (RA) step, the need for an equimolar amount of acetic acid was noted as this resulted in the efficient conversion of ketone **13** into the piperidineamine precursor **14** in the presence of sodium triacetoxyborohydride (Table 1, entry 5) [33,34]. Carrying out the reductive amination under the same conditions but switching the hydride source to either sodium cyanoborohydride or sodium borohydride resulted in significant loss of yield at room temperature (Table 1, entries 6 and 7). However, use of the latter hydride reagents under refluxing conditions (80°C) increased their yields significantly (Table 1, entries 8 and 9). Lastly, for the acylation step of the sequence, the use of either propanoyl chloride

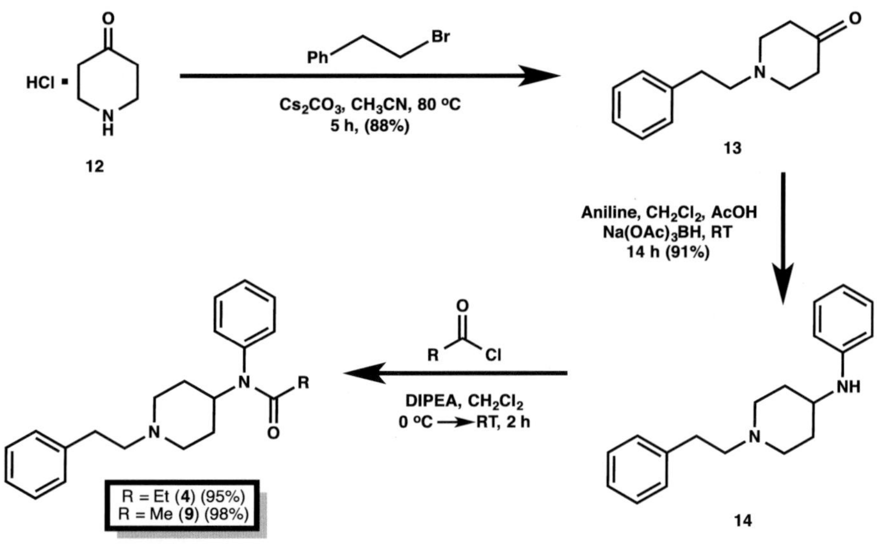

Figure 4. Synthesis of fentanyl and acetylthiofentanyl. Yields reflect the isolated materials by column chromatography after each step and using the optimized conditions (cf. Table 1). Citrate and hydrochloride salts for each analog were obtained in nearly quantitative yields by treating the free bases at the end of these routes with the corresponding acids.

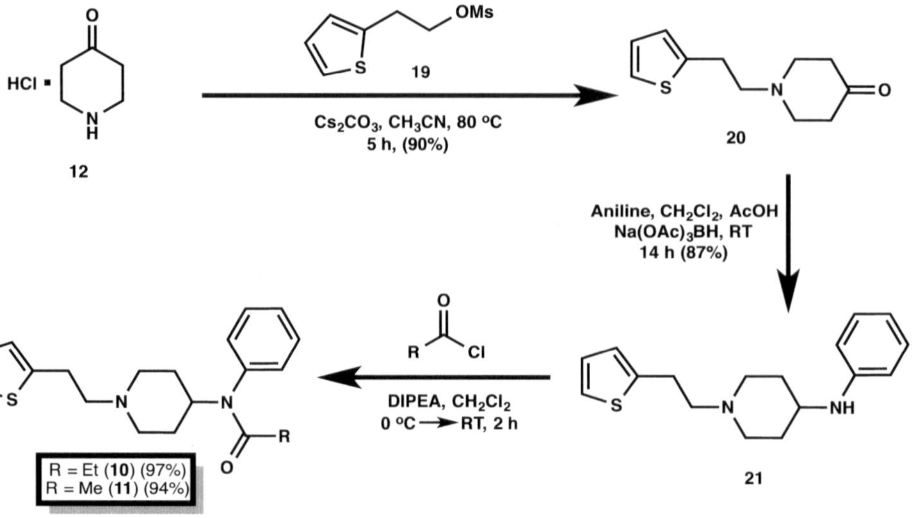

Figure 5. Synthesis of thiofentanyl and acetylthiofentanyl. Yields reflect the isolated materials by column chromatography after each step and using the optimized conditions (cf. Table 1). Citrate and hydrochloride salts for each analog were obtained in nearly quantitative yields by treating the free bases at the end of these routes with the corresponding acids.

or propanoic anhydride resulted in nearly identical yields (95% *vs.* 94%) regardless of the solvent to carry out the transformation (pyridine or dichloromethane) (Table 1, entries 10–12).

Synthesis

N-phenylethylpiperidin-4-one (13)

4-piperidone monohydrate hydrochloride (**12**) 22.0 g, 143.2 mmol) was dissolved in acetonitrile (400 mL) in a 1 L round-bottom flask equipped with a large stir bar and a condenser. The colorless solution was treated sequentially with cesium carbonate (Cs_2CO_3, 102.6 g, 315 mmol, 2.2 equiv.) and (2-bromoethyl)benzene (17.8 mL, 24.1 g, 130.2 mmol) at ambient temperature. The resulting suspension was vigorously stirred and refluxed at 80°C for 5 h. After 5 hours, the mixture was cooled to ambient temperature, transferred to a separatory funnel and partitioned (CH_2Cl_2//H_2O). The organic phase was washed with brine (NaCl/H_2O, 3×100 mL), satd. $NaHCO_3$ (2×100 mL), dried over Na_2SO_4 and concentrated *in vacuo* to give a yellow oil. The oily mixture was purified by flash column chromatography (1:1 → 7:3 EtOAc/hexanes) to give **13** as a light yellow oil (23.3 g, 88%). R_f = 0.25 (1:1 EtOAc/hexanes); ^1H NMR (600 MHz, $CDCl_3$) δ 7.31−7.28 (m, 2H), 7.22−7.19 (m, 3H), 2.85−2.83 (m, 2H), 2.82 (t, *J* = 6.0, 4H), 2.74−2.71 (m, 2H), 2.47 (t, *J* = 6.0, 4H); ^{13}C NMR (150 MHz, $CDCl_3$) δ 209.0, 140.0, 128.7, 128.4, 126.2, 59.3, 53.1, 41.2, 34.1; HRMS (CI) *m/z* calcd for $C_{13}H_{17}NO$ [M^+]: 203.1310; found 203.1309; Anal. Calcd for $C_{13}H_{17}NO$: C, 76.81; H, 8.43; N, 6.89. Found: C, 76.49; H, 8.71; N, 6.98.

N-[1-(2-phenylethyl)-4-piperidinyl]aniline (14)

Aniline (8.1 mL, 8.24 g, 88.5 mmol) was taken up in methylene chloride (240 mL) in a 500 mL round-bottom flask equipped with a stir bar. The light brown solution was placed on an ice bath and

Table 1. Optimization steps for the synthesis of fentanyl (**4**); [a]isolated yield; [b]alkylation in the synthesis of thiofentanyl derivatives; [c]reductive amination.

Entry	Synthetic Step	Reagents/Conditions	T (°C)	Yield[a] (%)
1	Alkylation	$PhCH_2CH_2Br$, Cs_2CO_3, DMF	80	72
2		$PhCH_2CH_2Br$, Cs_2CO_3, CH_3CN	80	88
3		R-OMs (**19**), Cs_2CO_3, DMF[b]	80	62
4		R-OMs (**19**), Cs_2CO_3, CH_3CN[b]	80	83
5	RA[c]	$Na(OAc)_3BH$, CH_2Cl_2, AcOH	25	91
6		$NaCNBH_3$, CH_2Cl_2, AcOH	25	64
7		$NaBH_4$, CH_2Cl_2, AcOH	25	52
8		$NaCNBH_3$, CH_2Cl_2, AcOH	80	86
9		$NaBH_4$, CH_2Cl_2, AcOH	80	84
10	Acylation	Propanoyl anhydride, pyridine	25	94
11		Propanoyl chloride, pyridine	25	95
12		Propanoyl chloride, DIPEA, CH_2Cl_2	25	95

treated dropwise with acetic acid (5.0 mL, 88.5 mmol). To the mixture, *N*-phenylethylpiperidin-4-one (**13**) (18.0 g, 88.5 mmol) was added as a solution in methylene chloride (60 mL), followed by the careful, slow addition of sodium triacetoxyborohydride (28.1 g, 132.8 mmol, 1.5 equiv.) in small portions. The reaction mixture was stirred at ambient temperature for 14 h. After this time, methanol (100 mL) was added to the mixture and all contents transferred to a separatory funnel. The mixture was partitioned (CH_2Cl_2//saturated $NaHCO_3$). Once neutralized, the organic phase was washed with brine ($NaCl/H_2O$, 3×100 mL), dried over Na_2SO_4 and concentrated *in vacuo* to give a light brown oil. The oily mixture was purified by flash column chromatography (1:1 → 9:1 EtOAc/hexanes) to give **14** as a light yellow oil (22.6 g, 91%). R_f = 0.22 (7:3 EtOAc/hexanes); ^{1}H NMR (600 MHz, $CDCl_3$) δ 7.28−7.27 (m, 2H), 7.21−7.18 (m, 3H), 7.16−7.15 (m, 2H), 6.68 (tt, *J* = 7.2, 1.2, 1H), 6.61−6.59 (m, 2H), 3.50 (br, 1H), 3.33−3.30 (m, 1H), 2.96−2.94 (m, 2H), 2.83−2.80 (m, 2H), 2.63−2.60 (m, 2H), 2.21 (t, *J* = 12.0, 2H), 2.10−2.07 (m, 2H), 1.53−1.47 (m, 2H); ^{13}C NMR (150 MHz, $CDCl_3$) δ 147.1, 140.4, 129.3, 128.7, 128.4, 126.0, 117.2, 113.3, 60.7, 52.5, 50.2, 33.9, 32.6; HRMS (CI) *m/z* calcd for $C_{19}H_{24}N_2$ [M$^+$]: 280.1939; found 280.1937; Anal. Calcd for $C_{19}H_{24}N_2$: C, 81.38; H, 8.63; N, 9.99. Found: C, 81.22; H, 8.68; N, 10.08.

Fentanyl (4)

N-[1-(2-phenylethyl)-4-piperidinyl]aniline (**14**) (1.35 g, 4.8 mmol) was dissolved in methylene chloride (40 mL) in a 100 mL round bottom flask equipped with a small stir bar and was treated with diisopropylethylamine (DIPEA, 1.68 mL, 1.24 g, 9.6 mmol, 2.0 equiv.). The solution was cooled with an ice bath and treated dropwise with propionyl chloride (0.83 mL, 0.88 g, 9.6 mmol, 2.0 equiv.). The resulting mixture was stirred for 2 h at ambient temperature. The mixture was transferred to a separatory funnel and partitioned (CH_2Cl_2//H_2O). The organic phase was washed with brine ($NaCl/H_2O$, 1×50 mL), satd. $NaHCO_3$ (1×50 mL), dried over anhydrous Na_2SO_4 and evaporated *in vacuo* at 40°C to give a yellow oil that was purified by flash column chromatography (3:7 → 7:3 EtOAc/hexanes) to furnish fentanyl (**4**) as a light yellow oil (1.53 g, 95%). R_f = 0.28 (1:1 EtOAc/hexanes); ^{1}H NMR (600 MHz, $CDCl_3$) δ 7.48−7.37 (m, 3H), 7.33−7.27 (m, 2H), 7.25−7.17 (m, 3H), 7.13−7.05 (m, 2H), 4.88−4.71 (br, 1H), 3.83−3.47 (br, 2H), 3.20−3.09 (br, 2H), 3.09−2.99 (br, 2H), 2.82−2.70 (br, 2H), 2.13−1.99 (br, 4H), 1.94 (q, *J* = 7.4, 2H), 1.01 (t, *J* = 7.4, 3H); ^{13}C NMR (150 MHz, $CDCl_3$) δ 174.0, 138.1, 137.0, 129.9, 129.8, 129.0, 128.9, 128.7, 127.0, 59.1, 52.6, 50.7, 31.3, 28.4, 28.0, 9.5; HRMS (CI) *m/z* calcd for $C_{22}H_{28}N_2O$ [M$^+$]: 336.2202; found 336.2201; Anal. Calcd for $C_{22}H_{28}N_2O$: C, 78.53; H, 8.39; N, 8.33. Found: C, 78.42; H, 8.05; N, 8.62.

Fentanyl hydrochloride (15)

Fentanyl (**4**) (138 mg, 0.41 mmol) was dissolved in diethyl ether (4 mL) in a 20 mL scintillation vial and treated at ambient temperature with 2.0 M HCl/Et_2O solution (205 µL, 0.41 mmol) using a pipette. Upon addition of the acid, the colorless solution became a white suspension. The resulting suspension was stirred at ambient temperature for 2 hours and then filtered using suction filtration. The white solid was washed with diethyl ether (3×10 mL) and placed under vacuum overnight. Fentanyl hydrochloride (**15**) was obtained as a white solid (148 mg, 97%). ^{1}H NMR (600 MHz, D_2O) δ 7.53−7.50 (m, 3H), 7.36 (m, 2H), 7.32−7.24 (m, 5H), 4.77−4.61 (m, 1H) (overlaps with HOD), 3.66−3.61 (m, 2H), 3.32 (d, *J* = 8.4, 2H), 3.15 (d, *J* = 12.6, 2H), 3.00 (d, *J* = 8.4, 2H), 2.12−2.10 (m, 2H), 2.00 (q, *J* = 7.2, 2H), 1.64−1.58 (m, 2H), 0.92 (t, *J* = 7.2, 3H); ^{13}C NMR (150 MHz, D_2O) δ 177.5, 137.2, 136.3, 129.8, 129.3, 129.1, 128.8, 127.4, 57.6, 52.1, 50.0, 29.8, 28.2, 27.5, 9.0; TOF-MS (ESI) *m/z* calcd for $C_{22}H_{29}N_2O$ [M+H$^+$]: 337.2274; found 337.2272; Anal. Calcd for $C_{22}H_{29}ClN_2O$: C, 70.85; H, 7.84; N, 7.51. Found: C, 70.51; H, 8.03; N, 7.53.

Fentanyl citrate (16)

Fentanyl (**4**) (148 mg, 0.44 mmol) was dissolved in MeOH (4 mL) in a 20 mL scintillation vial and treated with citric acid (85 mg, 0.44 mmol). The clear solution was stirred at ambient temperature for 2 hours. The methanol was removed *in vacuo* at 50°C to obtain a glassy solid that upon scrapping from the surface of the vial yielded a white solid that was placed under vacuum overnight. Fentanyl citrate (**16**) was obtained as a white solid (221 mg, 95%). ^{1}H NMR (600 MHz, D_2O) δ 7.51−7.46 (m, 3H), 7.35−7.32 (m, 2H), 7.28−7.27 (m, 1H), 7.25−7.23 (m, 2H), 7.22−7.20 (m, 1H), 4.77−4.61 (m, 1H) (overlaps with HOD), 3.60−3.57 (m, 2H), 3.30−3.27 (m, 2H), 3.11 (td, *J* = 12.6, 3.0, 2H), 2.98−2.96 (m, 2H), 2.94 (d, *J* = 15.6, 2H), 2.78 (d, *J* = 15.6, 2H), 2.09−2.08 (m, 2H), 1.97 (q, *J* = 7.2, 2H), 1.57 (qd, *J* = 13.2, 3.6, 2H), 0.89 (t, *J* = 7.2, 3H); ^{13}C NMR (150 MHz, D_2O) δ 177.5, 177.0, 173.6, 137.2, 136.3, 129.8, 129.3, 129.1, 128.8, 127.4, 73.4, 57.6, 52.1, 50.0, 43.3, 29.9, 28.2, 27.5, 9.0; HRMS (CI) *m/z* calcd for $C_{22}H_{29}N_2O$ [M+H$^+$]: 337.2274; found 337.2284; Anal. Calcd for $C_{28}H_{36}N_2O_8$: C, 63.62; H, 6.86; N, 5.30. Found: C, 63.88; H, 7.02; N, 5.66.

Acetylfentanyl (9)

N-[1-(2-phenylethyl)-4-piperidinyl]aniline (**14**) (1.50 g, 5.34 mmol) was dissolved in methylene chloride (50 mL) in a 100 mL round bottom flask with a small stir bar and was treated with diisopropylethylamine (DIPEA, 1.86 mL, 1.38 g, 10.7 mmol, 2.0 equiv.). The solution was cooled with an ice bath and treated dropwise with acetic anhydride (1.0 mL, 1.1 g, 10.7 mmol, 2.0 equiv.). The resulting mixture was stirred for 2 h at ambient temperature. The mixture was transferred to a separatory funnel and partitioned (CH_2Cl_2//H_2O). The organic phase was washed with brine ($NaCl/H_2O$, 1×50 mL), satd. $NaHCO_3$ (1×50 mL), dried over anhydrous Na_2SO_4 and evaporated *in vacuo* at 40°C to give a yellow oil that was purified by flash column chromatography (3:7 → 7:3 EtOAc/hexanes) to furnish acetylfentanyl (**9**) as a light yellow oil (1.68 g, 98%). R_f = 0.28 (1:1 EtOAc/hexanes); ^{1}H NMR (600 MHz, $CDCl_3$) δ 7.45−7.36 (m, 3H), 7.30−7.25 (m, 2H), 7.20−7.16 (m, 3H), 7.11−7.09 (m, 2H), 4.69 (tt, *J* = 12.0, 4.2, 1H), 3.42−3.36 (br, 1H), 3.04−3.00 (m, 2H), 2.80−2.73 (m, 2H), 2.60−2.55 (m, 2H), 2.20 (td, *J* = 12.0, 2.4, 2H), 1.86−1.82 (m, 2H), 1.77 (s, 3H), 1.47 (qd, *J* = 12.6, 4.2, 2H); ^{13}C NMR (150 MHz, $CDCl_3$) δ 170.3, 140.2, 139.3, 130.3, 129.4, 128.6, 128.4, 128.4, 126.1, 60.4, 53.0, 52.1, 33.7, 30.4, 23.5; HRMS (CI) *m/z* calcd for $C_{21}H_{26}N_2O$ [M$^+$]: 322.2045; found 322.2043; Anal. Calcd for $C_{21}H_{26}N_2O$: C, 78.22; H, 8.13; N, 8.69. Found: C, 78.26; H, 8.11; N, 8.75.

Acetylfentanyl hydrochloride (17)

Acetylfentanyl (**9**) (156 mg, 0.48 mmol) was dissolved in diethyl ether (4 mL) in a 20 mL scintillation vial and treated at ambient temperature with 2.0 M HCl/Et_2O solution (242 µL, 0.48 mmol) using a pipette. Upon addition of the acid, the colorless solution became a white suspension. The resulting suspension was stirred at ambient temperature for 2 hours and then filtered using suction filtration. The white solid was washed with diethyl ether (3×10 mL) and placed under vacuum overnight. Acetylfentanyl hydrochloride (**17**) was obtained as a white solid (165 mg, 96%).

^{1}H NMR (600 MHz, D_2O) δ 7.65−7.44 (m, 3H), 7.33−7.30 (m, 2H), 7.27−7.24 (m, 1H), 7.23−7.20 (m, 4H), 4.77−4.61 (m, 1H) (overlaps with HOD), 3.60−3.54 (m, 2H), 3.30−3.24 (m, 2H), 3.13−3.10 (m, 2H), 3.07−2.90 (m, 2H), 2.09−2.04 (m, 2H), 1.72 (s, 3H), 1.60−1.53 (m, 2H); ^{13}C NMR (150 MHz, D_2O) δ 174.1, 137.6, 136.2, 129.8, 129.7, 129.3, 129.1, 128.8, 127.4, 57.6, 52.1, 50.0, 29.9, 27.4, 22.5; TOF-MS (ESI) *m/z* calcd for $C_{21}H_{27}N_2O$ [M+H$^+$]: 323.2118; found 323.2124; Anal. Calcd for $C_{21}H_{27}ClN_2O$: C, 70.28; H, 7.58; N, 7.81. Found: C, 69.97; H, 7.72; N, 7.91.

Acetylfentanyl citrate (18)

Acetylfentanyl (**9**) (150 mg, 0.46 mmol) was dissolved in MeOH (4 mL) in a 20 mL scintillation vial and treated with citric acid (90 mg, 0.46 mmol). The clear solution was stirred at ambient temperature for 2 hours. The methanol was removed *in vacuo* at 50°C to obtain a glassy solid that upon scrapping from the surface of the vial yielded a white solid that was placed under vacuum overnight. Fentanyl citrate (**18**) was obtained as a white solid (225 mg, 95%). ^{1}H NMR (600 MHz, D_2O) δ 7.53−7.47 (m, 3H), 7.36−7.33 (m, 2H), 7.30−7.26 (m, 1H), 7.26−7.22 (m, 4H), 4.77−4.61 (m, 1H) (overlaps with HOD), 3.62−3.58 (m, 2H), 3.31−3.28 (m, 2H), 3.11 (td, *J* = 13.2, 2.4, 2H), 2.99−2.96 (m, 2H), 2.87 (d, *J* = 15.6, 2H), 2.73 (d, *J* = 15.6, 2H), 2.12−2.10 (m, 2H), 1.74 (s, 3H), 1.58 (qd, *J* = 14.4, 3.0, 2H); ^{13}C NMR (150 MHz, D_2O) δ 178.3, 174.5, 174.1, 137.6, 136.3, 129.8, 129.7, 129.3, 129.1, 128.8, 127.4, 73.7, 57.6, 52.1, 49.9, 48.9, 43.6, 29.8, 27.4, 22.5; TOF-MS (ESI) *m/z* calcd for $C_{21}H_{27}N_2O$ [M+H$^+$]: 323.2118; found 323.2127; Anal. Calcd for $C_{27}H_{34}N_2O_8$: C, 63.02; H, 6.66; N, 5.44. Found: C, 63.38; H, 6.69; N, 5.78.

2-(Thiophen-2-yl)ethyl methanesulfonate (19) [32]

2-Thiophene ethanol (5.0 g, 39 mmol) was taken up in methylene chloride (50 mL) in a 250 mL round bottom flask and treated with triethylamine (TEA, 6.5 mL, 46.8 mmol). The resulting dark brown solution was cooled with an ice bath and treated with mesyl chloride (MsCl, 3.7 mL, 46.8 mmol, 1.2 equiv.). The ice bath was removed and the resulting brown solution was allowed to warm to ambient temperature where it was stirred overnight. The brown solution was transferred to a separatory funnel and partitioned (CH_2Cl_2//H_2O). The organic phase was washed with brine ($NaCl/H_2O$, 3×50 mL), satd. $NaHCO_3$ (1×50 mL), dried over anhydrous Na_2SO_4 and evaporated *in vacuo* at 50°C to give a brown oil that was purified by flash column chromatography (hexanes → 3:7 EtOAc/hexanes) to furnish thiophene mesylate **19** as a light brown oil (6.76 g, 84%). R_f = 0.54 (3:7 EtOAc/hexanes); ^{1}H NMR (600 MHz, $CDCl_3$) δ 7.91 (dd, *J* = 4.8, 0.6, 1H), 6.95 (dd, *J* = 5.4, 3.6, 1H), 6.91−6.90 (m, 1H), 4.42 (t, *J* = 6.6, 2H), 3.27 (t, *J* = 6.6, 2H), 2.92 (s, 3H); ^{13}C NMR (150 MHz, $CDCl_3$) δ 138.1, 127.1, 126.2, 124.5, 69.7, 37.4, 29.8; HRMS (CI) *m/z* calcd for $C_7H_{10}O_3S_2$ [M$^+$]: 206.0071; found 206.0070.

N-[2-(2-thienyl)ethyl]-4-piperidinone (20)

4-piperidone monohydrate hydrochloride (**12**) (2.22 g, 14.5 mmol) was dissolved in acetonitrile (80 mL) in a 250 mL round-bottom flask equipped with a stir bar and a condenser. The colorless solution was treated sequentially with cesium carbonate (Cs_2CO_3, 10.4 g, 31.9 mmol, 2.2 equiv.) and 2-(thiophen-2-yl)ethyl methanesulfonate (**19**) (3.0 g, 14.5 mmol) at ambient temperature. The resulting suspension was vigorously stirred and refluxed at 80°C for 5 h. After 5 hours, the mixture was cooled to ambient temperature, transferred to a separatory funnel and partitioned (CH_2Cl_2//H_2O). The organic phase was washed with brine ($NaCl/H_2O$, 3×50 mL), saturated $NaHCO_3$ (2×50 mL), dried over Na_2SO_4 and concentrated *in vacuo* to give a yellow oil. The oily mixture was purified by flash column chromatography (1:1 → 7:3 EtOAc/hexanes) to give **20** as a light yellow oil (2.7 g, 90%). R_f = 0.25 (1:1 EtOAc/hexanes); ^{1}H NMR (600 MHz, $CDCl_3$) δ 7.14 (dd, *J* = 5.4, 1.2, 1H), 6.92 (dd, *J* = 5.4, 3.6, 1H), 6.84 (dq, *J* = 3.6, 1.2, 1H), 3.04 (t, *J* = 7.2, 2H), 2.82 (t, *J* = 6.0, 4H), 2.77 (t, *J* = 7.2, 2H), 2.48 (t, *J* = 6.0, 4H); ^{13}C NMR (150 MHz, $CDCl_3$) δ 209.0, 142.4, 126.6, 124.7, 123.7, 60.4, 53.0, 41.3, 28.3; HRMS (CI) *m/z* calcd for $C_{11}H_{15}NOS$ [M$^+$]: 209.0874; found 209.0872; Anal. Calcd for $C_{11}H_{15}NOS$: C, 63.12; H, 7.22; N, 6.69; Found: C, 63.01; H, 7.16; N, 6.77.

N-phenyl-1-(2-(thiophen-2-yl)ethyl)piperidin-4-amine (21)

Aniline (0.53 mL, 5.7 mmol) was taken up in methylene chloride (50 mL) in a 250 mL round-bottom flask equipped with a stir bar. The light brown solution was placed on an ice bath and treated dropwise with acetic acid (0.32 mL, 5.7 mmol). To the mixture, *N*-[2-(2-thienyl)ethyl]-4-piperidinone (**20**) (1.2 g, 5.7 mmol) was added as a solution in methylene chloride (30 mL), followed by the careful, slow addition of sodium triacetoxyborohydride (1.8 g, 8.6 mmol, 1.5 equiv.) in small portions. The reaction mixture was stirred at ambient temperature for 14 h. After this time, methanol (40 mL) was added to the mixture and all contents transferred to a separatory funnel. The mixture was partitioned (CH_2Cl_2//saturated $NaHCO_3$). Once neutralized, the organic phase was washed with brine ($NaCl/H_2O$, 3×50 mL), dried over Na_2SO_4 and concentrated *in vacuo* to give a light brown oil. The oily mixture was purified by flash column chromatography (1:1 → 9:1 EtOAc/hexanes) to give **21** as a light yellow oil (1.42 g, 87%). R_f = 0.33 (7:3 EtOAc/hexanes); ^{1}H NMR (600 MHz, $CDCl_3$) δ 7.18−7.15 (m, 2H), 7.13 (dd, *J* = 5.4, 1.2, 1H), 6.92 (dd, *J* = 5.4, 3.6, 1H), 6.84−6.82 (m, 1H), 6.69 (tt, *J* = 7.2, 0.6, 1H), 6.62−6.58 (m, 1H), 3.52 (br, 1H), 3.34−3.31 (m, 1H), 2.13 (t, *J* = 6.6, 2H), 2.95−2.93 (m, 2H), 2.68 (t, *J* = 6.6, 2H), 2.22 (td, *J* = 13.2, 2.4, 2H), 2.10−2.07 (m, 2H), 1.54−1.51 (m, 2H); ^{13}C NMR (150 MHz, $CDCl_3$) δ 147.1, 142.9, 129.3, 126.6, 124.6, 123.5, 117.2, 113.3, 60.0, 52.4, 49.9, 32.6, 28.0; HRMS (CI) *m/z* calcd for $C_{17}H_{22}N_2S$ [M$^+$]: 286.1504; found 286.1503; Anal. Calcd for $C_{17}H_{22}N_2S$: C, 71.29; H, 7.74; N, 9.78; Found: C, 71.16; H, 7.75; N, 9.66.

Thiofentanyl (10)

N-phenyl-1-(2-(thiophen-2-yl)ethyl)piperidin-4-amine (**21**) (2.21 g, 7.74 mmol) was dissolved in methylene chloride (50 mL) in a 100 mL round bottom flask equipped with a stir bar and was treated with diisopropylethylamine (DIPEA, 2.0 mL, 1.5 g, 11.6 mmol, 1.5 equiv.). The solution was cooled with an ice bath and treated dropwise with propionyl chloride (0.99 mL, 11.6 mmol). The resulting mixture was stirred for 2 h at ambient temperature. The mixture was transferred to a separatory funnel and partitioned (CH_2Cl_2//H_2O). The organic phase was washed with brine ($NaCl/H_2O$, 1×50 mL), satd. $NaHCO_3$ (1×50 mL), dried over anhydrous Na_2SO_4 and evaporated *in vacuo* at 40°C to give a yellow oil that was purified by flash column chromatography (3:7 → 7:3 EtOAc/hexanes) to furnish thiofentanyl (**10**) as a light yellow oil (2.57 g, 97%). R_f = 0.28 (1:1 EtOAc/hexanes); ^{1}H NMR (600 MHz, $CDCl_3$) δ 7.38−7.33 (m, 3H), 7.09−7.06 (m, 2H), 6.88 (dd, *J* = 4.8, 3.0, 1H), 6.77−6.75 (m, 1H), 4.67 (tt, *J* = 12.0, 4.2, 1H), 2.97−2.92 (m, 4H), 2.61−2.58 (m, 2H), 2.17 (td, *J* = 12.0, 1.8, 2H), 1.91 (q, *J* = 7.8, 2H), 1.81−1.78 (br s, 1H), 1.40 (qd, *J* = 11.4, 3.6, 2H), 1.00 (t, *J* = 7.8, 3H); ^{13}C NMR (150 MHz, $CDCl_3$) δ 173.5, 142.6, 138.8, 130.4, 129.3, 128.3, 126.6, 124.5, 123.4, 60.0, 53.0, 52.1, 30.5, 28.5, 27.8, 9.6; HRMS (CI) *m/*

z calcd for $C_{20}H_{26}N_2OS$ [M^+]: 342.1766; found 342.1765; Anal. Calcd for $C_{20}H_{26}N_2OS$: C, 70.14; H, 7.65; N, 8.18; Found: C, 70.11; H, 7.63; N, 8.10.

Thiofentanyl hydrochloride (23)

Thiofentanyl (**10**) (300 mg, 0.87 mmol) was dissolved in diethyl ether (6 mL) in a 20 mL scintillation vial and treated at ambient temperature with 2.0 M HCl/Et_2O solution (435 μL, 0.87 mmol) using a pipette. Upon addition of the acid, the colorless solution became a white suspension. The resulting suspension was stirred at ambient temperature for 2 hours and then filtered using suction filtration. The white solid was washed with diethyl ether (3×10 mL) and placed under vacuum overnight. Thiofentanyl hydrochloride (**23**) was obtained as a white solid (319 mg, 97%). ^{1}H NMR (600 MHz, D_2O) δ 7.52−7.47 (m, 3H), 7.30 (dd, J = 5.4, 1.2, 1H), 7.25−7.22 (m, 2H), 6.98 (dd, J = 4.8, 3.0, 1H), 6.94−6.93 (m, 1H), 3.59−3.57 (m, 2H), 3.35 (t, J = 7.2, 2H), 3.23 (t, J = 7.2, 2H), 3.17−3.15 (m, 2H), 2.09−2.08 (m, 2H), 1.98 (q, J = 7.8, 2H), 1.62−1.58 (m, 2H), 0.90 (t, J = 7.8, 3H); ^{13}C NMR (150 MHz, D_2O) δ 177.5, 138.1, 137.2, 129.8, 129.3, 127.6, 126.5, 125.3, 57.6, 50.0, 28.2, 27.4, 24.2, 9.0; TOF-MS (ESI) m/z calcd for $C_{20}H_{26}N_2OS$ [$M+H^+$]: 343.1839; found 343.1812; Anal. Calcd for $C_{20}H_{27}ClN_2OS$: C, 63.39; H, 7.18; N, 7.39; Found: C, 63.14; H, 7.25; N, 7.42.

Thiofentanyl citrate (24)

Thiofentanyl (**10**) (360 mg, 1.05 mmol) was dissolved in MeOH (5 mL) in a 20 mL scintillation vial and treated with citric acid (201 mg, 1.05 mmol). The clear solution was stirred at ambient temperature for 2 hours. The methanol was removed *in vacuo* at 50°C to obtain a glassy solid that upon scrapping from the surface of the vial yielded a white solid that was placed under vacuum overnight. Thiofentanyl citrate (**24**) was obtained as a white solid (538 mg, 96%). ^{1}H NMR (600 MHz, D_2O) δ 7.51−7.49 (m, 3H), 7.30 (dd, J = 4.8, 1.2, 1H), 7.23 (m, 2H), 6.98 (dd, J = 4.8, 3.6, 1H), 6.94−6.93 (m, 1H), 3.60−3.58 (m, 2H), 3.35 (t, J = 7.8, 2H), 3.24 (t, J = 7.8, 2H), 3.15−3.11 (m, 2H), 2.84 (d, J = 15.6, 2H), 2.72 (d, J = 15.6, 2H), 2.10−2.08 (m, 2H), 1.98 (q, J = 7.2, 2H), 1.59 (qd, J = 13.8, 3.6, 2H), 0.90 (t, J = 7.2, 3H); ^{13}C NMR (150 MHz, D_2O) δ 178.6, 177.5, 174.7, 138.1, 137.2, 129.8, 129.8, 129.3, 127.6, 126.5, 125.3, 73.8, 57.6, 52.1, 49.9, 28.2, 27.4, 24.1, 9.0; TOF-MS (ESI) m/z calcd for $C_{20}H_{26}N_2OS$ [$M+H^+$]: 343.1839; found 343.1842; Anal. Calcd for $C_{20}H_{27}ClN_2OS$: C, 58.41; H, 6.41; N, 5.24; Found: C, 58.70; H, 6.55; N, 5.41.

Acetylthiofentanyl (11)

N-phenyl-1-(2-(thiophen-2-yl)ethyl)piperidin-4-amine (**21**) (1.2 g, 4.2 mmol) was dissolved in methylene chloride (50 mL) in a 100 mL round bottom flask equipped with a stir bar and was treated with diisopropylethylamine (DIPEA, 0.98 mL, 0.72 g, 8.4 mmol). The solution was cooled with an ice bath and treated dropwise with acetic anhydride (0.52 mL, 0.56 g, 8.4 mmol). The resulting mixture was stirred for 2 h at ambient temperature. The mixture was transferred to a separatory funnel and partitioned ($CH_2Cl_2//H_2O$). The organic phase was washed with brine ($NaCl/H_2O$, 1×10 mL), satd. $NaHCO_3$ (1×10 mL), dried over anhydrous Na_2SO_4 and evaporated *in vacuo* at 40°C to give a yellow oil that was purified by flash column chromatography (3:7 → 7:3 EtOAc/hexanes) to furnish acetylthiofentanyl (**11**) as a light yellow oil (1.3 g, 94%). R_f = 0.28 (1:1 EtOAc/hexanes); ^{1}H NMR (600 MHz, $CDCl_3$) δ 7.40−7.34 (m, 3H), 7.09−7.07 (m, 3H), 6.88 (d, J = 5.4, 3.6, 1H), 6.77−6.75 (m, 1H), 4.66 (tt, J = 12.0, 4.2, 1H), 2.99−2.93 (m, 4H), 2.62−2.58 (m, 2H), 2.19 (td, J = 12.6, 2.4, 2H), 1.81−1.79 (m, 2H), 1.74 (s, 3H), 1.43 (qd, J = 12.0, 3.6, 2H); ^{13}C NMR (150 MHz, $CDCl_3$) δ 170.3, 142.5, 139.4, 130.2, 129.4, 128.4, 126.7, 124.6, 123.4, 59.9, 52.9, 52.1, 30.4, 27.7, 23.5; HRMS (CI) m/z calcd for $C_{19}H_{24}N_2OS$ [M^+]: 328.1609; found 328.1613; Anal. Calcd for $C_{19}H_{24}N_2OS$: C, 69.48; H, 7.36; N, 8.53; Found: C, 69.44; H, 7.28; N, 8.46.

Acetylthiofentanyl hydrochloride (25)

Acetylthiofentanyl (**11**) (260 mg, 0.79 mmol) was dissolved in diethyl ether (3 mL) in a 20 mL scintillation vial and treated at ambient temperature with 2.0 M HCl/Et_2O solution (396 μL, 0.79 mmol) using a pipette. Upon addition of the acid, the colorless solution became a white suspension. The resulting suspension was stirred at ambient temperature for 2 hours and then filtered using suction filtration. The white solid was washed with diethyl ether (2×5 mL) and placed under vacuum overnight. Acetylthiofentanyl hydrochloride (**25**) was obtained as a white solid (273 mg, 95%). ^{1}H NMR (600 MHz, D_2O) δ 7.50−7.45 (m, 3H), 7.27 (dd, J = 5.4, 2.1, 1H), 7.22−7.21 (m, 2H), 6.95 (dd, J = 4.8, 3.6, 1H), 6.92−6.90 (m, 1H), 3.57−3.56 (m, 2H), 3.33 (t, J = 7.2, 2H), 3.21 (t, J = 7.2, 2H), 3.13−3.10 (m, 2H), 2.08−2.06 (m, 2H), 1.72 (s, 3H), 1.61−1.56 (m, 2H); ^{13}C NMR (150 MHz, D_2O) δ 174.1, 138.0, 137.6, 129.8, 129.6, 129.3, 127.5, 126.4, 125.3, 57.5, 52.1, 49.9, 27.3, 24.1, 22.4; TOF-MS (ESI) m/z calcd for $C_{19}H_{25}N_2OS$ [$M+H^+$]: 329.1682; found 329.1666; Anal. Calcd for $C_{19}H_{25}ClN_2OS$: C, 62.53; H, 6.91; N, 7.68; Found: C, 62.25; H, 7.00; N, 7.63.

Acetylthiofentanyl citrate (26)

Acetylthiofentanyl (**11**) (282 mg, 0.86 mmol) was dissolved in MeOH (3 mL) in a 20 mL scintillation vial and treated with citric acid (165 mg, 0.86 mmol). The clear solution was stirred at ambient temperature for 2 hours. The methanol was removed *in vacuo* at 50°C to obtain a white solid that was placed under vacuum overnight. Acetylthiofentanyl citrate (**26**) was obtained as a white solid (438 mg, 98%). ^{1}H NMR (600 MHz, D_2O) δ 7.49−7.44 (m, 3H), 7.26 (dd, J = 4.8, 1.2, 1H), 7.20−7.19 (m, 2H), 6.94 (dd, J = 4.8, 3.0, 1H), 6.91−6.90 (m, 1H), 3.56−3.54 (m, 2H), 3.31 (t, J = 7.8, 2H), 3.20 (t, J = 7.2, 2H), 3.11−3.07 (m, 2H), 2.80 (d, J = 15.6, 2H), 2.68 (d, J = 15.6, 2H), 2.07−2.04 (m, 2H), 1.70 (s, 3H), 1.58−1.52 (m, 2H); ^{13}C NMR (150 MHz, D_2O) δ 178.3, 174.4, 174.1, 138.1, 137.5, 129.8, 129.6, 129.3, 127.5, 126.4, 125.2, 73.7, 57.5, 52.0, 49.3, 43.5, 27.3, 24.1, 22.4; TOF-MS (ESI) m/z calcd for $C_{19}H_{25}N_2OS$ [$M+H^+$]: 329.1682; found 329.1688; Anal. Calcd for $C_{25}H_{32}N_2O_8S$: C, 57.68; H, 6.20; N, 5.38; Found: C, 57.83; H, 6.52; N, 5.53.

Conclusion

The efficient syntheses of fentanyl and three other analogs (along with their hydrochloride and citric acid salts) have been accomplished. The three-step synthetic route was subject to optimization studies furnishing a process that generates the target fentanyls in high yields (73−78%). Thus, the syntheses described herein provide an efficient protocol for the construction of these interesting opioids for in depth biochemical as well as crystallographic studies.

Supporting Information

Information S1 Proton (^{1}H) and Carbon (^{13}C) NMR spectra for the fentanyl panel (free bases and salts) and their synthetic intermediates. A more specific table of contents can be located in the document.

Acknowledgments

Disclaimer: This document (LLNL-JRNL-656516) was prepared as an account of work sponsored by an agency of the United States government. Neither the United States government nor Lawrence Livermore National Security, LLC, nor any of their employees makes any warranty, expressed or implied, or assumes any legal liability or responsibility for the accuracy, completeness, or usefulness of any information, apparatus, product, or process disclosed, or represents that its use would not infringe privately owned rights. Reference herein to any specific commercial product, process, or service by trade name, trademark, manufacturer, or otherwise does not necessarily constitute or imply its endorsement, recommendation, or favoring by the United States government or Lawrence Livermore National Security, LLC. The views and opinions of authors expressed herein do not necessarily state or reflect those of the United States government or Lawrence Livermore National Security, LLC, and shall not be used for advertising or product endorsement purposes.

Author Contributions

Conceived and designed the experiments: CAV BPM. Performed the experiments: CAV BPM RNL. Analyzed the data: CAV BPM RNL. Contributed reagents/materials/analysis tools: CAV BPM RNL. Contributed to the writing of the manuscript: CAV BPM.

References

1. Friedrichsdorf SJ, Postier A (2014) Management of breakthrough pain in children with cancer. J. Pain Res. 7: 117–123.
2. Lee SK, Dawson J, Lee JA, Osman G, Levitin MO, et al. (2014) Management of cancer pain: 1. Wider implications of orthodox analgesics. Int. J. Gen. Med. 7: 49–58.
3. Grass JA (1992) Fentanyl: clinical use as postoperative analgesic: epidural/intrathecal route. J. Pain Symptom Manag. 7: 419–430.
4. Grass JA (1992) Sufentanil: clinical use as postoperative analgesic: epidural/intrathecal route. J. Pain Symptom Manag. 7: 271–286.
5. Grass JA (2000) The role of epidural anesthesia and analgesia in postoperative outcome. Anesthesiol. Clin. North America. 18(2): 407–428.
6. Lehmann KA (2005) Recent developments in patient-controlled analgesia. J. Pain Symptom Manag. 29: S72–S89.
7. Mercadante S (2011) New opioids. Curr. Pain Headache R. 15: 244–249.
8. Janssen PAJ, Eddy NB (1960) Compounds related to pethidine-IV. New general chemical methods of increasing the analgesic activity of pethidine. J. Med. Chem. 2: 31–45.
9. Janssen PAJ (1961) Pirinitramide (R 3365), a potent analgesic with unusual chemical structure. J. Pharm. Pharmacol. 13: 513–530.
10. Stanley TH (2005) Fentanyl. J. Pain Symptom Manag. 29: S67–S71.
11. Stanley TH (1992) The history and development of the fentanyl series. J. Pain Symptom Manag. 7: S3–S7.
12. Maciejewski D (2012) Sufentanil in anaesthesiology and intensive therapy. Anasthesiol. Intensive Ther. 44: 35–41.
13. Vardanyan RS, Hruby VJ (2014) Fentanyl-related compounds and derivatives: current status and future prospects for pharmaceutical applications. Future Med. Chem. 6: 385–412.
14. Gordon DB (2006) Oral transmucosal fentanyl citrate for cancer breakthrough pain: a review. Oncol. Nurs. Forum 33: S6–S13.
15. Kronstrand R, Druid H, Holmgren P, Rajs J (1997) A cluster of fentanyl-related deaths among drug addicts in Sweden. Forensic Sci. Int. 88: 185–195.
16. Between March–May of 2013, acetylfentanyl, an analog six times more potent than morphine was linked to 14 overdose deaths in Rhode Island, while on February of this year, this designer opioid drug was the cause of 3 overdose deaths in North Carolina. For the Rhode Island case please see: Centers for Disease Control and Prevention (2013) MMWR Morb. Mortal Wkly. Rep. 62: 703–704.
17. Chauhan S, Chauhan S, D'Cruz R, Faruqi S, Singh KK, et al. (2008) Chemical warfare agents. Environ. Tox. Pharm. 26: 113–122.
18. Wax PM, Becker CE, Curry SC (2003) Unexpected "gas" casualties in Moscow: a medical toxicology perspective. Ann. Emerg. Med. 41: 700–705.
19. Rieder J, Keller C, Hoffmann G, Lirk P (2003) Moscow theatre siege and anaesthetic drugs. Lancet 361: 1131.
20. Coupland RM (2003) Incapacitating chemical weapons: a year after the Moscow theatre siege. Lancet 362: 1346.
21. George AV, Lu JJ, Pisano MV, Metz J, Erickson TB (2010) Carfentanil–an ultra potent opioid. Am. J. Emerg. Med. 28: 530–532.
22. Sirohi S, Dighe SV, Walker EA, Yoburn BC (2008) The analgesic efficacy of fentanyl: relationship to tolerance and mu-opioid receptor regulation. Pharmacol. Biochem. Behav. 91: 115–120.
23. Duttaroy A, Yoburn BC (1995) The effect of intrinsic efficacy on opioid tolerance. Anesthesiology 82: 1226–1236.
24. Manglik A, Kruse AC, Kobilka TS, Thian FS, Mathiesen JM, et al. (2012) Crystal structure of the µ-opioid receptor bound to a morphinan antagonist. Nature 485: 321–326.
25. Wu H, Wacker D, Mileni M, Katritch V, Han GW, et al. (2012) Structure of the human κ-opioid receptor in complex with JDTic. Nature 485: 327–332.
26. Thompson AA, Liu W, Chun E, Katritch V, Wu H, et al. (2012) Structure of the nociceptin/orphanin FQ receptor in complex with a peptide mimetic. Nature 485: 395–399.
27. Granier S, Manglik A, Kruse AC, Kobilka TS, Thian FS, et al. (2012) Structure of the δ-opioid receptor bound to naltrindole. Nature 485: 400–405.
28. Gupta PK, Kumaran G, Ambuja P, Malhotra RC (2005) A convenient one pot synthesis of fentanyl. J. Chem. Res. 7: 452–453.
29. Watson AJA, Maxwell AC, Williams JMJ (2011) Borrowing hydrogen methodology for amine synthesis under solvent-free microwave conditions. J. Org. Chem. 76: 2328–2331.
30. Ghaffarzadeh M, Joghan SS, Faraji F (2012) A new method for the synthesis of amides from imines. Tetrahedron Lett. 53: 203–206.
31. Gant TG, Sarshar S (2010) US Patent 20100016365.
32. Albanese D, Ghidoli C, Zenoni M (2008) Concise Synthesis of Vinylheterocycles through β-Elimination under Solventless Phase Transfer Catalysis Conditions. Org. Process Res. Dev. 12: 736–739.
33. Burova SA, Davis R, Fitzgerald RN, Johnson BS, Matsuoka RT (2007) General Synthesis of 1-Substituted 2-Methylbenzimidazoles from Ketones and 2-Aminoacetanilide. Synth. Commun. 37: 3029–3039.
34. Balannik V, Wang J, Ohigashi Y, Jing X, Magavern E, et al. (2009) Design and Pharmacological Characterization of Inhibitors of Amantadine-Resistant Mutants of the M2 Ion Channel of Influenza A Virus. Biochemistry 48: 11872–11882.

3

Surgical Decompression of Painful Diabetic Peripheral Neuropathy: The Role of Pain Distribution

Chenlong Liao, Wenchuan Zhang*, Min Yang, Qiufeng Ma, Guowei Li, Wenxiang Zhong

Department of Neurosurgery, XinHua Hospital, affiliated to Shanghai JiaoTong University School of Medicine, Shanghai, P. R. China

Abstract

Objective: To investigate the effect of surgical decompression on painful diabetic peripheral neuropathy (DPN) patients and discuss the role which pain distribution and characterization play in the management of painful DPN as well as the underlying mechanism involved.

Methods: A total of 306 patients with painful diabetic lower-extremity neuropathy were treated with Dellon surgical nerve decompression in our department. Clinical evaluation including Visual analogue scale (VAS), Brief Pain Inventory Short Form for diabetic peripheral neuropathy (BPI-DPN) questionnaire, two-point discrimination (2-PD), nerve conduction velocity (NCV) and high-resolution ultrasonography (cross-sectional area, CSA) were performed in all cases preoperatively, and at 6 month intervals for 2 years post-decompression. The patients who underwent surgery were retrospectively assigned into two subgroups (focal and diffuse pain) according to the distribution of the diabetic neuropathic pain. The control group included 92 painful DPN patients without surgery.

Results: The levels of VAS, scores in BPI-DPN, 2-PD, NCV results and CSA were all improved in surgical group when compared to the control group ($P<0.05$). More improvement of VAS, scores in BPI-DPN and CSA was observed in focal pain group than that in diffuse group ($P<0.05$).

Conclusions: Efficacy of decompression of multiple lower-extremity peripheral nerves in patients with painful diabetic neuropathy was confirmed in this study. While both focal and diffuse group could benefit from surgical decompression, pain relief and morphological restoration could be better achieved in focal group.

Editor: Massimo Pietropaolo, University of Michigan Medical School, United States of America

Funding: This study was supported by the grant from the National Science Foundation of China. The grant number: 81371373. The URL of the funder's website: http://isisn.nsfc.gov.cn/egrantindex/funcindex/prjsearch-list.

Competing Interests: The authors have declared that no competing interests exist.

* Email: zhangwench88@hotmail.com

Introduction

There are over 250 million people in the world with type 1 and 2 diabetes mellitus. [1] Neuropathy is one of the most common complications of diabetes mellitus and leads to increasingly high morbidity and mortality, resulting in a huge economic burden for diabetes care. [2] Diabetic neuropathy is a heterogeneous condition containing symmetrical neuropathies and focal neuropathies, [3] presenting diverse clinical manifestations. Of all the neuropathies in diabetes, chronic diabetic peripheral neuropathy (DPN) is the commonest. [4] Of all the symptoms in DPN, pain is the most distressing and is the main factor that prompts the patients to seek medical advice. [5] One-third of diabetic patients have symptoms of neuropathic pain according to a recent community-based study [6] and up to 15–20% of patients with DPN may experience painful symptoms. [7] Therefore, a high proportion of patients are suffering from neuropathic pain as well as the relative depression, anxiety and sleep deprivation.

The management of neuropathic pain in diabetes still remains challenging mainly due to its various clinical features, wide spectrum severity and different distribution involved. Descriptions of pain can be burning, prickling, lancinating, shooting, cramping, aching, and also contact hypersensitivity (allodynia) and "dead feeling" (numbness) in their legs. [5] The severity may range from mild symptoms in one toe or two to continuous painful symptoms involving both legs and may even extend to the upper limbs. The extent involved may be focal or diffuse. One additional factor that contributes to the treatment dilemma of neuropathic pain is the varied response to the currently different treatments. The diverse manifestations of neuropathic pain in diabetes and various responses to current interventions imply that a number of mechanisms could contribute. Therefore, the management of painful DPN may not be one single intervention and a series of factors should be taken into consideration, one of which, as Vinik, A. and his colleagues put it in one guideline, [8] may be the distribution of pain. According to our clinical experience with management of painful diabetic neuropathy, features and severity of pain may change during the course of diabetic neuropathy while the distribution of pain is relatively invariable, which may be of some value for patient selection for surgical decompression. Thus we carry out this retrospective study to investigate the effects of surgical decompression on the outcome of painful diabetic patients and discuss the role which pain distribution plays in the management of painful diabetic neuropathy as well as the underlying mechanism involved.

Aside from traditional management including glucose control, lifestyle modification and pharmacological treatment, surgical decompression is recommended for pain relief in the recent reports [9–15] based on the "double crush" hypothesis. [16] Clinical observations revealed that many of the symptoms of diabetic neuropathy, including pain, are similar to those of chronic nerve compression, suggesting that entrapment of nerves may happen in the patients with diabetic neuropathy. Allowing for the currently traditional treatment dilemma on pain relief in patients with diabetic neuropathy, surgical decompression targeting superimposed compression, as an newly emerging promising approach, should be impartially taken into account.

Methods

This study is approved by the Xinhua Hospital Ethics Review Board and the forms of consent were obtained from all patients involved in this study.

Patients

A consecutive series of 306 patients (108 males and 198 females) with painful diabetic lower-extremity neuropathy, who underwent Dellon surgical nerve decompression [17] in our department from January 2008 to December 2011 was collected in this study. The control group included 92 painful DPN patients (38 males and 54 females) without surgery. The control group was mainly made up of the outpatients who refused hospitalization for surgical intervention owing to various personal reasons, most of which included fear of surgery and economic issues. Patients in the control group were all qualified for the inclusion criteria described below. According to the Wagner classification, 77 patients in surgical group (25.2%) and 26 patients in control group (28.3%) were rated as class 1 (surface ulcers and no clinical infection) before surgery. All patients had a history of type II diabetes mellitus according to 1999 WHO diagnostic criteria and showed symptoms of neuropathic pain, with high Toronto clinical scoring system (TCSS) scores. According to the definition proposed by the International Association for the Study of Pain, neuropathic pain in diabetes is "pain arising as a direct consequence of abnormalities in the somatosensory system in people with diabetes". [18] After reviewed the histories, we retrospectively defined the focal pain (the pain mainly confined to one to three scattered areas of the legs, dorsum of feet, the heels, the toes, or the plantar aspect of feet) and the diffuse pain (the pain is so dispersed along the affected extremities that exactly position can not be localized) and then divide the surgical group into two subgroups according to this definition. The focal pain was observed in 145 patients and the diffuse pain in the remaining 161 patients. The baseline characteristics of patients are displayed in Table 1.

Inclusion criteria include (1) history of pain in the distribution of the posterior tibial (medial and lateral plantar surface), common and superficial peroneal (lateral calf and dorsum of the foot), or deep peroneal nerves (dorsum of the foot, first web space), (2) positive Tinel sign presented at a known site of nerve entrapment including the fibular tunnel at the lateral side of the knee, for the common peroneal nerve, the tarsal tunnel at the ankle for the tibial nerve, and the junction between the first and second metatarsals and the cuneiforms for the deep peroneal nerve, (3) Decreased two-point discrimination: the big toe pulp two-point discrimination was greater than 9 mm [19].

Exclusion criteria include (1) presence of defined risk factors such as alcohol, nutrition, uremia and peripheral vascular disease, as demonstrated by absence of a palpable pulse, (2) previous history of cervical and lumbar spondylosis, (3) radiculopathy, (4) pedal edema.

Surgical Technique

The decompression surgery adopting Dellon triple procedures [17] were performed by the same senior surgeon (Zhang WC), with the use of microscope under continuous epidural anesthesia.

A 3 cm-long incision was made below the fibular head and the skin, superficial and deep fascia was cut. After excision of fascia above the common peroneal nerve and the peroneus longus muscle tendon, the common peroneal nerve trunk was exposed and decompressed.

A 6 cm-long curved incision was made along the medial malleolus and the skin, superficial and deep fascia was cut. After excision of the flexor retinaculum, the posterior tibial artery and veins and the tibal nerve were indentified and decompressed. Following this, the abductor halluces brevis was cut and spread to expose and divide the roof of the medial and of the lateral plantar tunnels. The medial calcaneal tunnel was then identified and decompressed. Epineurium decompression was performed if there was evidence of epineurial thickening.

A 2 cm-long incision was made longitudinally between the first and second metatarsal heads and the skin, superficial and deep fascia were cut to expose the tendon of the extensor hallucis brevis muscle. This tendon was then excised to decompress the deep peroneal nerve.

During the perioperative period, blood glucose was controlled at 6.2–8.0 mmol/L. After the patients were discharged, they were required to monitor their fasting plasma glucose every week and control their blood glucose levels to <8.0 mmol/L.

Clinical evaluation

Careful history taking and peripheral neurological/vascular examination were completed in all patients at admission. Aside from pain as a chief complaint, some of them simultaneously presented with other sensory symptoms including numbness, tingling and so forth. Patients were additionally inquired about their functional status, normal activities, ability to work, walking distance, family history of diabetes and the use of medications.

Assessment of pain including visual analogue scale (VAS) and Brief Pain Inventory Short Form for diabetic peripheral neuropathy (BPI-DPN), of sensation including plantar big toe and small toe two-point discrimination (2-PD), of morphological changes of nerves employing high-resolution ultrasound, of electrophysiological changes performing nerve conduction velocity (NCV) on admission prior to surgery and then at 6 months intervals for two years after surgery. The follow-up was conducted mainly on an outpatient basis.

Pre and post operative evaluations were performed by two clinical residents (in charge of history taking and peripheral neurological/vascular examination), one sonographer (undertaking high-resolution ultrasound of peripheral nerves) and one technician of electrophysiology (performing the NCV tests).

The visual analogue scale (VAS) [20], which is one of the oldest and best validated measurement (0 = no pain to 10 = worst possible pain), was used to assess the severity of diabetic neuropathic pain. All patients were asked to complete Brief Pain Inventory Short Form for diabetic peripheral neuropathy (BPI-DPN) to assess pain severity and pain interference with daily functioning. The BPI-DPN includes the four-item pain Severity scale (Worst Pain, Least Pain, Average Pain, and Pain Now) and

Table 1. Baseline of characteristics of patients.

	Control(n = 92)	Focal(n = 145)	Diffuse(n = 161)	*P*(a, b)*
Patient characteristics				
Median age(yr) (%)	57±13.62(36–86)	60±11.59(34–86)	58±11.36(36–85)	0.08, 0.93
Age in years, n (%)				
<40	9(9.7)	7(4.8)	11(6.8)	
40–49	21(22.8)	26(17.9)	31(19.3)	
50–59	25(27.1)	36(24.8)	39(24.2)	
60–69	22(23.9)	62(42.8)	67(41.6)	
>70	15(16.3)	14(9.7)	13(8.1)	
Sex, n (%)				0.29, 0.84
Male	38(41.3)	52(35.9)	56(34.8)	
Female	54(58.7)	93(64.1)	105(65.2)	
Course of DM(yr)	7.2±1.62	7.7±2.72	8.1±1.85	0.83, 0.78
Course of pain(mo)	47±5.38	43±5.61	57±6.32	0.80, 0.74

All variables were expressed in mean ± SD.
DM = Diabetes Mellitus.
*a: control group vs. focal & diffuse (surgical group), b: focal group vs. diffuse group.

the seven-item pain Interference scale (General Activity, Mood, Walking Ability, Normal Work, Relations with Others, Sleep, Enjoyment of Life). Each items of BPI uses a 0 to 10 numeric rating scale anchored at "no pain," and 10 for "pain as bad as you can imagine" for Severity, and "does not interfere" to "completely interferes" for Interference [21].

Neurosensory examination mainly included percussion over a distribution of the affected peripheral nerve (Tinel sign) and two-point discrimination (2-PD) using the Disk-Criminator at the big and small toes for medial and lateral plantar nerves, respectively. A positive Tinel sign was taken to be a positive response that indicated either a tingling or radiating electriclike perception either into the heel, the arch, or the toes (the most common responses), or proximally up the inside of the ankle (the least common response) [22].

Nerve conduction velocity was detected with the employment of a Denmark Medtronic EMG (DK 1 2740). The testing was performed under a quiet indoor environment with a room temperature of 25°C and skin temperature of 30°C, using surface electrodes for stimulation and recording. Bilateral motor NCVs of tibial nerve and sensory NCVs of the common peroneal nerve and superficial peroneal nerve were recorded in all patients.

High-resolution ultrasound of peripheral nerves was performed employing a Sequoia 512 ultrasound device (Siemens) with a 8–14 MHz transducer. Multislice, longitudinal, and transverse scans were made through the common peroneal nerve and the posterior tibial nerve to observe the continuity and echogeneity of the nerves. The anteroposterior diameter (Da) and transverse diameter (Dt) of the nerves were measured at the cross-section of 1.5 cm below the distal tip of fibular head (common peroneal nerve) and distal tip of medial malleolus (posterior tibial nerve). And then cross-sectional area (CSA) was calculated by the formula of $S = \pi(Da*Dt/4)$ [23].

Statistical Methods

Analysis was performed separately for patients comparing the change from preoperative levels to that of last visit (BPI-DPN, 2-PD, NCV, CSA). Data were expressed as the mean ± standard deviation. Pearson's χ^2 test and student's t-test were used with the employment of SPSS 18.0. A P value <0.05 was considered statistically significant.

Results

Twenty-five patients in surgical groups and six patients in control group were lost during the follow-up. The differences of age, sex, course of diabetes and pain symptom between the two groups were not statistically significant ($P>0.05$). The average courses of diabetes mellitus were longer than the average courses of pain symptom in all groups. In some individuals, however, the onset of pain symptom came before the diagnosis of diabetes, some may even lead to the diagnosis of diabetes, in which situation other potential diseases had been excluded before the diagnosis of diabetic neuropathy. There is no statistically significant difference between surgical and control groups and, also no statistically significant difference among the three groups (focal pain group, diffuse pain group and control group) after dividing the surgical group into two subgroups regarding to the initial VAS level, 2-PD, scores in BPI-DPN, NCV and CSA ($P>0.05$).

Visual Analogue Scales

The VAS levels in different time points were recorded and comparison was made among the three groups to assess the outcome of surgery. (Figure 1) In focal pain group, the average score of VAS was 8.20 on admission and at 6 months after surgery decreased to 2.28 ($P<0.01$). The average pain level remained between 2 and 1 for the remainder of the study. The mean VAS pain level of patients with diffuse pain was 8.32 and decreased to 3.43 ($P<0.01$) 6 months after surgery, higher than that of patients with focal pain ($P<0.05$). The mean pain level of diffuse pain group remained between 4 and 2 with fluctuation for the remainder of the study. The average VAS of patients in control group was 8.03 at first visit and remained around 8.0 during the two-year follow-up ($P>0.05$). There was a statistically significant difference as to VAS level between surgical and control groups after surgery ($P<0.01$). The results show pain relief can be achieved through surgical decompression, especially in the patients with focal pain.

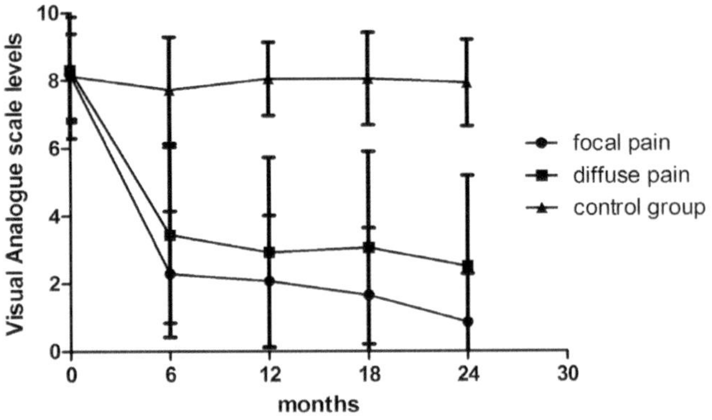

Figure 1. The figure displays the records of VAS levels at different time points. The VAS scores in both surgical groups showed notable decline with the time course while no changes occurred in control group during the follow-up. The overall postoperative VAS levels of focal pain group were much lower than that of diffuse pain group ($P<0.01$).

Two-point discrimination

In focal pain group, the postoperative (two years later) average big toe 2-PD (6.43±1.46 mm) and small toe 2-PD (6.24±1.72 mm) showed a statistically significant improvement ($P<0.05$) comparing to those before surgery (17.4±1.86 mm, 16.7±1.71 mm). Analogously, markedly improvement can also be observed when comparison was made between preoperative (18.7±1.68 mm, 19±1.34 mm) and postoperative (7.34±1.54 mm, 10.24±1.94 mm) big toe and small toe 2-PD in diffuse pain group ($P<0.05$). There is no statistically significant difference between two groups with regard to both big toe 2-PD ($P = 0.73$) and small 2-PD ($P = 0.77$) after decompression. In control group, no statistically significant difference could be seen between preoperative and postoperative 2-PD of big toe (pre: 16.3±1.77 mm, post: 17.8±1.72 mm, $P>0.05$) and small toe (pre: 16.3±1.77 mm, post: 16.8±1.57 mm, $P>0.05$). A statistically significant improvement in both small toe and big toe 2-PD could be observed between surgical and control groups ($P<0.05$) (Figure 2 A, B).

BPI-DPN questionnaire

The scores of all items in BPI-DPN were recorded, and the "Mean severity" as well as the "Mean interference" was compared in this study. (Figure 2 C, D) In the focal pain group, the preoperative scores of "Mean severity" (5.56±1.14) decreased greatly after two years (0.52±0.78) ($P<0.05$). There is also an observable decline (5.64±1.07, 1.12±1.01) in "Mean severity" two years after surgery in the diffuse pain group ($P<0.05$). Initial "Mean interference" of focal and diffuse pain group is 4.75±0.86 and 4.73±0.82, which decreased to 1.88±1.15 ($P<0.05$) and 2.00±1.07 ($P<0.05$) respectively. Statistically significant difference existed between the two groups regarding both postoperative "Mean severity" ($P<0.05$) and "Mean interference" ($P<0.05$). As respect to "Mean severity" (preoperative: 5.77±1.05, postoperative: 5.37±0.83) and "Mean interference" (preoperative: 4.69±0.88, postoperative: 4.36±0.83), there was almost no changes in control group.

Nerve conduction velocity (NCV) study

Two years after surgery, NCVs of all the patients increased significantly compared to that before surgery ($P<0.05$) while NCVs of patients in control group remained almost unchanged. Statistically significant difference could be observed between the surgical and control groups ($P<0.05$) while no statistically significant difference existed between the focal and diffuse pain group ($P = 0.84$) two years after surgery (Table 2).

High-resolution ultrasonography

In all groups, fusiform swelling of the nerves, intraneural hypoecho and, disappearance of intraneural parallel and linear structure were observed by high-resolution ultrasonography. Two years after surgery, the restoration of nerve structure can be seen in both focal and diffuse pain group. More decrease of CSA was seen in patients with focal pain ($P<0.05$). (Figure 3) The CSA of patients in control group remained larger than that of both focal ($P<0.05$) and diffuse ($P<0.05$) pain group after surgery (Table 3).

All patients underwent surgical decompression recovered well except that three patients suffered from surgical complications. Wound dehiscence in two patients healed within 2 months after strict blood glucose control, antibiotics administration and daily dressing change. One patient with extensive lower-leg subcutaneous hemorrhage was treated by surgical incision and drainage. In the control group, ten patients developed superficial ulcers in the lower-limb and two underwent surgical amputation during this period. None of the operated patients had developed new ulcer, ulcer progression or amputation in two-year follow-up.

Discussion

Diabetic neuropathy has traditionally been considered as an irreversible condition and the treatments are mostly symptomatic aiming to prevent the development of complications rather than to target the underlying pathologic mechanisms. [24] However, the proposal of "double crush" hypothesis contributed by the combination of increase endoneurial water content [25,26] and consequent slow axoplasmic flow [27–29] offers hope to people with diabetic neuropathy and superimposed nerve compression since neurolysis of these entrapped nerves may give symptomatic relief and possess potential for reversibility. As such, over the past two decades, surgical decompression of peripheral nerves has become an increasingly popular method for treating patients suffering from painful diabetic neuropathy.

Painful DPN can be divided into two varieties: acute and chronic painful DPN. Here we mainly focus on chronic painful DPN due to its highly prevalence and the facts that acute painful DPN is relatively rare and the acute symptoms may resolve within a year. [30,31] According to our clinical experience with management of painful diabetic neuropathy, pain is a heterogenous sensation and patients may describe their symptoms in markedly different ways. Features and severity of the pain may change with the development of diabetic neuropathy while the extent of pain is relatively invariable, which may be of somewhat value. We observed that some patients with painful DPN localized their pain mainly to the scattered areas of the legs, dorsum of feet, the heels, the toes, or the plantar aspect of feet while some others complained the pain was so dispersed that it even involved the whole lower limbs and the exact position could not be localized. Inspired by one previous guideline [8], we retrospectively defined the former as focal pain and the later as diffuse pain, and divided a series of 306 painful diabetic patients who underwent decompression surgery into two subgroups in the light of this definition. In this study we firstly compared the surgical result between surgical group and control group and, confirmed the efficacy of these decompression surgeries. Then we compared the surgical result of pain relief in patients of surgical group, revealing different responses of patients with focal and diffuse pain to the surgical decompression: people with focal painful DPN show a greater

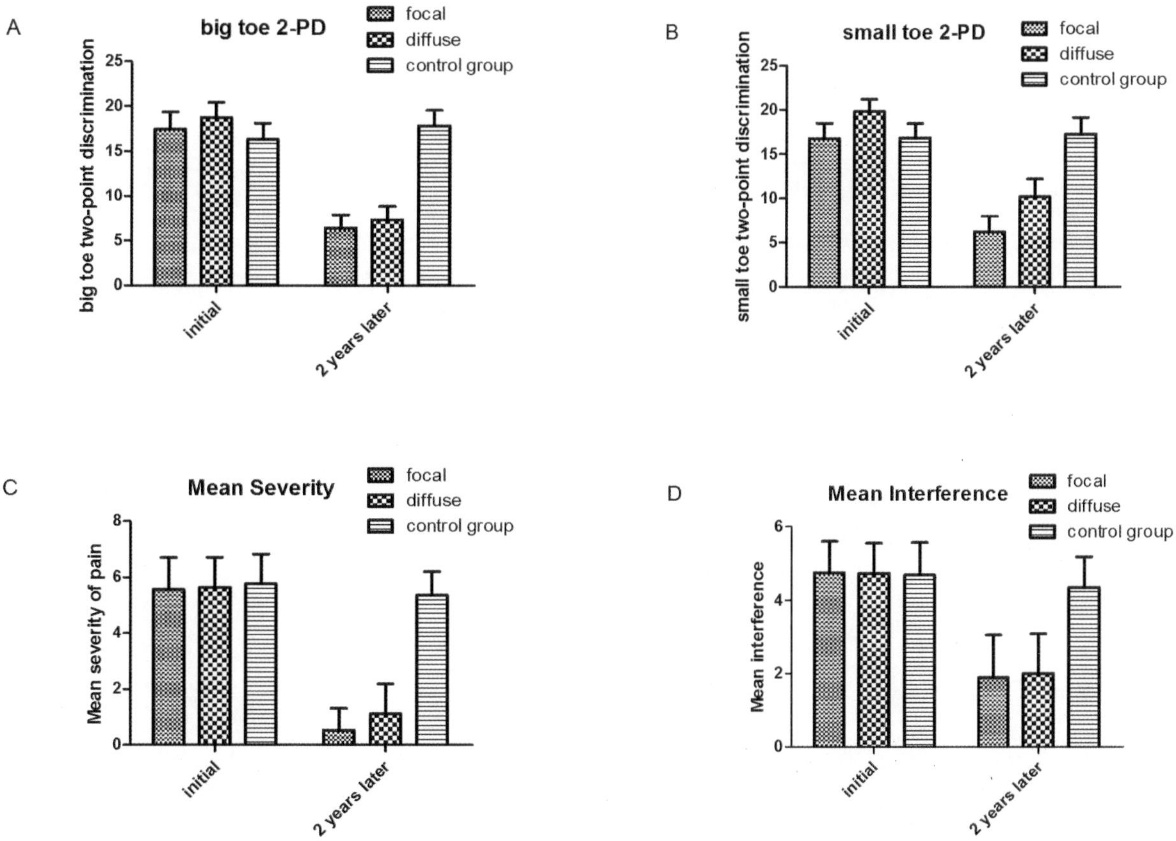

Figure 2. Graphs illustrate results of two-point discrimination and BPI-DPN in all groups. A, B, both surgical groups show marked decline in plantar big toe and small toe 2-PD while no apparent improvement can be observed in the control group; C, both surgical groups exhibit significant alleviation in pain severity through surgery while the control group remained at nearly the same level of mean severity of pain; D, decrease in the mean activity interference was displayed in both surgical groups and almost no changes existed in the control group.

potential to achieve pain relief. Morphologically, in addition, better ultrasound restoration could be observed in focal pain group than diffuse pain group.

The answer to the question of "what is the pathophysiology behind the distinct reaction to the decompression between patients with focal or diffuse painful DPN" should be started with the mechanisms of neuropathic pain in diabetes. Although the exact pathophysiological mechanisms of neuropathic pain in diabetes remain enigmatic, several mechanisms including peripheral and central mechanisms have been postulated based on the result of experiments in animal model of neuropathic pain. [32–36] It is suggested that all levels of the nervous system, from peripheral nerve to the brain, were affected by the diabetic neuropathy. [37] Both metabolic and mechanical (compressive) mechanism may be the source of the painful symptom.

Diabetes causes deposition of collagen in the small arteries that supply the peripheral nerves, hypothetically resulting in a length-dependent sensorimotor neuropathy. Increased aldose reductase

Table 2. Pre and post operative NCVs of DPN patients ($\overline{x}\pm S$).

	Preoperative NCV(ms)			Postoperative NCV(ms)		
	Control Group	Focal Group	Diffuse Group	Control Group	Focal Group	Diffuse Group
Posterior tibial nerve	36.7±3.4	33.5±3.1	35.5±3.6	31.6±3.5	41.8±2.6	42.0±2.8
Common peroneal nerve	33.8±2.8	37.8±3.4	36.8±1.9	28.6±3.3	42.5±2.4	42.2±2.9
Superficial peroneal nerve	38.6±3.7	35.8±2.5	37.6±2.9	34.4±3.6	42.2±3.1	43.6±2.3
Sural nerve	37.4±2.8	37.8±3.4	37.7±3.9	37.0±2.5	43.6±2.7	43.2±3.6

All variables were expressed in mean ± SD.
NCV: nerve conduction velocity.
Nerve decompression increases NCV in operated cases by 15–20%.

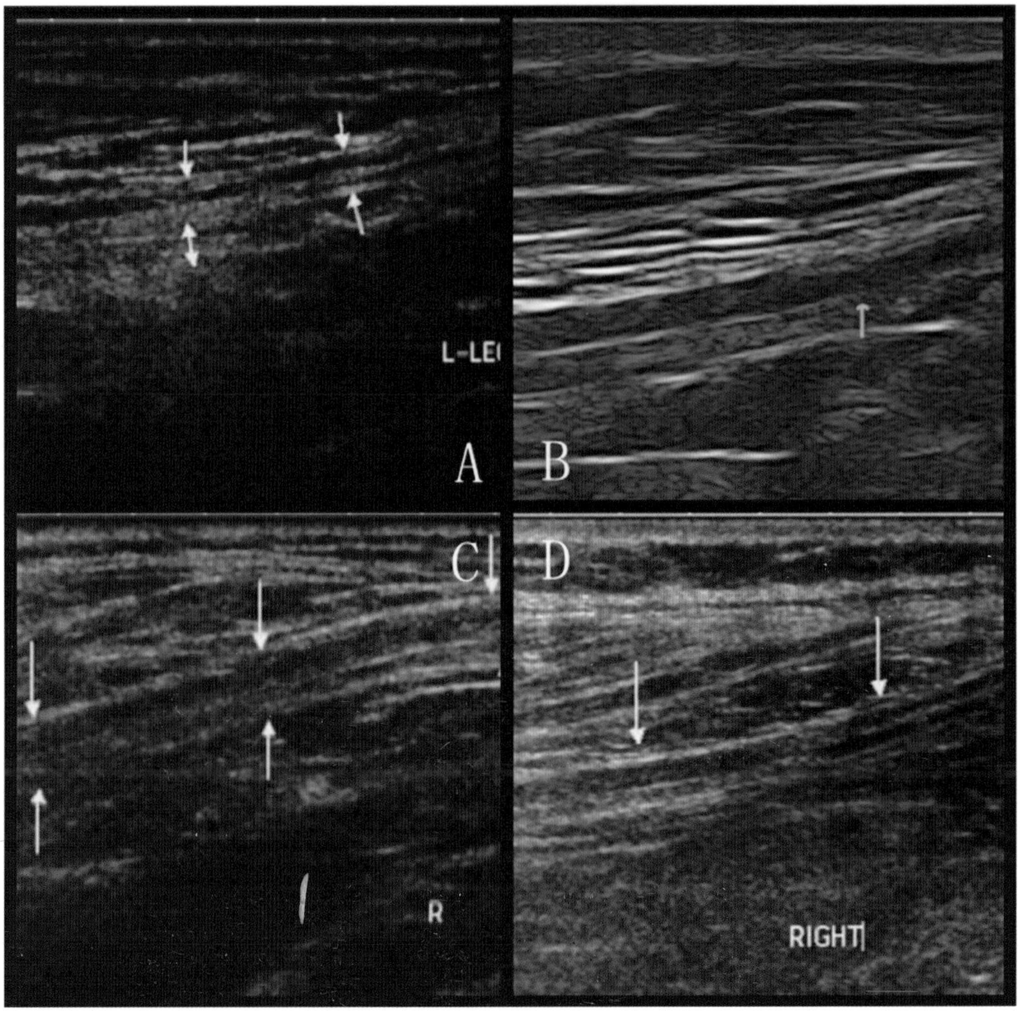

Figure 3. Longitudinal sonograms showing difference of morphological changes after surgical decompression between two patients with focal and diffuse painful DPN. A and B represent the preoperative (Da: 4.4 mm, Dt: 7.6 mm) and postoperative (Da: 2.9 mm, Dt: 6.3 mm) sonograms of the common peroneal nerve at the level of knee joint of patient with focal painful DPN. C and D represent the preoperative (Da: 4.2 mm, Dt: 7.0 mm) and postoperative (Da: 3.7 mm, Dt: 6.8 mm) sonograms of the common peroneal nerve at the level of knee joint of patient with diffuse painful DPN.

activity in diabetes converts glucose to sorbitol, which is hydrophilic and draws water into the nerve, rendering the peripheral nerve susceptible to mechanical compression and decreasing the slow axoplasmic transport in the diabetic nerve. As a consequence, proteins for structural repairs could not be transported to the impaired site within the diabetic nerve. [38] Injured peripheral nerve fibers give rise to the intense and prolonged input of ectopic activity to the central nervous system. After that, neurons in the spinal and the brain may change their response characteristics and exhibit signs of hyperexcitability in a fashion, mimicking that presented after peripheral nerve injury [39].

Table 3. Pre and post operative CSA of DPN patients ($\overline{x}\pm s$).

	Preoperative CSA			Postoperative CSA		
	Control Group	**Focal Group**	**Diffuse Group**	**Control Group**	**Focal Group**	**Diffuse Group**
Tibial nerve CSA(mm^2)	24.4±4.2	25.3±3.5	25.1±4.1	25.1±3.6	16.9±3.2	19.7±3.8
Common peroneal nerve CSA(mm^2)	21.6±3.7	20.8±3.5	21.2±4.0	21.9±3.2	14.6±2.8	15.9±3.5

All variables were expressed in mean ± SD.
CSA: cross-sectional area.

Given all that above, in the early stage of some cases, nerve thickening is suggested to play a fundamental role in the pathophysiology of painful diabetic neuropathy, with a manifestation of focal pain. As such, it is conceivable that entrapment of affected nerves at sites of anatomic narrowness may occur, which could be treated through surgical decompression. As the compression continues, however, neuroplastic changes in central nervous system happen after reorganization of structures participating in the processing of noxious information, which may present with diffuse pain in certain patients. The management is rather complicated. Aside from the current medical therapies including tricyclic antidepressants, the serotonin and noradrenaline re-uptake inhibitor and anti-convulsants, and so forth, an unmet need still exists for pharmacological agents targeting the underlying mechanisms due to the ineffectiveness and the side effects of the available drugs. In this study, the severity of pain, two-point discrimination, NCV results and morphological changes (SCA) of compressed nerve were all improved in surgical group when compared to the control group. Furthermore, there is no significant difference between the focal and diffuse pain groups regarding the results of two-point discrimination and NCV testing, which was increased by 15–20% after nerve decompression. (Table 2) Therefore, surgical decompression is also encouraged among the patients with diffuse painful DPN when the Tinel sign is positive, which indicates the existence of entrapment and regeneration of axons [40].

The limitations in our study include: (1) although being queried on admission, non-surgical treatment such as pharmacotherapy of neuropathic pain was not precisely measured among all the patients due to the retrospective nature of this study. For this reason, preoperative evaluation including pain levels was performed with both VAS and BPI-DPN and no significant difference was observed. (2) The specific definition of the focal and diffuse pain. Although extent of pain in most patients is relatively invariable, parts of patients would experience both focal and diffuse pain during the course of painful DPN. The phenotype of pain was decided on admission prior to surgery. Further prospective, randomized and controlled trial with blinded study executers and observers is needed to verify the role of peripheral nerve decompression in patients with painful DPN and further elucidate the role which pain distribution and characterization play in managing painful diabetic neuropathy as well as the underlying mechanism involved.

Allowing for the mixed results reported and the continuing controversy among researchers as to the effectiveness of nerve decompression surgery on DPN, [9,10,12,13,15,17,41–46] patient selection for surgery becomes increasingly critical through the long march to definitely delineate and confirm the place for nerve decompression. Distribution of pain indeed plays a practical role in predicting the response of painful DPN to the surgery according to the result of this study.

Conclusions

The results of this study continue to support the efficacy of decompression of multiple lower-extremity peripheral nerves in patients with painful diabetic neuropathy who presented with a positive Tinel sign. Favorable outcomes could be achieved in treating focal painful DPN through surgical decompression, which would also be helpful and should not be abandoned in diffuse painful DPN in the presence of Tinel sign.

Author Contributions

Conceived and designed the experiments: CLL WCZ. Performed the experiments: CLL MY. Analyzed the data: CLL QFM GWL WXZ. Contributed reagents/materials/analysis tools: MY WXZ QFM. Contributed to the writing of the manuscript: CLL.

References

1. Shaw JE, Sicree RA, Zimmet PZ (2010) Global estimates of the prevalence of diabetes for 2010 and 2030. Diabetes Res Clin Pract 87: 4–14.
2. Vinik AI, Park TS, Stansberry KB, Pittenger GL (2000) Diabetic neuropathies. Diabetologia 43: 957–973.
3. Thomas PK (1973) Metabolic neuropathy. J R Coll Physicians Lond 7: 154–160.
4. Boulton AJ, Malik RA, Arezzo JC, Sosenko JM (2004) Diabetic somatic neuropathies. Diabetes Care 27: 1458–1486.
5. Quattrini C, Tesfaye S (2003) Understanding the impact of painful diabetic neuropathy. Diabetes Metab Res Rev 19 Suppl 1: S2–8.
6. Abbott CA, Malik RA, van Ross ER, Kulkarni J, Boulton AJ (2011) Prevalence and characteristics of painful diabetic neuropathy in a large community-based diabetic population in the U.K. Diabetes Care 34: 2220–2224.
7. Tesfaye S, Boulton AJ, Dickenson AH (2013) Mechanisms and management of diabetic painful distal symmetrical polyneuropathy. Diabetes Care 36: 2456–2465.
8. Vinik AI, Casellini CM (2013) Guidelines in the management of diabetic nerve pain: clinical utility of pregabalin. Diabetes Metab Syndr Obes 6: 57–78.
9. Wieman TJ, Patel VG (1995) Treatment of hyperesthetic neuropathic pain in diabetics. Decompression of the tarsal tunnel. Ann Surg 221: 660–664; discussion 664–665.
10. Aszmann O, Tassler PL, Dellon AL (2004) Changing the natural history of diabetic neuropathy: incidence of ulcer/amputation in the contralateral limb of patients with a unilateral nerve decompression procedure. Ann Plast Surg 53: 517–522.
11. Biddinger KR, Amend KJ (2004) The role of surgical decompression for diabetic neuropathy. Foot Ankle Clin 9: 239–254.
12. Rader AJ (2005) Surgical decompression in lower-extremity diabetic peripheral neuropathy. J Am Podiatr Med Assoc 95: 446–450.
13. Siemionow M, Alghoul M, Molski M, Agaoglu G (2006) Clinical outcome of peripheral nerve decompression in diabetic and nondiabetic peripheral neuropathy. Ann Plast Surg 57: 385–390.
14. Karagoz H, Yuksel F, Ulkur E, Celikoz B (2008) Early and late results of nerve decompression procedures in diabetic neuropathy: a series from Turkiye. J Reconstr Microsurg 24: 95–101.
15. Wood WA, Wood MA (2003) Decompression of peripheral nerves for diabetic neuropathy in the lower extremity. J Foot Ankle Surg 42: 268–275.
16. Upton AR, McComas AJ (1973) The double crush in nerve entrapment syndromes. Lancet 2: 359–362.
17. Dellon AL (1992) Treatment of symptomatic diabetic neuropathy by surgical decompression of multiple peripheral nerves. Plast Reconstr Surg 89: 689–697; discussion 698–689.
18. Treede RD, Jensen TS, Campbell JN, Cruccu G, Dostrovsky JO, et al. (2008) Neuropathic pain: redefinition and a grading system for clinical and research purposes. Neurology 70: 1630–1635.
19. Bril V, Perkins BA (2002) Validation of the Toronto Clinical Scoring System for diabetic polyneuropathy. Diabetes Care 25: 2048–2052.
20. Scott J, Huskisson EC (1976) Graphic representation of pain. Pain 2: 175–184.
21. Zelman DC, Gore M, Dukes E, Tai KS, Brandenburg N (2005) Validation of a modified version of the Brief Pain Inventory for painful diabetic peripheral neuropathy. J Vasc Nurs 23: 97–104.
22. Lee CH, Dellon AL (2004) Prognostic ability of Tinel sign in determining outcome for decompression surgery in diabetic and nondiabetic neuropathy. Ann Plast Surg 53: 523–527.
23. Zhang W, Zhong W, Yang M, Shi J, Guowei L, et al. (2013) Evaluation of the clinical efficacy of multiple lower-extremity nerve decompression in diabetic peripheral neuropathy. Br J Neurosurg.
24. Melenhorst WB, Overgoor ML, Gonera EG, Tellier MA, Houpt P (2009) Nerve decompression surgery as treatment for peripheral diabetic neuropathy: literature overview and awareness among medical professionals. Ann Plast Surg 63: 217–221.
25. Gabbay KH (1973) The sorbitol pathway and the complications of diabetes. N Engl J Med 288: 831–836.
26. Jakobsen J (1978) Peripheral nerves in early experimental diabetes: expansion of the endoneurial space as a cause of increased water content. Diabetologia 14: 113–119.
27. Medori R, Autilio-Gambetti L, Monaco S, Gambetti P (1985) Experimental diabetic neuropathy: impairment of slow transport with changes in axon cross-sectional area. Proc Natl Acad Sci U S A 82: 7716–7720.
28. Dahlin LB, Meiri KF, McLean WG, Rydevik B, Sjostrand J (1986) Effects of nerve compression on fast axonal transport in streptozotocin-induced diabetes

mellitus. An experimental study in the sciatic nerve of rats. Diabetologia 29: 181–185.
29. Fink DJ, Purkiss D, Mata M (1987) Alterations in retrograde axonal transport in streptozocin-induced diabetic rats. Diabetes 36: 996–1000.
30. Tesfaye S, Malik R, Harris N, Jakubowski JJ, Mody C, et al. (1996) Arterio-venous shunting and proliferating new vessels in acute painful neuropathy of rapid glycaemic control (insulin neuritis). Diabetologia 39: 329–335.
31. Vinik A (2010) The approach to the management of the patient with neuropathic pain. J Clin Endocrinol Metab 95: 4802–4811.
32. Tesfaye S, Kempler P (2005) Painful diabetic neuropathy. Diabetologia 48: 805–807.
33. Ueda H (2006) Molecular mechanisms of neuropathic pain-phenotypic switch and initiation mechanisms. Pharmacol Ther 109: 57–77.
34. DeJong RN (1977) CNS manifestations of diabetes mellitus. Postgrad Med 61: 101–107.
35. Suzuki C, Ozaki I, Tanosaki M, Suda T, Baba M, et al. (2000) Peripheral and central conduction abnormalities in diabetes mellitus. Neurology 54: 1932–1937.
36. Eaton SE, Harris ND, Rajbhandari SM, Greenwood P, Wilkinson ID, et al. (2001) Spinal-cord involvement in diabetic peripheral neuropathy. Lancet 358: 35–36.
37. Kapur D (2003) Neuropathic pain and diabetes. Diabetes Metab Res Rev 19 Suppl 1: S9–15.
38. Barrett SL, Dellon AL, Fleischli J, Gould JS, Wang C (2010) Metabolic and compressive neuropathy. Foot Ankle Spec 3: 132–139.
39. Jensen TS, Baron R (2003) Translation of symptoms and signs into mechanisms in neuropathic pain. Pain 102: 1–8.
40. Dellon AL, Muse VL, Scott ND, Akre T, Anderson SR, et al. (2012) A positive Tinel sign as predictor of pain relief or sensory recovery after decompression of chronic tibial nerve compression in patients with diabetic neuropathy. J Reconstr Microsurg 28: 235–240.
41. Valdivia Valdivia JM, Weinand M, Maloney CT Jr, Blount AL, Dellon AL (2013) Surgical treatment of superimposed, lower extremity, peripheral nerve entrapments with diabetic and idiopathic neuropathy. Ann Plast Surg 70: 675–679.
42. Hollis Caffee H (2000) Treatment of diabetic neuropathy by decompression of the posterior tibial nerve. Plast Reconstr Surg 106: 813–815.
43. Aszmann OC, Kress KM, Dellon AL (2000) Results of decompression of peripheral nerves in diabetics: a prospective, blinded study. Plast Reconstr Surg 106: 816–822.
44. Therapeutics, Technology Assessment Subcommittee of the American Academy of N, Chaudhry V, Stevens JC, Kincaid J, et al. (2006) Practice Advisory: utility of surgical decompression for treatment of diabetic neuropathy: report of the Therapeutics and Technology Assessment Subcommittee of the American Academy of Neurology. Neurology 66: 1805–1808.
45. Cornblath DR, Vinik A, Feldman E, Freeman R, Boulton AJ (2007) Surgical decompression for diabetic sensorimotor polyneuropathy. Diabetes Care 30: 421–422.
46. Chaudhry V, Russell J, Belzberg A (2008) Decompressive surgery of lower limbs for symmetrical diabetic peripheral neuropathy. Cochrane Database Syst Rev: CD006152.

4

Primary Reasons for Osteopathic Consultation: A Prospective Survey in Quebec

Chantal Morin[1,2]*, Andrée Aubin[1]

1 Centre ostéopathique du Québec, Montréal, Québec, Canada, **2** School of Rehabilitation, Faculty of Medicine and Health Sciences, University of Sherbrooke, Sherbrooke, Québec, Canada

Abstract

Background: Osteopathy is an increasingly popular health care modality to address pain and function in the musculoskeletal system, organs and the head region, as well as functional somatic syndromes. Although osteopathy is recommended principally in guidelines for management of back pain, osteopaths' scope of practice is wide, albeit poorly defined. In order to understand better the practice of osteopathy, this study aimed to investigate the most common reasons for osteopathic consultations in clinical settings in Quebec.

Methods: A prospective survey of members of the Registre des ostéopathes du Québec was conducted to examine demographics in osteopathic practices, as well as patients' primary reasons for consultations over a two-week period. The questionnaire was devised following a literature review and refined and verified with two stages of expert input.

Results: 277 osteopaths (60.1% response rate) responded to the survey notice. 14,002 patients' primary reasons for consultations were reported in completed questionnaires and returned by practicing osteopaths. Musculoskeletal pain located in the spine, thorax, pelvis and limbs was the most common reason for consultations (61.9%), with females consulting most commonly for cervical pain and males for lumbar pain. Perinatal and paediatric (11.8%), head (9.1%), visceral (5.0%) and general concerns (4.8%) were the other most common reasons for consultations. Preventive care represented the remaining 0.3%.

Interpretation: The nature of primary reasons for osteopathic consultations, coupled with documented satisfaction of patients with this approach, suggest a future for multidisciplinary collaborative health care including osteopathy. Results of this survey may contribute to informing physicians and others pending regulation of Quebec osteopaths, and also provide direction for future clinical research and guidelines development.

Editor: Hamid Reza Baradaran, Iran University of Medical Sciences, Iran, Islamic Republic of

Funding: This study received funding from the Registre des ostéopathes du Québec (now Ostéopathie Québec); the first author received PhD scholarships from the Fonds de recherche en santé du Québec and the Faculty of Medicine and Health Sciences of the Université de Sherbrooke; and Ostéopathie Québec provided a grant to authors for publication. The funders had no role in the study concept and design, data collection and analysis, decision to publish, or preparation of the manuscript for submission.

Competing Interests: The authors have declared that no competing interests exist.

* Email: Chantal.Morin@USherbrooke.ca

Introduction

Osteopathy is based on manual contact for medical assessment and treatment. According to Benchmarks for training in osteopathy guidelines published by the World Health Organization (WHO), the osteopathic practitioners use a wide variety of therapeutic manual techniques to improve physiological function and/or support homeostasis that has been altered by somatic (body framework) dysfunction. Examples include impaired or altered function of components of the somatic system; skeletal, arthrodial and myofascial structures; and vascular, lymphatic, and neural elements [1]. Osteopathy is based on the principle that the structure and functions of the body are closely integrated, and that a person's wellbeing requires the neurological, musculoskeletal, circulatory and visceral structures to work in balance together. Osteopathic practice thus aims to restore (and maintain) a person's body to its overall natural state of wellbeing [2]. Osteopathy is an increasingly popular approach for somatic dysfunctions [1]. Disordered physiology may manifest as functional somatic syndromes, characterised by patterns of persistent bodily complaints that may occur independently from pathological changes [3].

Canadians' use of osteopathy doubled between 1997 and 2006; much of this occurred in Quebec, where utilization increased from 3% to 11% during this period [4]. Osteopathy is also the complementary therapy that is the most frequently recommended by general practitioners in Quebec [5].

In light of increasing use of osteopathy by Quebecers, including as a front line services, regulation seems desirable, and indeed the Office des professions du Québec intends to regulate the osteopathic profession in the province [6], to protect the osteopath's title, define reserved acts and shift education from private schools to a university Master's degree. Non-physician osteopaths are already regulated in many countries (United Kingdom (UK), Australia, Finland, New

Zealand, France and Switzerland) [7]. Osteopathy is recommended mainly in guidelines for management of back pain [8,9,10,11,12], but the scope of practice of osteopaths is wide, albeit poorly defined. Only a few studies in countries where osteopathy is a regulated profession reported results of surveys about profiles of practice including primary reasons for osteopathic consultations [13,14,15,16,17]. These recent surveys are one day snap shots documenting many aspects of osteopathic practice at the same time. They have limited rates of participation (3.4% to 38.9%), and report on small numbers of patients for each osteopath participant. The total number of patients reporting a primary reason for consultation is limited (799 to 2238 patients). To our knowledge, no published study has reported the most common reasons for osteopathic consultation for all patients seen over more than one day, for more than few patients per osteopath, or in relation to gender. As well, no study has been conducted specifically in Quebec, or in Canada. With the prospect of regulation and the increasing popularity of osteopathy, there is a need to better understand its practice in Quebec, in particular the most common reasons for consultation.

Although effectiveness of osteopathy for various conditions needs to be further documented, the aim of this study was to investigate the most common reasons for osteopathic consultations in clinical settings in Quebec for all patients seen during a two-week period. This knowledge is needed to inform not only regulatory bodies, but also health care providers in order to promote patient centered care including open physician-patient communication related to osteopathic consultations, and to establish research priorities.

Methods

Setting and participants

All members of the Registre des Osteopathes du Québec (ROQ) practicing in the province were eligible to participate. The ROQ (now known as Ostéopathie Québec) was the largest professional body of osteopaths in Quebec in 2011–2012, representing the majority of provincial osteopaths with training according to the WHO Benchmarks for training in osteopathy [1]. The Human Research and Ethics Committee of the Centre Hospitalier Universitaire de Sherbrooke provided approval for the study. Precise written instructions provide along with the questionnaire included reassurance that information provided was only to examine the most common reasons for osteopathic consultation in Quebec, and that all data would be treated and reported anonymously. The only patient data collected were gender, age category (children from birth to 14 years, or adult 15 years and older) and the leading reason for consulting in osteopathy.

Study design

For this descriptive study, a prospective self-administrated survey was devised based upon a literature review, and adapted for the Quebec provincial context. The questionnaire captured demographic information about osteopaths, limited patient data (age category, gender) and the primary reason for consultation for each patient. The use of anatomical sites of symptoms as categories for adult patients and concerns for paediatric patients is consistent with the standardised data collection in Part two (presenting symptoms) of the tool developed by the National Council for Osteopathic Research (NCOR) in UK [14,17,18]. Although the NCOR data collection tool was regarded as being useful for a cross-sectional survey, clinicians expressed the view that the whole tool was too long to use on a daily basis in practice [18]. The current study was designed to optimize the participation rate with a short questionnaire to be completed on a day-to day basis in clinic, to capture the most common reasons for consultation over a two-week period, with a sample allowing comparisons between genders.

Questionnaires were completed during a consecutive two-week working period at the convenience of each osteopath, between October 2011 and March 2012. The survey was announced in a communication by the ROQ, and the questionnaire was distributed to all osteopathic practitioners registered with the ROQ. The first postal mailing occurred in October 2011 ($n = 454$), followed by an email reminder two weeks later. The questionnaire was attached to an email reminder in December 2011 and again in February 2012. The completed survey was returned either by postal mail or by email to the principal investigator. In addition to the primary reason for consultation of each patient, osteopaths had to indicate the total number of females, males and children seen in the two-week period of the survey. A research assistant verified the equivalence of the total numbers indicated, and the data provided regarding individual patients.

Primary measurements

The questionnaire sought demographic information about the osteopath, years of experience, time spent with patients for a single consultation, practice profiles (type of practice), percentage of the practice that entails an exclusive osteopathic approach, and each patient's primary reason for the consultation. Primary reasons of consultation were categorized according to the anatomical site of the symptom (pain or dysfunction) except for perinatal and paediatric which were categorized according to the concern. Categories are: 1) Upper limb; 2) Lower limb; 3) Spine or pelvis; 4) Visceral; 5) Head; 6) Perinatal and paediatric concerns; 7) General concerns; or 8) Any other reasons (Questionnaire in French, Appendix S1). These eight categories included finer sub-categories, differentiated according to patient gender. This straightforward classification scheme avoided relying on a variety of practitioners' categories, on the results of physical assessment, or on the presumed origin of the symptoms [19]. Osteopathic practitioners could add items as needed.

A preliminary version of the questionnaire included socio-demographic information, and areas of symptoms relevant defined in other similar surveys including the standardised data collection tool developed by the NCOR [18]. Two experts, each with more than 10 years of clinical experience in osteopathy, one of whom also had a research background, established face validity of the initial version of the questionnaire. Each expert also provided feedback and participated in discussions to improve the questionnaire. It was further refined in accordance with clarifications recommended by four osteopaths, who pre-tested the instrument for a typical week of work.

Statistical analysis

Descriptive statistics (frequencies and percentages) were used to analyse demographics of respondents and to explore data on common reasons for consultations. Demographics (gender and years of experience) of respondents were compared to those of non-respondent members of the ROQ using chi-square and T-tests. Chi-square tests were further used to compare reasons for consulting between patients' gender in the entire sample (regardless of their osteopath). Statistical significance was set at $p<0.001$ after the Bonferroni correction was applied for multiple comparisons. Analyses were conducted using SPSS (version 17.0, SPSS Inc, Chicago, IL, USA).

Results

Of the 454 osteopaths initially mailed, 274 (60.1%) responded to the survey notice, of whom 245 were currently working and completed the prospective two week questionnaire. Four questionnaires were completed incorrectly and rejected in the analysis (multiple primary reasons for consulting were given per patient (n = 3); or data collection was only a one week period rather than a 2 week working period (n = 1)). Gender (p = 0.97) and years of experience (p = 0.17) were similar between osteopath respondents and non-respondents (data not shown). Characteristics of osteopath respondents are shown in Table 1. Osteopaths spent a mean of 55 minutes (range 30 to 75 minutes standard deviation (SD) = 8.79) with each patient. On average, they devoted 92.9% of their practice specifically to osteopathy. The total number of females, males and children treated indicated by each osteopath, and the data provided regarding individual patients were consistent in all questionnaires included in the analysis.

Overall, respondents treated a total of 14002 patients during the two-week working period, including 8739 females (62.4%), 3826 males (27.3%) and 1437 children (10.3%). A very high percentage (98.3%) of osteopaths had a general type of practice and nearly half treat children. Spinal, thorax and pelvic symptoms (42.4%) were the predominant primary reasons for osteopathic consultation, followed by lower limb (13.4%) and upper limb (13.3%) symptoms (Figure 1). Thus, musculoskeletal symptoms located in the spine, pelvis, thorax or limbs represented 69.1% of the primary reasons to consult an osteopath. Although those musculoskeletal symptoms were the leading reasons for both males and females, some differences were observed between genders (Table 2), with females consulting significantly more frequently for cervical and hip symptoms than males, while males consulted more frequently for lumbar, as well as shoulder and elbow symptoms.

Perinatal and paediatric concerns combined (11.8%), including consultations both for pain or discomfort experienced by pregnant women (n = 211) and for children below 15 years of age (n = 1437), was the second most common category of reasons for osteopathic consultations, after musculoskeletal complaints located in the spine, thorax, pelvis or limbs. Paediatric consultations were for a wide range of concerns; proportions of each of these categories are presented in Figure 2.

Table 1. Characteristics of osteopath respondents (N = 241).

	Frequency	(%)
Gender		
Female	160	(66.4)
Experience		
0–5 years	69	(28.6)
5–10 years	54	(22.4)
10–15 years	50	(20.7)
15 and more years	68	(28.2)
Areas of practice*		
General	237	(98.3)
Perinatal	106	(44.0)
Sports	68	(28.2)
Urogynecology	48	(20.0)

* An osteopath may cover more than one area of practice.

Symptoms localized in the head region (9.1%) were the third most common reason for osteopathic consultations, followed by visceral (5.0%), general concerns (4.7%) and preventive care (0.3%) (Table 3). For those categories, females consulted significantly more frequently for migraine, headache, urogenycological concerns and chronic pain associated with systemic dysfunction (e.g. fibromyalgia) than did males. Urogenycological concerns refer to urinary problems such as incontinence and perineal re-education for both females and males. In addition, some female patients also consulted for reproductive system dysfunction.

If a significance level of 5% is used instead of the 0.1% threshold, females also consult more than males for fatigue, temporomandibular disorders, pelvic pain, digestive problems and other general questions whereas males consult more than females for pain in ankles or feet and back or chest. The dataset is available upon request.

Interpretation

This first survey of osteopaths in Quebec reports on 241 practitioners and 14002 patients, seen over a two-week period. The high initial response rate (60.1% of the ROQ membership), with no significant differences in gender and years of experience between respondents and non-respondents, indicate that findings are representative of the most common reasons for consultation among osteopath members of the ROQ, the largest professional body of osteopaths in Quebec in 2011–2012.

Osteopaths were predominately consulted for musculoskeletal pain and dysfunction located in the spinal, pelvis, thorax and limbs. Lumbar (particularly in males) and cervical (particularly in females) regions were the most frequent pain locations, followed by shoulder, dorsal and costal regions. Perinatal and paediatric concerns were also frequent; principally for head shape, as well as torticollis. Patients also consulted for a variety of other concerns in the head region as well as for visceral, general and prevention purposes.

The finding that musculoskeletal pain and dysfunction in the spine, pelvis, thorax, and limbs was the primary reason for osteopathic consultation is consistent with recent surveys on osteopathic practices in general populations, across the UK, France and Australia [13,14,15,16,17]. None of previous surveys compared male's and female's reasons for consultation in osteopathy.

The trends observed for osteopathic consultation in the present study mirror known patterns of symptoms and physician consultation. In Quebec, males are more likely than females to consult a physician repeatedly for low back pain [20], while cervical pain was more frequently documented in females than in males [21]. A higher prevalence of headache [22,23] and chronic pain [24] have also been observed in Canadian females than males.

Paediatric osteopathic consultations ranged from 8% to 12% across previous surveys [13,14,15] but few details are available on primary reasons for consultation. An American study using administrative data on clinical diagnosis of paediatric patients [25] yielded similar observations, with consultations predominantly for torticollis and skull/face deformity, otitis media, infant feeding problems, muscle spasms and gastrointestinal concerns.

International recommendations for early management of musculoskeletal symptoms [26] and potentially severe impacts of spinal problems on health status [27] necessitate consideration of options for complementary care. Multidisciplinary care including professionals such as osteopaths, whose clinical interests and expertise focus on specific treatments for musculoskeletal and functional

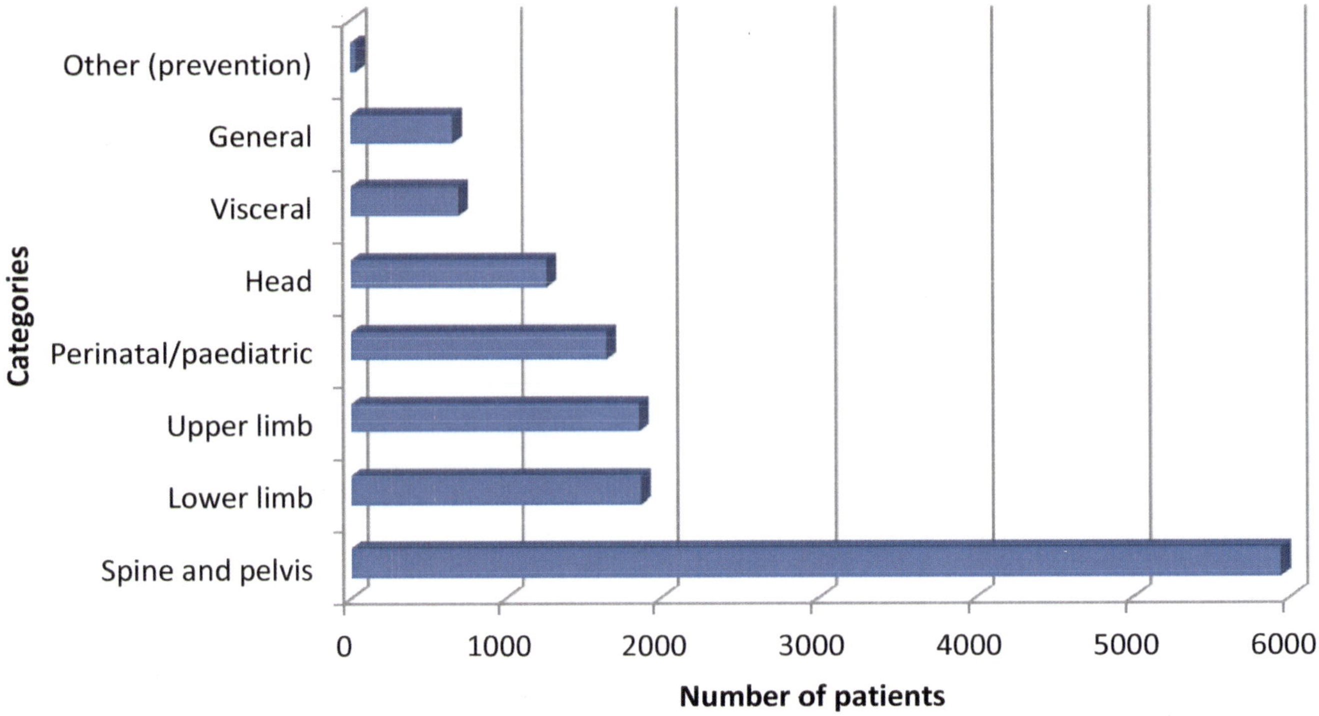

Figure 1. Frequencies of primary reason of consultation for all patients (n = 14002).

Table 2. Reasons for osteopathic consultation related to pain and dysfunction in spine, pelvis and limbs.

Location	All* (N = 14002)	Female (n = 8739)	Male (n = 3826)	
	Frequency (%; 95%CI)	Frequency (%; 95%CI)	Frequency (%; 95%CI)	*P* value†
Spine and pelvis	**5940 (42.4; 41.6–43.2)**	**3997 (45.7; 44.7–46.8)**	**1943 (50.8; 49.2–52.4)**	
Cervical	1796 (12.8; 12.3–13.4)	1321 (15.1; 14.4–15.9)	475 (12.4; 11.4–13.5)	<0.001
Dorsal or thorax	993 (7.1; 6.7–7.5)	656 (7.5; 7.0–8.1)	337 (8.8; 7.9–9.8)	0.013
Lumbar	2025 (14.5; 13.9–15.1)	1202 (13.8; 13.0–14.5)	823 (21.5; 20.2–22.8)	<0.001
Pelvis	662 (4.7; 4.4–5.1)	484 (5,5; 5.1–6.0)	178 (4.7; 4.0–5.4)	0.041
Spine, general	439 (3.1; 2.9–3.4)	316 (3.6; 3.2–4.0)	123 (3.2; 2.7–3.8)	0.260
Hernia or scoliosis	25 (0.2; 0.1–0.3)	18 (0.2; 0.1–0.3)	7 (0.2; 0.09–0.4)	0.790
Lower limb	**1873 (13.4; 12.8–14.0)**	**1262 (14.4; 13.7–15.2)**	**611 (16.0; 14.8–17.2)**	
Hip	452 (3.2; 3.0–3.5)	352 (4.0; 3.6–4.5)	100 (2.6; 2.2–3.2)	<0.001
Knee	489 (3.5; 3.2–3.8)	300 (3.4; 3.1–3.8)	189 (4.9; 4.3–5.7)	<0.001
Ankle and foot	441 (3.2; 2.9–3.5)	278 (3.2; 2.8–3.6)	163 (4.3; 3.7–5.0)	0.002
Lower limb, general	141 (1.0; 0.9–1.1)	99 (1.1; 0.9–1.4)	42 (1.1; 0.8–1.5)	0.864
Referred pain	350 (2.5; 2.3–2.7)	233 (2.7; 2.4–3.0)	117 (3.1; 2.6–3.7)	0.219
Upper limb	**1863 (13.3; 12.8–13.9)**	**1198 (13.7; 13.0–14.4)**	**665 (17.4; 16.2–18.6)**	
Shoulder	1108 (7.9; 7.5–8.3)	696 (8.0; 7.4–8.6)	412 (10.8; 9.8–11.8)	<0.001
Elbow	199 (1.4; 1.2–1.6)	106 (1.2; 1.0–1.5)	93 (2.4; 2.0–3.0)	<0.001
Wrist and hand	202 (1.4; 1.2–1.6)	145 (1.7; 1.4–2.0)	57 (1.5; 1.1–1.9)	0.487
Upper limb, general	147 (1.1; 0.9–1.2)	105 (1.2; 1.0–1.4)	42 (1.1; 0.8–1.5)	0.619
Referred pain	207 (1.5; 1.3–1.7)	146 (1.7; 1.4–2.0)	61 (1.6; 1.2–2.0)	0.757

95%CI: 95% confidence interval.
* All includes adults and children.
†*P*-value for differences between frequency of consultation according to patient gender. Statistically significant difference between genders' was defined as $p<0.001$ using the Bonferroni correction due to multiple comparisons.

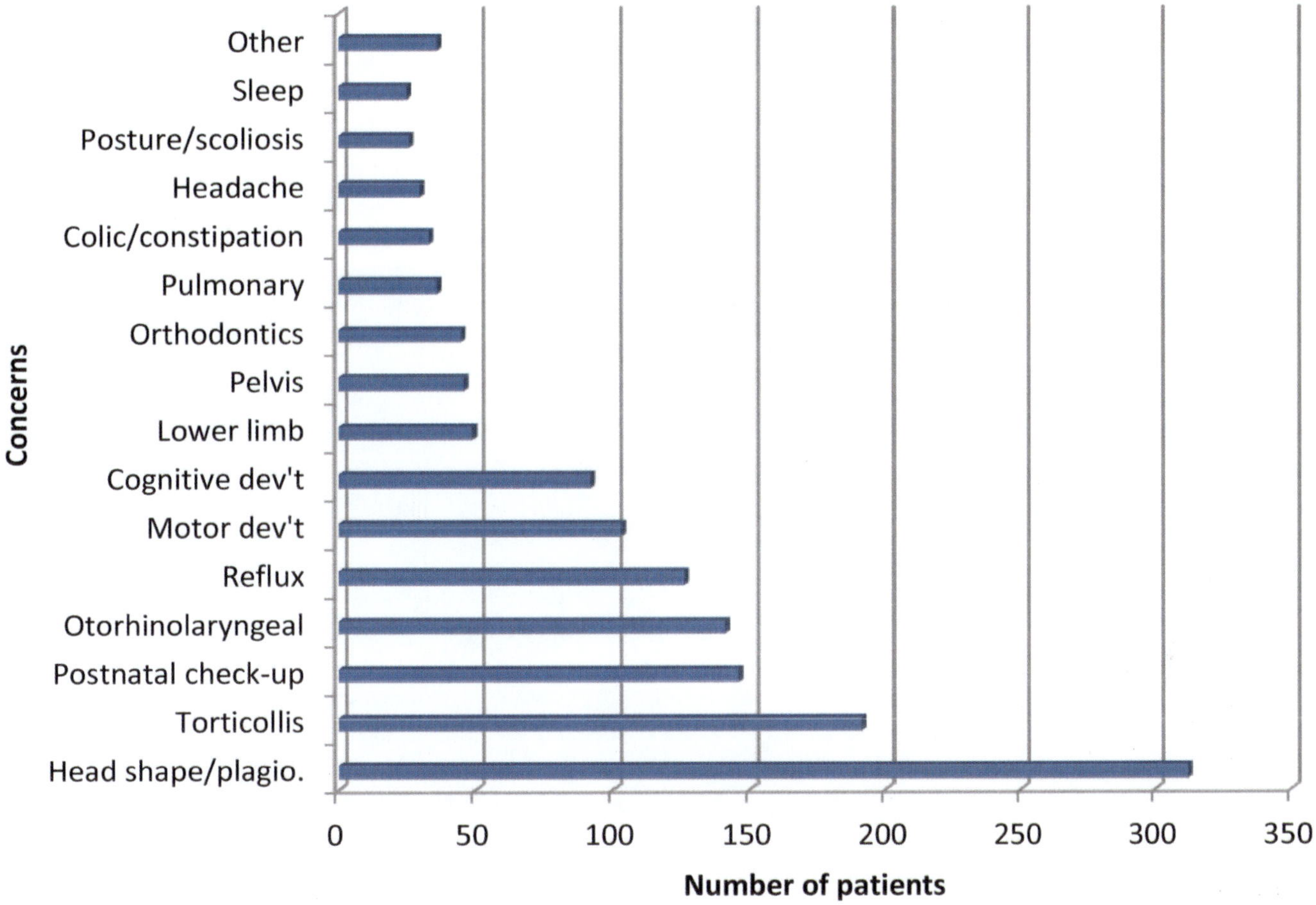

Figure 2. Frequencies of primary reason for paediatric consultations (Children <15 y, n = 1437).

problems, must be pursued, along with ongoing research to document efficacy and cost-effectiveness of interventions [26,28]. Knowledge of common reasons for osteopathic consultation may facilitate open physician-patient communication about best approaches for musculoskeletal and functional problems in multidisciplinary care. While patients express satisfaction with osteopathic treatment results, explanations given by osteopaths and overall health outcomes [14,29], physicians should be able to help patients to make the best choices in health care, including consideration of complementary therapies like osteopathy [30,31,32,33].

Limitations and strengths

The chief limitation of the questionnaire design was that only the primary reason for each consultation was collected. We were concerned that documentation of multiple reasons, requiring more time for questionnaire completion by osteopaths, might have reduced the participation rate.

Patients are seldom seen twice in the same month in osteopathic care, so the questionnaire did not capture if a patient was treated more than once during the two-week working period. Thus, a small amount of duplication may have occurred. Although surveys were verified for accuracy, it is possible that osteopaths may have omitted some patients during the two-week working period. This is a possible source of bias, although the scale is unknown alongside the 14002 documented reasons for consultation. Finally, given the number of statistical tests carried out, it is possible that type I errors occurred; however, the Bonferroni correction was applied to minimize this likelihood.

The main strengths of this study are the prospective design to reduce inaccuracies with recall, a high response rate, and inclusion of patient gender. The results of our survey provide the first general clinical overview of patients' reasons to consult an osteopath member of the ROQ.

Conclusion and future direction

Osteopaths treat both adults and children, mainly for musculoskeletal pain and dysfunction located in the spine, pelvis, thorax and limbs, but also for head region complaints, visceral and general concerns, as well as prevention, for both adults and children. The nature of primary reasons for osteopathic consultations, coupled with documented satisfaction of patients with this approach, suggest a future for multidisciplinary collaborative health care including osteopathy. With regulation of osteopathic practice pending in Quebec, results of this survey could contribute to informing regulators, to developing clinical guidelines and establishing clinical research priorities. Further research is needed to investigate safety and effectiveness of osteopathic practice for a variety of conditions, including patients' outcomes and satisfaction. Studies of effective interprofessional collaboration between physicians and osteopaths will facilitate safe and efficient patient centered care.

Table 3. Reasons for osteopathic consultation related to visceral region, head region, general concerns, preventive care, and perinatal and paediatric concerns.

Location or concern	All* (N = 14002)	Female (n = 8739)	Male (n = 3826)	
	Frequency (%; 95%CI)	Frequency (%; 95%CI)	Frequency (%; 95%CI)	*P* value[†]
Visceral	**703 (5.0; 4.7–5.4)**	**549 (6.3; 5.8–6.8)**	**154 (4.0; 3.4–4.7)**	
Digestive	371 (2.7; 2.4–2.9)	276 (3.2; 2.8–3.6)	95 (2.5; 2.0–3.0)	0.040
Pulmonary	96 (0.7; 0.6–0.8)	67 (0.8; 0.6–1.0)	29 (0.8; 0.5–1.1)	0.959
Urogynecology	199 (1.4; 1.2–1.6)	180 (2.1; 1.8–2.4)	19 (0.5; 0.3–0.8)	<0.001
Other visceral concerns[‡]	37 (0.3; 0.2–0.4)	26 (0.3; 0.2–0.4)	11 (0.3; 0.2–0.5)	0.924
Head	**1269 (9.1; 8.6–9.6)**	**972 (11.1; 10.5–11.8)**	**297 (7.8; 7.0–8.6)**	
Migraine	235 (1.7; 1.5–1.9)	194 (2.2; 1.9–2.5)	41 (1.1; 0.8–1.4)	<0.001
Headache	377 (2.7; 2.4–3.0)	297 (3.4; 3.0–3.8)	80 (2.1; 1.7–2.6)	<0.001
Dizziness, vertigo	153 (1.1; 0.9–1.3)	110 (1.3; 1.1–1.5)	43 (1.1; 0.8–1.5)	0.526
Facial pain	72 (0.5; 0.4–0.6)	53 (0.6, 0.5–0.8)	19 (0.5; 0.3–0.8)	0.453
Otorhinolaryngeal	161 (1.2; 1.0–1.4)	114 (1.3; 1.1–1.6)	47 (1.2; 0.9–1.6)	0.727
Orthodontics	34 (0.2; 0.1–0.3)	26 (0.3; 0.2–0.4)	8 (0.2; 0.1–0.4)	0.380
Temporomandibular joint	195 (1.4; 1.2–1.6)	151 (1.7; 1.5–2.0)	44 (1.2; 0.9–1.5)	0.016
Commotion or eye-related	42 (0.3; 0.2–0.4)	27 (0.3; 0.2–0.4)	15 (0.4; 0.2–0.6)	0.458
General concerns	666 (4.8; 4.4–5.1)	526 (6.0; 5.5–6.5)		
Fatigue	233 (1.7; 1.5–1.9)	184 (2.1; 1.8–2.4)	49 (1.3; 1.0–1.7)	0.002
Mood	58 (0.4; 0.3–0.5)	42 (0.5; 0.4–0.6)	16 (0.4; 0.3–0.7)	0.635
Sleep	85 (0.6; 0.5–0.7)	59 (0.7; 0.5–0.9)	26 (0.7; 0.5–1.0)	0.978
Chronic pain	226 (1.6; 1.4–1.8)	189 (2.2; 1.9–2.5)	37 (1.0; 0.7–1.3)	<0.001
Other general concerns[§]	64 (0.5; 0.4–0.6)	52 (0.6; 0.5–0.8)	12 (0.3; 0.2–0.5)	0.041
Preventive care	40 (0.3; 0.2–0.4)	24 (0.3; 0.2–0.4)	16 (0.4; 0.2–0.7)	0.189
Perinatal and paediatric concerns	1648 (11.8; 11.3–12.3)	211 (2.4; 2.1–2.7)		

95%CI: 95% confidence interval.
* All includes men, women and children.
[†]*P*-value for differences in frequency of reason for consultation according to patient gender. Statistically significant difference between genders' was defined as $p<0.001$ using the Bonferroni correction due to multiple comparisons.
[‡]Abdominal pain, post-surgical adhesions, skin problems.
[§]Hormonal balance, degenerative diseases, homeostasis and vitality, circulatory problems and depression.

Acknowledgments

We would like to thank our colleagues, Louise Collette and Stéphane Tremblay, who established face validity of the survey, Isabelle Gaboury and Meg Sears for manuscript revisions, and Jean-Pierre Bellerive and Nicole Spino for their dedicated work. The first author received scholarships from the Fonds de recherche en santé du Québec and the Faculty of Medicine and Health Sciences of the Université de Sherbrooke. Authors received a grant from Ostéopathie Québec for this publication.

Author Contributions

Conceived and designed the experiments: CM AA. Performed the experiments: CM. Analyzed the data: CM. Contributed reagents/materials/analysis tools: CM AA. Wrote the paper: CM AA.

References

1. WHO (2010) Benchmarks for training in traditional/compementary and alternative medicine: Benchmarks for training in osteopathy. apps.who.int/medicinedocs/documents/s17555en/s17555en.pdf. Accessed 2014 Jun 23.
2. OIA (2014) Osteopathy and osteopathic medicine: A global view of practice, patients, education and contribution to healthcar delivery. Chicago: http://wp.oialliance.org/?page_id = 3741. Accessed 2014 May 19.
3. Williams N, Wilkinson C, Stott N, Menkes DB (2008) Functional illness in primary care: dysfunction versus disease. BMC Family Practice 9: 1–8.
4. Esmail N (2007) Complementary and Alternative Medicine in Canada: Trends in Use and Public Attitudes, 1997–2006. Vancouver: The Fraser Institute. pp. 53.
5. O'Connor D (2009) Étude sur les perspectives des omnipraticiens du Québec quant à leur rôle-conseil concernant l'utilisation des médecines alternatives et complémentaires (MAC). Sherbrooke: Université de Sherbrooke. 136 p.
6. Fiore F (2013) Les "mdecines douces": atout supplémentaire en médecine? Le Médecin du Québec 48: 14–18.
7. OIA (2012) History and Current Context of Osteopathic Profession. Osteopathic International Alliance.
8. van Tulder M, Becker A, Bekkering T (2006) European guidelines for the management of acute nonspecific low back pain in primary care. European Spine Journal: S169–S191.
9. Airaksinen O, Brox JL, Cedraschi C (2006) European guidelines for the management of chronic non-specific low back pain. European Spine Journal: S192–S300.
10. (2006) Musculoskeletal Services Framework. A joint responsibility: doing it differently. In: Health Do, editor. London: http://webarchive.nationalarchives.gov.uk/20130124073659/http://www.dh.gov.uk/prod_consum_dh/groups/dh_digitalassets/@dh/@en/documents/digitalasset/dh_4138412.pdf. Accessed 2014 Aug 7.

11. Chou R, Qaseem A, Snow V (2007) Diagnosis and treatment of low back pain: a joint clinical practice guideline from the American College of Physicians and the American Pain Society. Annals of Internal Medicine 147: 478–491.
12. Savigny P, Kuntze S, Watson P (2009) Low back pain: early management of persistent non-specific low back pain. In: Practitioners NCCfPCaRCoG, editor. London.
13. Dubois T, Coatmellec J (2012) Osteopathy in France: A demographic and epidemiologic descriptive analysis of french osteopaths' patients. OIA. Paris.
14. Fawkes C, Leach J, Mathias S, Moore AP (2010) Standardised data collection within osteopathic practice in the UK: development and first use of a tool to profile osteopathic care in 2009. In: Research NCfO, editor. University of Brighton: Clinical Research Centre for Health Professions. pp. 1–176.
15. Orrock PJ (2009) Profile of members of the Australian Osteopathic Association: Part 2 – The patients. International Journal of Osteopathic Medicine: 128–139.
16. Burke SR, Myers R, Zhang AL (2013) A profile of osteopathic practice in Australia 2010–2011: a cross sectional survey. BMC Musculoskeletal Disorders 14.
17. Fawkes CA, Leach CM, Mathias S, Moore AP (2014) A profile of osteopathic care in private practices in the United Kingdom: A national pilot using standardised data collection. Manual Therapy 19: 125–130.
18. Fawkes CA, Leach CM, Mathias S, Moore AP (2014) Development of a data collection tool to profile osteopathic practice: Use of a nominal group technique to enhance clinician involvement. Manual Therapy 19: 119–124.
19. McIllwraith B (2003) A survey of 1200 osteopathic patients in the United Kingdom. Journal of Osteopathc Medicine 6: 7–12.
20. Beaudet N, Courteau J, Sarret P, Vanasse A (2013) Prevalence of claims-based recurrent low back pain in a Canadian population: A secondary analysis of an administrative database. BMC Musculoskeletal Disorders 14: 1–8.
21. Hogg-Johnson S, van der Velde G, Carroll LJ, Holm LW, Cassidy JD, et al. (2008) The Burden and Determinants of Neck Pain in the General Population. Eur Spine: S39–51.
22. O'Brien B, Goeree R, Streiner D (1994) Prevalence of Migraine Headache in Canada: A Population-Based Survey. International Journal of Epidemiology 23: 1020–1026.
23. Cooke LJ, Becker WJ (2010) Migraine Prevalence, Treatment and Impact: The Canadian Women and Migraine Study. Can J Neurol Sci: 580–587.
24. Meana M, Cho R, DesMeules M (2004) Chronic Pain: The Extra Burden on Canadian Women. BMC Women's Health 4: 1–11.
25. Lund G, Carreiro J (2010) Characteristics of Pediatric Patients Seen in Medical School–Based Osteopathic Manipulative Medicine Clinics. JAOA 110: 376–380.
26. Foster NE, Hartvinsen J, Croft PR (2012) Taking responsibility for the early assessment and treatment of patients with musculoskeletal pain: a review and critical analysis. Arthritis Research & Therapy: 205.
27. Fanuele JC, Birkmeyer NJO, Abdu WA, Tosteson TD, Weinstein JN (2000) The Impact of Spinal Problems on the Health Status of Patients. Spine 25: 1509–1514.
28. Gurden M, Morelli M, Sharpe G, Baker K, Betts N, et al. (2012) Evaluation of a general practitioner referral service for manual treatment of back and neck pain. Primary Health Care Research & Development: 204–210.
29. Strutt R, Shaw Q, Leach J (2008) Patients' perceptions and satisfaction with treatment in a UK osteopathic training clinic. Manual Therapy: 456–467.
30. Jean D, Cyr C (2007) Use of Complementary and Alternative Medicine in a General Pediatric Clinic. Pediatrics 120: e138–e141.
31. Pélissier-Simard L, Xhignesse M (2008) Les approches complémentaires en santé: comprendre pour bien conseiller. Le Médecin du Québec 43: 23–30.
32. Cheshire A, Polley M, Peters D, Ridge D (2011) Is it feasible and effective to provide osteopathy and acupuncture for patients with musculoskeletal problems in a GP setting? A service evaluation. BMC Family Practice: 1–10.
33. Metcalfe A, Williams J, McChesney J, Patten SB, Jetté N (2010) Use of complementary and alternative medicine by those with a chronic disease and the general population - results of a national population based survey. BMC Complementary and Alternative Medicine 10: 1–6.

5

Differential Expressions of the Alternatively Spliced Variant mRNAs of the μ Opioid Receptor Gene, *OPRM1*, in Brain Regions of Four Inbred Mouse Strains

Jin Xu[1], Zhigang Lu[1], Mingming Xu[1], Grace C. Rossi[2], Benjamin Kest[3], Amanda R. Waxman[3], Gavril W. Pasternak[1], Ying-Xian Pan[1]*

1 Department of Neurology and Molecular Pharmacology and Chemistry Program, Memorial Sloan Kettering Cancer Center, New York, New York, United States of America, **2** Department of Psychology, Long Island University, Post Campus, Brookville, New York, United States of America, **3** Department of Psychology and Center for Developmental Neuroscience, City University of New York, Staten Island, New York, United States of America

Abstract

The μ opioid receptor gene, *OPRM1*, undergoes extensive alternative pre-mRNA splicing in rodents and humans, with dozens of alternatively spliced variants of the *OPRM1* gene. The present studies establish a SYBR green quantitative PCR (qPCR) assay to more accurately quantify mouse *OPRM1* splice variant mRNAs. Using these qPCR assays, we examined the expression of *OPRM1* splice variant mRNAs in selected brain regions of four inbred mouse strains displaying differences in μ opioid-induced tolerance and physical dependence: C56BL/6J, 129P3/J, SJL/J and SWR/J. The complete mRNA expression profiles of the *OPRM1* splice variants reveal marked differences of the variant mRNA expression among the brain regions in each mouse strain, suggesting region-specific alternative splicing of the *OPRM1* gene. The expression of many variants was also strain-specific, implying a genetic influence on *OPRM1* alternative splicing. The expression levels of a number of the variant mRNAs in certain brain regions appear to correlate with strain sensitivities to morphine analgesia, tolerance and physical dependence in four mouse strains.

Editor: Tuck Wah Soong, National University of Singapore, Singapore

Funding: This work was supported, in part, by research grants DA13997 & DA029244 (to YXP) and DA02615, DA06241 and DA07242 (to GWP) from the National Institute on Drug Abuse and a core grant from the National Cancer Institute to MSKCC (CA08748). The funders had no role in study design, data collection and analysis, decision to publish, or preparation of the manuscript.

Competing Interests: The authors have declared that no competing interests exist.

* Email: pany@mskcc.org

Introduction

Morphine and most clinical analgesic agents, as well as heroin, act primarily through μ opioid receptors [1]. However, their actions, such as analgesia, tolerance, physical dependence and other side-effects vary among patients [2–4]. Similar effects have been observed in animal models [5–9]. These observations are consistent with the concept of subtypes of μ opioid receptors that was initially proposed by pharmacological studies [10–12] and subsequently confirmed with the isolation of a multitude of μ opioid receptor variants generated by alternative splicing [13–17] in rodents and humans despite the presence of a single μ opioid receptor gene, as determined by chromosomal mapping [18–21] and genomic sequencing. Alternative pre-mRNA splicing is a major mechanism for generating protein diversity and is extensively used by the μ opioid receptor gene. To date, studies show that the mouse, rat and human *OPRM1* genes generate 29, 16 and 19 splice variants, respectively, with similar patterns (Fig. 1) (see reviews: [16,22]). These splice variants can be categorized into three major groups based upon receptor structure: 1) Full-length carboxyl (C-) terminal variants with 7-transmembrane (7-TM) domains; 2) Truncated variants containing 6-TM domains; and 3) Truncated variants containing a single TM. The full length 7-TM C-terminal variants differ in their region-specific expressions, receptor phosphorylation, internalization, and post-endocytic sorting [23–31]. Furthermore, the intrinsic activities of μ drugs vary from variant to variant [32]. The significance of the exon 11-associated 6-TM variants is illustrated by their role in the analgesic actions of opioids such as morphine-6β-glucuronide (M6G), fentanyl and heroin [33], as a novel new class of opioid analgesics lacking many of the side-effects of traditional opiates [34].

The sensitivity of mice towards μ opioids on a variety of phenotypic measures is genotype dependent [35–40]. For example, surveys of inbred mouse strains reveal differences in morphine dependence, assessed with naloxone-precipitated withdrawal jumping scores, and tolerance, as seen by analgesic potency shifts after chronic morphine administration [35,36,41]. 129P3/J mice are highly refractory to morphine tolerance and naloxone-precipitated withdrawal, whereas C57BL/6J and SWR/J mice develop significant morphine tolerance and physical dependence. These inbred mouse strains also show similar differences in naloxone-precipitated withdrawal jumping scores toward other μ opioids including heroin [37], M6G and methadone [42].

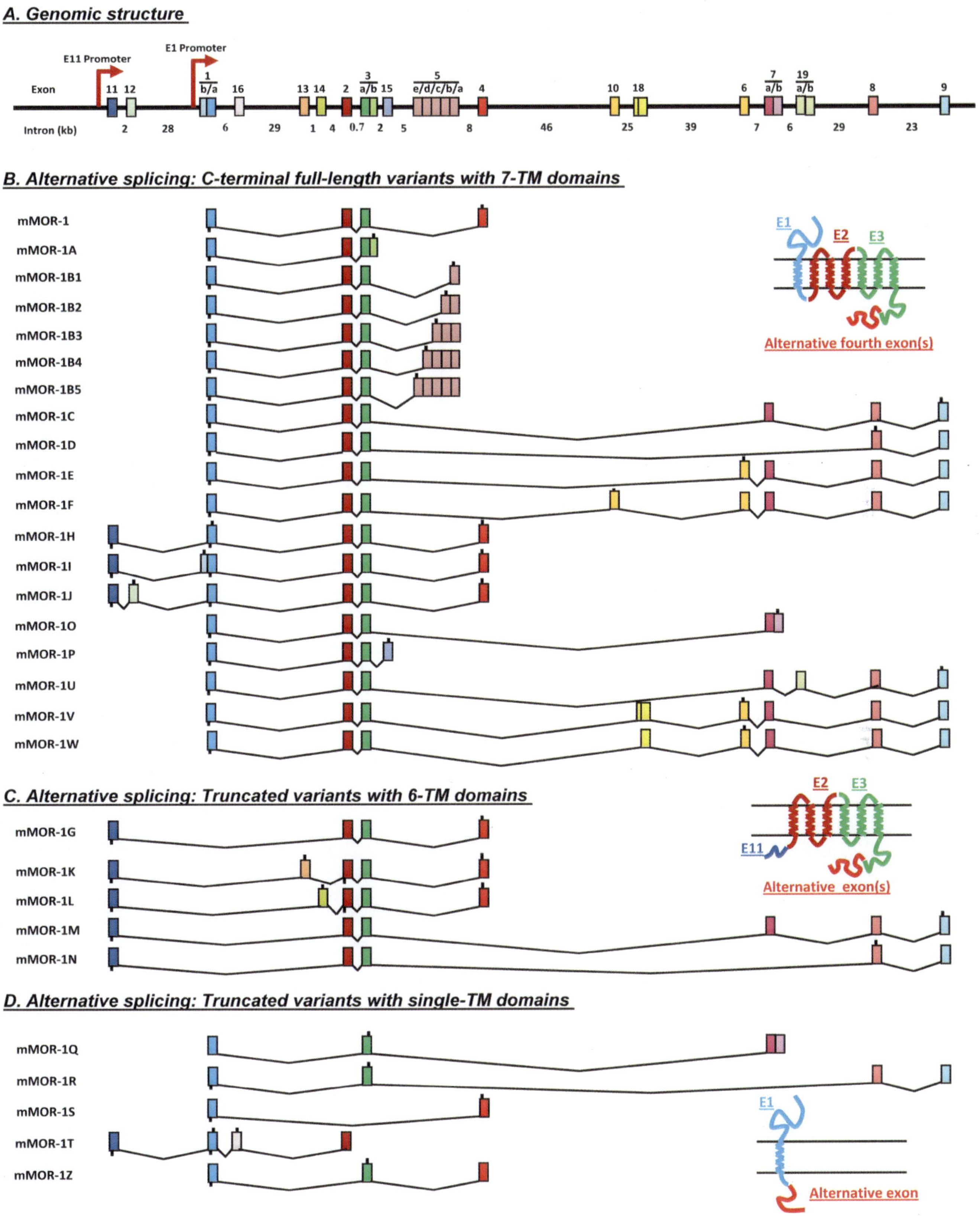

Figure 1. Schematic of the mouse *OPRM1* gene structure, alternative splicing and predicted protein structures. A, Genomic structure of the mouse *OPRM1*gene. Exons and introns are showed by boxes and horizontal lines, respectively. Intron size is indicated below the introns as kilobases (kb). Promoters are showed by arrows. Exons are numbered based upon the published data. B, Alternative splicing of C-terminal splice variants with 7-TM domains. Translational start and termination sites are indicated by downward and upward lines on exon boxes, respectively. The

lines between exons are introns that are spliced out during splicing. Predicted receptor structures are inserted at the right with colored bars indicating different coding exons. C, Alternative splicing of truncated variants with 6-TM domains. D, Alternative splicing of truncated variants with 1-TM domain.

However, it is not clear how the genetic background of these strains influences the expression of the *OPRM1* gene, a primary candidate responsible for the actions of μ drugs seen in these strains.

Our previous studies suggested region-specific alternative splicing of the *OPRM1* gene among brain regions using regular RT-PCR approaches [25–28]. However, regular PCR can only provide estimates of quantification due to technical limitations. To establish more accurate, reliable and sensitive assays for quantifying *OPRM1* variant mRNAs we have established SYBR green quantitative PCR (qPCR) assays for the *OPRM1* splice variants. Using these qPCR assays, we examined the expression levels of *OPRM1* splice variant mRNAs in selected brain regions of four inbred mouse strains: C56BL/6J (B6), 129P3/J (129), SJL/J (SJL) and SWR/J (SWR).

Materials and Methods

Animal

C56BL/6J (B6, stock #: 000664), 129P3/J (129, stock#: 000690), SJL/J (SJL, stock #: 000686) and SWR/J (SWR, stock #: 000689) male mice at 7–8 weeks of age were obtained from Jackson Laboratory. All mice were housed in groups of five, maintained on a 12-h light/dark cycle and given ad libitum access to food and water. All animal studies were approved by the Institutional Animal Care and Use Committee of the Memorial Sloan-Kettering Cancer Center.

Tissue dissection, RNA extraction and reverse-transcription (RT)

Brain regions including the prefrontal cortex (Pfc), striatum (Str), thalamus (Tha), hypothalamus (Hyp), hippocampus (Hip), brain stem (BS), periaqueductal gray (PAG), and cerebellum (Cb) were dissected on a mouse Plexiglas brain mold using the atlas of Paxinos and Franklin [43] as a reference. The spinal cord (Spc) from L1 to L5 and whole brain were also dissected. The dissected tissues were immediately homogenized in QiAzol Reagent (Qiagen). The homogenates were stored at $-80°C$ until further RNA isolation. 2–3 mice were pooled for each region, and a total of 8–10 mice used for each strain. Total RNAs were extracted using miRNeasy kit (Qiagen) following manufacture protocol. RNA concentrations were determined using a Qubit 2.0 Fluorometer (Invitrogen). RNAs were first treated with Turbo-DNA free reagent (Ambion) following the manufacture's protocol to remove potentially contaminating genomic DNA, and reverse transcribed with Superscript II reverse transcriptase (Invitrogen) and random hexmers. The first-strand cDNA was then used as templates in SYBR qPCRs.

Primer design and SYBR green qPCR

Since many exons are shared by different variants, it is difficult to design the short amplicon required for an efficient qPCR using the TaqMan assay for most of the splice variants. SYBR Green qPCR offers more flexibility in terms of amplicon size and thermocycle conditions. Using primer design tools in GeneRunner and VectorNTI, we designed appropriate primers for each splice variants, optimized qPCR parameters, such as annealing temperature and extension time, and obtained reasonable amplification efficiency by generating standard curves using 5–7 serial 10-fold dilutions of corresponding cDNAs as templates (Table S1). In most cases, we designed primers targeting exon-exon junctions or crossing at least two exons to obtain specific amplification. Specificities of the primers were verified by qPCRs using plasmid constructs containing corresponding variant cDNAs, and by melting curve analysis and agarose gel analysis after qPCR. Table S1 lists the names, sequences and location of primers, as well as amplicon size, efficiency and PCR parameters, for all 29 splice variants. Two workstations in two separate rooms were used exclusively for qPCR to avoid cross contamination. Three reference genes, succinate dehydrogenase subunit A (SDHA), TATA box binding protein (TBP) and glycerakdehyde 3-phosphate dehydrogenase (G3PDH), were selected to obtain normalization factors using the formula[44–46]: Normalization factor $(NF) = (C(t)_{SDHA} \times C(t)_{TBP} \times C(t)_{G3PDH})^{1/3}$. All qPCRs were performed using HotStart-IT SYBR Green qPCR Master Mix (USB, Affymetrix, INC) with Opticon 2 DNA Engine System (Bio-Rad). Normalized expression (NE) or expression level for each variant was calculated using the formula [44]: $NE_{variant} = E^{-(C(t)\text{-}variant - C(t)NF)}$ $(E^{-\Delta C(t)})$, where E is efficiency. Fold change (FC) was calculated using the formula [44]: $FC = NE_{variant}/NE_{reference}$, where a reference was mE1/2 and is was defined as 100%. mE1/2 amplified with primers from exon 1 to exon 2 represented all C-terminal variants, including the original mMOR-1. Although the original mMOR-1 transcribed through the exon 1 promoter is by far the most abundant, it is difficult to design a pair of specific primers for amplifying the exon 1 promoter-driven mMOR-1, since exons 1–4 are shared by several other variants as well.

Statistical analysis

Data are represented as the mean ± S.E.M. from at least three independent experiments. Two-way ANOVA with Tukey's multiple comparisons test was used for analyzing qPCR data. Statistical significance was set at $p<0.05$. The results are listed in Table S3.

Results

Expression levels of *OPRM1* splice variant mRNAs in four inbred mouse strains

Using the established RT-SYBR green qPCR assays, we examined the expression levels of *OPRM1* splice variant mRNAs in nine brain regions of four inbred mouse strains. The overall expression levels among the variants are shown in a heatmap clustered based upon Z-scores from the values (Log_2 $(E^{-\Delta C(t)})$ of individual variants across different strains/regions, plotting from the highest level (left, red) to the lowest level (right, green) (Fig. 2) (All $E^{-\Delta C(t)}$ values are listed in Table S2). The heatmap reveals a wide range of expression levels among the variants, as indicated by Z-score values from <-4 to >4. mE1-2, which represents the entire repertoire of full-length 7-TM variants, was expressed at the highest level in all brain regions and strains. The expression of the other splice variants differed dramatically among the regions and strains.

To visualize expression patterns more closely, we compared five C-terminal splice variants and two 6-TM and two 1-TM variants, as well as mE1-2, by plotting their $(-1)/log_2(E^{-\Delta C(t)})$ values in the brain regions (Fig. 3). The various splice variant expression levels among the brain regions ranged widely. For example, in the

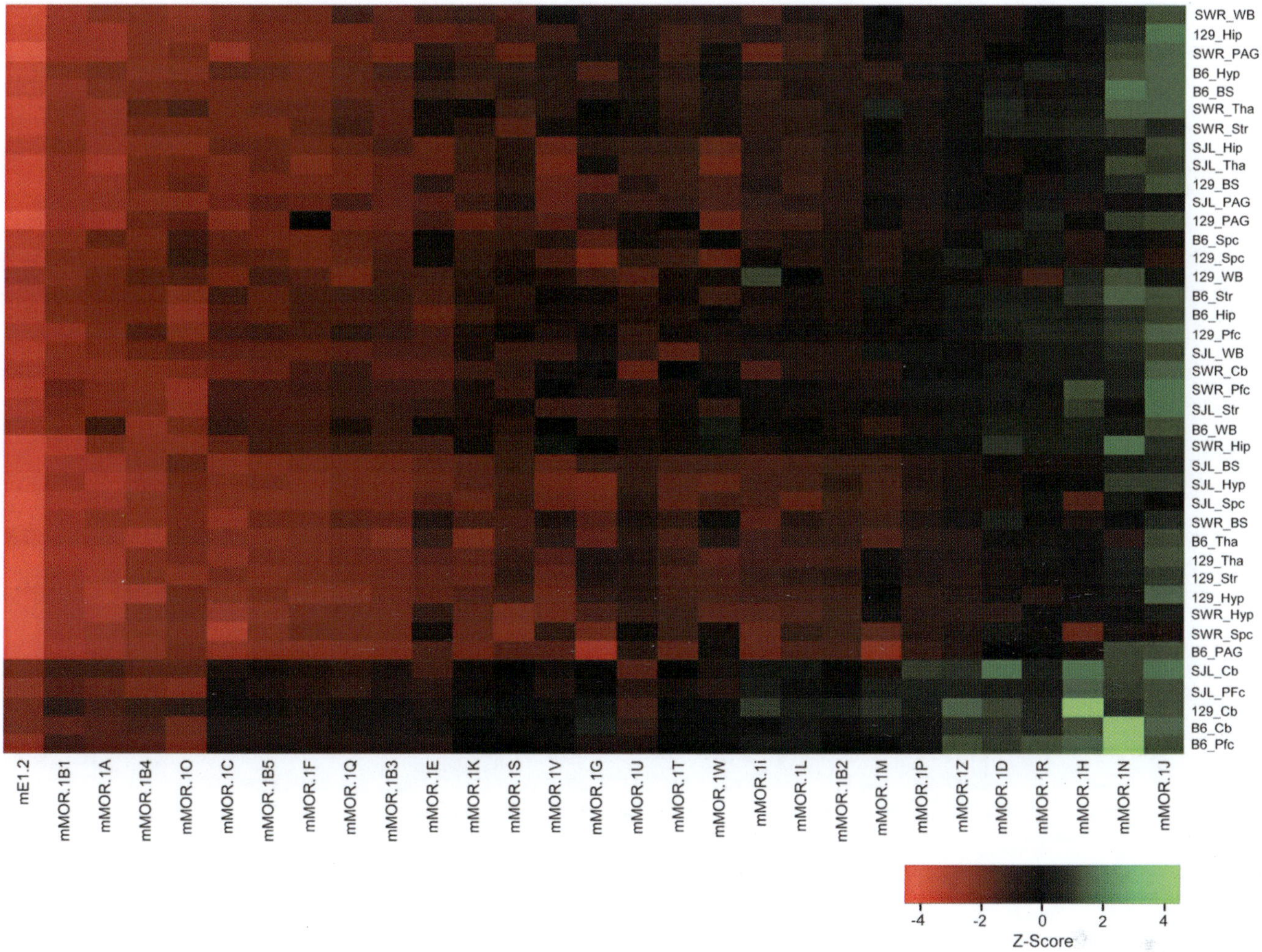

Figure 2. Heatmap of expression levels of *OPRM1* splice variant mRNAs. The heatmap was generated by clustering Z-scores calculated from the values (Log$_2$ ($E^{-\Delta C(t)}$) of individual variants across different strains/regions using R statistical language (2.15.0) (www.r-project.org), and plotting based upon expression levels among the variants with enhanced heatmap function heatmap.2 from gplots package. Pfc: prefrontal cortex; Str: striatum; Tha: thalamus; Hyp: hypothalamus; Hip: hippocampus; PAG: periaqueductal gray; BS: brainstem; Cb: cerebellum; Spc: spinal cord; WB: whole brain. 129:129P3/J; B6: C56BL/6J; SJL: SJL/J; SWR: SWR/J. Expression level was indicated by Z-score.

hypothalamus of 129 mice, the relative expression levels ranged from 0.1% for mMOR-1M to 22% for mMOR-1A, when their $E^{-\Delta C(t)}$ values were used to compare with those of mE1-2 designated as 100% (Fig. 3 & Table S2). The full length C-terminal splice variants mMOR-1A and mMOR-1B1 in 129 mice were highly expressed among most brain regions, corresponding to approximately 10–20% of mE1-2 levels in their $E^{-\Delta C(t)}$ values (Fig. 3 & Table S2). On the other hand, in 129 mice the levels of the truncated 6-TM variant mMOR-1G and mMOR-1M and single TM variants, mMOR-1S and mMOR-1T, and the full length mMOR-1D, ranged from about 0.1% to 5% of mE1-2 levels (Fig. 3 & Table S2). Similar expression patterns were observed in other mouse strains (Fig. 3 & Table S2).

Region-specific expressions of *OPRM1* splice variant mRNAs in four inbred mouse strains

Overall, expression levels in whole brain were not predictive of strain differences in specific regions. Within each strain, there are major differences in the regional expression of the variants. The heatmap segregating the different strains shows the overall differential expression pattern of all variants across the brain regions (Fig. 4). Plotting the expression level ($E^{-\Delta C(t)}$) for each variant among the regions illustrates the differences quantitatively and provides a visual pattern of regional expression (Figs. 5, S1 & S2). For example, the expression pattern of the full length variant mMOR-1A differed among the four strains. Its levels were high in the thalamus and PAG of B6 mice, with lower levels in the hippocampus and hypothalamus. In contrast, mMOR-1A expression in 129 mice was highest in the hypothalamus with similar high levels in the striatum, thalamus, hippocampus and PAG. In SWR mice mMOR-1A levels were highest in the hypothalamus with lowest levels in the hippocampus.

Within a strain, the regional expression patterns of some of the variants were similar. For example, mMOR-1A, mMOR-1B1, mMOR-1C, mMOR-1G, mMOR-1S and mMOR-1T expression in the B6 mice was highest in the PAG and thalamus (Fig. 5). A similar expression pattern in B6 mice was observed in other eleven variants including mMOR-1B2, mMOR-1B3, mMOR-1B5, mMOR-1F, mMOR-1i, mMOR-1K, mMOR-1L, mMOR-1M, mMOR-1P, mMOR-1Q and mMOR-1Z (Figs. S1 & S2).

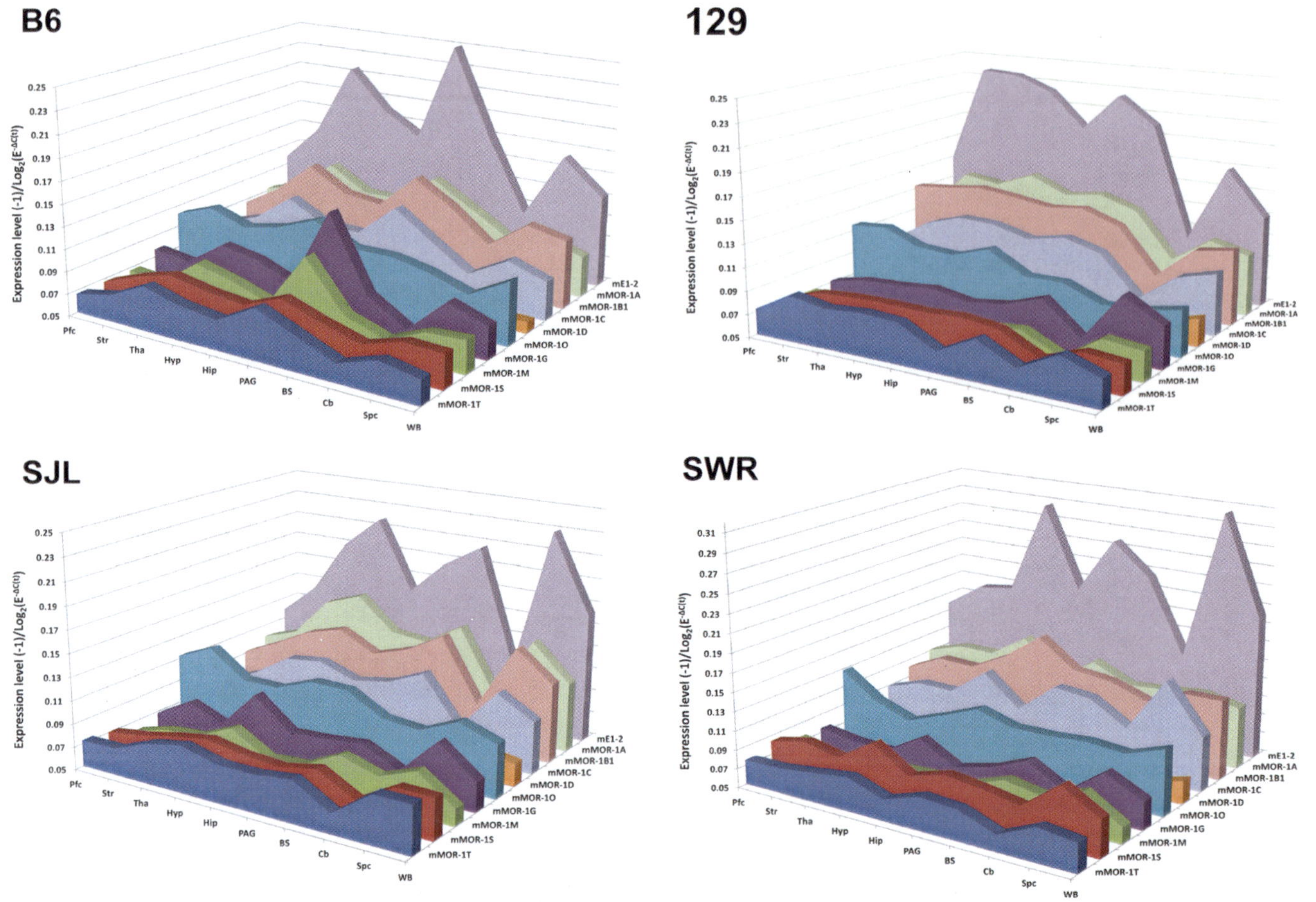

Figure 3. Expression levels of selected ten splice variants in brain regions of four mouse strains. Expression levels of $(-1)/(\text{Log}_2\,(E^{-\Delta C(t)}))$ of selected variants is plotted across regions using MS excel. Pfc: prefrontal cortex; Str: striatum; Tha: thalamus; Hyp: hypothalamus; Hip: hippocampus; PAG: periaqueductal gray; BS: brainstem; Cb: cerebellum; Spc: spinal cord; WB: whole brain. 129:129P3/J; B6: C56BL/6J; SJL: SJL/J; SWR: SWR/J.

However, other strains showed different patterns of variant expression among the regions. For example, in SJL mice, mMOR-1*O* expression was highest in the striatum with low levels in the brainstem while mMOR-1C expression levels in these same regions were opposite (Fig. 5).

In general, variant expression was low in the cerebellum and prefrontal cortex, consistent prior *in situ* hybridization studies with the full-length MOR-1 probe [47]. However, this was not uniformly the case. In SWR mice, mMOR-1U expression was greatest in the cerebellum (Fig. S2) while mMOR-1*O* was highest in the prefrontal cortex (Fig. 5).

Strain-specific expression of *OPRM1* splices variant mRNAs in selected brain regions

Segregating variant expression by individual regions provides another approach to visualize strain differences in different splice variants, and reveals interesting comparisons (Figs. 6, 7, S3 & S4). The heatmap shows broad differences in expression of individual variants among the strains in most brain regions (Fig. 6), as does quantitative graphing where the expression level ($E^{-\Delta C(t)}$) of each variant was plotted by strains within each region (Figs. 7, S3 & S4). Within a region on the heatmap, each column provides the relative expression of the different variants within the strain whereas the horizontal comparisons reveal interstrain differences for a specific variant.

Overall, the expression level of the variants varied among the mouse strains. For example, in the spinal cord, the expression of mMOR-1A in SJL mice was higher than the other strains (Fig. 7). However, in the striatum, 129 mice had the highest expression level. In the thalamus the 6-TM variant mMOR-1N expression was much higher in B6 mice than in other tree mouse strains, contrasting to its expression in the PAG where SJL levels were greater than other three strains (Fig. 7). The expression of the single TM variant mMOR-1S was higher in SWR mice in most brain regions including the spinal cord, hypothalamus, prefrontal cortex, striatum, PAG and brainstem. Although this single TM variant does not directly bind opioid receptors, it is pharmacologically relevant in that it stabilizes the full length mMOR-1 variant and significantly contributes to morphine analgesia [48].

Finally, the expression patterns of the variants within a brain region varied among the strains. For example, the spinal expression of mMOR-1C, mMOR-1i and mMOR-1S in SWR mice was far higher than other strains, while in SJL mice the expression of mMOR-1A, mMOR-1E and mMOR-1L predominated spinally (Figs. 7, S3 & S4). A similar scenario was observed in the PAG where the expressions of mMOR-1B2, mMOR-1G, mMOR-1M, mMOR-1P and mMOR-1T were much greater in

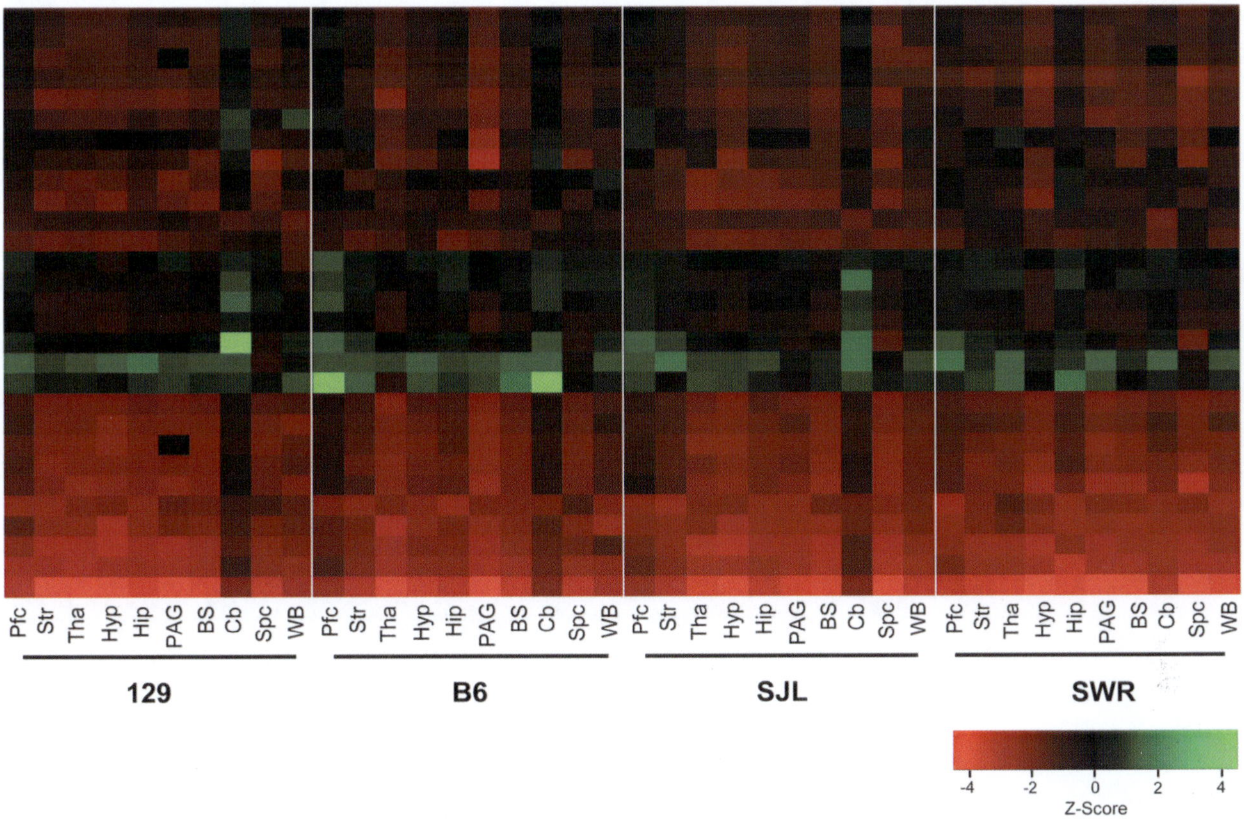

Figure 4. Heatmap of regional expression *OPRM1* splice variant mRNAs. The heatmap was generated by clustering Z-scores calculated from the values (Log$_2$ (E$^{-\Delta C(t)}$) of individual variants across different strains/regions using R statistical language (2.15.0) (www.r-project.org), and plotting based upon individual brain regions within each mouse strain with enhanced heatmap function heatmap.2 from gplots package. Pfc: prefrontal cortex; Str: striatum; Tha: thalamus; Hyp: hypothalamus; Hip: hippocampus; PAG: periaqueductal gray; BS: brainstem; Cb: cerebellum; Spc: spinal cord; WB: whole brain. 129:129P3/J; B6: C56BL/6J; SJL: SJL/J; SWR: SWR/J. Expression level was indicated by Z-score.

B6 mice than the other strains, whereas mMOR-1N had its highest expression in SJL mice (Figs. 7 & S4). In the striatum, mMOR-1A, mMOR-1B2, mMOR-1B3, mMOR-1B5, mMOR-1D, mMOR-1F, mMOR-1Q, mMOR-1T, mMOR-1V and mMOR-1Z were most highly expressed in 129 mice (Figs. 7, S3 & S4). However, mMOR-1N and mMOR-1S were predominately expressed in the striatum of SJL and SWR mice, respectively (Fig. 7). In the thalamus, mMOR-1B3, mMOR-1B4, mMOR-1K, mMOR-1N and mMOR-1R were most highly expressed in B6 mice, whereas the thalamus expression of mMOR-1V and mMOR-1W in SJL mice was much higher than other strains (Figs. 7, S3 & S4). Together, these results suggested strain-specific alternative splicing of the *OPRM1* gene.

Discussion

The identification of a vast array of splice variants of the μ opioid receptor gene has shown a complexity in opioid pharmacology far beyond what had previously been imagined. Autoradiography provided the earliest means of examining the anatomical distribution of μ binding sites [49–52]. The distribution of μ opioid receptors was then examined immunohistochemically and with in situ hybridation following the cloning of the receptor [53–63]. While these studies have provided valuable insights into opioid action, they all have limitations. Autoradiographic approaches are functional in the sense that they require active binding of ligand. Since the early studies utilized traditional μ radioligands, they detected all the full length 7-TM variants, but none of the truncated ones, and were not able to distinguish among the 7-TM variants. The early immunohistochemical studies targeted the C-terminus of MOR-1, with most using an epitope encoded by exon 4. These probes will detect the full length variants MOR-1, MOR-1H, MOR-1i and MOR-1J, as well as the 6-TM variant MOR-1G which all share the exon 4 epitope, but none of the other variants. Some studies have examined epitopes from alternatively spliced C-terminals, but they, too, may have labeled more than one species. For example, early studies examined the labeling of a 7/8/9 epitope, assuming it corresponded to mMOR-1C. Yet, subsequent cloning studies identified mMOR-1M, a truncated 6-TM variant that also contains the 7/8/9 epitope. The *in situ* hybridization studies using probes targeting exons 2 and 3 detected all the 7-TM and 6-TM splice variants, but not the single TM ones. Thus, each approach gives a unique set of labeling. Theoretically, qPCR offers the ability to identify an individual mRNA, but even PCR faces selectivity challenges due to both 3′ and 5′ splicing and extensive overlap in sequence among the variants.

We previously used traditional RT-PCR approaches to examine the expression of *OPRM1* splice variant mRNAs in brain regions [25–28]. However, these early approaches provided only an approximation of levels since they were not quantitative. Many of these studies also were carried out prior to the identification of additional variants with overlapping sequences. The present study using SYBR green qPCR overcomes these limitations and more

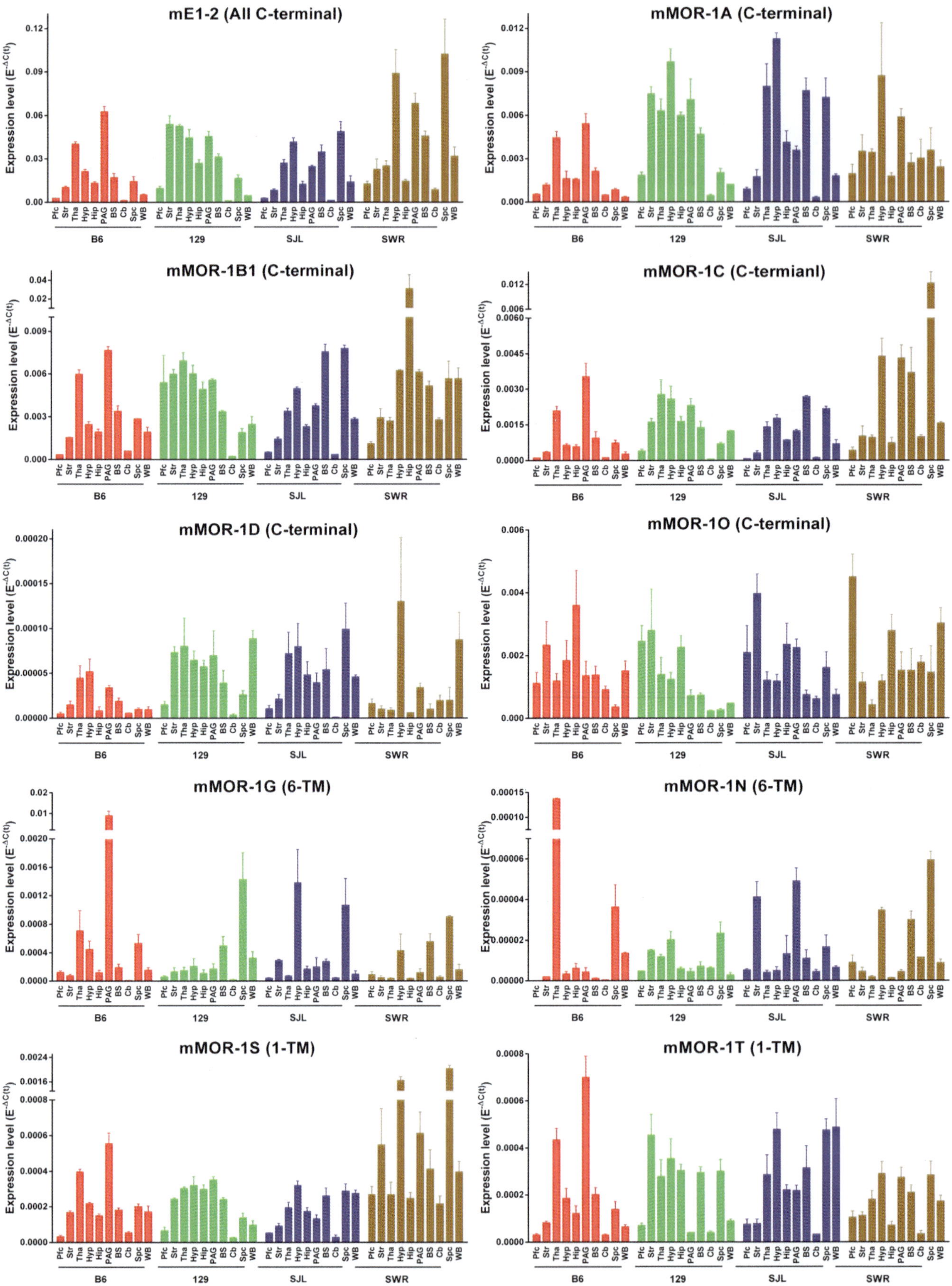
mE1-2 (All C-terminal)
mMOR-1A (C-terminal)
mMOR-1B1 (C-terminal)
mMOR-1C (C-termianl)
mMOR-1D (C-terminal)
mMOR-1O (C-terminal)
mMOR-1G (6-TM)
mMOR-1N (6-TM)
mMOR-1S (1-TM)
mMOR-1T (1-TM)
Expression level ($E^{-\Delta C(t)}$)
Pfc Str Tha Hyp Hip PAG BS Cb Spc WB
B6
129
SJL
SWR

Figure 5. Region-specific expressions of ten-selected *OPRM1* splice variants. Each panel represents the regional expression of one variant in four inbred mouse strains. Red bar: B6 mice; Green bar: 129 mice; Blue bar: SJL mice; Brown bar: SWR mice. Bars represent the mean of $E^{-\Delta C(t)}$ values ± S.E.M. Pfc: prefrontal cortex; Str: striatum; Tha: thalamus; Hyp: hypothalamus; Hip: hippocampus; PAG: periaqueductal gray; BS: brainstem; Cb: cerebellum; Spc: spinal cord; WB: whole brain. mE1-2 represents all full-length 7-TM variants. Significant difference was calculated by Two-way ANOVA with Tukey's multiple comparisons test for each variant (Prism 5.0). The results of the statistical analysis were listed in Table S3. The expression profiles of the other 19 *OPRM1* splice variants are shown in Figures S1 & S2.

precisely quantifies the expression of *OPRM1* splice variant mRNAs. Using these assays, we investigated the expression profiles of all *OPRM1* splice variant mRNAs in various brain regions of four inbred mouse strains, for the first time, a complete expression mRNA profile. However, even this approach does not address their expression at the protein level.

Although our current approach provides selectivity, dissecting tissues from a limited of brain regions does not provide anatomical resolution at the cellular level and provides only an incomplete assessment of variant expression. Future studies using single cell qPCR or more sophisticated *in situ* hybridization approaches may overcome these limitations. However, the current studies provide the first step toward our understanding of *OPRM1* splice variant expression in brain.

The abundance of the *OPRM1* splice variant mRNAs covers a wide range. These mRNA levels presumably reflect steady-state levels that depend upon many factors that may vary over time, including transcription, post-transcriptional modification and mRNA degradation. The *OPRM1* gene has two distinct promoters, exon 1 and exon 11 promoters. Most of the exon 1 promoter-controlled variants involve 3′ splicing, yielding unique C-terminal sequences, and are quite abundant. They include mMOR-1A, mMOR-1B1, mMOR-1C, mMOR-1*O* and mMOR-1V. In contrast, the exon 11 promoter-controlled variants generate 6-TM variants and are expressed at lower levels. While the promoters may influence mRNA expression, they cannot explain all the differences. Within each promoter group, mRNA levels vary, as shown by the far lower levels of mMOR-1B2 and mMOR-1P levels than those of mMOR-1A, mMOR-1B1 and mMOR-1C in the PAG, hypothalamus and hippocampus of B6 mice and the differences in the exon 11 promoter-controlled 6-TM variants mMOR-1G, mMOR-1K and mMOR-1N.

mRNA stability also may impact expression levels. Of particular interest is nonsense-mediated decay (NMD) that targets an mRNA containing a premature stop codon located more than 50 nt upstream of the last exon-exon junction [64,65]. Eight variants, including mMOR-1E, mMOR-1F, mMOR-1Q, mMOR-1R, mMOR-1T, mMOR-1V, mMOR-1W, and mMOR-1Z, are

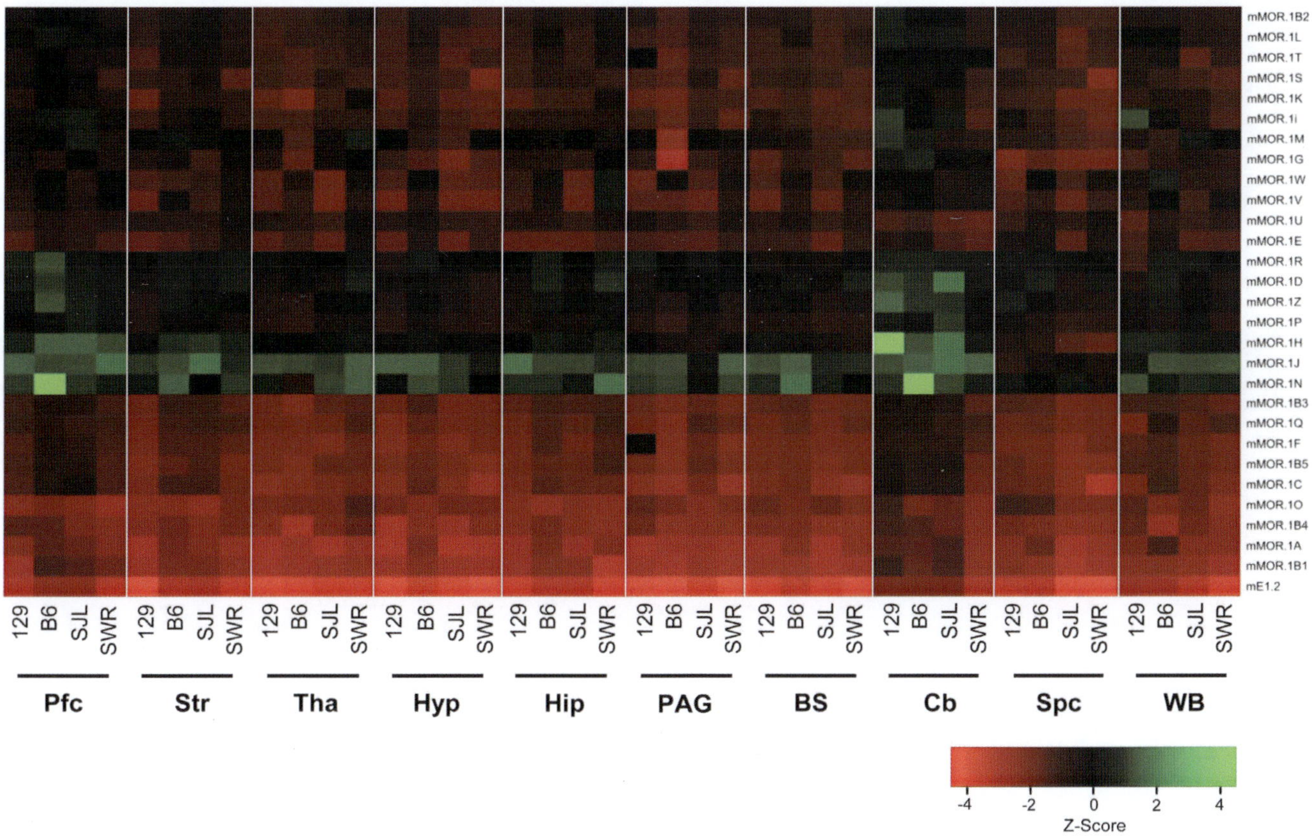

Figure 6. Heatmap of expression of *OPRM1* splice variant mRNAs among four inbred mouse strains. The heatmap was generated by clustering Z-scores calculated from the values (Log_2 ($E^{-\Delta C(t)}$) of individual variants across different strains/regions using R statistical language (2.15.0) (www.r-project.org), and plotting based upon individual strains within each brain region with enhanced heatmap function heatmap.2 from gplots package. Pfc: prefrontal cortex; Str: striatum; Tha: thalamus; Hyp: hypothalamus; Hip: hippocampus; PAG: periaqueductal gray; BS: brainstem; Cb: cerebellum; Spc: spinal cord; WB: whole brain. 129:129P3/J; B6: C56BL/6J; SJL: SJL/J; SWR: SWR/J. Expression level was indicated by Z-score.

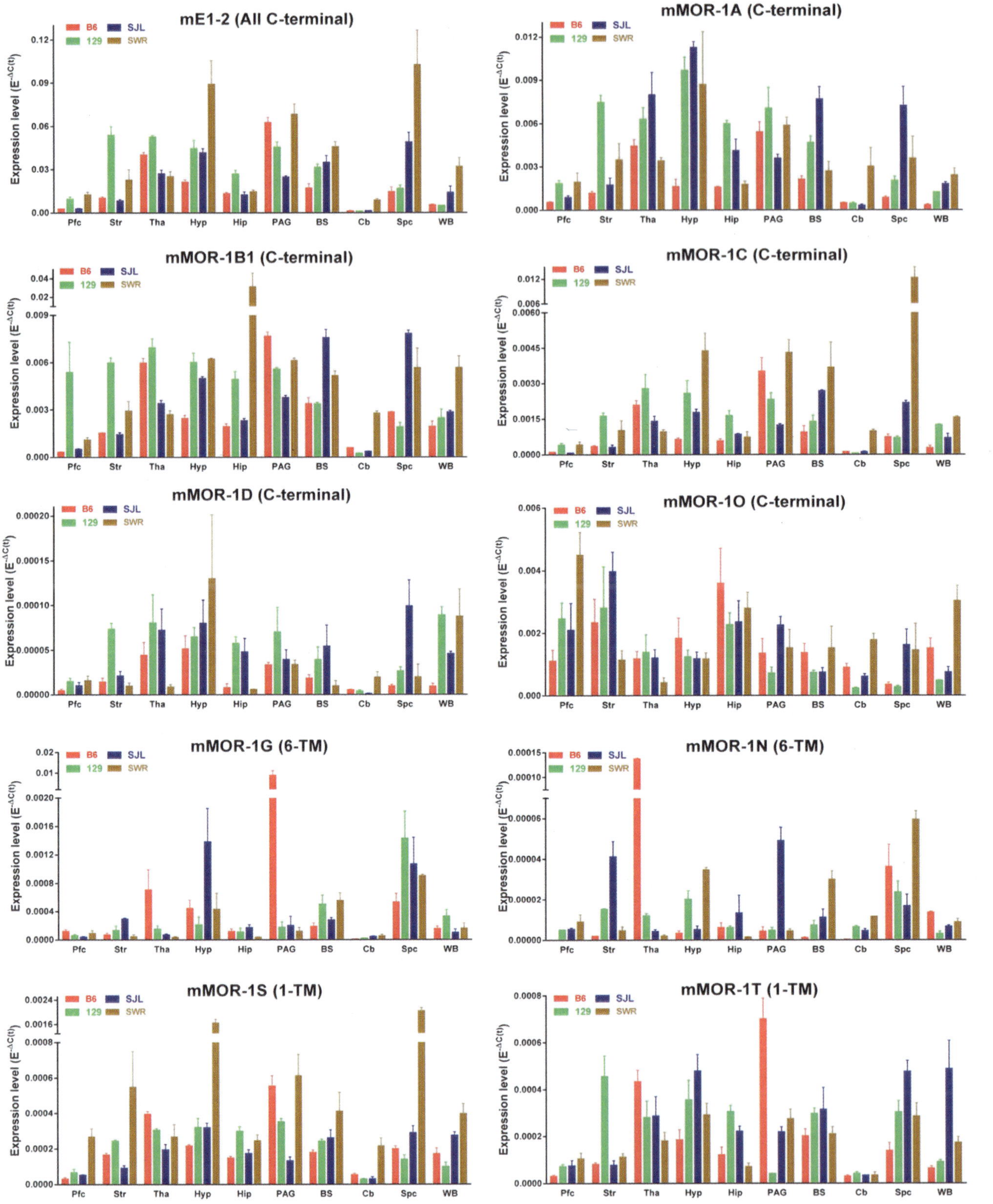

Figure 7. Strain-specific expressions of *OPRM1* splice variants. Each panel represents the expression of one variant in 10 regions of 4 inbred mouse strains. Red bar: B6 mice; Green bar: 129 mice; Blue bar: SJL mice; Brown bar: SWR mice. Bars represent the mean of $E^{-\Delta C(t)}$ values ± S.E.M. Pfc: prefrontal cortex; Str: striatum; Tha: thalamus; Hyp: hypothalamus; Hip: hippocampus; PAG: periaqueductal gray; BS: brainstem; Cb: cerebellum; Spc: spinal cord; WB: whole brain. Significant difference was calculated by Two-way ANOVA with Tukey's multiple comparisons test for each variant. The results of the statistical analysis were listed in Table S3. The expression profiles of the other 19 *OPRM1* splice variants are shown in Figures S3 & S4.

potential targets of NMD. However, the variability of expression among these variants implies that NMD is not solely one factor among many influencing expression levels.

mRNA levels may not correlate with either their corresponding protein expression or with their pharmacological importance. For example, immunostaining by an exon 7/8/9-specific antisera that label mMOR-1C and mMOR-1M was as robust as that seen with the exon 4-specific antisera labeling mMOR-1, mMOR-1H, mMOR-1i and mMOR-1J despite great differences in their respective mRNA levels [23,24]. The lack of correlation between mRNA and protein levels also may involve many factors. The association of the different mRNAs with polyribosomes can vary widely (Z. Lu, J. Xu, G.W. Pasternak, and Y.X. Pan, unpublished data), suggesting the differential regulation of the variants at the translational level. Other evidence indicates that the stability of the variants at the protein level is dependent upon a range of factors. For example, internalization and recycling of the receptors varies among the variants [31] and co-expression of single TM splice variants stabilizes MOR-1 protein levels, decreasing its degradation, extending its half-lives and thereby increasing its overall levels [48]. Therefore, it will be important to develop a reliable and an accurate method for determining protein expression of these OPRM1 splice variants in the future.

mRNA levels do not necessarily correlate with pharmacological relevance. For example, mMOR-1D has been implicated in morphine-induced itch through its dimerization with gastrin-releasing peptide receptor (GRPR) [66] despite its low mRNA levels. Exon 11-associated 6-TM variants are also among the low abundant transcripts. Yet, an exon 11 knockout mouse model indicates a key role of these 6-TM variants in the analgesic actions of a range of opioids, including heroin, morphine-6β-glucuronide, fentanyl, levorphanol and buprenorphine [33,34]. These 6-TM variants also are critical in the actions of a novel class of opioid analgesic exemplified by 3′-iodobenzoyl-6β-naltexamide (IBNtxA), which is interesting since IBNtxA produces potent analgesia without many traditional opioid side-effects such as respiratory depression, physical dependence and reward behavior [34]. The importance of 6-TM variants is further supported by recent studies showing the rescue of IBNtxA analgesia in knockout mice lacking 6-TM variants that are insensitive to IBNtxA by the lentiviral-mediated delivery of a 6-TM variant, mMOR-1G (Z. Lu, J. Xu, G. Rossi, G.W. Pasternak, and Y.X. Pan, unpublished observations).

Our data also demonstrate variability in the expression of *OPRM1* splice variants in different strains. The importance of genetic backgrounds in opioid pharmacology is becoming increasingly appreciated. The four strains chosen for evaluation differ in their sensitivity to morphine analgesia, with AD_{50} values ranging from 6.8 mg/kg in C57BL/6 and 7.2 mg/kg in SJL to 13.7 mg/kg in 129P3 and 18.7 mg/kg in SWR mice [36]. They also differ in the development of tolerance to chronic morphine dosing of over three days, with analgesic shifts of 0.8 in the 129P3 mice to 2.2 in the SJL mice, 5 in SWR mice and 7.2 in the C56BL/6 mice [36]. Dependence, measured by jumping following naloxone precipitated withdrawal, also varies with the 129P3 and SJL mice showing virtually no jumping with moderate levels of jumping in the C57BL/6 mice and the most in the SWR mice [35]. Although four strains is a very limited sample, it is interesting that linear regression analysis correlating mRNA expression levels with 1) morphine analgesia using half-maximal analgesic doses (AD_{50}), 2) morphine tolerance using the shift in AD_{50} fold with chronic dosing over three days or [36] or 3) physical dependence determined by jump scores from naloxone-precipitated withdrawal [35] revealed strong correlations for some of the variants ($r^2>0.90$; Fig. S5), raising questions regarding the functional relevance of the variants in these brain regions. While intriguing, these correlations must be interpreted cautiously and require additional studies. Recently, we observed that long-term morphine treatment in CD-1 mice markedly upregulates a number of OPRM1 splice variants in various brain regions, as determined by the qPCR assays described here (J. Xu, A.J. Faskowitz, G.C. Rossi, M. Xu, Z. Lu, Y.-X Pan and G.W. Pasternak, submitted). Considering the variability in mRNA expression among the current strains of mice, it will be interesting to compare morphine effects on the expression of OPRM1 splice variants in these inbred mice.

Why the pattern of the variant expression in these four inbred mouse strains containing the same single-copy *OPRM1* gene varies is not clear. Presumably, the strains differ in their modulation of the promoters and alternative splicing machinery. These may reflect genetic variations, such as single nucleotide polymorphisms (SNPs), deletions, insertions and transposon elements. Recently, we identified a heroin addiction severity-associated intronic SNP that modulates alternative splicing of the human *OPRM1* variants via hnRNPH interaction [67]. Further identifying the genetic variations that modulate the strain-specific *OPRM1* alternative splicing will greatly advance our knowledge not only on the *OPRM1* alternative splicing, but also on alternative splicing in general.

Supporting Information

Figure S1 Expression levels of additional ten *OPRM1* splice variants in brain regions of B6, SJL and SWR mice. Each panel represents the regional expressions of one variant in four inbred mouse strains. Red bar: B6 mice; Green bar: 129 mice; Blue bar: SJL mice; Brown bar: SWR mice. Bars represent the mean of $E^{-\Delta C(t)}$ values ± S.E.M. Pfc: prefrontal cortex; Str: striatum; Tha: thalamus; Hyp: hypothalamus; Hip: hippocampus; PAG: periaqueductal gray; BS: brainstem; Cb: cerebellum; Spc: spinal cord; WB: whole brain. Significant difference was calculated by Two-way ANOVA with Tukey's multiple comparisons test for each variant. The results of the statistical analysis were listed in Table S3.

Figure S2 Expression levels of additional nine *OPRM1* splice variants in brain regions of B6, SJL and SWR mice. Each panel represents the regional expressions of one variant in four inbred mouse strains. Red bar: B6 mice; Green bar: 129 mice; Blue bar: SJL mice; Brown bar: SWR mice. Bars represent the mean of $E^{-\Delta C(t)}$ values ± S.E.M. Pfc: prefrontal cortex; Str: striatum; Tha: thalamus; Hyp: hypothalamus; Hip: hippocampus; PAG: periaqueductal gray; BS: brainstem; Cb: cerebellum; Spc: spinal cord; WB: whole brain. Significant difference was calculated by Two-way ANOVA with Tukey's multiple comparisons test for each variant. The results of the statistical analysis were listed in Table S3.

Figure S3 Strain-specific expressions of additional ten *OPRM1* splice variants. Each panel represents the expression of one variant among four mouse strains in ten brain regions. Red bar: B6 mice; Green bar: 129 mice; Blue bar: SJL mice; Brown bar: SWR mice. Bars represent the mean of $E^{-\Delta C(t)}$ values ± S.E.M. Pfc: prefrontal cortex; Str: striatum; Tha: thalamus; Hyp: hypothalamus; Hip: hippocampus; PAG: periaqueductal gray; BS: brainstem; Cb: cerebellum; Spc: spinal cord; WB: whole brain. mE1-2 represents all full-length 7TM variants. Significant difference was calculated by Two-way ANOVA with Tukey's multiple comparison for each variant. The results of the statistical analysis were listed in Table S3.

Figure S4 Strain-specific expressions of additional nine *OPRM1* splice variants. Each panel represents the expression of one variant among four mouse strains in ten brain regions. Red bar: B6 mice; Green bar: 129 mice; Blue bar: SJL mice; Brown bar: SWR mice. Bars represent the mean of $E^{-\Delta C(t)}$ values ± S.E.M. Pfc: prefrontal cortex; Str: striatum; Tha: thalamus; Hyp: hypothalamus; Hip: hippocampus; PAG: periaqueductal gray; BS: brainstem; Cb: cerebellum; Spc: spinal cord; WB: whole brain. Significant difference was calculated by Two-way ANOVA with Tukey's multiple comparison for each variant. The results of the statistical analysis were listed in Table S3.

Figure S5 Correlation of the expression levels of *OPRM1* splice variant mRNAs with morphine-induced analgesia, tolerance and physical dependence in four inbred mouse strains. A & B: Correlation of the expression levels of *OPRM1* splice variant mRNAs with morphine analgesia in four inbred mouse strains. The square of the correlation coefficient (r^2) listed was obtained from linear regression analysis (Prizm 5.0) between expression level ($E^{-\Delta C(t)} * 10^4$) values (mean ± S.E.M.) for each variant in the indicated brain region and morphine analgesia potency (log (AD_{50})). The AD_{50} (mg/kg) values in B6, SJL, 129 and SWR mice were 6.8, 7.2, 13.7 and 18.7, respectively [36]. C & D: Correlation of the expression levels of *OPRM1* splice variant mRNAs with morphine tolerance in four inbred mouse strains. The square of the correlation coefficient (r^2) listed was obtained from linear regression analysis (Prizm 5.0) between expression level ($E^{-\Delta C(t)} * 10^4$) values (mean ± S.E.M.) for each variant in the indicated brain region and morphine AD_{50} shift before and after chronic morphine treatment (log (Morphine AD_{50} shift)). The AD_{50} shift values in 129, SJL, SWR and B6 mice were 0.8, 2.2, 5 and 7.2, respectively [36]. E & F: Correlation of the expression levels of *OPRM1* splice variant mRNAs with morphine-induced physical dependence in four inbred mouse strains. The square of the correlation coefficient (r^2) listed was obtained from linear regression analysis (Prizm 5.0) between expression level ($E^{-\Delta C(t)} * 10^4$) values (mean ± S.E.M.) for each variant in the indicated brain region and jumping scores after chronic morphine treatment followed by naloxone precipitated withdrawal (log (Jumps/15 min)). The jumping scores in 129, SJL, B6 and SWR mice were 7, 16, 60 and 200, respectively [35]. All the variants listed have an r^2 value over 0.90. A positive slope indicates that the more expression of the variants, the more AD_{50} values (the less potent) or the more AD_{50} value shifts (the more tolerant) or the more jumps (the more dependent) are. A negative slope shows opposite relationships. Pfc: prefrontal cortex; Str: striatum; Hyp: hypothalamus; Hip: hippocampus; PAG: periaqueductal gray; BS: brainstem; Spc: spinal cord; WB: whole brain.

Table S1 SYBR green qPCR assay. SYBR green qPCR assay for each variant was established as described in Materials and Methods. Optimized conditions including primers and their locations, thermal cycle condition, amplicon size and efficiency are listed. SP: sense primer; AP: antisense primer.

Table S2 Expression levels of OPRM1 splice variants. Normalized expression level for each variant was calculated as $E^{-\Delta C(t)}$, where E is efficiency listed in Table S1, as described in Materials and Methods. The mean of $E^{-\Delta C(t)}$ values ± S.E.M. is listed.

Table S3 Two-Way ANOVA analysis. Two-Way ANONVA analysis with Tukey's multiple comparisons test was performed as described in Materials and Methods. Pfc: prefrontal cortex; Str: striatum; Tha: thalamus; Hyp: hypothalamus; Hip: hippocampus; PAG: periaqueductal gray; BS: brainstem; Cb: cerebellum; Spc: spinal cord; WB: whole brain. For each variant, left tables are regional comparisons in each inbred mouse strain, and right tables, strain comparisons in each brain region. *p* values listed in tables are: *: $p<0.05$; **: $p<0.01$; ***: $p<0.001$; ****: $p<0.0001$.

Author Contributions

Conceived and designed the experiments: JX BK GWP YXP. Performed the experiments: JX ZL MX GCR BK ARW YXP. Analyzed the data: JX ZL BK ARW GWP YXP. Contributed reagents/materials/analysis tools: JX ZL GWP YXP. Contributed to the writing of the manuscript: JX GCR BK GWP YXP.

References

1. Pasternak GW (1993) Pharmacological mechanisms of opioid analgesics. Clin Neuropharmacol 16: 1–18.
2. Foley KM (1985) Management of Cancer Pain. In: DeVita VT, Hellman S, Rosenberg SA, editors. Cancer: Principles and Practice of Oncology. New York: Lippincott. 1940–1961.
3. Payne R, Pasternak GW (1992) Pain. In: Johnston MV, Macdonald RL, Young AB, editors. Principles of drug therapy in neurology. Philadelphia: F.A. Davis. 268–301.
4. Portenoy RK (1996) Opioid Analgesics. In: Portenoy RK, Kanner RM, editors. Pain management: Theory and practice. Philadelphia: F.A. Davis. 248–276.
5. Ling GSF, MacLeod JM, Lee S, Lockhart SH, Pasternak GW (1984) Separation of morphine analgesia from physical dependence. Science 226: 462–464.
6. Ling GSF, Spiegel K, Lockhart SH, Pasternak GW (1985) Separation of opioid analgesia from respiratory depression: evidence for different receptor mechanisms. J Pharmacol Exp Ther 232: 149–155.
7. Moulin DE, Ling GSF, Pasternak GW (1988) Unidirectional analgesic cross tolerance between morphine and levorphanol in the rat. Pain 33: 233–239.
8. Chang A, Emmel DW, Rossi GC, Pasternak GW (1998) Methadone analgesia in morphine-insensitive CXBK mice. Eur J Pharmacol 351: 189–191.
9. Pasternak GW (2004) Multiple opiate receptors: deja vu all over again. Neuropharmacology 47 Suppl 1: 312–323.
10. Leipzig J, Pevzner P, Heber S (2004) The Alternative Splicing Gallery (ASG): bridging the gap between genome and transcriptome. Nucleic Acids Res 32: 3977–3983.
11. Rossi GC, Pan YX, Brown GP, Pasternak GW (1995) Antisense Mapping the Mor-1 Opioid Receptor - Evidence for Alternative Splicing and A Novel Morphine-6-Beta-Glucuronide Receptor. FEBS Lett 369: 192–196.
12. Rossi GC, Leventhal L, Pan YX, Cole J, Su W, et al. (1997) Antisense mapping of MOR-1 in the rat: Distinguishing between morphine and morphine-6b-glucuronide antinociception. J Pharmacol Exp Ther 281: 109–114.
13. Chen Y, Mestek A, Liu J, Hurley JA, Yu L (1993) Molecular cloning and functional expression of a m-opioid receptor from rat brain. Mol Pharmacol 44: 8–12.
14. Wang JB, Imai Y, Eppler CM, Gregor P, Spivak CE, et al. (1993) m opiate receptor: cDNA cloning and expression. Proc Natl Acad Sci USA 90: 10230–10234.
15. Thompson RC, Mansour A, Akil H, Watson SJ (1993) Cloning and pharmacological characterization of a rat m opioid receptor. Neuron 11: 903–913.
16. Pan YX (2005) Diversity and complexity of the mu opioid receptor gene: alternative pre-mRNA splicing and promoters. DNA Cell Biol 24: 736–750.
17. Pan Y-X, Pasternak GW (2010) Molecular Biology of Mu Opioid Receptors. In: Pasternak GW, editors. Opiate. Humana Press. 121–160.
18. Kozak CA, Filie J, Adamson MC, Chen Y, Yu L (1994) Murine chromosomal location of the m and kappa opioid receptor genes. Genomics 21: 659–661.
19. Giros B, Pohl M, Rochelle JM, Seldin MF (1995) Chromosomal localization of opioid peptide and receptor genes in the mouse. Life Sci 56: PL369–PL375.
20. Belknap JK, Mogil JS, Helms ML, Richards SP, O'Toole LA, et al. (1995) Localization to chromosome 10 of a locus influencing morphine analgesia in crosses derived from C57BL/6 and DBA/2 strains. Life Sci 57: L117–L124.

21. Wang JB, Johnson PS, Persico AM, Hawkins AL, Griffin CA, et al. (1994) Human m opiate receptor: cDNA and genomic clones, pharmacologic characterization and chromosomal assignment. FEBS Lett 338: 217–222.
22. Pasternak GW, Pan YX (2013) Mu opioids and their receptors: evolution of a concept. Pharmacol Rev 65: 1257–1317. 65/4/1257 [pii];10.1124/pr.112.007138 [doi].
23. Abbadie C, Pan YX, Pasternak GW (2000) Differential distribution in rat brain of mu opioid receptor carboxy terminal splice variants MOR-1C-like and MOR-1-like immunoreactivity: Evidence for region-specific processing. J Comp Neurol 419: 244–256.
24. Abbadie C, Pan YX, Drake CT, Pasternak GW (2000) Comparative immunohistochemical distributions of carboxy terminus epitopes from the mu-opioid receptor splice variants MOR-1D, MOR-1 and MOR-1C in the mouse and rat CNS. Neuroscience 100: 141–153.
25. Pan YX, Xu J, Bolan EA, Abbadie C, Chang A, et al. (1999) Identification and characterization of three new alternatively spliced mu opioid receptor isoforms. Mol Pharmacol 56: 396–403.
26. Pan YX, Xu J, Bolan E, Chang A, Mahurter L, et al. (2000) Isolation and expression of a novel alternatively spliced mu opioid receptor isoform, MOR-1F. FEBS Lett 466: 337–340.
27. Pan YX, Xu A, Mahurter L, Bolan E, Xu MM, et al. (2001) Generation of the mu opioid receptor (MOR-1) protein by three new splice variants of the Oprm gene. Proc Natl Acad Sci USA 98: 14084–14089.
28. Pan L, Xu J, Yu R, Xu MM, Pan YX, et al. (2005) Identification and characterization of six new alternatively spliced variants of the human mu opioid receptor gene, Oprm. Neuroscience 133: 209–220.
29. Koch T, Schulz S, Schroder H, Wolf R, Raulf E, et al. (1998) Carboxyl-terminal splicing of the rat mu opioid receptor modulates agonist-mediated internalization and receptor resensitization. J Biol Chem 273: 13652–13657.
30. Abbadie C, Pasternak GW (2001) Differential in vivo internalization of MOR-1 and MOR-1C by morphine. Neuroreport 12: 3069–3072.
31. Tanowitz M, Hislop JN, von ZM (2008) Alternative splicing determines the post-endocytic sorting fate of G-protein-coupled receptors. J Biol Chem 283: 35614–35621.
32. Bolan EA, Pasternak GW, Pan Y-X (2004) Functional analysis of MOR-1 splice variants of the mu opioid receptor gene, *Oprm*. Synapse 51: 11–18.
33. Pan YX, Xu J, Xu M, Rossi GC, Matulonis JE, et al. (2009) Involvement of exon 11-associated variants of the mu opioid receptor MOR-1 in heroin, but not morphine, actions. Proc Natl Acad Sci U S A 106: 4917–4922. 0811586106 [pii];10.1073/pnas.0811586106 [doi].
34. Majumdar S, Grinnell S, Le RV, Burgman M, Polikar L, et al. (2011) Truncated G protein-coupled mu opioid receptor MOR-1 splice variants are targets for highly potent opioid analgesics lacking side effects. Proc Natl Acad Sci U S A 108: 19778–19783. 1115231108 [pii];10.1073/pnas.1115231108 [doi].
35. Kest B, Palmese CA, Hopkins E, Adler M, Juni A, et al. (2002) Naloxone-precipitated withdrawal jumping in 11 inbred mouse strains: evidence for common genetic mechanisms in acute and chronic morphine physical dependence. Neuroscience 115: 463–469.
36. Kest B, Hopkins E, Palmese CA, Adler M, Mogil JS (2002) Genetic variation in morphine analgesic tolerance: a survey of 11 inbred mouse strains. Pharmacol Biochem Behav 73: 821–828.
37. Klein G, Juni A, Waxman AR, Arout CA, Inturrisi CE, et al. (2008) A survey of acute and chronic heroin dependence in ten inbred mouse strains: evidence of genetic correlation with morphine dependence. Pharmacol Biochem Behav 90: 447–452.
38. Metten P, Crabbe JC, Belknap JK (2009) Genetic correlates of morphine withdrawal in 14 inbred mouse strains. Drug Alcohol Depend 99: 123–131.
39. Schlussman SD, Zhang Y, Hsu NM, Allen JM, Ho A, et al. (2008) Heroin-induced locomotor activity and conditioned place preference in C57BL/6J and 129P3/J mice. Neurosci Lett 440: 284–288.
40. Belknap JK, Riggan J, Cross S, Young ER, Gallaher EJ, et al. (1998) Genetic determinants of morphine activity and thermal responses in 15 inbred mouse strains. Pharmacol Biochem Behav 59: 353–360. S0091-3057(97)00421-8 [pii].
41. Kolesnikov Y, Jain S, Wilson R, Pasternak GW (1998) Lack of morphine and enkephalin tolerance in 129/SvEv mice: evidence for a NMDA receptor defect. J Pharmacol Exp Ther 284: 455–459.
42. Xu J, Xu M, Rossi GC, Kest B, Pasternak GW, Pan Y-X (2009) Differential expression of alternatively spliced variant mRNAs from the mu opioid receptor (OPRM1) gene in brain regions of four inbred mouse strains. Soc Neurosci 232.1/D14.
43. Paxinos G, Franklin K (2000) Mouse brain in stereotaxic coordinates. 2d.
44. Pfaffl MW (2001) A new mathematical model for relative quantification in real-time RT-PCR. Nucleic Acids Res 29: e45.
45. Vandesompele J, De PK, Pattyn F, Poppe B, Van RN, et al. (2002) Accurate normalization of real-time quantitative RT-PCR data by geometric averaging of multiple internal control genes. Genome Biol 3: RESEARCH0034.
46. Pfaffl MW, Tichopad A, Prgomet C, Neuvians TP (2004) Determination of stable housekeeping genes, differentially regulated target genes and sample integrity: BestKeeper–Excel-based tool using pair-wise correlations. Biotechnol Lett 26: 509–515.
47. Kaufman DL, Keith DE Jr, Anton B, Tian J, Magendzo K, et al. (1995) Characterization of the murine m opioid receptor gene. J Biol Chem 270: 15877–15883.
48. Xu J, Xu M, Brown T, Rossi GC, Hurd YL, et al. (2013) Stabilization of the mu opioid receptor by truncated single transmembrane splice variants through a chaperone-like action. JBC 288: 21211–21227.
49. Atweh SF, Kuhar MJ (1983) Distribution and physiological significance of opioid receptors in the brain. British Medical Bulletin 39: 47–52.
50. Atweh SF, Kuhar MJ (1977) Autoradiographic localization of opiate receptors in rat brain. III. The telencephalon. Brain Res 134: 393–405.
51. Atweh SF, Kuhar MJ (1977) Autoradiographic localization of opiate receptors in rat brain. I. Spinal cord and lower medulla. Brain Res 124: 53–67.
52. Atweh SF, Kuhar MJ (1977) Autoradiographic localization of opiate receptors in rat brain. II. The brain stem. Brain Res 129: 1–12.
53. Mansour A, Khachaturian H, Lewis ME, Akil H, Watson SJ (1987) Autoradiographic differentiation of mu, delta, and kappa opioid receptors in the rat forebrain and midbrain. J Neurosci 7: 2445–2464.
54. Mansour A, Fox CA, Burke S, Akil H, Watson SJ (1995) Immunohistochemical localization of the cloned m opioid receptor in the rat CNS. J Chem Neuroanat 8: 283–305.
55. Mansour A, Fox CA, Burke S, Watson SJ (1994) Immunohistochemical localization of the mu opioid receptors. Regul Pept 54: 179–180.
56. Mansour A, Fox CA, Burke S, Meng F, Thompson RC, et al. (1994) Mu, delta, and kappa opioid receptor mRNA expression in the rat CNS: An in situ hybridization study. J Comp Neurol 350: 412–438.
57. Mansour A, Fox CA, Akil H, Watson SJ (1995) Opioid-receptor mRNA expression in the rat CNS: Anatomical and functional implications. Trends Neurosci 18: 22–29.
58. Mansour A, Fox CA, Thompson RC, Akil H, Watson SJ (1994) m-Opioid receptor mRNA expression in the rat CNS: comparison to m-receptor binding. Brain Res 643: 245–265.
59. Arvidsson U, Riedl M, Chakrabarti S, Lee J-H, Nakano AH, et al. (1995) Distribution and targeting of a m-opioid receptor (MOR1) in brain and spinal cord. J Neurosci 15: 3328–3341.
60. Honda CN, Arvidsson U (1995) Immunohistochemical localization of delta- and mu-opioid receptors in primate spinal cord. Neuroreport 6: 1025–1028.
61. Ding YQ, Kaneko T, Nomura S, Mizuno N (1996) Immunohistochemical localization of m-opioid receptors in the central nervous system of the rat. J Comp Neurol 367: 375–402.
62. Moriwaki A, Wang JB, Svingos A, Van Bockstaele E, Cheng P, et al. (1996) m Opiate receptor immunoreactivity in rat central nervous system. Neurochem Res 21: 1315–1331.
63. Wang H, Moriwaki A, Wang JB, Uhl GR, Pickel VM (1997) Ultrastructural immunocytochemical localization of mu-opioid receptors in dendritic targets of dopaminergic terminals in the rat caudate- putamen nucleus. Neuroscience 81: 757–771.
64. Lejeune F, Maquat LE (2005) Mechanistic links between nonsense-mediated mRNA decay and pre-mRNA splicing in mammalian cells. Current Opinion in Cell Biology 17: 309–315.
65. Chang YF, Imam JS, Wilkinson MF (2007) The nonsense-mediated decay RNA surveillance pathway. Annu Rev Biochem 76: 51–74. 10.1146/annurev.biochem.76.050106.093909 [doi].
66. Liu XY, Liu ZC, Sun YG, Ross M, Kim S, et al. (2011) Unidirectional cross-activation of GRPR by MOR1D uncouples itch and analgesia induced by opioids. Cell 147: 447–458. S0092-8674(11)01064-6 [pii];10.1016/j.cell.2011.08.043 [doi].
67. Xu J, Lu Z, Xu M, Pan L, Deng Y, et al. (2014) A Heroin Addiction Severity-Associated Intronic Single Nucleotide Polymorphism Modulates Alternative Pre-mRNA Splicing of the mu Opioid Receptor Gene OPRM1 via hnRNPH Interactions. J Neurosci 34: 11048–11066. 34/33/11048 [pii];10.1523/JNEUROSCI.3986-13.2014 [doi].

6

Assessing and Responding to Palliative Care Needs in Rural Sub-Saharan Africa: Results from a Model Intervention and Situation Analysis in Malawi

Michael E. Herce[1,2,3*❡], Shekinah N. Elmore[4❡], Noel Kalanga[2,3], James W. Keck[2,3¤a], Emily B. Wroe[2,3,5], Atupere Phiri[2,3], Alishya Mayfield[5], Felix Chingoli[6], Jason A. Beste[2,3¤b], Listern Tengatenga[6], Junior Bazile[2,3], Eric L. Krakauer[3,4,7¶], Jonas Rigodon[2,3¤c¶]

1 Department of Medicine, Division of Infectious Diseases, University of North Carolina School of Medicine, Chapel Hill, North Carolina, United States of America, **2** Abwenzi Pa Za Umoyo, Neno, Malawi, **3** Partners in Health, Boston, Massachusetts, United States of America, **4** Department of Global Health and Social Medicine, Harvard Medical School, Boston, Massachusetts, United States of America, **5** Department of Medicine, Brigham and Women's Hospital, Boston, Massachusetts, United States of America, **6** Neno District Health Office, Neno District Hospital, Ministry of Health, Government of the Republic of Malawi, Neno, Malawi, **7** Department of Medicine, Division of Palliative Care, Massachusetts General Hospital, Boston, Massachusetts, United States of America

Abstract

Introduction: Palliative care is rarely accessible in rural sub-Saharan Africa. Partners In Health and the Malawi government established the Neno Palliative Care Program (NPCP) to provide palliative care in rural Neno district. We conducted a situation analysis to evaluate early NPCP outcomes and better understand palliative care needs, knowledge, and preferences.

Methods: Employing rapid evaluation methodology, we collected data from 3 sources: 1) chart review of all adult patients from the NPCP's first 9 months; 2) structured interviews with patients and caregivers; 3) semi-structured interviews with key stakeholders.

Results: The NPCP enrolled 63 patients in its first 9 months. Frequent diagnoses were cancer (n = 50, 79%) and HIV/AIDS (n = 37 of 61, 61%). Nearly all (n = 31, 84%) patients with HIV/AIDS were on antiretroviral therapy. Providers registered 112 patient encounters, including 22 (20%) home visits. Most (n = 43, 68%) patients had documented pain at baseline, of whom 23 (53%) were treated with morphine. A majority (n = 35, 56%) had ≥1 follow-up encounter. Mean African Palliative Outcome Scale pain score decreased non-significantly between baseline and follow-up (3.0 vs. 2.7, $p = 0.5$) for patients with baseline pain and complete pain assessment documentation. Providers referred 48 (76%) patients for psychosocial services, including community health worker support, socioeconomic assistance, or both. We interviewed 36 patients referred to the NPCP after the chart review period. Most had cancer (n = 19, 53%) or HIV/AIDS (n = 10, 28%). Patients frequently reported needing income (n = 24, 67%) or food (n = 22, 61%). Stakeholders cited a need to make integrated palliative care widely available.

Conclusions: We identified a high prevalence of pain and psychosocial needs among patients with serious chronic illnesses in rural Malawi. Early NPCP results suggest that comprehensive palliative care can be provided in rural Africa by integrating disease-modifying treatment and palliative care, linking hospital, clinic, and home-based services, and providing psychosocial support that includes socioeconomic assistance.

Editor: Sam Eldabe, The James Cook University Hospital, United Kingdom

Funding: The True Colours Trust/ Waterloo Coalition and the Diana Princess of Wales Memorial Fund provided generous financial support for key components of the Neno Palliative Care Program. Grant funding from these organizations was provided under awards TCT 833 and URN6650/3423, respectively. Additional information about these organizations may be found at the following URLs: http://www.truecolourstrust.org.uk; http://www.dianaprincessofwalesmemorialfund.org. This work was supported in part by the US National Institutes of Health, grants T32 AI007001-36 (MH) and CTSA UL1TR000083 (MH). The funders had no role in study design, data collection and analysis, decision to publish, or preparation of the manuscript.

Competing Interests: The authors have declared that no competing interests exist.

* Email: michael_herce@med.unc.edu

¤a Current address: Department of Family Medicine, Tufts University School of Medicine, Boston, Massachusetts, United States of America
¤b Current address: Department of Medicine, Division of Allergy and Infectious Diseases, University of Washington School of Medicine, Seattle, Washington, United States of America
¤c Current address: Haiti Assistance Program, American Red Cross, Washington, D.C., United States of America

❡ These authors contributed equally to this work.

¶ These authors also contributed equally to this work.

Introduction

Palliative care encompasses assessment and relief of suffering of all kinds including pain, other physical and psychological symptoms, and social distress along the entire course of the patient's disease process [1]. Palliative care has been shown to improve patient outcomes, including mortality, when integrated with disease-modifying therapy [2]. The integration of palliative care with routine treatment for HIV/AIDS, cancer and other serious chronic illnesses is an important strategy for increasing access to palliative care and improving the quality of health care [3–6]. Despite the documented benefits, however, access to comprehensive, integrated palliative care remains limited in most developing countries, where the global burden of chronic disease is greatest [7,8].

Worldwide, 80% of patients lack access to adequate pain control–the cornerstone of palliative care [9]. In sub-Saharan Africa (SSA), only 5% of people in need of palliative care receive it despite the growing availability of palliative care programs [10]. The demand for palliative care in SSA is expected to increase over the next 20 years as more persons living with HIV (PLHIV) access life-prolonging antiretroviral therapy (ART) and develop long-term complications of HIV disease, and as non-communicable diseases (NCDs), including cancer, become more prevalent [10–12].

Malawi, a densely populated sub-Saharan African country with low per capita health expenditure, offers palliative care services at 21 sites–a fraction of the over 600 public and non-governmental health facilities located throughout the country [13,14]. Despite recent increases in palliative care service availability, major challenges remain in making these services accessible to all Malawians in need, particularly in rural areas. Geographical coverage of palliative care remains concentrated in urban and peri-urban locales, often out of reach for the 80% of the population who reside in less densely populated areas [15–18]. In rural settings where health infrastructure and human resources are limited, HIV and NCDs strain the capacity of health systems to deliver palliative care services. Based on recent estimates, over 1 million Malawians are living with HIV/AIDS and more than 25,000 have cancer [13,19,20]. Many Malawian patients and their family caregivers endure these illnesses at home–where they may prefer to receive care. Yet their needs, knowledge, and preferences regarding palliative care are not well characterized.

Qualitative research provides insight into palliative care needs, knowledge, and preferences, identifies causes of suffering, and guides local responses to recognized needs [16,21–25]. Available evidence from SSA indicates that the greatest needs of patients facing serious chronic illnesses and their caregivers may be psychosocial with basic socioeconomic necessities–including food, adequate shelter, and help with school fees–featuring prominently [1,16]. However, few published accounts describe palliative care needs, knowledge, and preferences in rural areas [1,26–27]. Fewer still detail efforts to translate identified needs into programmatic action and describe effective models of palliative care service delivery, particularly community- and home-based models that integrate palliative care with health services relevant to the SSA context, including treatment for HIV/AIDS [26,28–29].

Since 2007, Partners In Health (PIH), a non-governmental organization based in Boston, USA, has partnered with its Malawian sister organization, Abwenzi Pa Za Umoyo (APZU), and the Malawi Ministry of Health (MoH) to provide comprehensive healthcare to the people of Neno, a rural and impoverished district in the country's Southern region. In early 2012, APZU/PIH launched the Neno Palliative Care Program (NPCP) in order to integrate pain and symptom relief and psychosocial support with disease modifying treatment for patients with serious chronic illnesses and their families. As part of APZU/PIH's ongoing palliative care work, we conducted a situation analysis of the palliative care needs, knowledge, preferences, and services available in Neno district, aiming to improve the NPCP in a manner responsive to identified needs. We report here the results of the situation analysis, including early outcomes from the NPCP.

Methods

We performed a situation analysis employing rapid evaluation methodology (REM). First developed by the World Health Organization (WHO), REM involves collecting data through field-based interviews and observations to assist ministries of health and implementing partners in rapidly and efficiently taking programmatic action [30]. In SSA, REM has been used to evaluate health services, including palliative care services, and to guide quality improvement efforts [16,30–32].

Setting

We carried out the situation analysis in Neno district, Malawi. Neno district, with a population of 130,612, is a rural, hard-to-reach area bordered by Mozambique to the West and six Malawi districts along its remaining boundaries (Figure 1) [33]. The district's main health and economic indicators are representative of national averages, with male and female life expectancy slightly higher in Neno at 48.6 and 53.1 years, respectively, than Malawi overall, and 56% of the population living below the World Bank poverty line of 116 USD of income per person per year [33,34]. The Malawi Ministry of Health, through the Neno District Health Office (DHO), provides essential health services free of charge at 13 public health facilities, including Neno District Hospital situated in the administrative capital of the district–Neno boma [33].

Data Collection Overview

Employing REM, we collected data from three principal sources: 1) chart review of paper-based and electronic medical records for adult palliative care patients enrolled in the NPCP during its first 9 months; 2) structured interviews with patients and their caregivers; and 3) semi-structured interviews with key stakeholders. Collecting data from three sources enabled verification of information through triangulation [25,35]. We defined caregivers to be any accompanying family member, friend, or life partner identified by the patient as their primary custodian or "guardian" at the time of NPCP enrollment. We defined key stakeholders as frontline health workers and leaders of organizations involved in any aspect of palliative care delivery in Neno district or those involved in palliative care policy at the national level.

Chart Review

We reviewed paper-based medical records and registers for all adult patients enrolled in the NPCP during its first 9 months of existence (mid-January through early October 2012). We assessed the first 9 months to better understand our patient population and referral practices and to evaluate the quality of service delivery at the start of the program. We used the APZU OpenMRS-based electronic medical record to augment data abstracted from paper-based records [36]. We collected de-identified data on the following patient dimensions: demographic information, primary diagnosis, HIV status, pain, other symptoms, psychosocial distress, encounter location (i.e. in the outpatient clinic, hospital ward,

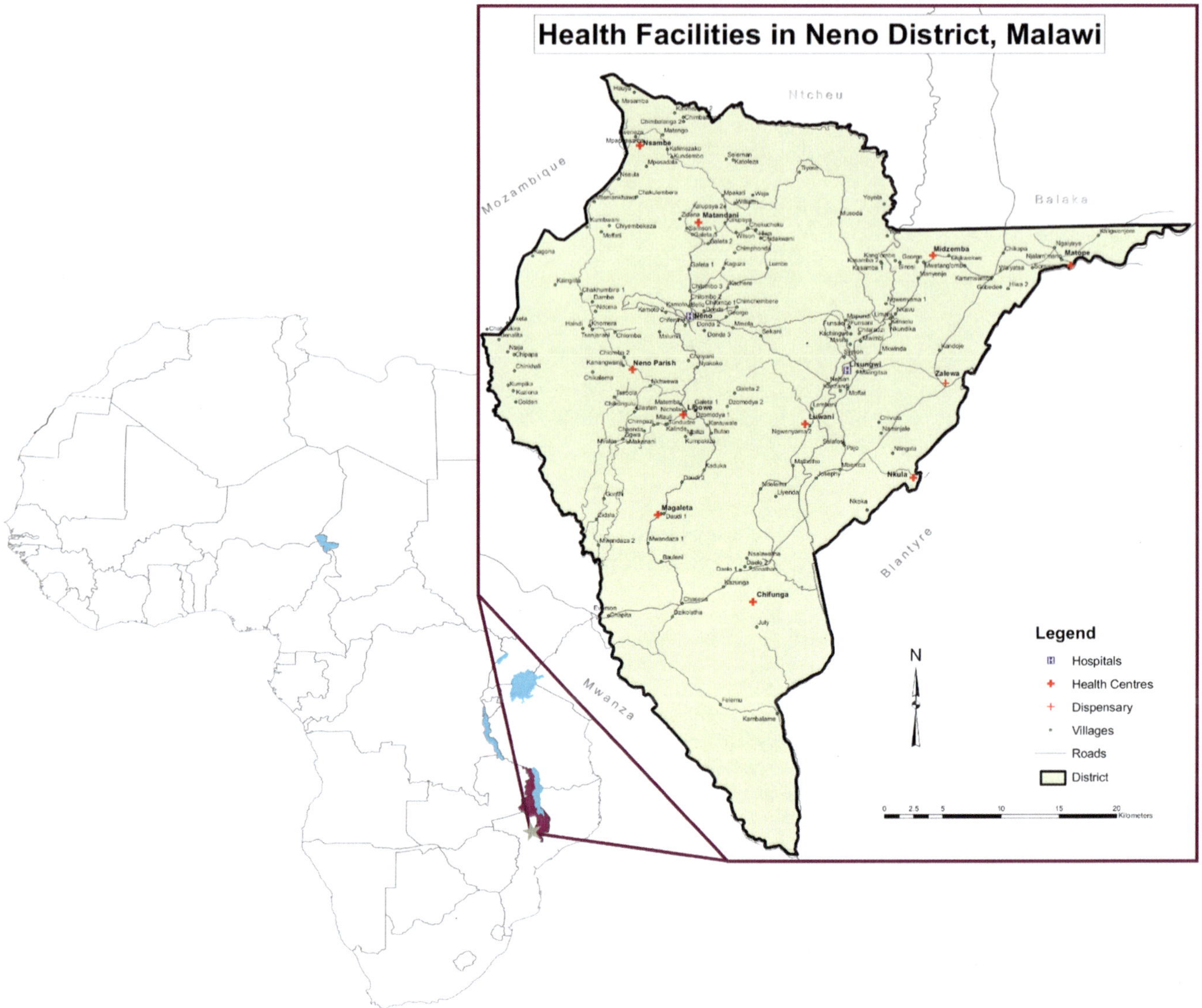

Figure 1. Map of Neno District, Republic of Malawi. The inset picture depicts Neno district, located in the southwestern portion of the country. The district shares an international border with Mozambique to the west and borders with Ntcheu district to the north; Balaka and Zomba districts to the northeast; Blantyre district to the east; Chikwawa to the south; and Mwanza district to the southwest. The inset legend illustrates the locations of major health facilities, including the district's two hospitals–Neno District Hospital and Lisungwi Community Hospital–as well as the remaining 11 health centers.

and/or home visit in the patient's home), retention-in-care, and referral for psychosocial support services. Palliative care providers documented the severity and quality of patient pain, other symptoms, and psychosocial distress at the time of each clinical encounter using a visual hand-scale representation of the African Palliative Care Association (APCA) African Palliative Outcome Scale (African POS) [37–40]. The African POS is a multidimensional palliative care scale designed for and validated in African palliative care populations [38,39]. Responses to African POS questions are scored using a 6-point Likert scale ranging from 0 to 5 [39]. When used to assess pain in adults, an African POS score of 3 or greater suggests moderate-to-severe pain, with a score of 5 representing the most severe or worst pain.

Structured Interviews: Patients and Caregivers

We developed two interview instruments–one for patients and a second for caregivers–to qualitatively assess the following participant domains: 1) awareness of diagnosis and preferences for palliative care; 2) pain and other physical symptoms; and 3) psychological, social, and spiritual needs and sources of support. Both instruments incorporated structured items and open-ended questions with interviewee prompts. The patient and caregiver interview instruments included all items intended for patients and caregivers, respectively, of the African POS [37,39]. The African POS has been used to measure patient outcomes on the three domains enumerated above; to evaluate caregiver knowledge, confidence, and anxiety; and to assess the quality of palliative care services [37]. The structured interview instrument was translated from English into the local language of patient and caregiver participants, Chichewa. The translation and preparation of the final Chichewa version of the instrument were performed at the APZU field office by trained local staff fluent in both English and Chichewa.

We planned to interview a sample of 80 individuals, comprising 5 patient participants at each of 4 antiretroviral therapy clinics (20 total), 10 hospitalized patients, and 10 patients receiving chemotherapy for Kaposi sarcoma, along with a matching number of accompanying caregivers (i.e. 40 caregiver participants total). We devised this sampling strategy in an attempt to capture a diverse range of patient and caregiver perspectives regarding palliative care services and experiences with serious chronic illness in Neno, Malawi. With this strategy in place, we recruited and interviewed a consecutive sample of patients and their caregivers 18 years of age or older who presented for routine HIV care, in-patient hospital care, or chemotherapy for Kaposi sarcoma, and who were newly referred for enrollment in the NPCP at 4 public health facilities in Neno District on selected days from January 14 to February 27, 2013. The facilities included one district hospital, one community hospital, and two health centers, chosen to represent the breadth of facility-based healthcare delivery in the district. We approached potential participants face-to-face at health facilities to maximize the efficiency of the recruitment process given the accessibility of the target population at health facilities and the cost and logistical limitations involved with alternative recruitment approaches (e.g. telephone, paper flier, etc.). While study investigators helped recruit interview participants, they had not met any participants prior to the time of the interview. Recruitment was stopped at 47 participants (36 patient and 11 caregiver participants) after an interim analysis revealed that saturation of major themes had been achieved. No patients or caregivers declined study participation.

Study investigators with formal medicine and public health training (S.N.E., E.B.W., and A.M.) conducted patient and caregiver interviews with the assistance of an independent, trained study interpreter fluent in both English and Chichewa. We obtained written informed consent from all participants prior to commencing interviews. As part of the informed consent process and prior to the structured interviews, study investigators (S.N.E., E.B.W., and A.M.) explained the rationale for the study but did not disclose any personal information regarding their interests in the research topic or their assumptions about possible study findings. Patient and caregivers were interviewed separately in the absence of the other person, whenever possible. However, at the discretion of patient participants, caregivers were allowed to be present during interview sessions and vice versa. All interviews were conducted in private areas at one of the four health facilities described above in a single session lasting approximately 30 to 45 minutes. An investigator led each interview session and read questions aloud sequentially, allowing enough time to fully capture participant responses and adhering to the format of the interview instrument as it progressed through the following sections: 1) Patient demographics, knowledge about their diagnosis and treatment, and medical care preferences; 2) African POS items; and 3) Psychosocial support and relevant information–needs, preferences, and ongoing sources of support (Appendix S1). For each participant, the study interpreter translated all questions aloud into the local language, Chichewa, and subsequently translated participant responses into English. The investigator then transcribed English-translated responses verbatim. No audiovisual recording equipment was used during interviews because of local restrictions on the use of such technology in patient care areas. No repeat interviews were carried out at any time during the study period.

Semi-structured Interviews: Key Stakeholders

We interviewed a purposive sample of key local and national stakeholders, including at least one individual from all organizations in Neno district working in the palliative care arena. The specific sites were as follows: 1) an integrated cancer and palliative care clinic at Neno District Hospital; 2) a MoH ART clinic; 3) the Neno District Health Office home-based care program; 4) the APZU/PIH Program on Social and Economic Rights (POSER); 5) the APZU/PIH Village Health Worker Program; 6) Chiyembekezo Community-based Organization (CBO); and 7) the Palliative Care Association of Malawi (PACAM).

Stakeholders were interviewed at each site by one of the study investigators (S.N.E.) and asked to discuss the palliative care infrastructure and service delivery practices at their institution or organization. Transcripts were reviewed with key stakeholder participants for comment and correction. Palliative care policy documents, clinical encounter forms, data recording tools, and training materials were reviewed by the investigator prior to stakeholder interviews to provide context, among them the *NPCP Initial Assessment Form* (Appendix S2), *Malawi National Palliative Care Guidelines* (Appendix S3), the *Introduction to Palliative Care: Health Care Workers' Service Providers Manual* (Appendix S4), and the *Malawi Guidelines for the Clinical Management of HIV in Children and Adults* (Appendix S5) [13,41–43]. To minimize the influence of palliative care documents on stakeholder responses, these materials were not provided to stakeholders before or during study interviews. Preliminary study findings were shared at a dissemination meeting to refine our understanding and representation of perspectives expressed by key stakeholders during interviews.

Data Analysis and Reporting

For qualitative data we employed content analysis methodology to develop thematic codes for patient, caregiver, and stakeholder interview responses using Dedoose software (SocioCultural Research Consultants, LLC, Manhattan Beach, CA, USA) [44,45]. Two study investigators (S.N.E., E.B.W.) coded participant responses together (beginning with "participant 0" as designated automatically by Dedoose software) and reconciled differences by consensus. We calculated frequencies and simple proportions for all thematic codes generated, including root and child codes. We then used this information to develop a taxonomy of themes, providing a structure to interpret patient and caregivers' experiences with illness and to describe palliative care knowledge and preferences among all interview participants. The results of structured interviews are reported in accordance with accepted criteria for qualitative research [46]. For quantitative survey and chart review data we calculated frequencies, proportions, means or medians, and measures of dispersion. For continuous variables, we compared means between two independent groups using the two-sample t-test and means of repeated measurements in the same group using the paired t-test. For variables with more than two categories, we compared means with the one-way analysis of variance. We considered a two-sided p-value$<$0.05 to be statistically significant. All quantitative analyses were performed in SPSS (Version 20, 2011, IBM, Armonk, NY, USA) or Stata (Version 12.1, 2011, StataCorp, College Station, TX, USA).

Ethics Statement

All components of this study were conducted in accordance with the principles expressed in the Declaration of Helsinki. All patient and caregiver interview participants provided written informed consent prior to participation in the study. All key stakeholder interview participants, who were asked generic questions about palliative care programs and policies only and not about themselves or individual patients, provided verbal informed consent, which was documented on de-identified semi-structured interview instruments. All individuals depicted in this manuscript are NPCP service providers, not study participants, and have given written informed consent (as outlined in the PLOS consent form) to publish their likeness in photograph form. Human subjects research approval for all study procedures was granted by the National Health Sciences Research Committee of Malawi and by the Institutional Review Boards of the University of North Carolina, Chapel Hill, USA, Partners Healthcare System, Boston, USA and Harvard Medical School, Boston, USA.

Results

Overview

We first describe the Neno Palliative Care Program (NPCP) model and early results from the NPCP. We then report major characteristics of patient and caregiver interview participants. Lastly, we present the results of patient, caregiver, and key stakeholder interviews, organized by our taxonomy of major and minor interview themes (Figure 2).

The Neno Palliative Care Program Model

The joint MoH–APZU/PIH Neno palliative care team, first formed in late 2011 to implement the NPCP, consists of: 1) 1 physician; 2) 2 clinical officers (mid-level health workers common in Malawi); 3) 1 palliative care coordinator; 4) 1 nurse; 5) approximately 150 MoH home-based care volunteers; and 6) 691 community health workers, known locally as village health workers (VHWs), paid and trained by APZU/PIH to provide health-related services throughout the district. An experienced international palliative care physician-educator provides longitudinal training and clinical mentorship to NPCP clinical providers [47,48]. All clinical providers received a week-long palliative care training in early January 2012 prior to NPCP implementation, followed by a week-long advanced training in March 2012.

NPCP clinical providers train VHWs to recognize pain, other symptoms, treatment side effects, major disease complications, and psychosocial distress, and to request an immediate home visit for patients with one of these issues (Figure 3). The palliative care clinical team manages a weekly outpatient clinic at Neno District Hospital, conducts daily inpatient hospital consultations, and oversees a weekly district-wide mobile outreach clinic. Clinical officers working closely with the supervising palliative care physician conduct clinical evaluations, administer disease-modifying chemotherapy for Kaposi sarcoma, and prescribe symptom-relieving medications (including morphine), following MoH guidelines and the three-step WHO pain relief ladder [13,40,41,43,49]. The Malawi MoH, with support from APZU/PIH, procures essential palliative care medicines and supplies for the NPCP and all district health facilities–including morphine liquid, slow-release morphine tablets, codeine phosphate tablets, ibuprofen, amitriptyline, diazepam, anti-emetics, antibiotics, incontinence pads, sterile gauze, and bandages, among other commodities–in accordance with local regulations, including the Malawi Controlled Drug Act [13]. MoH and APZU/PIH health workers and programmatic staff refer patients to the NPCP from patient support programs and health facilities located throughout Neno district, including the wards and clinical departments of the district's two hospitals–Neno District Hospital and Lisungwi Community Hospital (Figure 1). At the discretion of the referring health worker, patients may start analgesia before or at the time of NPCP referral, or during the first NPCP encounter. For patients living with HIV, clinical officers provide integrated HIV treatment and primary care services, including assessment for ART initiation and evaluation for possible ART side effects in accordance with national guidelines [43].

The NPCP responds to patient and family psychosocial needs through the APZU/PIH Program on Social and Economic Rights (POSER). POSER provides counseling and emotional support, as well as socioeconomic assistance for selected patients, in partnership with local community-based and faith-based organizations and government Ministries, including the Ministry of Gender, Child Development and Community Development and the Neno Office of Social Welfare. POSER staff evaluate the vulnerability of referred patients using a standardized assessment tool, and provide qualifying patients with one or more of the following types of socioeconomic assistance: food packages, home repairs, transportation reimbursement, and school support for children.

Early Results from the Neno Palliative Care Program

Over a 9-month period from mid-January through early October 2012, the NPCP enrolled 63 patients with serious chronic illnesses (Table 1). Most patients had cancer as a primary diagnosis ($n = 50$, 79%), and 32 of these (64%) had Kaposi sarcoma (Table 1). The majority of patients were HIV-infected (37 of 61, 61%). Of those with HIV infection, 31 (84%) lived in Neno district and received ART at 1 of the district's 13 public clinics.

Neno palliative care providers conducted 112 patient encounters during the 9-month evaluation period. Most encounters occurred in the outpatient palliative care clinic based at Neno District Hospital ($n = 57$, 51%) (Table 2). NPCP providers conducted 22 home visits, comprising 20% of all patient encounters. Complementing clinical service delivery, APZU/PIH VHWs provided longitudinal psychosocial support to 35 (56%) patients in the form of counseling during regularly scheduled home visits. Similarly, 34 (54%) patients were referred to POSER for psychosocial support, which included emotional support and socioeconomic assistance (Table 2). In total, providers referred 48 (76%) patients for psychosocial services in the form of VHW home visits, POSER support, or both.

Overall, 56 (89%) patients had a documented baseline pain assessment from their initial NPCP encounter, which included a record of the presence and severity of pain (Table 3). Among these 56 patients, 13 (23%) patients were found to be pain free (i.e. African POS score = 0) and 43 (77%) reported the presence of *any* pain (i.e. African POS score>0) (Table 3). Among the 43 patients reporting any pain at baseline, the mean African POS pain score was 3.2 (standard error, SE: 0.2), and 31 (72%) patients reported moderate-to-severe pain (i.e. African POS score≥3). Of the 43 patients with documented pain at baseline, 35 (81%) had a cancer diagnosis. Patients with documented baseline pain and cancer had a significantly higher mean African POS pain score than those without cancer (3.3 with cancer vs. 2.4 without cancer, $p = 0.04$) (Table 3). Among patients with baseline pain, pain severity did not differ significantly by age, gender, HIV status, or presence of Kaposi sarcoma (Table 3).

Among the 43 patients with documented pain at NPCP intake, 29 (67%) reported ongoing use of pain medications initiated by a referring health worker (Table 3). Of these 29 patients: 13 (45%) described using non-opioid analgesics exclusively, such as ibuprofen, paracetamol, aspirin, amitriptyline or some combination thereof; 2 (7%) reported taking codeine–a weak opioid–with or without an accompanying non-opioid agent; and 14 (48%) reported using oral morphine–a strong opioid–with or without a co-administered non-opioid medication (Table 3).

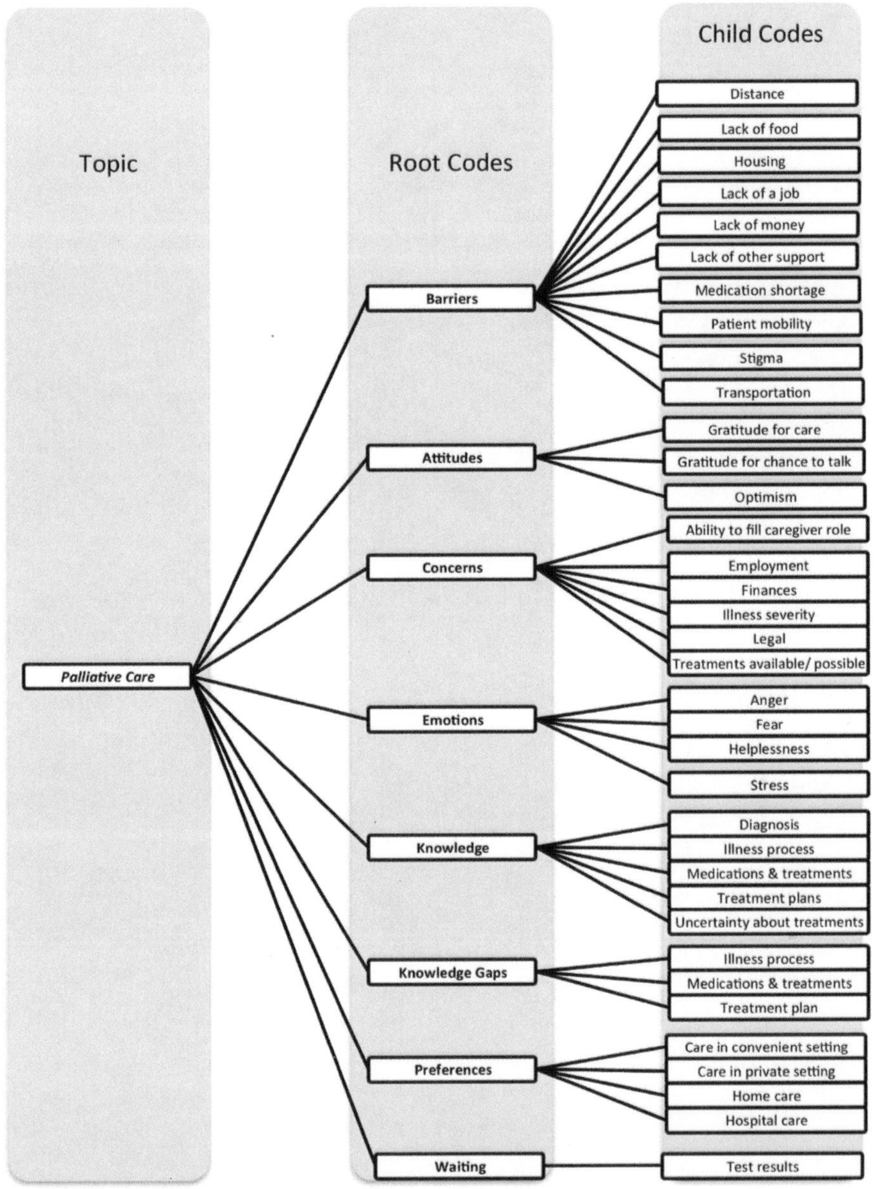

Figure 2. Major thematic codes generated from patient and caregiver interviews. The coding tree depicts major themes identified from structured patient and caregiver interviews. Codes relate to patient and family caregivers' experiences with illness, palliative care services provided, and palliative care services desired. Subordinate child codes elaborate descriptions for each root code. All root and child codes were generated using content analysis methodology and Dedoose software (SocioCultural Research Consultants, LLC., Manhattan Beach, CA, USA).

For the 43 patients with documented pain at baseline, NPCP providers newly started 10 (23%) patients on analgesia, added a drug or changed the current analgesic regimen for 15 (35%) patients, and continued the previously prescribed pain medications in 9 (21%) patients; 9 (21%) patients had no documentation of receiving a prescription for an analgesic agent during their initial NPCP encounter (Table 3). Morphine–available free of charge from the Malawi MoH–was prescribed for 23 of 43 (53%) patients with documented baseline pain. Having documented moderate-to-severe baseline pain was significantly associated with receiving a prescription for morphine at the initial NPCP encounter ($p = 0.001$). The mean African POS pain score was significantly higher for patients prescribed morphine (3.7, SE: 0.2) than for patients prescribed codeine or a non-opioid analgesic (2.1, SE: 0.3) ($p<0.001$) (Table 3).

Most patients ($n = 35$, 56%) had at least one recorded follow-up encounter (Table 4). Of these, 26 (74%) patients had a documented pain assessment, with 5 (19%) noted to be pain free and 21 (81%) reporting *any* pain (Table 4). Among the 21 patients reporting any pain at follow-up, the mean African POS pain score was 2.9 (SE: 0.3) and 11 (52%) patients reported moderate-to-severe pain. Pain severity did not differ significantly by age, gender, HIV status, or the presence of cancer, including KS, for patients reporting pain at follow-up (Table 4). For patients with pain at baseline and documented pain assessment at enrollment and follow-up ($n = 18$), we observed a small, non-significant decrease in mean African POS pain score (3.0 vs. 2.7, $p = 0.5$)

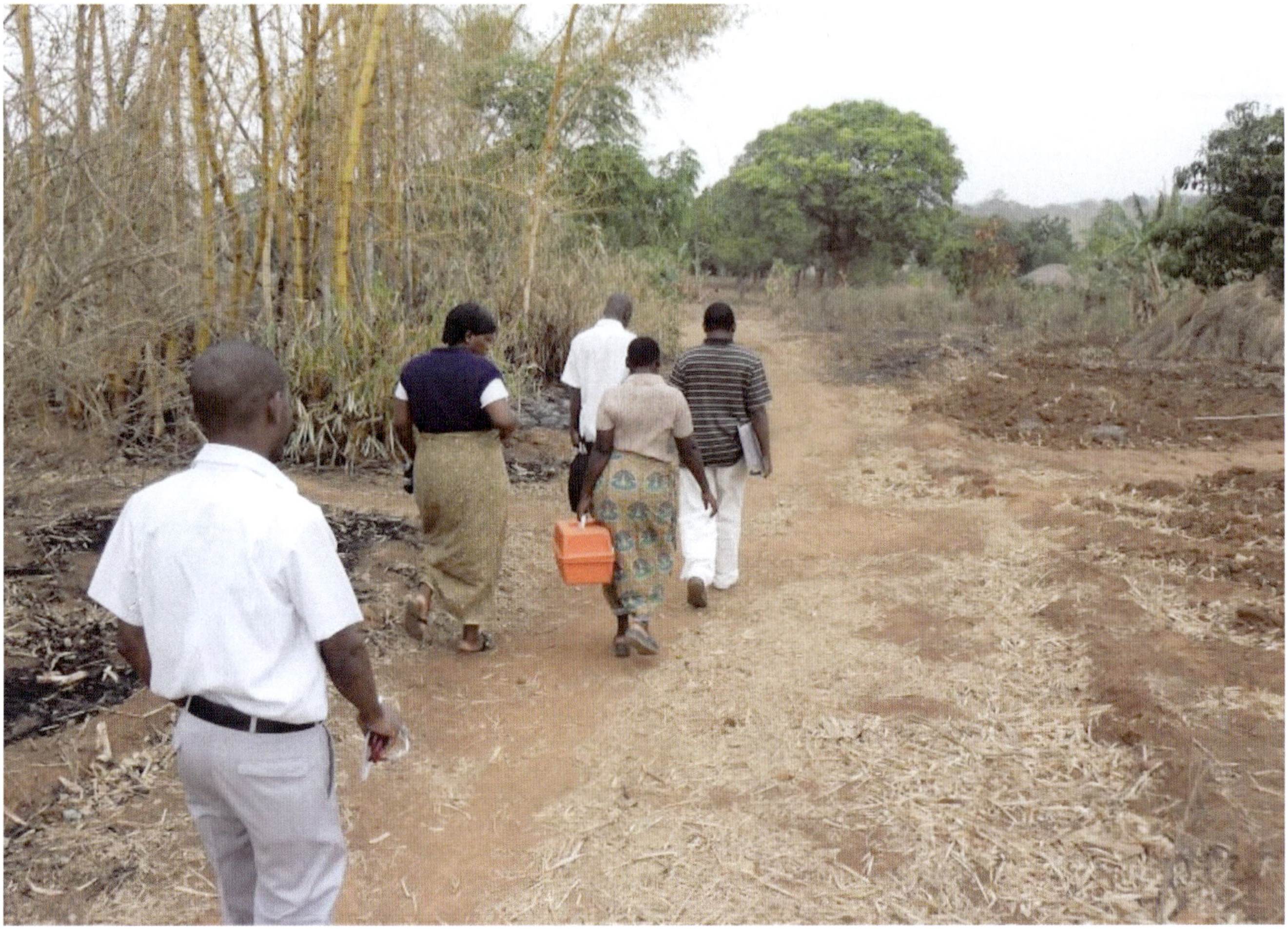

Figure 3. Neno Palliative Care Program team members conduct a home visit in a rural village. Five members of the Neno Palliative Care Program (NPCP) team travel by foot to reach the home of a palliative care patient living in rural Neno district, Malawi. An Abwenzi Pa Za Umoyo/ Partners In Health Medical Officer with specialized training in palliative care (foreground) leads the home visit. He is accompanied by (from left to right) a palliative care nurse, a Program on Social and Economic Rights social worker, a Village Health Worker and a NPCP clerk. NPCP team members work together to assess and treat patient pain and other physical symptoms, provide disease-specific care for serious chronic illnesses, and offer psychosocial support to patients and their families.

over the follow-up interval. We recorded 4 deaths (6%) that occurred before the patient's first scheduled follow-up encounter, each transpiring within 1 month of program enrollment (Table 4).

Characteristics of Patient and Caregiver Interview Participants

We interviewed 36 patients at the time of NPCP enrollment who were not in the early NPCP cohort, including 9 patients interviewed in the presence of their caregiver. Patients interviewed were, on average, 38 years old and 19 (53%) were female (Table 5). Most patients interviewed had cancer (n = 19, 53%), with Kaposi sarcoma being the most prevalent diagnosis in the sample (n = 13, 36%). HIV/AIDS was the primary diagnosis for 10 (28%) patients, with every known HIV-infected patient interviewed already enrolled in MoH HIV care. Those surveyed reported being ill for about 1 year, on average (median: 13 months; interquartile range, IQR: 0–156 months), at the time of the interview. Several patients (n = 7, 19%) were unable to work due to illness.

We interviewed 11 of the 12 (92%) caregivers who had accompanied a patient interview participant and were available for study recruitment (Table 5). All caregivers surveyed were family relatives of a patient enrolled in the study and were predominantly female (n = 8, 73%) (Table 5). Most caregivers reported working, typically having jobs as subsistence farmers or market vendors. Caregivers reported having served in this role for a median of 13 months (IQR: 0–54 months).

Prevalence of Pain and Other Symptoms among Patient Interview Participants

A majority of interviewed patients reported pain (n = 31, 86%), with 23 (64%) experiencing moderate-to-severe pain (African POS score≥3) (Table 6). Of those with moderate-to-severe pain, 13 (57%) had a cancer diagnosis. The mean African POS pain score of the 31 interview participants reporting pain was 3.3 (SE 0.2). Most interviewed patients reported additional physical symptoms, with numbness, cough, difficulty sleeping, and shortness of breath cited most frequently.

Table 1. Characteristics of patients at enrollment in the Neno Palliative Care Program (NPCP, January through October 2012).

Characteristic		n/N (%)
Total cohort		63/63 (100)
Gender		
	Male	37/63 (59)
Age (years)		
	Mean (standard error, SE)	48 (SE: 2.2)
Primary diagnoses		
Cancer		
	All cancers	50/63 (79)
	Kaposi sarcoma	32/50 (64)
	Cervical	7/50 (14)
	Other malignancy	11/50 (22)
Stroke		5/63 (8)
Cirrhosis		3/63 (5)
Peripheral Neuropathy		2/63 (3)
Other*		3/63 (5)
HIV[§] status[¶]		
	Sero-positive	37/61 (61)
HIV care		
Enrollment status		
	Documented in HIV care and receiving ART● in Neno District	31/37 (84)
	No documentation of HIV care	6/37 (16)[#]

*Includes the following conditions: anal fissure, paraplegia, and tuberculosis.
[§]HIV = Human immunodeficiency virus.
[¶]Documented HIV sero-status is missing for 2 patients.
●ART = Antiretroviral therapy.
[#]For 3 of 6 patients documentation could not be verified because patients presented for palliative care from districts other than Neno district.

Psychosocial Needs and Support Reported by Patient and Caregiver Interview Participants

In response to questions about desired psychosocial services, patients frequently mentioned socioeconomic needs (Table 7). Most patients cited a need for generating income (n = 24, 67%), receiving food (n = 22, 61%), or having their homes repaired (n = 22, 61%). Many patients mentioned poverty and lack of food as important barriers to their well-being:

Table 2. Summary of palliative care services provided by the Neno Palliative Care Program (NPCP, January through October 2012).

NPCP Services	n/N (%)
Clinical	
Total encounters	112/112 (100)
Patient encounter setting*	
Outpatient Clinic	57/112 (51)
Hospital	32/112 (29)
Patient Home Visit	22/112(20)
Non-Clinical[§]	
APZU/PIH Village Health Worker assigned	35/63 (56)
Referred for psychosocial services (includes socioeconomic assistance)[¶]	34/63 (54)

*Setting information is missing for 1 patient encounter.
[§]Describes non-clinical services provided to the 63 patients enrolled in the NPCP from January through October 2012. Non-clinical services were provided by the Abwenzi Pa Za Umoyo (APZU)/Partners In Health (PIH) Village Health Worker program and Program on Social and Economic Rights in collaboration with the Ministry of Health, Ministry of Gender, Child Development and Community Development, and the Neno Office of Social Welfare.
[¶]In addition to counseling and emotional support, psychosocial services include provision of in-kind support (soap, water collection receptacles, new shoes, etc.), food packages, housing repairs, and school tuition payments and school supplies for patients' children.

Table 3. Patient pain status, severity, and management at the initial Neno Palliative Care Program (NPCP) encounter (January through October 2012).

Variable		**n/N (%)**	**Mean African POS* Pain Score[§] (SE)[¶]**	**p-value**
Clinical status at initial encounter[●]				
	Pain assessed & documented	56/63 (89)		
	Pain free[#]	13/56 (23)		
	Any pain**	43/56 (77)	3.2 (0.2)	
	Moderate-to-severe pain[§§]	31/43 (72)	3.8 (0.1)	
Pain severity at initial encounter for patients with documented pain, by patient characteristic				
Age				0.8
	<50	24/43 (56)	3.2 (0.3)	
	≥50	19/43 (44)	3.1 (0.2)	
Gender				0.6
	Male	25/43 (58)	3.2 (0.2)	
	Female	18/43 (42)	3.1 (0.3)	
HIV status[¶¶]				0.5
	Sero-positive	26/41 (63)	3.2 (0.3)	
	Sero-negative	15/41 (37)	2.9 (0.3)	
Cancer				0.04
	With Cancer Diagnosis	35/43 (81)	3.3 (0.2)	
	Without Cancer Diagnosis	8/43 (19)	2.4 (0.3)	
Kaposi sarcoma (KS)				0.3
	With KS Diagnosis	21/43 (49)	3.4 (0.3)	
	Without KS Diagnosis	22/43 (51)	3.0 (0.2)	
Analgesia at NPCP intake				0.4
	None	14/43 (33)	2.9 (0.3)	
	Any analgesia[●●]	29/43 (67)	3.3 (0.2)	
	Non-opioids	13/43 (30)	3.0 (0.4)	
	Weak opioids (e.g. codeine)	2/43 (5)	3.5 (1.5)	
	Strong opioids (e.g. morphine)	14/43 (33)	3.5 (0.3)	
Pain management during initial encounter for patients with documented pain				
Provider prescribing actions				0.6
	Started analgesia	10/43 (23)	2.9 (0.4)	
	Adjusted analgesia	15/43 (35)	3.2 (0.4)	
	Continued previously prescribed analgesia	9/43 (21)	3.6 (0.4)	
	No documentation of analgesia prescription	9/43 (21)	3.0 (0.3)	
Morphine				<0.001
	Morphine prescribed	23/43 (53)	3.7 (0.2)	
	Other analgesia prescribed	11/43 (26)	2.1 (0.3)	

*African POS = African Palliative Care Association African Palliative Outcome Scale.
[§]Pain measured using the African POS, which scores pain in 1-point increments from 0 to 5 on a 6-point Likert scale. Harding R, Selman L, Agupio G, Dinat N, Downing J, et al. (2010) Validation of a core outcome measure for palliative care in Africa: the APCA African Palliative Outcome Scale. Health and Quality of Life Outcomes 8:10.

[¶]SE = standard error.
[●]Documented baseline pain assessment at initial encounter is missing for 7 patients.
[#]Indicated by African POS = 0.
**Indicated by African POS>0.
[§§]Indicated by African POS≥3.
[¶¶]Documented HIV sero-status is missing for 2 patients.
[●●]Includes any non-opioid (e.g. ibuprofen), weak opioid (e.g. codeine), or strong opioid (e.g. morphine) prescribed by the referring health worker prior to NPCP enrollment.

Table 4. Patient pain status, severity, and management at the first follow-up Neno Palliative Care Program (NPCP) encounter (May through October 2012).

Variable	n/N (%)	Mean African POS* Pain Score[§] (SE)[¶]	p-value
Patient follow-up			
≥1 Follow-up NPCP encounter	35/63 (56)		
Patient died before first follow-up (within 1 month of initial encounter)	4/63 (6)		
Clinical status at first follow-up encounter			
Pain assessed & documented[●]	26/35 (74)		
Pain free[#]	5/26 (19)		
Any pain**	21/26 (81)	2.9 (0.3)	
Moderate-to-severe pain[§§]	11/21 (52)	4.0 (0.2)	
Pain severity at first follow-up encounter for patients with documented pain, by patient characteristic[¶¶]			
Age			0.1
<50	13/21 (62)	2.5 (0.3)	
≥50	8/21 (38)	3.5 (0.5)	
Gender			0.6
Male	15/21 (71)	2.8 (0.3)	
Female	6/21 (29)	3.2 (0.6)	
HIV status[●●]			0.6
Sero-positive	13/20 (65)	3.0 (0.5)	
Sero-negative	7/20 (35)	2.7 (0.3)	
Cancer			0.5
With Cancer Diagnosis	17/21 (81)	3.0 (0.3)	
Without Cancer Diagnosis	4/21 (19)	2.5 (0.9)	
Kaposi sarcoma (KS)			0.5
With KS Diagnosis	11/21 (52)	2.7 (0.3)	
Without KS Diagnosis	10/21 (48)	3.1 (0.5)	
Pain management during first follow-up encounter for patients with documented pain[¶¶]			
Morphine			0.4
Morphine prescribed	14/21 (67)	3.1 (0.3)	
Other analgesia prescribed[##]	7/21 (33)	2.6 (0.5)	

*African POS = African Palliative Care Association African Palliative Outcome Scale.
[§]Pain measured using the African POS, which scores pain severity in 1-point increments from 0 to 5 on a 6-point Likert scale. Harding R, Selman L, Agupio G, Dinat N, Downing J, et al. (2010) Validation of a core outcome measure for palliative care in Africa: the APCA African Palliative Outcome Scale. Health and Quality of Life Outcomes 8:10.
[¶]SE = standard error.
[●]Documented follow-up pain assessment at first return encounter is missing for 9 patients.
[#]Indicated by African POS = 0.
**Indicated by African POS>0.
[§§]Indicated by African POS≥3.
[¶¶]For the 21 patients with documented pain at the first follow-up NPCP encounter.
[●●]Documented HIV sero-status is missing for 1 patient.
[##]Includes 2 patients without documented analgesia prescription with mean African POS pain score of 2.

'I was told to eat a well-balanced diet, which I can't do because of financial constraints.
First I was given food rations, but I'm not getting them now and I'm losing weight.' (Participant 20)
'[My house is] very debilitated. It was built by the church. [I am] happy to be in the hospital with rain coming because I won't get soaked. I sleep in mud at home.' (Participant 26)
'What I need most in my life is a job; I have always wanted to have a job. I would like help with that.' (Participant 0)

Most (n = 21, 58%) patients interviewed reported a desire for emotional support. Few patients (n = 2, 6%) mentioned HIV-related stigma when discussing their need for emotional support.

'There are people who still don't understand. Neighbors. And I was told I would not be hired for a landscaping job because of my status.' (Participant 19)

Similar to patients, most caregivers (n = 7, 64%) stated that they needed emotional support. A high percentage of caregivers

Table 5. Characteristics of patient and caregiver interview participants.

Characteristic		Patients (N = 36)	Caregivers (N = 11)
		n/N (%)	n/N (%)
Gender			
	Female	19/36 (53)	8/11 (73)
Age (years)			
	Mean (standard error, SE)	38 (SE: 1.8)	47 (SE: 5.1)
Highest Education Level Completed			
	None	8/36 (22)	3/11 (27)
	Primary	17/36 (47)	7/11 (64)
	Secondary	10/36 (28)	1/11 (9)
	University	1/36 (3)	0/11 (0)
Marital Status			
	Married	21/36 (58)	10/11 (91)
	Divorced	8/36 (22)	0/11 (0)
	Widowed	4/36 (11)	1/11 (9)
	Single	2/36 (6)	0/11 (0)
	Living as Married	1/36 (3)	0/11 (0)
Household Size	Median (IQR)*	6 (2–10)	6 (3–13)
Living Children per Household	Median (IQR)	3 (0–8)	4 (1–6)
Employment Status			
	Subsistence farmer	12/36 (33)	5/11 (45)
	Market vendor	7/36 (19)	4/11 (36)
	Unable to work due to illness	7/36 (19)	0/11 (0)
	Part-time unskilled labor	4/36 (11)	1/11 (9)
	Part-time skilled labor	4/36 (11)	0/11 (0)
	Unable to find work	2/36 (6)	1/11 (9)
Patient Primary Diagnosis			
HIV/AIDS[§]		10/36 (28)	
	In HIV care, on ART[¶]	9/10 (90)	
	In HIV care, HCC[●] Clinic	1/10 (10)	
Cancer		19/36 (53)	
	Kaposi sarcoma	13/36 (36)	
	Cervical cancer	4/36 (11)	
	Other malignancy	2/36 (6)	
Other serious chronic illness[#]		7/36 (19)	
Illness Duration (months)	Median (IQR)	13 (0–156)	
Caregiver Present at Visit/Hospital**		12/36 (33)	
Caregiver Relationship to Patient			
	Parent		3/11 (27)
	Spouse		3/11 (27)
	Sibling		3/11 (27)
	Other family		2/11 (18)
Time as caregiver (months)	Median (IQR)		13 (0–54)

*IQR = interquartile range.
[§]Indicates a primary diagnosis of HIV/AIDS, in the absence of Kaposi sarcoma.
[¶]ART = Antiretroviral Therapy.
[●]HCC = HIV Care Clinic.
[#]Other serious chronic illnesses include: multi-drug resistant tuberculosis (MDR-TB), end stage liver disease, and progressive neurological illness.
**One caregiver was ineligible for study inclusion because she was younger than 18.

Table 6. Patient symptom presence and severity over the three days prior to Neno Palliative Care Program enrollment (N = 36).

Symptom	Present*		African POS[¶]
	n	%[§]	Mean Score (SE)●
Pain	31	86	3.3 (0.2)
Numbness	13	36	3.5 (0.4)
Cough	12	33	3.5 (0.4)
Difficulty sleeping	12	33	3.5 (0.3)
Shortness of breath	12	33	3.7 (0.4)
Nausea/vomiting	8	22	3.4 (0.5)
Constipation	8	22	2.8 (0.7)

*Present indicates score of >0 on the African Palliative Care Association African Palliative Outcome Scale.
[¶]African POS = African Palliative Outcome Scale, which scores symptom severity in 1-point increments from 0 to 5 on a 6-point Likert scale. Harding R, Selman L, Agupio G, Dinat N, Downing J, et al. (2010) Validation of a core outcome measure for palliative care in Africa: the APCA African Palliative Outcome Scale. Health and Quality of Life Outcomes 8:10.
[§]Percentages do not sum to 100% as more than one symptom was reported per patient.
●SE = Standard error.

reported needs in helping meet the demands of caring for patients, including financial support (n = 10, 91%), food (n = 8, 73%), and physical assistance in providing care (n = 5 45%). A smaller number of caregivers reported the following additional needs: affordable medical care for the patient (n = 2, 18%) and help finding employment or help with transportation (n = 1, 9%).

All patients interviewed reported receiving some form of psychosocial support (Table 7). A majority of patients (n = 27, 75%) described receiving psychosocial support from family members. This most frequently consisted of emotional support, but often also included food, housing, caregiving, or financial support. Caregivers noted that close friends (n = 5, 45%), or a

Table 7. Patient-reported psychosocial needs and sources of psychosocial support (N = 36).

Psychosocial needs	n	%
Help getting a job/making money	24	67
Food support	22	61
Help with home repairs	22	61
Counseling/emotional support	21	58
Relief from other symptoms*	20	56
Help sending children to school	18	50
Doctor or nurse visit	12	33
Spiritual Advice	11	31
Care for children	9	25
Legal Advice	2	6
Other	7	19
Sources of Psychosocial Support		
Family	27	75
Church	18	50
Friends	14	39
APZU[§]/PIH[¶] Program on Social and Economic Rights	12	33
APZU/PIH Village Health Worker Program	12	33
Neighbors	8	22
Community-Based Organization	1	3
Social Welfare Office/District Assembly	1	3
Other	4	11

*"Other symptoms" include any physical symptom other than pain.
[§]APZU = Abwenzi Pa Za Umoyo.
[¶]PIH = Partners In Health.

parent or neighbor (n = 2, 18%) were important sources of assistance. Several caregivers (n = 4, 36%) reported that they had received material support in the form of food, sharing of caregiving duties, and financial support. When provided, this support came from immediate or extended family members.

Community churches provided many patients (n = 18, 50%) and caregivers (n = 6, 55%) with psychosocial support consisting of home visits by clergy or congregation members or, occasionally, housekeeping and cleaning services. APZU/PIH was also a frequently cited source of psychosocial support, with 12 (33%) patients reporting longitudinal assistance from a VHW and an equal number (n = 12, 33%) mentioning that they had received POSER services. POSER provided patients with emotional support and socioeconomic assistance in the form of food packages, income generating activities, school fee funding, and housing renovations. Patients reported that village health workers in their communities provided them with frequent counseling during home visits.

The Role of Caregivers

All caregivers reported that they took on the role because of familial obligation. However, a minority of caregivers interviewed also noted that volunteering, friendship, and being the only caregiver available (n = 1 for each response) were also valued reasons. All caregivers described a large time commitment involved in the caregiver role. Caregivers reported attending to patients from 6 to 24 hours per day (mean = 17 hours). Caregivers assisted with a variety of activities of daily living, including feeding, bathing and dressing. Caregivers also frequently gave medications (n = 7, 64%), offered emotional support (n = 7, 64%), and provided symptomatic care (n = 5, 45%). Transportation to the clinic and care for dependents were provided by most caregivers (n = 6, 55%), and several (n = 3, 27%) provided housing.

Caregivers reported considerable confidence in their abilities to provide care but also considerable worry (Table 8). Caregivers noted the following as their greatest fears: losing a loved one (n = 5, 45%); not having enough money or resources to care for the patient (n = 4, 36%); an undesirable future for the patient's children (n = 3, 27%); an unwanted future for themselves (n = 2, 18%); and discrimination or not receiving any assistance in caring for the patient (n = 1, 9%).

> *'I [as a caregiver] worry about the illness because I don't have enough money at home because I can't work and take care of my brother, and I'm also taking care of two orphaned children.' (Participant 7)*
>
> *'We cannot be open about this type of illness, so I am her only guardian.... Our neighbors think that they will get the disease if they come near, since they're not sure what type of illness she has.' (Participant 4)*

Palliative Care Knowledge

With respect to knowledge about their illness, most patients interviewed were able to describe the nature of their illness and the names of, or indications for, any treatments that they were receiving. The most frequent gaps in knowledge existed for hospitalized patients. These patients often had a new or still unconfirmed diagnosis. One patient–who knew that he was HIV-positive but was not aware that he had just been diagnosed with Kaposi sarcoma–illustrated this point as follows:

> *'I have some sores on the chest, edema in the legs, and some shortness of breath,*
> *and some bad pains. I haven't been told anything else.' (Participant 33)*

Despite attending to the many physical and psychosocial needs of patients, few caregivers (n = 2, 18%) had received formal training or counseling in palliative care. Most caregivers (n = 7, 64%) identified training in patient care as a major need.

We interviewed 7 key stakeholders. All key stakeholders reported being familiar with the concept of palliative care, even those working for organizations providing psychosocial support without an explicit palliative care mission. All were aware that national palliative care guidelines existed and that they had been updated in 2011. However, most stakeholders not directly involved with the NPCP had not seen the updated guidelines, and noted that they had not yet been fully disseminated at the district level. Stakeholders noted that additional training was needed for all levels of palliative care providers.

Preferences for Palliative Care Setting and Models of Service Delivery

Patient and caregiver interview participants were asked to select one or more settings where they would most like to receive palliative care from among five possibilities and to explain the rationale for their selections (Appendix S1). Patient responses most frequently included home-based care (46%), community-based care at a nearby health post or health center (30%), and hospital-based care (24%); only 1 response (2% of the 50 total responses) favored intensive palliative care provided in a designated hospital-based ward (a notion approximating the idea of a hospice). Caregivers reported split preferences for where they would most like patients to receive palliative care, with 46% of responses mentioning home-based care, 46% citing community-based care, and 36% referencing hospital-based care. Most caregivers (n = 9,

Table 8. Caregiver-reported confidence, worry, and information over the past three days (N = 11).

Dimension	Mean Africa POS* Score (SE)[§]
Caregiving confidence level	3.9 (0.5)
Level of worry	3.6 (0.5)
Degree to which caregiver felt adequate information was provided by the palliative care provider(s)	3.4 (0.6)

*African POS = African Palliative Outcome Scale, which scores caregiver dimensions in 1-point increments from 0 to 5 on a 6-point Likert scale. Harding R, Selman L, Agupio G, Dinat N, Downing J, et al. (2010) Validation of a core outcome measure for palliative care in Africa: the APCA African Palliative Outcome Scale. Health and Quality of Life Outcomes 8:10.

[§]SE = Standard error.

82%) reported wanting the support of a village health worker, home-based care volunteer, or other form of home-based care assistance.

> *'If I can get a doctor to visit at home that would be good because I came a very long way here and I have many other duties that I am missing at home.' (Participant 13)*
> *'Assuming I will be discharged, will I be able to get care at home? I cannot walk, or use my arms and legs, so it was very difficult to get here, and I need care at home.' (Participant 3)*

While most patients and caregivers expressed a preference for home-based care, hospital care was still important to many, particularly patients who felt that their illness was serious or required higher level care, and patients who expressed a distrust of the level of expertise that would be provided in a health center or in their home. For others, the convenience of receiving care in an easily accessible place was most important. Several patients noted that travel to the hospital could be difficult, time-consuming, and disruptive to work and home responsibilities. One caregiver summarized the conflicts between accessing healthcare and the other areas of his life this way:

> *'It would be good to have health care close to where we live, because then I would be able to take my brother for care and then go out and do my farming and work. Then I would be able to take care of our family.' (Participant 6)*

All stakeholders who identified as health workers expressed that palliative care should be widely accessible and integrated with inpatient and outpatient clinical services.

> *'Palliative care should be part of the routine services, not a separate project. It is part of essential healthcare delivery.' (Stakeholder 7)*

Health workers at public facilities noted that the integration of palliative care with other clinical services proved difficult because of limited health worker time and training. Most stakeholders favored a model in which a mobile palliative care team combined home-based care–where symptom assessment and psychosocial support would be provided by home-based care volunteers or village health workers in the community–with a dedicated hospital-based palliative care clinic or inpatient service for very sick or complex patients. They stated that a major success of palliative care in Neno District was the linking of palliative care in the home, the community, and health facilities. All stakeholders noted that trained village health workers and home-based care volunteers had been crucial in making palliative care, and healthcare in general, accessible to vulnerable patients in Neno district.

Future Palliative Care Priorities

Opinions about future palliative care priorities varied widely among key stakeholders. Policy-makers felt that the integration of palliative care into national policy would assure its eventual implementation in all districts. Health workers prioritized development and scale up of new models of palliative care service delivery, particularly mobile teams. Psychosocial service providers from APZU/PIH and Chiyembekezo CBO cited the need to further integrate clinical and non-clinical palliative care services and reinforce existing referral systems between these services. Most stakeholders noted that improving coordination–both among palliative care-relevant governmental and non-governmental organizations and across tiers of the public health system–should be a priority for future palliative care activities in Neno district. All stakeholders cited a lack of consistent funding for palliative care activities, amidst competing health priorities, as a threat to the sustainability and scale-up of palliative care services.

> *'When donors provide money for certain activities, priorities shift and old plans can be forgotten. We need to have money [for palliative care] that is stable from year to year.' (Stakeholder 5)*

Discussion

We present the results of the first palliative care situation analysis, to our knowledge, from rural Malawi and one of the first from a rural setting in Sub-Saharan Africa. Using rapid evaluation methodology, we describe the scope of needs among patients, family caregivers, and key stakeholders, the availability of integrated palliative care services in Neno district, and a model for palliative care service delivery applicable to rural resource-poor settings. We report a high prevalence of pain, other physical symptoms, and psychosocial needs among patients with serious chronic illnesses, indicating a large need for palliative care in one rural district. Early results from the NPCP suggest that comprehensive palliative care can be provided and integrated with disease-modifying treatment even in the most challenging settings by creating a network of hospital, clinic, and home-based services that include psychosocial support incorporating socioeconomic assistance.

In sub-Saharan Africa, and Malawi in particular, there have been few published evaluations of palliative care programs and limited accounts of successful models of palliative care service delivery relevant to rural areas [27–29,50–52]. Indeed, the African Palliative Care Research Network has identified describing and evaluating innovative models of palliative care service delivery as a priority area for palliative care research [29]. We describe an innovative district-wide palliative care program employing a tiered network of providers, integrated with HIV/AIDS and Kaposi sarcoma treatment, and providing novel linkages to psychosocial support services, which achieved several favorable outcomes despite the challenges posed by a rural, resource-limited setting. First, a majority of NPCP patients with pain at baseline successfully accessed oral morphine and NPCP's trained palliative care providers generally prescribed morphine appropriately to those patients with the highest African POS pain scores. Previous accounts of palliative care services in SSA have highlighted the limited accessibility of strong opioids like morphine and the need for health worker training in pain management, particularly in rural areas [8,25,27]. Second, 56% of patients received at least one NPCP follow-up evaluation. This compares favorably to a hospital-based program in urban Malawi where only 40% of palliative care patients had a recorded follow-up visit [15]. We hypothesize that the higher retention we observed was due to patient home visits made by the Neno palliative care clinical team and the work of VHWs and home-based care volunteers who actively linked patients to palliative care services and provided psychosocial support. Moreover, an effective national ART program, supported in Neno by PIH community-based interventions, also may have contributed to favorable retention among HIV-infected NPCP patients. Third, we found that a high proportion of HIV-infected NPCP patients were enrolled in

HIV care and on ART, suggesting integration of palliative care services with HIV/AIDS treatment in Neno district. Lastly, we observed a small, non-significant decrease in patient pain severity between the initial and follow-up NPCP encounters for patients with complete pain assessment documentation as well as a decrease in the proportion of patients experiencing moderate-to-severe pain at follow-up. However, inferences about the effectiveness of pain management in our program are limited by missing chart information and insufficiently granular prescribing data. We postulate that several patients experienced moderate-to-severe pain at follow-up either because providers were hesitant to start or escalate opioid therapy at the initial NPCP encounter or because of progression of their chronic disease.

Previous studies of palliative care programs in Malawi have reported the young age and high HIV prevalence of adult patients with serious chronic illnesses accessing palliative care services [15,16]. We present similar findings for patients from rural Neno district, most of whom were young and HIV-infected. These data reflect the demographics of the generalized HIV epidemic in Malawi [19]. Unlike the national epidemic, however, in which women are affected disproportionately, most patients in the NPCP cohort were men–a gender composition similar to that of a hospital-based program in urban Malawi, but differing from female-predominant gender distributions reported by other palliative care centers in SSA [15,53]. For patients with pain in our cohort, African POS pain scores did not differ significantly by gender at either the initial or fist follow-up encounter. Limited cross-sectional data suggest there may be an association between gender and pain, as well as between gender and overall symptom burden in the African context [27,53,54]. Additional observational studies from SSA are needed to better understand the effect of gender on symptom frequency, physical and psychological symptom burden, other palliative care outcomes, and care seeking behavior.

We identified Kaposi sarcoma (KS) as the most prevalent diagnosis among patients interviewed at the time of NPCP enrollment and the most common cancer among the first patients cared for in the NPCP. Kaposi sarcoma was also the most common diagnosis among palliative care patients at one center in Salima district, highlighting the burden that KS and other cancers place on patients and the health system in Malawi [17,20]. We observed NPCP cancer patients to have a significantly higher baseline African POS pain score than patients without a cancer diagnosis. However, this difference was not observed when comparing patients with and without KS. While differences in needs and perspectives between cancer patients and PLHIV (without cancer) did not emerge as a theme in our qualitative analyses, ours is among the few studies from SSA to quantitatively evaluate adult cancer pain or compare pain by patient diagnosis [25,27].

Our study also presents one of the largest samples of patients and caregivers from a single SSA country interviewed about palliative care needs, knowledge, and preferences. We report a high prevalence of patient pain, shortness of breath, and cough, reflecting a symptom profile similar to that of AIDS patients from rural Uganda and patients accessing palliative care services at a referral hospital in urban Malawi [15,26]. Neno patients and caregivers expressed a strong desire for psychosocial support at the time of NPCP enrollment, with unmet socioeconomic needs cited most frequently. In an evaluation of an independent, home-based care program serving peri-urban areas outside Blantyre, Malawi, patients expressed a desire to have basic necessities met, including the need for employment, food, and shelter [16]. Patients in Neno reported similar needs at NPCP enrollment, requesting support for income generation, food, and home repairs.

Numerous Neno patients detailed how the effects of poverty exacerbated the physical and psychological symptoms of their chronic illness. Similar findings have been described elsewhere in SSA [25,54–55]. In South Africa, for example, food insecurity was associated with greater HIV symptom severity, and in a survey of PLHIV from four Southern African countries, fewer disease symptoms were reported among study participants who had a modicum of socioeconomic security [54,55]. Basic unmet socioeconomic needs also affected caregivers in Neno, contributing to caregiver worry and shaping perceptions about their ability to manage the caregiver role. Taken together, these findings underscore the importance of including socioeconomic interventions as a core component of palliative care.

Despite the well-documented socioeconomic needs reported by palliative care patients and caregivers, however, few programs have been described that provide integrated, psychosocial interventions to mitigate the adverse effects of poverty. One of the few programs to effectively incorporate such psychosocial support, Hospice Africa Uganda, uses a "comfort fund" to pay for patient transportation expenses and to cover the costs of basic patient necessities [56]. We report that 76% of patients in our NPCP cohort were referred for psychosocial services, including 54% linked directly to socioeconomic assistance, including food packages, transportation vouchers, and other forms of material support. Socioeconomic assistance, as well as counseling and emotional support, was provided by the APZU/PIH Program on Social and Economic Rights–a partnership with the Government of Malawi that enables integration of psychosocial and clinical palliative care services.

While the burden of caring for patients with serious, chronic illnesses in resource-limited settings often falls to caregivers [57], limited evidence describes their palliative care needs [58]. We report that caregivers are considerably worried about their loved ones and have fears about the future wellbeing of themselves, the patient, and the patient's children. We found that caregivers were the primary providers of nursing care and emotional support, helping patients with activities of daily living 17 hours per day, on average. Caregivers expressed a desire for receiving assistance in the home from either a community health worker or home-based care volunteer to enable them to meet competing familial obligations while still providing direct care to the patient. Given the extent of their involvement in palliative care, we identified a need to improve caregiver training and psychosocial support to enable them to continue functioning in the caregiver role.

Due to funding and time constraints, our study was not designed to identify predictors of pain control, assess longitudinal patient outcomes, or explore all themes surrounding palliative care in the African context. Instead, structured interviews provided a comprehensive assessment of patient symptoms and support at the time of NPCP enrollment and the chart review described patient characteristics and changes in pain level over a short follow-up period. The qualitative components of our study may have been limited by information bias arising from the interview translation process or the presence of an accompanying counterpart during patient and caregiver interviews, recall bias as participants generated their responses, or selection bias due to the palliative care referral practices of health workers or the recruitment process for interview participants. In particular, selection bias may have been introduced by enrolling fewer than the targeted number of caregivers. While no caregivers refused study participation, only 25% of patient interview participants had an accompanying caregiver available for study recruitment, potentially limiting the breadth of caregiver perspectives represented in our study. We attempted to limit the systematic bias presented by these issues by employing a dedicated, trained study interpreter, incorporating the African POS into our structured interview instrument, sensitizing health workers throughout Neno district about appropriate indications for NPCP referral, and conducting an interim analysis to ensure that we had achieved saturation of major themes before concluding participant recruitment. Owing to the immediate de-identification of study data, it was not possible to obtain feedback on our findings from patient and caregiver interview participants, which may have limited full understanding of the meanings and perspectives derived from participant responses [46]. For the chart review, missing data due to patient loss to follow-up and incomplete documentation by palliative care providers limit the inferences that may be drawn regarding the effectiveness of pain management, clinical predictors of pain control, and provider analgesia-prescribing practices. While a prospective study design would have obviated many of these limitations, using routinely collected clinical data in our analyses provided a 'real-world' operational perspective on palliative care service delivery in rural Malawi.

Since completing data collection for the situation analysis, we have enrolled 105 additional patients in the NPCP (through December 31, 2013). We have applied our findings to recruit and train more village health workers, now numbering 820, to provide additional community-based psychosocial support to patients and their caregivers throughout Neno district, and we have further harmonized their services with those of home-based care volunteers. We have also worked to improve patient pain and symptom management by disseminating the most recent MoH palliative care guidelines, providing longitudinal mentorship to health workers on palliative care practice, including use of the WHO pain relief ladder, and strengthening analgesic supply chain management at all Neno health facilities. In the future, we plan to identify designated personnel to offer intensive caregiver counseling and to further integrate palliative care with non-communicable disease treatment provided at the district's two hospitals. Notably, all components of the Neno Palliative Care Program continue to be jointly implemented by APZU/PIH in partnership with the government of Malawi, including the Ministry of Health and the Ministry of Local Government and Rural Development–distinguishing the Neno model from other palliative care programs and increasing the potential for replication in other Malawi districts.

In summary, pain, other physical symptoms and psychosocial distress are highly prevalent among patients with cancer, HIV/AIDS, and other serious chronic illnesses in rural Malawi. Patient suffering and caregiver anxiety are exacerbated by poverty and a lack of access to psychosocial support, particularly socioeconomic assistance. However, early results from the NPCP suggest it is possible to provide comprehensive palliative care integrated with disease-modifying treatment in a rural, resource-limited setting through public-private partnership and by establishing a network of community-based village health workers and home-based care volunteers that links households with health centers and hospitals. This network can provide care where most patients live and want services–in their homes–while providing a safety net of facility-based palliative care for patients with severe or refractory symptoms or who lack adequate family support. Further research is needed to assess the effect of comprehensive community-based palliative care on longitudinal patient clinical outcomes, including control of pain and other physical and psychological symptoms, and to assess the cost and scalability of our model. In Neno District, and likely other comparable rural settings in sub-Saharan Africa, palliative care can be improved by integrating palliative care with disease-specific therapies, aggressively treating pain and other symptoms, providing support for caregivers in the home, and pragmatically addressing the issues of poverty that exacerbate symptoms of chronic disease and patient and caregiver distress.

Acknowledgments

The authors acknowledge the contributions of the patients and staff of Neno District Hospital, Lisungwi Community Hospital, Nsambe Health Center, and Matope Health Center. In particular, we thank the District Nursing Officer, Mr. Stanislous Kutsamba, for his important leadership on palliative care in Neno district. The authors also recognize the dedicated front-line service providers and managers of the APZU/PIH Program on Social and Economic Rights (POSER), the APZU/PIH Office of HIV and Nutrition, and the APZU/PIH Village Health Workers Program. The authors thank the many village health workers and home-based care volunteers who make community-based palliative care possible in Neno district. We also thank Mr. Blessings Banda for his help translating important study documents. We acknowledge the local leadership of the Neno District Health Office, the Neno District Commissioner, the Ministry of Gender, Child Development and Community Development, and the Neno Office of Social Welfare for supporting this work and promoting a rights-based approach to comprehensive palliative care in Neno District.

Author Contributions

Conceived and designed the experiments: MEH SNE NK JWK FC JAB LT ELK JR. Performed the experiments: MEH SNE NK JWK EBW AP AM FC JAB LT JB ELK JR. Analyzed the data: MEH SNE JWK EBW. Contributed reagents/materials/analysis tools: MEH SNE JWK EBW FC JB ELK JR. Wrote the paper: MEH SNE JWK ELK.

References

1. Harding R, Higginson IJ (2005) Palliative care in sub-Saharan Africa. Lancet 365(9475): 1971–1977.
2. Temel JS, Greer JA, Muzikansky A, Gallagher ER, Admane S, et al. (2010) Early palliative care for patients with metastatic non-small-cell lung cancer. NEJM 363(8): 733–742.
3. Eramova I, Matic S, Munz M (2007) HIV/AIDS treatment and care: clinical protocols for the WHO European Region. Available: http://www.euro.who.int/__data/assets/pdf_file/0004/78106/E90840.pdf. Accessed 2013 Dec 13.
4. Simms V, Higginson IJ, Harding R (2012) Integration of palliative care throughout HIV disease. Lancet Infect Dis 12: 571–575.
5. Harding R, Simms V, Krakauer E, DeLima L, Downing J, et al. (2011) Quality HIV care to the end of life. Clinical Infectious Diseases 52(4): 553–554.

6. Stjernswärd J, Foley KM, Ferris FD (2007) The public health strategy for palliative care. J Pain Symptom Manage 33: 486–493.
7. World Health Organization (2011) Global status report on noncommunicable diseases 2010. Geneva: World Health Organization. Available: http://whqlibdoc.who.int/publications/2011/9789240686458_eng.pdf. Accessed 2014 Jan 22.
8. Human Rights Watch (9 September 2010). Needless Pain: Government Failure to Provide Palliative Care for Children in Kenya. Human Rights Watch. Available: http://www.hrw.org/reports/2010/09/09/needless-pain-0. Accessed 2014 Jun 26.
9. Lamas D, Rosenbaum L (2012) Painful inequalities–Palliative care in developing countries. N Engl J Med 366(3): 199–201.
10. Grant L, Downing J, Namukwaya E, Leng M, Murray S (2011). Palliative care in Africa since 2005: good progress, but much further to go. BMJ Supportive & Palliative Care 1(2): 118–122.
11. de-Graft Aikins A, Unwin N, Agyemang C, Allotey P, Campbell C, et al. (2010) Tackling Africa's chronic disease burden: from the local to the global. Globalization and Health 6: 5.
12. Kanavos P (2006) The rising burden of cancer in the developing world. Ann Oncol (Suppl 8): viii15–viii23.
13. Government of Malawi Ministry of Health (2011). National Palliative Care Guidelines. Lilongwe: Ministry of Health. 29 p.
14. Ministry of Health, Department of Planning (2004). A joint programme of work for a health sector wide approach (SWAp), 2004–2010. Lilongwe: Government of the Republic of Malawi. Available: http://gametlibrary.worldbank.org/FILES/466_Health%20Sector%20SWAp%20Malawi.pdf. Accessed 2013 Oct 20.
15. Tapfield JB, Bates MJ (2011) Hospital based palliative care in sub-Saharan Africa; a six month review from Malawi. BMC Palliative Care 10: 12.
16. Grant L, Brown J, Leng M, Bettega N, Murray SA (2011) Palliative care in rural Uganda, Kenya and Malawi: three rapid evaluation field studies. BMC Palliative Care 10: 8. Available: http://www.biomedcentral.com/content/pdf/1472-684X-10-8.pdf. Accessed 2012 Mar 25.
17. Finch T (2008) Palliative care in Salima district. Malawi Medical Journal 20(4): 118–119.
18. World Bank (2013). Rural population databank. Washington, D.C.: World Bank. Available: http://data.worldbank.org/indicator/SP.RUR.TOTL.
19. United Nations Joint Programme on HIV and AIDS (UNAIDS) (2013). Global Report: UNAIDS report on the global AIDS epidemic 2013. Geneva: Joint United Nations Programme on HIV/AIDS. Available: http://www.unaids.org/en/media/unaids/contentassets/documents/epidemiology/2013/gr2013/UNAIDS_Global_Report_2013_en.pdf. Accessed 2013 Nov 20.
20. Msyamboza KP, Dzamalala C, Mdokwe C, Kamiza S, Lemerani M, et al. (2012) Burden of cancer in Malawi; common types, incidence and trends: National population-based cancer registry. available care. BMC Research Notes 5: 149. Available: http://www.biomedcentral.com/content/pdf/1756-0500-5-149.pdf. Accessed 2012 Mar 31.
21. Krakauer EL (2008). Just palliative care: responding responsibly to the suffering of the poor. J Pain Symptom Manage 36(5): 505–512.
22. Bruera E, De Lima L, Wenk R, Farr W (2004) In: Palliative care in developing countries: principles and practice. Houston: IAHPC Press. 9, 23–37.
23. Murray SA, Grant E, Grant A, Kendall M (2003) Dying from cancer in developed and developing countries: lessons from two qualitative interview studies of patients and their carers. BMJ 326(7385): 368.
24. Wright M, Clark M (2006) Hospice and palliative care in Africa: a review of development and challenges. Oxford: Oxford University Press. 528 p.
25. Selman L, Simms V, Penfold S, Powell RA, Mwangi-Powell F, et al. (2013) 'My dreams are shuttered down and it hurts lots'–a qualitative study of palliative care needs and their management by HIV outpatient services in Kenya and Uganda. BMC Palliat Care 12: 35.
26. Wakeham K, Harding R, Bamukama-Namakoola D, Levin J, Kissa J, et al. (2010) Symptom burden in HIV-infected adults at time of HIV diagnosis in rural Uganda. J Palliat Med 13(4): 375–380.
27. Dekker AM, Amon JJ, le Roux KW, Gaunt CB (2012) "What is killing me most": Chronic pain and the need for palliative care in the Eastern Cape, South Africa. J Pain Palliat Care Pharmacother 26(2): 334–340.
28. Harding R, Powell RA, Downing J, Connor SR, Mwangi-Powell F, et al. (2008) Generating an African palliative care evidence base: the context, need, challenges, and strategies. J Pain Symptom Manage 36(3): 304–309.
29. Powell RA, Harding R, Namisango E, Katabira E, Gwyther L, et al. (2013) Palliative care research in Africa: Consensus building for a prioritized agenda. J Pain Symptom Manage. doi:10.1016/j.jpainsymman.2013.03.022.
30. Anker M, Guidotti RJ, Orzeszyna S, Sapirie SA, Thuriaux MC (1993) Rapid evaluation methods (REM) of health services performance: methodological observations. Bull World Health Organ 71(1): 15–21.
31. Annett H, Rifkin SB (1995). Guidelines for rapid participatory appraisals to assess community health needs: A focus on health improvements for low-income urban and rural areas. Geneva: World Health Organization. 60 p.
32. Anker M (1991) Epidemiological and statistical methods for rapid health assessment introduction. World Health Statistics Quarterly 44: 94–97.
33. Neno District Executive Committee (2013) Neno District Socioeconomic Profile: 2013. Neno, Malawi: Ministry of Local Government and Rural Development. 86 p.
34. World Bank (2007) Malawi poverty and vulnerability assessment: Investing in our future. Washington, D.C.: World Bank. 304 p.
35. Murray SA, Tapson J, Turnbull L, McCallum J, Little A (1994) Listening to local voices: adapting rapid appraisal to assess health and social needs in general practice. BMJ 308: 698–700.
36. Wolfe BA, Mamlin BW, Biondich PG, Fraser HSF, Jazayeri D, et al. (2006) The OpenMRS system: Collaborating toward an open source EMR for developing countries. AMIA Annual Symposium Proceedings 1146.
37. Powell RA, Downing J, Harding R, Mwangi-Powell F, Connor S (2007) Development of the APCA African Palliative Outcome Scale. Journal of Pain and Symptom Management 33(2): 229–232.
38. Harding R, Selman L, Simms VM, Penfold S, Agupio G, et al. (2013) How to analyze palliative care outcomes data for patients in sub-Saharan Africa: An international, multicenter, factor analytic examination of the APCA African POS. J Pain Symptom Manage 45(4): 746–752.
39. Harding R, Selman L, Agupio G, Dinat N, Downing J, et al. (2010) Validation of a core outcome measure for palliative care in Africa: the APCA African Palliative Outcome Scale. Health and Quality of Life Outcomes 8: 10. doi:10.1186/1477-7525-8-10.
40. African Palliative Care Association (2010) Beating pain: A pocket guide for pain management in Africa. Kampala: African Palliative Care Association. 99 p. Available: http://apps.who.int/medicinedocs/documents/s19114en/s19114en.pdf. Accessed 2014 Jun 28.
41. Government of Malawi Ministry of Health (2011) Introduction to palliative care: Health Care Workers' Service Providers Manual. Lilongwe: Ministry of Health. 136 p. Available: http://palliativecareassociationofmalawi.org/media/data/palliative_care_service_providers_manual_for_health_care_workers.pdf. Accessed 2014 Jun 26.
42. Government of Malawi Ministry of Health (2009) Palliative Care Training Manual for Home Based Care Volunteers in Malawi. Lilongwe: Ministry of Health. 56 p.
43. Government of Malawi Ministry of Health (2011) Malawi Guidelines for the Clinical Management of HIV in Children and Adults. Lilongwe: Ministry of Health. 79 p.
44. Arnold BL (2011) Mapping hospice patients' perceptions and verbal communication of end-of-life needs: an exploratory mixed methods inquiry. BMC palliative care 10: 1.
45. Fleming DA, Sheppard VB, Mangan PA, Taylor KL, Tallarico M, et al. (2006) Caregiving at the end of life: Perceptions of health care quality and quality of life among patients and caregivers. Journal of pain and symptom management 31(5): 407–420.
46. Tong A, Sainsbury P, Craig J (2007) Consolidated criteria for reporting qualitative research (COREQ): a 32-item checklist for interviews and focus groups. Int J Qual Health Care 19(6): 349–357.
47. Krakauer EL, Minh Ngoc NT, Green K, Van Kham L, Ngoc Khue L (2007) Vietnam: integrating palliative care into HIV/AIDS and cancer care. J Pain and Symptom Manage 33(5): 578–583.
48. Krakauer EL, Phuong Cham NT, Ngoc Khue L (2010) Vietnam's palliative care initiative: successes and challenges in the first five years. J Pain Symptom Manage 40(1): 27–30. doi:10.1016/j.jpainsymman.2010.04.009.
49. Mlombe Y (2008) Management of HIV associated Kaposi's sarcoma in Malawi. Malawi Med J 20(4): 129–132.
50. Robinson CA, Pesut B, Bottorff JL, Mowry A, Broughton S, et al. (2009) Rural palliative care: a comprehensive review. J Palliat Med 12(3): 253–258.
51. Di Sorbo PG, Chifamba DD, Mastrojohn J, Sisimayi CN, Williams SH (2010) The Zimbabwe rural palliative care initiative: PCI-Z. J Pain Symptom Manage 40(1): 19–22.
52. Nanney E, Smith S, Hartwig K, Mmbando P (2010) Scaling up palliative care services in rural Tanzania. J Pain Symptom Manage 40(1): 15–18.
53. Harding R, Selman L, Agupio G, Dinat N, Downing J, et al. (2012) Prevalence, burden, and correlates of physical and psychological symptoms among HIV palliative care patients in Sub-Saharan Africa: An international multicenter study. J Pain Symptom Manage 44(1): 1–9.
54. Makoae LN, Seboni NM, Molosiwa K, Moleko M, Human S, et al. (2005) The symptom experience of people living with HIV/AIDS in Southern Africa. J Assoc Nurses AIDS Care 16(3): 22–32.
55. Peltzer K, Phaswana-Mafuya N (2008) The symptom experience of people living with HIV and AIDS in the Eastern Cape, South Africa. BMC Health Serv Res 8: 271.
56. Jagwe J, Merriman A (2007) Uganda: Delivering analgesia in rural Africa: Opioid availability and nurse prescribing. J Pain Symptom Manage 33(5): 547–551.
57. Grant E, Murray SA, Grant A, Brown J. (2003) A good death in rural Kenya? Listening to Meru patients and their families talk about care needs at the end of life. J Palliat Care 19(3): 159–67.
58. Olenja JM. (1999) Assessing community attitude towards home-based care for people with AIDS (PWAs) in Kenya. J Community Health 24: 187–199.

Effusanin E Suppresses Nasopharyngeal Carcinoma Cell Growth by Inhibiting NF-κB and COX-2 Signaling

Mingzhu Zhuang[1], Mouming Zhao[1,3], Huijuan Qiu[2], Dingbo Shi[2], Jingshu Wang[2], Yun Tian[2], Lianzhu Lin[1]*, Wuguo Deng[2]*

1 College of Light Industry and Food Sciences, South China University of Technology, Guangzhou, China, **2** State Key Laboratory of Oncology in South China, Sun Yat-Sen University Cancer Center, Guangzhou, China, **3** State Key Laboratory of Pulp and Paper Engineering, South China University of Technology, Guangzhou, China

Abstract

Rabdosia serra is well known for its antibacterial, anti-inflammatory and antitumor activities, but no information has been available for the active compounds derived from this plant in inhibiting human nasopharyngeal carcinoma (NPC) cell growth. In this study, we isolated and purified a natural diterpenoid from *Rabdosia serra* and identified its chemical structure as effusanin E and elucidated its underlying mechanism of action in inhibiting NPC cell growth. Effusanin E significantly inhibited cell proliferation and induced apoptosis in NPC cells. Effusanin E also induced the cleavage of PARP, caspase-3 and -9 proteins and inhibited the nuclear translocation of p65 NF-κB proteins. Moreover, effusanin E abrogated the binding of NF-κB to the COX-2 promoter, thereby inhibiting the expression and promoter activity of COX-2. Pretreatment with a COX-2 or NF-κB-selective inhibitor (celecoxib or ammonium pyrrolidinedithiocarbamate) had an additive effect on the effusanin E-mediated inhibition of proliferation, while pretreatment with an activator of NF-κB/COX-2 (lipopolysaccharides) abrogated the effusanin E-mediated inhibition of proliferation. Effusanin E also significantly suppressed tumor growth in a xenograft mouse model without obvious toxicity, furthermore, the expression of p50 NF-κB and COX-2 were down-regulated in the tumors of nude mice. These data suggest that effusanin E suppresses p50/p65 proteins to down-regulate COX-2 expression, thereby inhibiting NPC cell growth. Our findings provide new insights into exploring effusanin E as a potential therapeutic compound for the treatment of human nasopharyngeal carcinoma.

Editor: Peiwen Fei, University of Hawaii Cancer Center, United States of America

Funding: This work was supported by funds from the National Natural Science Foundation of China (81071687, 81272195), the State "863 Program" of China (SS2012AA0204030), the Doctoral Programs Foundation of Ministry of Education of China (20110171110077), and the State Key Laboratory of Oncology in Southern China and Fundamental Research Funds for the Central Universities (Project No. 2014ZB0010). The funders had no role in study design, data collection and analysis, decision to publish, or preparation of the manuscript.

Competing Interests: The authors have declared that no competing interests exist.

* Email: felzlin@scut.edu.cn (LL); dengwg@sysucc.org.cn (WD)

Introduction

Nasopharyngeal carcinoma (NPC) is a relatively uncommon, malignant, head and neck cancer that is found worldwide but is highly prevalent in South China and Southeast Asia [1]. It frequently occurs in the Guangdong area, China, where the annual incidence reaches 25 cases per 100,000 [2]. A combination of radiotherapy and adjuvant chemotherapy is now the standard treatment for NPC. However, the 5-year survival rate is only 50–60% due to the frequency of distant metastasis and local recurrence and the long-term secondary effects of radiotherapy and chemotherapy [3]. In addition, these methods may sometimes cause severe acute toxicity and even increased incidence of late complications without obvious survival benefits [4]. Currently, the use of natural, synthetic or biologic chemicals has been considered as effective cancer chemopreventions in the prevention, suppression or delay of the carcinogenesis process [5].

The plant *Rabdosia serra* (*R. serra*), which is called Xihuangcao in Chinese, has been used in traditional Chinese medicine for centuries as a characteristic plant resource in south China. The genus *R. serra* is well known for its antibacterial, antiviral, anti-inflammatory and antitumor activities [6], is a rich source of diterpenoids and is widely distributed in China. It has been shown that some chemicals isolated from this plant have inhibitory effects on cancer cell growth in vitro and tumor growth in vivo. The strong cytotoxicities of diterpenoids isolated from *R. serra*, such as nodosin, oridonin and lasiokaurin, against human cancer cells were verified in previous investigations. Diterpenoid could effectively reduce the accumulation of COX-2 protein to exhibit cytotoxicity against cancer cells [7]. It also has been shown that diterpenoids (quercetin and oridonin) derived from I. Japonicus exerted its anticancer properties by regulating the NF-κB signaling pathways [8-10]. Additionally, it is known that effusanin C inhibits inflammatory responses via blocking NF-κB signaling in monocytes [11].

COX-2 is an inducible enzyme that plays a critical role in multiple pathophysiological processes such as inflammation, atherosclerosis, tissue injury, angiogenesis and tumorigenesis [12,13]. COX-2 is chronically overexpressed in many premalignant, malignant, and metastatic human cancers, and its expression is tightly controlled by the binding of multiple transactivators such as NF-κB. The transcription factor NF-κB includes two important members: p50 and p65. NF-κB regulates the transcription of a large number of genes, particularly those involved in immune, inflammatory and antiapoptotic responses [14]. The well-known anti-inflammatory substances such as glucocorticoids or nonsteroidal antiinflammatory drugs (NSAIDs) exert at least a portion of their effects by inhibiting NF-κB activity [15–17].

In this study, we isolated and identified effusanin E from *R. Serra* and analyzed its anticancer activity and elucidated the underlying mechanisms of its antitumor activities in NPC cells.

Results

Isolation and identification of effusanin E from *R. serra*

Effusanin E was purified and characterized according to our previous report [18] and obtained as a white, amorphous powder. HPLC analysis showed that the compound purified from *R. Serra* was pure (Fig. 1A). The mass spectrum (MS) and ^{1}H and ^{13}C NMR assays identified the chemical structure of the compound as effusanin E (Fig. 1B). Based on our data previously reported [18], the amount of effusanin E ranked second to rosmarinic acid and higher than other diterpenoids in *R. serra*, so effusanin E was one of the main substance from *R. Serra* [18]. The data of mass spectrum and ^{1}H and ^{13}C NMR of effusanin E were indicated below. Positive ESI MS m/z 387.1 $[M+Na]^+$; ^{1}H NMR (400 MHz, DMSO-d_6): δ: 6.36 (1H, s, OH-7), 6.06 (1H, d, J = 10.3 Hz, OH-6), 5.78 (1H, s, H-17a), 5.50 (1H, s, H-17b), 5.34 (1H, d, J = 6.3 Hz, OH-11), 5.16 (1H, d, J = 4.5 Hz, OH-1), 4.33 (1H, m, H-11), 4.06 (1H, d, J = 10.4 Hz, H-20a), 3.87 (1H, dd, J = 1.74 Hz, J = 10.4 Hz, H-20b), 3.66 (1H, m, H-1), 3.58 (1H, dd, J = 5.9 Hz, J = 10.2 Hz, H-6), 3.10 (1H, dd, J = 4.1 Hz, J = 9.9 Hz, H-13), 2.60 (1H, m, H-12e), 2.12 (1H, d, J = 12.4 Hz, H-14e), 1.89 (1H, dd, J = 4.2 Hz, J = 12.4 Hz, H-14a), 1.54 (2H, m, H2-2), 1.43-1.38 (2H, m, H-3e and H-9), 1.24-1.19 (2H, m, H-3a and H-12a), 1.13 (1H, d, J = 5.6 Hz, H-5), 1.03 (3H, s, Me-18), 1.00 (3H, s, Me-19); ^{13}C NMR (100 MHz, DMSO-d_6): δ: 210.8 (C-15), 153.3 (C-16), 116.7 (C-17), 94.9 (C-7), 73.3 (C-6), 72.5 (C-1), 63.7 (C-20), 62.5 (C-11), 60.6 (C-5), 59.4 (C-8), 56.9 (C-9), 42.0 (C-10), 39.4 (C-3), 34.3 (C-13), 34.2 (C-4), 33.1 (C-19), 27.9 (C-2), 26.9 (C-14), 22.6 (C-18).

Effusanin E inhibited cell proliferation

The effect of effusanin E on the proliferation of NPC cells was investigated using MTS and colony formation assays. The result of the MTS assay showed that CNE1 and CNE2 cell viabilities were inhibited in a concentration-dependent manner in the presence of effusanin E while normal cell line NP69 cell viability was not affected (Fig. 1C). In addition, NPC cells became round, shrunken and detached from adjacent cells after 24 hours of treatment with effusanin E (Fig. 2A). To evaluate the long-term effects of effusanin E on NPC cell proliferation, colony formation was also carried out. The colony size (Fig. 2B) and number (Fig. 2C) were reduced by effusanin E in a dose-dependent manner. These results indicate that effusanin E inhibits cancer cell proliferation.

Effusanin E induced apoptosis

To determine whether the cytotoxic effect of effusanin E was mediated via apoptosis, annexin V-FITC/PI double staining was performed. As shown in Fig. 3A and Fig. 3B, the percentage of apoptotic NPC cells increased from approximately 0.8% to 20.3% in CNE1, and from 0.0% to 20.2% in CNE2 after treatment with effusanin E from 0 μM to 250 μM.

We speculated that effusanin E affected the level of apoptotic genes. We therefore measured the expression of cleaved caspase-3/9 and cleaved PARP as well as pro- caspase-3/9 and PARP, and found that the expression of these apoptotic, cleaved proteins were increased significantly while the expression of pro-caspase-3/9 and PARP were decreased in NPC cells that were treated with effusanin E (Fig. 3C).

Effusanin E inhibited COX-2 expression and promoter activity

COX-2 is an inducible enzyme that plays a critical role in multiple pathophysiological processes such as inflammation, atherosclerosis, tissue injury, angiogenesis and tumorigenesis. Effusanin E has antibacterial, antiviral, anti-inflammatory and antitumor activities. Therefore, we verified that effusanin E inhibited COX-2 expression and found that effusanin E decreased the expression of COX-2 (Fig. 4A).

We first determined the effects of effusanin E on COX-2 promoter activity. We transfected NPC cells with a luciferase expression vector containing a 459-bp, COX-2 5-flanking fragment. The results indicated that the promoter activity was comparably inhibited by effusanin E in a dose-dependent manner in CNE2 cells (Fig. 4B).

To validate the role of effusanin E in regulating COX-2 signaling, we analyzed the effect of effusanin E on inhibition of cell proliferation by celecoxib, which is a COX-2-selective inhibitor. Pretreatment of the cells with this COX-2-selective inhibitor (20 μM or 50 μM) dramatically affected the effusanin E-mediated inhibition of proliferation at 24 hours and 48 hours after treatment (Fig. 4C).

Effusanin E inhibited NF-κB signaling pathway

Many studies have demonstrated that diverse inflammatory processes are regulated through NF-κB signaling. NF-κB pathways are known to promote proinflammatory cytokine gene expression, and previous studies showed that COX-2 expression is tightly controlled by the binding of multiple transactivators such as NF-κB. We further examined whether the inhibition of COX-2 signaling by effusanin E was mediated through NF-κB signaling in NPC cells. We determined the expression of p50/p65. As shown in Fig. 5A, effusanin E effectively blocked the expression of p50 but did not alter the expression of p65. We then pretreated NPC cells with PDTC (100 μM), a NF-κB-selective inhibitor, after effusanin E had been added at 125 μM and 250 μM for 8 hours. After 24 hours or 48 hours, the cell viabilities of the PDTC-alone and PDTC with effusanin E-treated cells were nearly the same. The results indicated that effusanin E significantly altered PDTC-mediated inhibition of NF-κB signaling (Fig. 5C).

NF-κB/COX-2 can be activated by LPS; therefore, we evaluated the effect of effusanin E on NF-κB/COX-2 activated by LPS. We pretreated NPC cells with LPS (2 μg/ml) for 8 hours and then with effusanin E at 125 μM and 250 μM. 24 hours or 48 hours later, the effect of effusanin E was strongly blocked at a concentration of 125 μM, which was consistent with the effect by LPS, and cell viabilities of cells treated with effusanin E and LPS at 250 μM were higher than those treated with effusanin E alone (250 μM) (Fig. 5D). These results showed that the effect of effusanin E toward NPC cells was greatly offset by LPS.

We then found reduced nuclear translocation of p65 in NPC cells by immunofluorescence imaging (Fig. 5E). Therefore, we determined whether the effusanin E-induced suppression of cell proliferation and COX-2 expression was mediated by inhibition of the binding of NF-κB to the COX-2 promoter in NPC cells. We analyzed the binding of p50 and p65 NF-κB to a biotin-labeled, 479-bp COX-2 promoter region that corresponded to its 5-flanking sequence by streptavidin-agarose pulldown assays, and we confirmed that the expression of p50/p65 was decreased (Fig. 5B). These results indicated that effusanin E suppressed COX-2 promoter activity by inhibiting p50/p65 binding to the COX-2 promoter, thus leading to decreased cell survival, and proliferation of NPC cells. These results demonstrate the antitumor effects that are exerted by effusanin E through the modulation of the NF-κB/

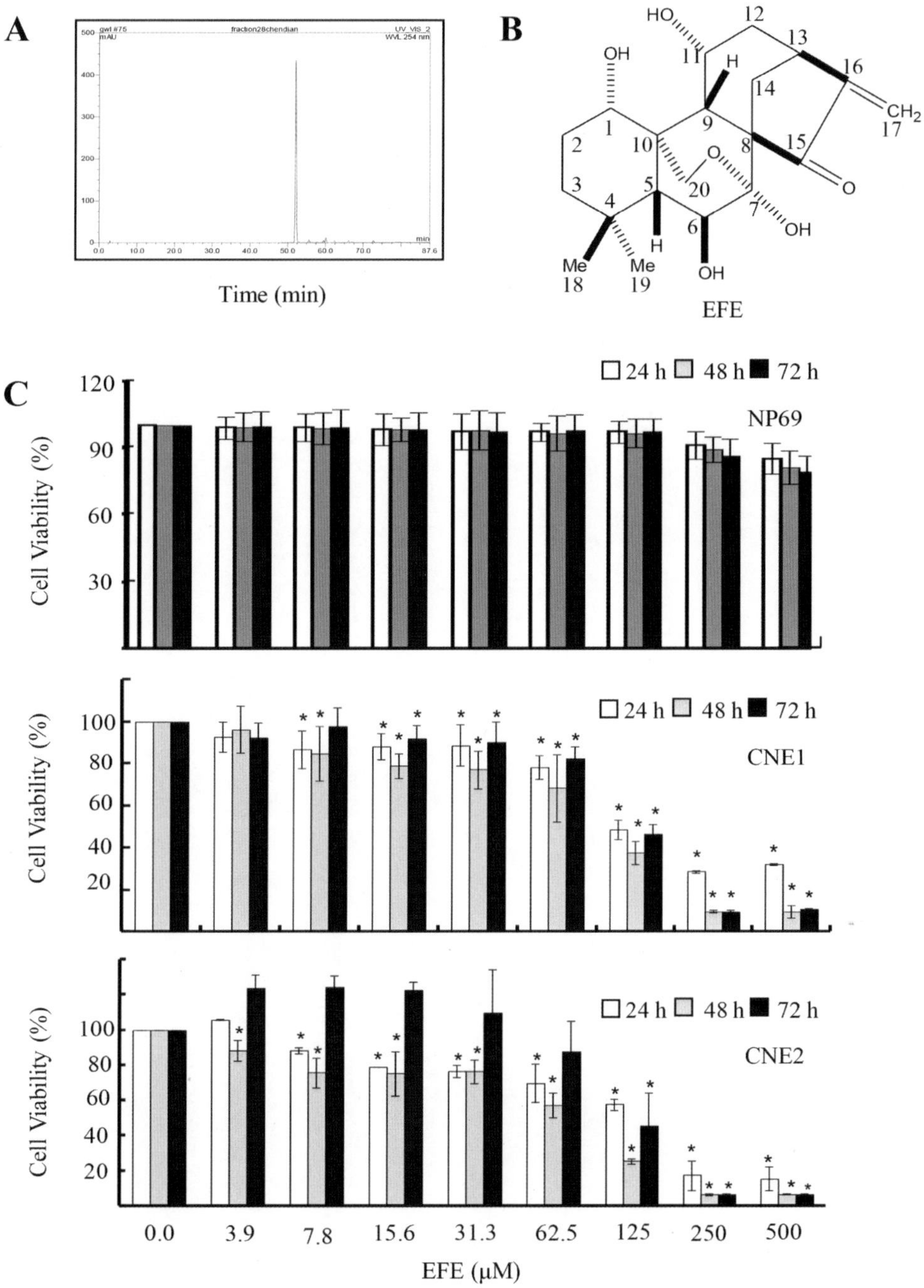

Figure 1. Purification and identification of effusanin E from *R. serra*. (**A**) HPLC analysis of effusanin E. (**B**) The structure of effusanin E (EFE). (**C**) Human CNE1 and CNE2 were treated with effusanin E (EFE) at 3.9–500 μM for 24 hours, 48 hours and 72 hours. The viability of the cells was determined using the MTS assay. Cells treated with the vehicle control (DMSO) were used as the reference group, with its cell viability set at 100%. The percent cell viability of each treatment group was calculated relative to that of cells treated with the vehicle control. The data are presented as the mean ± SD of three separate experiments. * represent $P<0.05$.

COX-2 signaling pathways in Human Nasopharyngeal Carcinomas.

Effusanin E inhibited tumor growth in a xenograft mouse model

To directly evaluate the effect of effusanin E on tumors in vivo, tumor growth of CNE2 cells in nude mice were tested using a tumor xenograft model. When the tumors became palpable (~200 mm^3), the mice were treated with either a vehicle control or effusanin E at 10.0 mg/kg/d or 30.0 mg/kg/d for 30 days. The results showed that tumor growth was decreased and slower after effusanin E treatment when compared with the vehicle control. During the analysis, no significant weight changes in the mice were observed (Fig. 6B). These results suggest that effusanin E did not induce significant weight loss and had no obvious toxicity. Greater and heavier in vivo tumor formation and volume were observed in the control mice compared to mice treated with effusanin E (Fig. 6A). After the mice were sacrificed, the tumors were removed

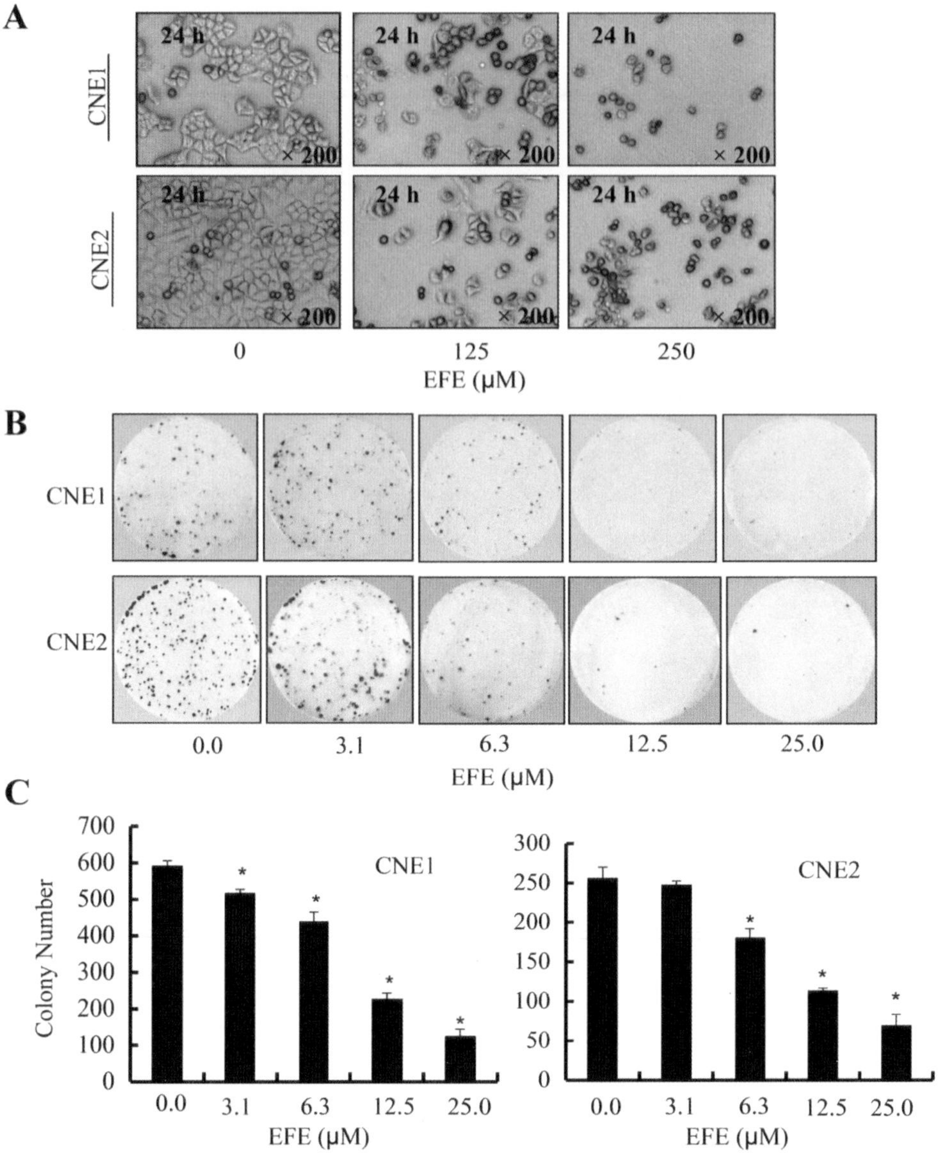

Figure 2. Effusanin E inhibits proliferation of NPC cells in vitro. (**A**) The cell morphology changes of human CNE1 and CNE2 cells after treatment with effusanin E (EFE) at 125 μM or 250 μM. (**B**) Colony formation assay of human CNE1 and CNE2 cells treated with effusanin E (EFE) at 3.1–25.0 μM. Cells were cultured as indicated in 6-well plates and treated with effusanin E for 10 days. After treament, the cells were dyed with crystal violet and took pictures. (**C**) The number of colony formation assay. The grown colonies of colony formation assay were scored. The data are presented as the mean ± SD of three separate experiments. * represent $P<0.05$.

from the mice and pictures were taken. The weight of the tumors was showed in Fig. 6C. Thus, effusanin E was able to inhibit the growth of NPC tumor in vivo. Furthermore, the expression of COX-2 and p50 were downregulated in the tumor, while the expression of p65 did not alter (Fig. 6D), these results are consistent with cell study.

Discussion

In this study, we demonstrate that effusanin E inhibited the proliferation and induced apoptosis of NPC cells in vitro. Our study showed that effusanin E inhibited NF-κB signaling, furthermore, effusanin E reduced the tumor volume and weight of treament mice compared with the control group. In detail, effusanin E inhibited the p50 protein level and reduced nuclear translocation of p65. Pretreatment with a NF-κB-selective inhibitor had an additive effect on the effusanin E-mediated inhibition of proliferation and the nuclear translocation of p65, while pretreatment with LPS abrogated the effusanin E-mediated inhibition of proliferation. We also found that effusanin E suppressed COX-2 promoter activity and inhibited p50/p65 binding to the COX-2 promoter, thus leading to decreased cell proliferation, and induced apoptosis. Also effusanin E stimulated PARP, caspase-3 and -9 cleavages. To our knowledge, this is the first report that demonstrated effusanin E-exerted antitumor effects through the modulation of NF-κB signaling pathways and induced apotosis in NPC cells.

The use of celecoxib is associated with a significant decrease in many cancer risk, including nasopharyngeal carcinoma. However, the long-term use of high-dose celecoxib might be limited owing to

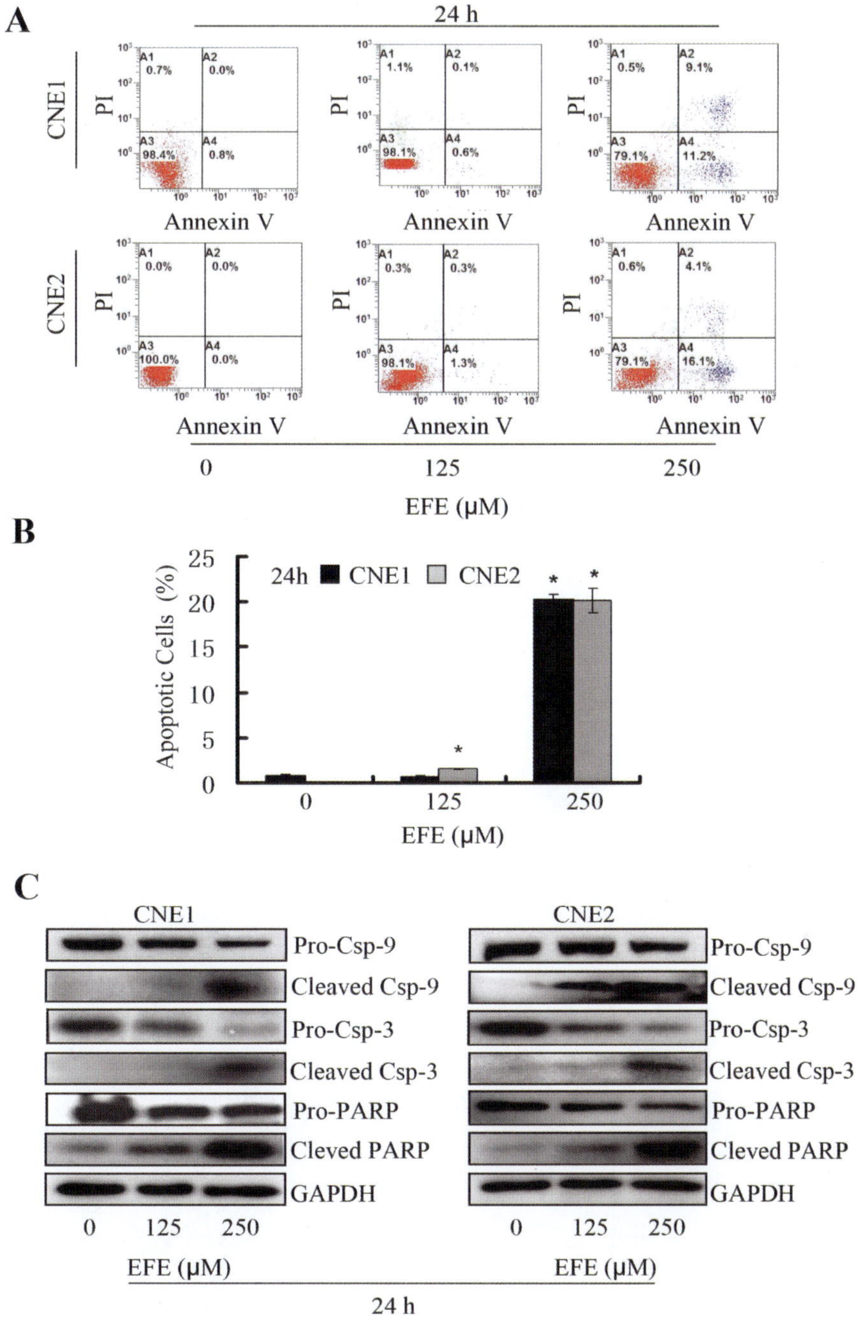

Figure 3. Effusanin E induced apoptosis. (**A**) Effusanin E (EFE) induced NPC cells apoptosis. Apoptosis was analyzed using TUNEL-based, fluorescence-activated cell sorter analysis and was represented by the relative percentages of TUNEL-positive cells versus those of DMSO-treated cells. (**B**) The percentages of apoptotic cells were calculated. (**C**) Western blotting of cleaved caspase-3, caspase-9 and PARP proteins in NPC cells. Total proteins isolated from the indicated cells were blotted with antibodies as labeled, and GAPDH was used as a control for sample loading.

cardiovascular side effects [19]. In this study, we found that effusanin E, extract from a Chinese herb, could reduce celecoxib dose and potentiate the growth-inhibitory effect in NPC cells.

The expression of COX-2 plays a key role in inflammatory disorders and cancers [20]. COX-2 expression is strongly correlated with prognosis in some cancers [21]. COX-2 inhibition may result in cell-growth suppression and apoptosis. A core promoter region that lies within 500 bp from the COX-2 transcription start site harbors several regulatory elements, notably the cyclic adenosine monophosphate response element, CCAAT/enhancer binding protein enhancer element and NF-κB binding sites, which are essential for COX-2 promoter activity in response to inflammatory signals [22]. The most abundant NF-κB dimer is the p65/p50 heterodimer followed by the p50/p50 and the p65/p65 homodimer complexes [23,24]. Aberrant regulation of NF-κB affects all six hallmarks of cancer through the regulation of genes that are associated with cell proliferation, angiogenesis, metastasis, tumor promotion, inflammation and the suppression of apoptosis [25]. Currently, a large number of natural compounds have been reported as NF-κB inhibitors [26,27]. It is known that oridonin,

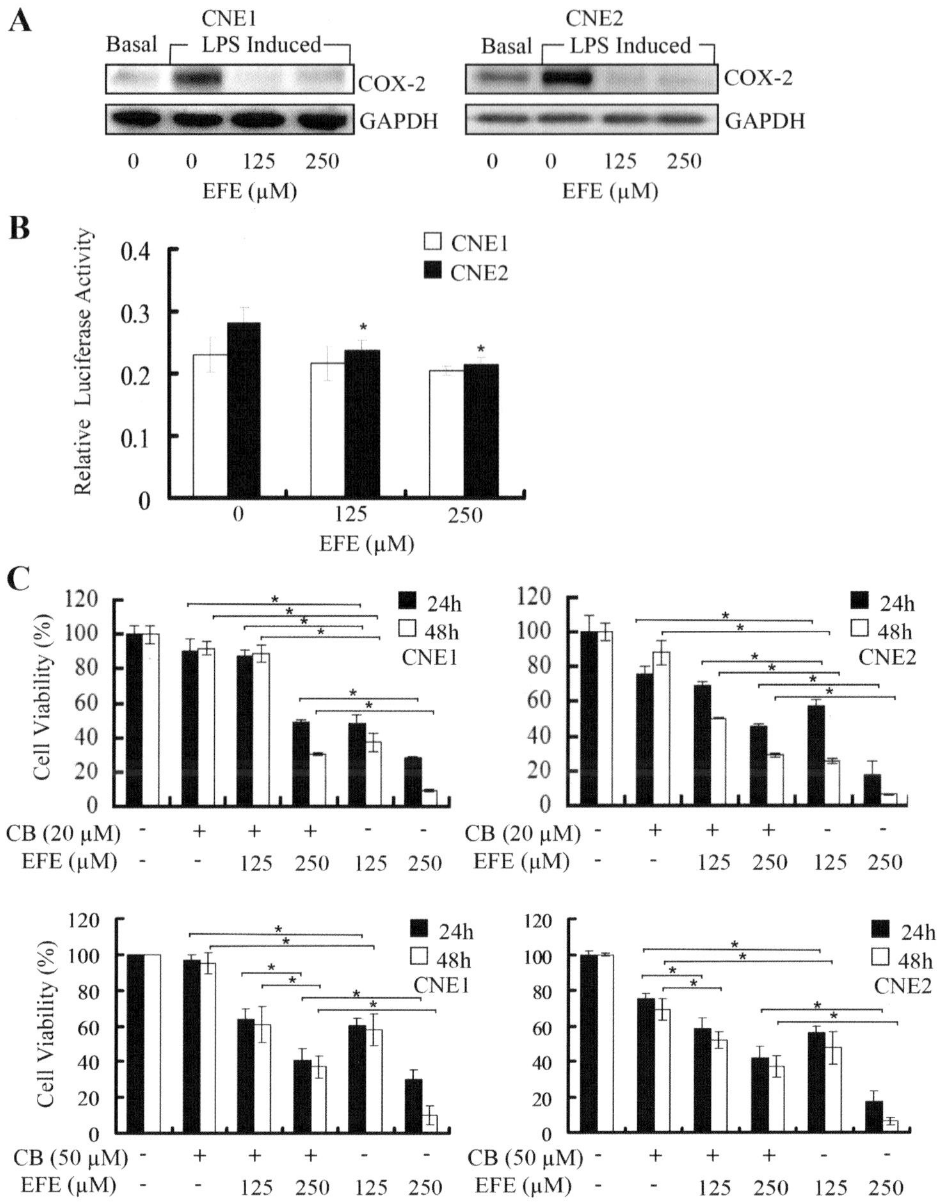

Figure 4. Effusanin E affects activity of the COX-2 pathway. (**A**) NPC cells were pretreated with lipopolysaccharides (LPS) (2 μg/ml) for 8 hours then treated with effusanin E at 125 μM and 250 μM (EFE 125 μM or EFE 250 μM). At 24 hours after treatment, COX-2 protein expression was determined by western blotting. (**B**) NPC cells were transfected with a luciferase expression vector containing a COX-2 5-flanking fragment for 8 hours and treated with effusanin E (EFE) at the indicated doses. At 24 hours after treatment, COX-2 promoter activities were determined. (**C**) The effect of effusanin E was inhibited by an inhibitor of COX-2 in NPC cells. NPC cells were treated with celecoxib (CB) (20 μM or 50 μM) for 8 hours followed by effusanin E at 125 μM and 250 μM (EFE 125 μM or EFE 250 μM) for up to 24 hours or 48 hours. At the indicated time points, the cells were analyzed using the MTS assay. The data are presented as the mean ± S.D. of three separate experiments. * represent $P<0.05$.

ponicidin (two 7,20-epoxy-*ent*-kaurenoids), xindongnin A and xindongnin B (two C-20-nonoxygenated-*ent*-kauranoids) could be potential inhibitors of NF-κB transcription activity by inhibiting the NF-κB DNA-binding activity and the expression of its downstream target COX-2 [28], this finding was consistent with our results . It is well known that p65 is a critical transactivation subunit of NF-κB [29,30], and our study showed that effusanin E apparently blocked with translocation of p65, which is supported by the report that oridonin, ponicidin, and kamebakaurin have an impact on the translocation of p65 to different degrees. It also had been reported that diterpenoids (oridonin) derived from I. Japonicus exert its anti-cancer properties by regulating NF-κB signaling pathways [8–10], which support our result suggesting that diterpenoids are a new class of NF-κB inhibitor. Moreover, it is known that effusanin C inhibits inflammatory responses via blocking NF-κB signaling in monocytes [11], which confirms that effusanin E could inhibit tumor cells by targeting NF-κB. To confirm the COX-2/NF-κB signaling pathway was involved in the effusanin E-mediated inhibition of cell viability, we pretreated the cells with COX-2 or NF-κB inhibitor (CB or PDTC) for 8 h, and then treated with effusanin E for 24 h. The results showed that the combined treatment of CB or PDTC with effusanin E did not

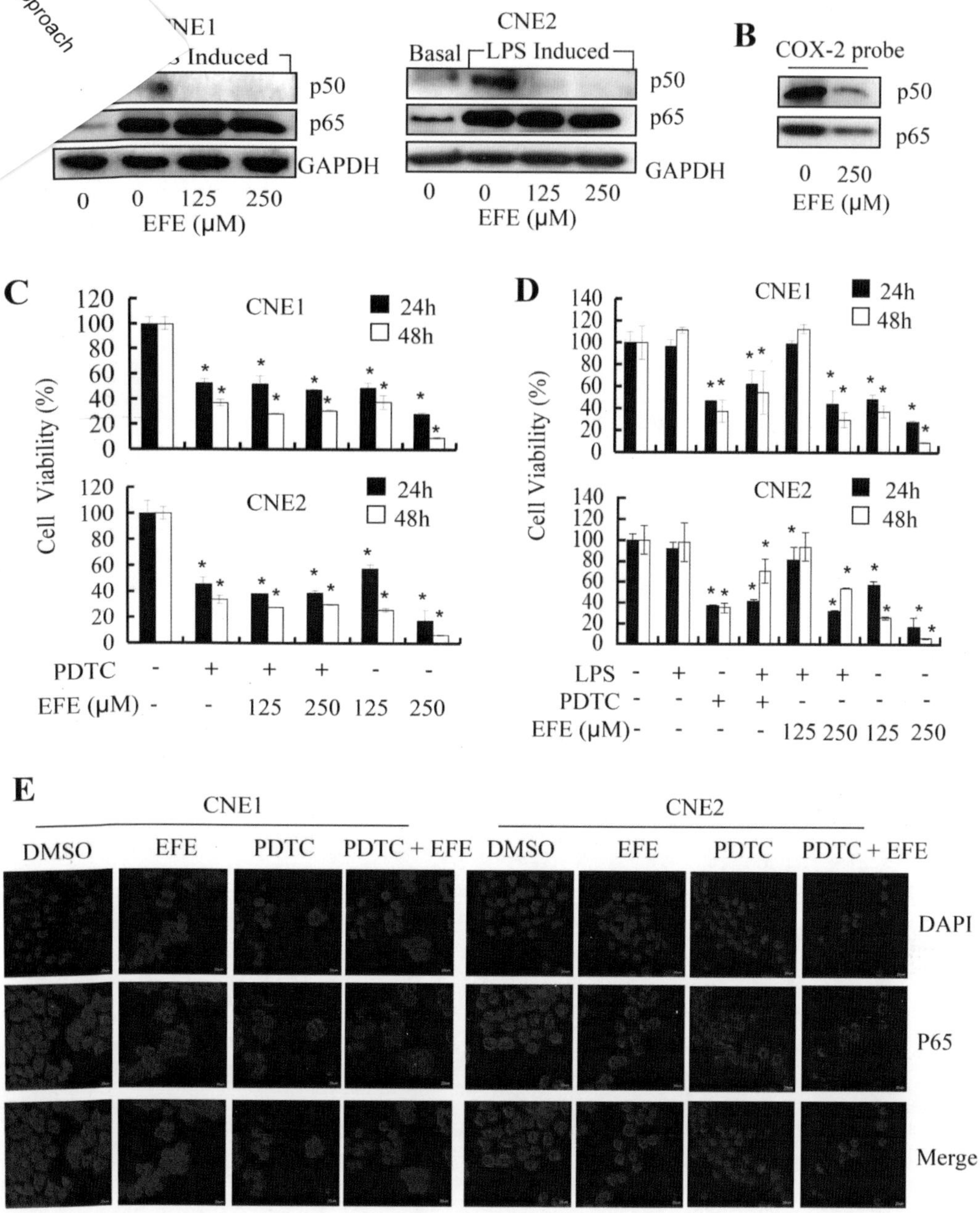

Figure 5. Effusanin E affects the activity of the NF-κB pathway. (**A**) Effusanin E inhibited the expression of p50 and p65. NPC cells were treated with DMSO (basal) or LPS (2 μg/ml) for 8 hours followed by effusanin E treatment at125 μM or 250 μM (EFE 125 μM or EFE 250 μM) for up to 24 hours. At the indicated time points, the cells were detected by Western blot analysis. (**B**) The binding of p50 and p65 NF-κB to the biotin-labeled, COX-2 promoter probe was analyzed by streptavidin-agarose pulldown assays, and the levels of p50 and p65 protein expression were detected by Western blot analysis. (**C**) The effect of effusanin E was inhibited by an inhibitor of NF-κB in NPC cells. NPC cells were treated with PDTC (100 μM) for 8 hours followed by effusanin E at 125 μM and 250 μM (EFE 125 μM or EFE 250 μM) treatment for up to 24 hours or 48 hours. At the indicated time points, the cells were analyzed using the MTS assay. (**D**) The effect of effusanin E was blocked by an activator of NF-κB. NPC cells were treated with LPS (2 μg/ml) or ammonium pyrrolidinedithiocarbamate (PDTC) (100 μM) for 8 hours followed by effusanin E at125 μM or 250 μM (EFE 125 μM or EFE 250 μM) treatment for up to 24 hours or 48 hours. At the indicated time points, the cells were analyzed using the MTS assay. (**E**) Analysis of the reduced nuclear translocation of NF-κB p65 by immunofluorescence imaging (IFI). CNE1 and CNE2 cells were treated with effusanin E at 125 μM (EFE) or PDTC (100 μM) or PDTC (100 μM) for 8 hours followed by effusanin E at 125 μM (PDTC + EFE), and NF-κB nuclear translocation in CNE1 and CNE2 cells was determined by immunofluorescence imaging analysis. * represent $P<0.05$.

significantly increase the inhibition of cell viability as compared with the effusanin E alone. This maybe because pretreatment with CB or PDTC effectively abrogated or completely blocked the COX-2 and NF-κB signaling, and while effusanin E (125 μM or 250 μM) was added after CB or PDTC treatment, effusanin E at this concentration could not function to inhibit cell viability by suppressing the COX-2 and NF-κB signaling. These results suggested that effusanin E inhibits tumor cell growth partially through the inhibition of the NF-κB/COX-2 signaling pathway in NPC cell signaling pathways. *R. serra* is famous for its

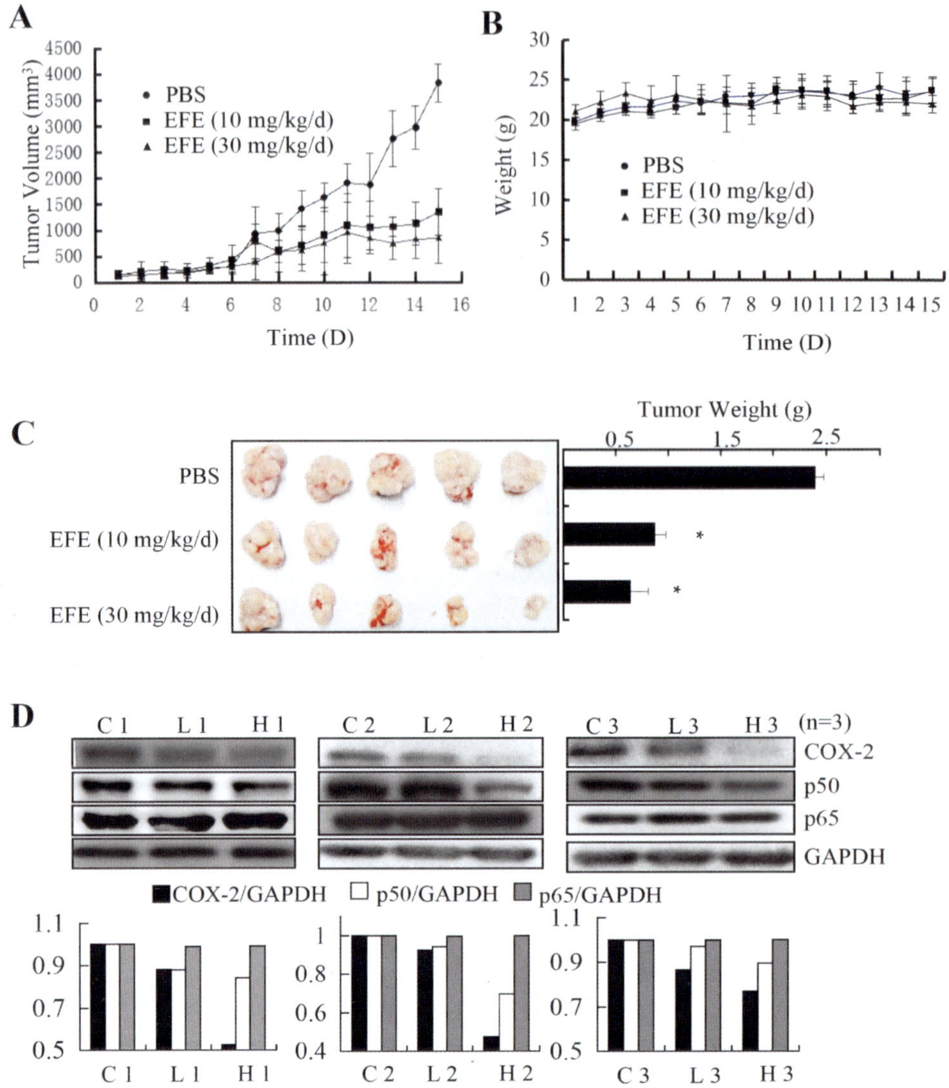

Figure 6. Effusanin E suppressed tumor growth in a human NPC nude mice model. (**A**) Tumor volumes measured *in situ* and images of the mice that were treated with the negative control (20 µl DMSO and 80 µl PBS) or effusanin E (EFE) at the indicated doses. The mice were randomly separated into three groups and treated with the negative control or effusanin E, and the tumor volumes were measured every other day. (**B**) Weight changes of the nude mice were measured after treatment every other day. (**C**) The weight of the tumors from the mice and images of tumors that were removed from the mice. After the mice were sacrificed, the tumors were removed from the mice and pictures were taken. (**D**) Representative Western blot showing the expression of COX-2, p50 and p65 in the tumors from nude mice. C1, C2 and C3 represent tumor 1, tumor 2 and tumor 3 from negative control. L1, L2 and L3 represent tumor 1, tumor 2 and tumor 3 from effusanin E-treated mice at 10 mg/kg/d. H1, H2 and H3 represent tumor 1, tumor 2 and tumor 3 from effusanin E-treated mice at 30 mg/kg/d. * represent $P<0.05$.

antibacterial, antiviral, anti-inflammatory and antitumor activities, and effusanin E, a compound from natural herb, inhibited NPC cells via disrupting NF-κB signaling and induced apotosis in NPC cells, meanwhile, effusanin E significantly suppressed tumor growth in a xenograft mouse model of NPC cells without obvious toxicity, moreover, the expression of p50 and COX-2 were downregulated in the tumors of nude mice, which are consistent with cell study, so these findings evidenced the antitumor activities of *R. serra*. However, the upstream of NF-κB remains unknown, and needs further study to research. We also selected the 500-bp COX-2 promoter probe which included two conserved NF-κB-binding sites and found that effusanin E decreased the binding of NF-κB on the COX-2 promoter. We will use ChIP assays to confirm this in our further study.

In summary, this report is to study the anticancer mechanism of effusanin E from *R. serra*, and the results showed that effusanin E suppresses nasopharyngeal carcinoma growth by inhibiting NF-κB signaling. Therefore, effusanin E is a promising natural compound for assisting NPC treatment. Furthermore, this study confirms that Xihuangcao, an herbal tea, is capable of anticancer activity.

Materials and Methods

Ethics Statement

The study was approved by the Ethics Committee of Sun Yatsen University Cancer Center. The aerial parts of R. serra were collected from Luofu mountain (GPS coordinates: 23.29522, 114.105266), Huizhou, Guangdong, China on September 14th, 2011, and were authenticated by Professor Huagu Ye of South

China Botanical Garden, Chinese Academy of Sciences, where voucher specimens (voucher specimen number 21373) were kept. R. serra leaf was separated from stem, cleanly washed without any damage, and sun-dried and ground into fine powder by laboratory mill (FW100, Taisite Instrument Co., Ltd, Tianjin, China). And this study was carried out in strict accordance with the recommendations in the Guide for the Care and Use of Laboratory Animals of the National Institutes of Health. The protocol was approved by the Committee on the Ethics of Animal Experiments of Sun Yat-Sen University (Permit Number: SCXK (yue) 2008–0002). All efforts were made to minimize suffering. The nude mice were employed for tumorigenicity analysis. No specific permissions were required for these locations/activities. In addition, the field studies did not involve endangered or protected species.

Cell lines and cell culture

The human nasopharyngeal high differentiated squamous epithelium carcinoma cell (CNE1), human nasopharyngeal low differentiated squamous epithelium carcinoma cell (CNE2) lines and normal nasopharyngeal epithelial cell line NP69 were provided by Sun Yat-Sen University Cancer Center (China) and were cultured in DMEM medium (Invitrogen, US) that was supplemented with 10% fetal bovine serum (FBS) (HyClone, Logan, UT) and were maintained in an incubator with a humidified atmosphere of 95% air and 5% CO_2 at 37°C.

Reagents

Ammonium pyrrolidinedithiocarbamate (PDTC), celecoxib (CB) and lipopolysaccharides (LPS) were purchased from Sigma (St. Louis, MO). Effusanin E was purified from *R. serra* by column chromatography in our previous study. The purity of the compound exceeds 95%.

Plant material

The aerial portions of *R. serra* were collected from Luofu mountain (GPS coordinates: 23.29522, 114.105266), Huizhou, Guangdong, China on September 14th, 2011, and were authenticated by Professor Huagu Ye of South China Botanical Garden, Chinese Academy of Sciences, where voucher specimens (voucher specimen number 21373) were kept. *R. serra* leaf was separated from stem, cleanly washed without any damage, and sun-dried and ground into fine powder by laboratory mill (FW100, Taisite Instrument Co., Ltd, Tianjin, China). No specific permissions were required for these locations or activities. In addition, the field studies did not involve endangered or protected species.

Cell viability assay

The cell viability was determined using the MTS assay. Cells were plated in 96-well plates (2000 cells/well) and were treated with the tested samples at the indicated doses. At 24, 48 or 72 hours after treatment, 10 μl of MTS was added into each well, and the cell viability was determined at 490 nm.

Cellular morphology observation

Cells were treated with effusanin E at the indicated doses. After 24 hours, cellular morphology was observed using an Olympus microscope that was fitted with a digital camera.

Colony formation assay

Cells were seeded into a 6-well culture dish (800 cells/well). After incubation for 24 hours, effusanin E was added to the cells. Once colony formation was observed visually, the cells were washed twice with PBS, fixed for 30 min at room temperature with 4% paraformaldehyde and stained with Crystal Violet Staining Solution for 10 min. Subsequently, the cells were washed an additional two times with PBS. Colonies of >50 cells were counted and analyzed using a microscope, and the plate colony formation efficiency was calculated using the following formula: plate colony formation efficiency = (number of colonies/number of cells inoculated) ×100%.

Apoptosis assay

The effusanin E-treated cells (2×10^4) were stained with AnnexinV-FITC using an Annexin V/Dead Cell Apoptosis Kit (Invitrogen, USA). The cells were washed twice in PBS and re-suspended in binding buffer. The suspension (100 μl) was then stained with 5 μl of Annexin V-FITC and gently vortexed and incubated in the dark for 15 minutes at room temperature. Last, 10 μl of Propidium Iodide (PI) was added, and the suspension was incubated in the dark for 5 minutes at room temperature. After the addition of 400 μl of binding buffer to each tube, the cells were analyzed by flow cytometry (Cytomics FC500 Flow Cytometry; Beckman Coulter).

Western blot analysis

Cells were treated with effusanin E at the indicated doses for 24 hours, and cell lysates were subjected to Western blot analysis using antibodies for GAPDH, p50 and p65 NF-κB (Santa Cruz Biotechnology, Santa Cruz, CA) and antibodies for caspase-3, caspase-9, PARP, cleaved caspase-3, cleaved caspase-9, cleaved PARP and COX-2 from Cell Signaling Technology (Beverly, MA).

The tumor of nude mice were dissected and homogenized, then the sample of protein were subjected to Western blot analysis using antibodies for GAPDH, p50 and p65 NF-κB from Santa Cruz Biotechnology (Santa Cruz, USA) and COX-2 from Cell Signaling Technology (Beverly, MA, USA).

Validation of the regulation of COX-2 and NF-κB signaling by effusanin E

To validate the role of effusanin E in regulating NF-κB signaling, the effect of effusanin E on the PDTC- (a NF-κB-selective inhibitor), celecoxib- (a COX-2-selective inhibitor) or LPS-mediated inhibition of cell proliferation was analyzed. NPC cells plated in 96-well plates (2000 cells/well) were pretreated with PDTC (100 μM), celecoxib (20 μM or 50 μM) or LPS (2 μg/mL) for 8 hours and then treated with effusanin E at 125 μM or 250 μM. After treatment for 24 hours, cell viability was determined using MTS analysis.

Analysis of reduced nuclear translocation of p65 by immunofluorescence imaging (IFI)

Cells were seeded in six-well chamber slides at a density of 1×10^5 cells per well and treated with effusanin E (125 μM) or PDTC or PDTC followed by effusanin E at 125 μM. After 24 hours, the cells were washed in PBS, fixed at room temperature with 4% paraformaldehyde, and permeabilized with 0.2% Triton X-100. Immunofluorescence staining was performed according to standard procedures. Briefly, the treated cells were first stained with the anti-p65 antibody followed by incubation with FITC-conjugated anti-rabbit IgG secondary antibody and co-staining with DAPI.

Analysis of promoter activity

A promoter region of the human COX-2 gene (459 bp) and its fragment deletions were cloned into the luciferase reporter vector pGL3. COX-2 promoter activity was determined by transient expression of the luciferase vectors in cells using Lipofectamine 2000 (Invitrogen). Luciferase activity was measured using an assay kit (Promega, Madison, WI, USA).

DNA–protein binding by streptavidin-agarose pulldown assay

Transactivator binding to COX-2 core promoter probes were determined using a streptavidin-agarose pulldown assay as previously described [31]. A 479-bp, biotin-labeled, double-stranded probe corresponding to the COX-2 promoter sequence (−30 to −508) was used for the experiments, and DNA-bound NF-κB was analyzed by Western blotting.

Animal assays

This study was carried out in strict accordance with the recommendations in the Guide for the Care and Use of Laboratory Animals of the National Institutes of Health. The protocol was approved by the Committee on the Ethics of Animal Experiments of Sun Yat-Sen University (Permit Number: SCXK (yue) 2008-0002). All efforts were made to minimize suffering. The nude mice were employed for tumorigenicity analysis. Male, nude mice, 4-5 weeks old, weighting 17–22 g were housed in filter-capped cages kept in a sterile facility and maintained in a specific, pathogen-free barrier system. CNE2 cells were harvested by 0.25% trypsinization, washed twice with sterile PBS and resuspended at a concentration of 1×10^7 cells/ml. CNE2 cells (100 μl) were injected subcutaneously into the flank of nude mice, and the mice were randomly assigned to receive either 20 μl DMSO and 80 μl PBS (control; 5 mice) or effusanin E (10 mg/kg/d or 30 mg/kg/d, 20 μl effusanin E solution and 80 μl PBS; 10 mice). Treatment was administered through intraperitoneal injection, and tumor growth was measured after the injection and then every day. The tumor volume (V) was monitored by measuring its length (L) and width (W) with calipers and calculated using the following formula: $V = (L\times W^2)\times 0.5$. Photographs were taken 16 days after the injection. Finally, animals were euthanized by CO_2 asphyxiation.

Statistical analysis

The significance was evaluated by the paired *t* test, and * represent $P<0.05$, they were considered to be a statistically significant difference between the treatment and control groups. SPSS 11.0 software was used for all statistical analysis. All the experiments were performed three times, and the mean values and standard deviations were calculated.

Acknowledgments

The authors thank Dr. Tiebang Kang (Sun Yat-Sen University Cancer Center) for helpful comments on the article.

Author Contributions

Conceived and designed the experiments: M. Zhuang LL WD M. Zhao. Performed the experiments: M. Zhuang HQ DS JW YT. Analyzed the data: M. Zhuang LL WD. Contributed reagents/materials/analysis tools: WD M. Zhao. Wrote the paper: M. Zhuang LL WD.

References

1. Wu E, Golitz LE (2000) Primary noncutaneous melanoma. Clin Lab Med 20: 731–744.
2. Busson P, Keryer C, Ooka T, Corbex M (2004) EBV-associated nasopharyngeal carcinomas, from epidemiology to virus-targeting strategies. Trends Microbiol 12: 356–360.
3. Xu Y, Zhang J, Shi W, Liu Y (2013) Anticancer effects of 3,3'-diindolylmethane are associated with G1 arrest and mitochondria-dependent apoptosis in human nasopharyngeal carcinoma cells. Oncol lett 5: 655–662.
4. Xiao WW, Huang SM, Han F, Wu SX, Lu LX, et al. (2011) Local Control, Survival, and Late Toxicities of Locally Advanced Nasopharyngeal Carcinoma Treated by Simultaneous Modulated Accelerated Radiotherapy Combined With Cisplatin Concurrent Chemotherapy Long-Term Results of a Phase 2 Study. Cancer 117: 1874–1883.
5. Huang J, Liang ZD, Wu TT, Hoque A, Chen H, et al. (2007) Tumor-suppressive effect of retinoid receptor-induced gene-1 (RRIG1) in esophageal cancer. Cancer Res 67: 1589–1593.
6. China Flora Editorial Committee of Flora of Chinese Academy of Sciences (1977) The flora of China : Beijing: Science Press. pp. 433–434.
7. Fang HY, Hsu CH, Chao CH, Wen ZH, Wu YC, et al. (2013) Cytotoxic and Anti-Inflammatory Metabolites from the Soft Coral Scleronephthya gracillimum. Mar Drugs 11: 1853–1865.
8. Nitoda T, Isobe T, Kubo I (2008) Effects of phenolic compounds isolated from Rabdosia japonica on B16-F10 melanoma cells. Phytother Res 22: 867–872.
9. Hu HZ, Yang YB, Xu XD, Shen HW, Shu YM, et al. (2007) Oridonin induces apoptosis via PI3K/Akt pathway in cervical carcinoma HeLa cell line. Acta Pharmacol Sin 28: 1819–1826.
10. Cui Q, Tashiro S, Onodera S, Minami M, Ikejima T (2007) Oridonin induced autophagy in human cervical carcinoma HeLa cells through Ras, JNK, and P38 regulation. J Pharmacol Sci 105: 317–325.
11. Kim JY, Kim HS, Kim YJ, Lee HK, Kim JS, et al. (2013) Effusanin C inhibits inflammatory responses via blocking NF-κB and MAPK signaling in monocytes. Int. Immunopharmacol 15: 84–88.
12. Sinicrope FA, Gill S (2004) Role of cyclooxygenase-2 in colorectal cancer. Cancer Metastasis Rev 23: 63–75.
13. Singh B, Lucci A (2002) Role of cyclooxygenase-2 in breast cancer. J Surg Res 108: 173–179.
14. Ghosh S, May MJ, Kopp EB (1998) NF-κB and Rel proteins: evolutionarily conserved mediators of immune responses. Annu Rev Immunol 16: 225–260.
15. De Bosscher K, Schmitz ML, Plaisance S, Vanden Berghe W, Fiers W, et al. (1997) Glucocorticoid-mediated repression of nuclear factor-κB-dependent transcription involves direct interference with transactivation. Proc Natl Acad Sci USA 94: 13504–13509.
16. Yin MJ, Yamamoto Y, Gaynor RB (1998) The anti-inflammatory agents aspirin and salicylate inhibit the activity of IkB kinase-b. Nature 396: 77–80.
17. Yamamoto Y, Yin MJ, Lin KM, Gaynor RB (1999) Sulindac inhibits activation of the NF-κB pathway. J Biol Chem 274: 27307–27314.
18. Lin L, Gao Q, Cui C, Zhao H, Fu L, et al. (2012) Isolation and identification of ent-kaurane-type diterpenoids from Rabdosia serra (MAXIM.) HARA leaf and their inhibitory activities against HepG-2, MCF-7, and HL-60 cell lines. Food Chem 131: 1009–1014.
19. Liu B, Wen JK, Li BH, Fang XM, Wang JJ, et al. (2011) Celecoxib and acetylbritannilactone interact synergistically to suppress breast cancer cell growth via COX-2-dependent and -independent mechanisms. Cell death Dis 2: 1–9.
20. Wang J, Xiao X, Zhang Y, Shi D, Chen W, et al. (2012) Simultaneous modulation of COX-2, p300, Akt, and Apaf-1 signaling by melatonin to inhibit proliferation and induce apoptosis in breast cancer cells. J Pineal Res 53: 77–90.
21. Kang CH, Chiang PH, Huang SC (2008) Correlation of COX-2 expression in stromal cells with high stage, high grade, and poor prognosis in urothelial carcinoma of upper urinary tracts. Urology 72: 153–157.
22. Deng WG, Zhu Y, Wu KK (2003) Up-regulation of p300 binding and p50 acetylation in tumor necrosis factor-alpha-induced cyclooxygenase-2 promoter activation. J Biol Chem 278: 4770–4777.
23. Hayden MS, Ghosh S (2008) Shared principles in NF-kappa B signaling. Cell 132: 344–362.
24. Mankan AK, Lawless MW, Gray SG, Kelleher D, McManus R (2009) NF-kappa B regulation: the nuclear response. J Cell Mol Med 13: 631–643.
25. Baud V, Karin M (2009) Is NF-kappa B a good target for cancer therapy? Hopes and pitfalls. Nat Rev Drug Discov 8: 33–40.
26. Karin M, Yamamoto Y, Wang QM (2004) The IKKNF-kappa B system: A treasure trove for drug development. Nat Rev Drug Discov 3: 17–26.
27. Newman DJ, Cragg GM (2007) Natural products as sources of new drugs over the last 25 years. J Nat Prod 70: 461–477.
28. Leung CH, Grill SP, Lam W, Han QB, Sun HD, et al. (2005) Novel mechanism of inhibition of nuclear factor-kappa B DNA-binding activity by diterpenoids isolated from Isodon rubescens. Mol Pharmacol 68: 286–297.
29. Schmitz ML, Baeuerle PA (1991) The p65 subunit is responsible for the strong transcription activating potential of NF-kappa B. EMBO J 10: 3805–3817.

30. Ballard DW, Dixon EP, Peffer NJ, Bogerd H, Doerre S, et al. (1992) The 65-kDa subunit of human NF-kappa B functions as a potent transcriptional activator and a target for v-Rel-mediated repression. Proc Natl Acad Sci USA 89: 1875–1879.

31. Deng WG, Zhu Y, Montero A, Wu KK (2003) Quantitative analysis of binding of transcription factor complex to biotinylated DNA probe by a streptavidin-agarose pulldown assay. Anal Biochem 323: 12–18.

8

Morphine and Clonidine Combination Therapy Improves Therapeutic Window in Mice: Synergy in Antinociceptive but Not in Sedative or Cardiovascular Effects

Laura S. Stone[1,2,3,4,5*], Jonathan P. German[7], Kelly F. Kitto[7], Carolyn A. Fairbanks[6,7,8], George L. Wilcox[7,8,9]

1 Alan Edwards Centre for Research on Pain, McGill University, Montreal, Quebec, Canada, **2** Faculty of Dentistry, McGill University, Montreal, Quebec, Canada, **3** Department of Anesthesiology, Faculty of Medicine, McGill University, Montreal, Quebec, Canada, **4** Department of Pharmacology and Therapeutics, Faculty of Medicine, McGill University, Montreal, Quebec, Canada, **5** Department of Neurology and Neurosurgery, Faculty of Medicine, McGill University, Montreal, Quebec, Canada, **6** Department of Pharmaceutics, College of Pharmacy, University of Minnesota, Minneapolis, Minnesota, United States of America, **7** Department of Neuroscience, Medical School, University of Minnesota, Minneapolis, Minnesota, United States of America, **8** Department of Pharmacology, Medical School, University of Minnesota, Minneapolis, Minnesota, United States of America, **9** Department of Dermatology, Medical School, University of Minnesota, Minneapolis, Minnesota, United States of America

Abstract

Opioids are used to manage all types of pain including acute, cancer, chronic neuropathic and inflammatory pain. Unfortunately, opioid-related adverse effects such as respiratory depression, tolerance, physical dependence and addiction have led to an underutilization of these compounds for adequate pain relief. One strategy to improve the therapeutic utility of opioids is to co-administer them with other analgesic agents such as agonists acting at α_2-adrenergic receptors (α_2ARs). Analgesics acting at α_2ARs and opioid receptors (ORs) frequently synergize when co-administered *in vivo*. Multimodal analgesic techniques offer advantages over single drug treatments as synergistic combination therapies produce analgesia at lower doses, thus reducing undesired side effects. This inference presumes, however, that the synergistic interaction is limited to the analgesic effects. In order to test this hypothesis, we examined the effects of α_2AR/OR combination therapy in acute antinociception and in the often-undesired side effects of sedation and cardiovascular depression in awake unrestrained mice. Morphine, clonidine or their combination was administered by spinal or systemic injection in awake mice. Antinociception was determined using the warm water tail flick assay (52.5°C). Sedation/motor impairment was evaluated using the accelerating rotarod assay and cardiovascular function was monitored by pulse oximetry. Data were converted to percent maximum possible effect and isobolographic analysis was performed to determine if an interaction was subadditive, additive or synergistic. Synergistic interactions between morphine and clonidine were observed in the antinociceptive but not in the sedative/motor or cardiovascular effects. As a result, the therapeutic window was improved ~200-fold and antinociception was achieved at non-sedating doses with little to no cardiovascular depression. In addition, combination therapy resulted in greater maximum analgesic efficacy over either drug alone. These data support the utility of combination adrenergic/opioid therapy in pain management for antinociceptive efficacy with reduced side-effect liability.

Editor: Prasun K. Datta, Temple University, United States of America

Funding: This work was supported by the National Institute of Health (www.nih.gov), National Institute of Drug Abuse grants to LSS [R21-DA-017075], GLW [R01-DA-04274, R01-DA-15438] and CAF [K01-DA-00509], Canadian Institutes for Health Research (www.cihr-irsc.gc.ca) Operating Grant [MOP-86691] to LSS and a Fonds de la Recherche en Santé Québec (www.frsq.gouv.qc.ca) Salary Award to LSS. The funders had no role in study design, data collection and analysis, decision to publish, or preparation of the manuscript.

Competing Interests: The authors have declared that no competing interests exist.

* Email: laura.s.stone@mcgill.ca

Introduction

Opioid receptor agonists have analgesic properties following both spinal and systemic administration [1,2]. Opioid analgesics remain the mainstay for the treatment of moderate to severe pain [3]. However, the utility of opioid analgesics is limited by the incidence and prevalence of well-known problematic effects, including respiratory and cardiovascular depression [4], sedation, constipation, nausea, cognitive impairment, itch, and the development of analgesic tolerance [1].

Agonists acting at α_2ARs have analgesic properties in multiple species including humans [5–15]. Therapeutic development of α_2AR agonists for the treatment of pain is particularly important for the management of patients who are under-responsive to conventional opioid therapy [10,12,16–23]. The prototypic α_2AR agonist, clonidine, is currently approved for spinal delivery in intractable cancer pain. However, the therapeutic utility of α_2AR agonists has been hampered by their side-effect profile, with sedation and hypotension being of particular concern [24–26].

Co-administration of α_2AR agonists with opioids often results in a greater-than-additive (i.e. synergistic) interaction following either

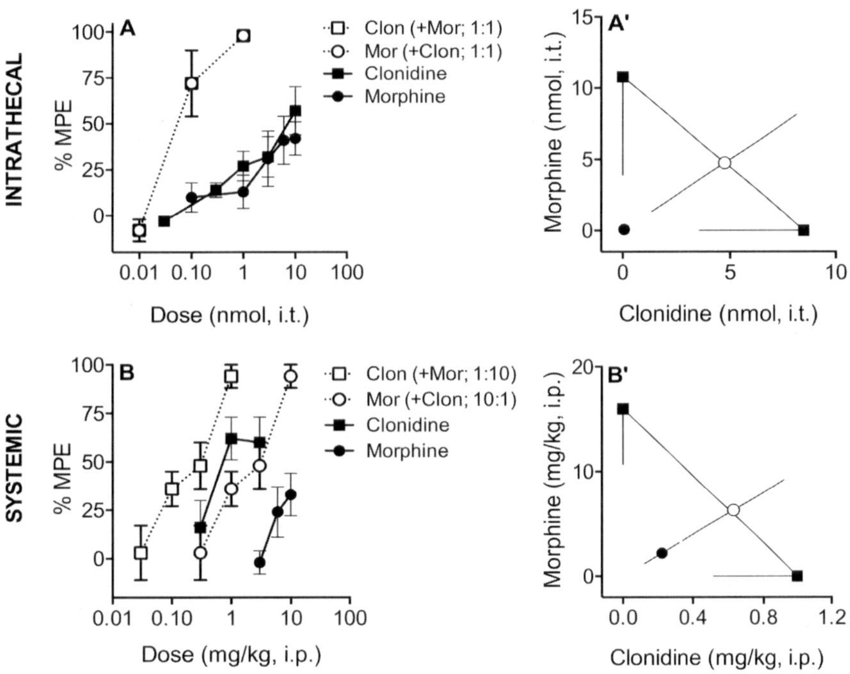

Figure 1. Effects of Morphine and Clonidine in the Tail Flick Antinociception Assay. A: Intrathecally delivered morphine (●) and clonidine (■) dose-dependently inhibited thermal nociception with similar potency and efficacy. When co-administered at a constant dose ratio of 1:1 (○ morphine; □ clonidine), both potency and efficacy were increased. **A′**: Isobolographic analysis applied to the data from Figure 1A. The y-intercept represents the ED_{50} for morphine and the x-intercept represents the ED_{50} for clonidine. The lines directed from each ED_{50} value toward zero represent the lower 95% confidence limits of each ED_{50}. The line connecting these two points is the theoretical additive line. The unfilled circle on the theoretical additive line represents the calculated theoretical ED_{50} value of the combination if the interaction is additive. The observed combination ED_{50} (●) was significantly ($p<0.05$; t-test) lower than the theoretical additive ED_{50} (○), indicating that the interaction is synergistic. **B.** Systemically administered morphine (●) and clonidine (■) dose-dependently inhibited thermal nociception when administered either alone or in combination at a constant morphine:clonidine dose ratio of 10:1 (○ morphine; □ clonidine). **B′**: Isobolographic analysis applied to the data from Figure 1B. The y-intercept represents the ED_{50} for morphine and the x-intercept represents the ED_{50} for clonidine. The observed combination ED_{50} (●) was significantly ($p<0.05$; t-test) lower than the theoretical additive ED_{50} (○), indicating that the interaction is synergistic. Data pictured were obtained 10 minutes following intrathecal (Figures 1A, A′) and 15 minutes following systemic administration (Figures 1B, B′). Error bars represent ±SEM for each dose point ($n=6$–10 animals/dose). See Table 1 for ED_{50} values.

spinal or systemic delivery [27–36], although the interaction is of greater magnitude in the spinal cord [28,29]. Synergistic drug interactions result in enhanced potency and/or efficacy when one agent is given together with another. Therapeutic application of synergistic adrenergic-opioid combinations is important in pain management because of the expectation of improved efficacy and reduced doses, and theoretically, reduced side effects [13,25,37]. This inference presumes, however, that the synergistic interaction is limited to the desired analgesic effect and not the undesired side effect(s), which may not always be the case [38]. The objective of the current study is to address this presumption.

The potential for adrenergic-opioid combination therapy to improve clinical utility depends on the potentiation of analgesia without similar potentiation of the side effects. The effects of co-administered morphine and clonidine on antinociception, sedation/motor impairment, heart rate and a surrogate of blood pressure were examined to determine if combination therapy could be used to increase the therapeutic window. The present study therefore assessed effects on these variables in unrestrained, awake, behaving mice to test for both sedative/motor and cardiovascular side effects of adrenergic-opioid combination therapy.

Methods

Animals

Male CD-1 ICR mice (20±5 g; Harlan, Madison, WI) were maintained on a 12-hour light/dark cycle with unlimited access to food and water. All experiments were approved by the Institutional Animal Care and Use Committee of the University of Minnesota (Permit #0407A62285) and conformed to the ethical guidelines of the Guide for the Care and Use of Laboratory Animals of the National Institutes of Health and the guidelines of the Committee for Research and Ethical Issues of the International Association for the Study of Pain [39].

Drug Preparation and Administration

Morphine sulfate (NIDA) and clonidine (Sigma; St. Louis, MO) were dissolved in 0.9% saline. Intrathecal (i.t.) drug administration was done by direct lumbar puncture in a volume of 5 μL according to the method of Hylden and Wilcox in conscious mice [2]. Following i.t. administration, tail flick latencies, heart rate and carotid distension were obtained at 10 and 30 minutes and rotarod retention times were obtained 15 and 35 minutes post-injection. Intraperitoneal injections (i.p.) were administered in a total volume of 100 μL per 25 g. Following i.p. administration, tail flick latencies, heart rate and carotid blood flow were obtained 15 and

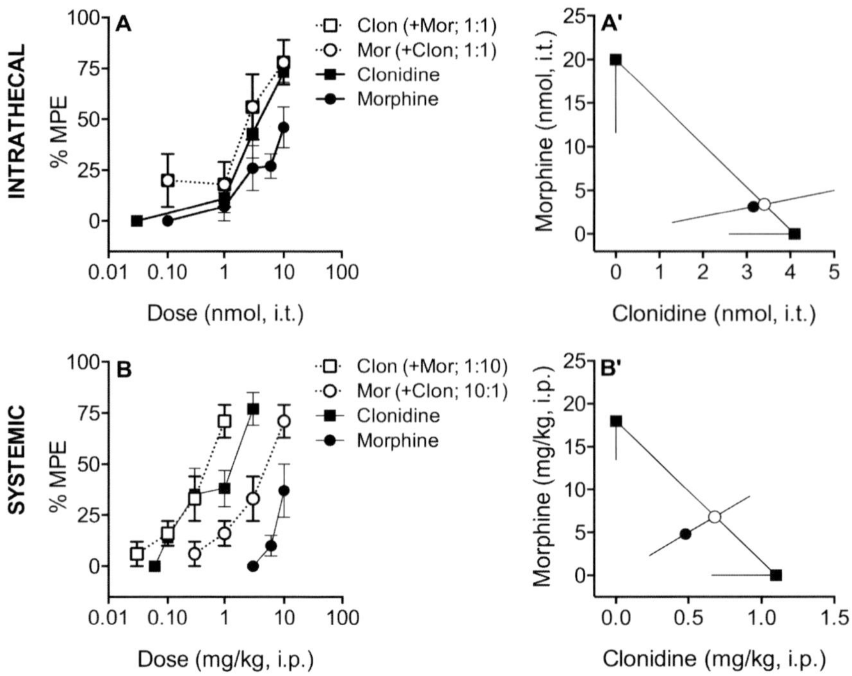

Figure 2. Effects of Morphine and Clonidine in the Rotarod Sedation Assay. A. Rotarod retention was challenged by intrathecal morphine, clonidine or both. Morphine (●) and clonidine (■) inhibited rotarod performance in a dose-dependent manner with similar potency. When the agonists were co-administered at a constant ratio of 1:1 (○ morphine; □ clonidine), no increases in potency or efficacy were observed. **A′**. Isobolographic analysis applied to the data from Figure 2A. The y-intercept represents the ED_{50} for morphine and the x-intercept represents the ED_{50} for clonidine. The lines directed from each ED_{50} value toward zero represent the lower 95% confidence limits of each ED_{50}. The line connecting these two points is the theoretical additive line. The unfilled circle on the theoretical additive line represents the calculated theoretical ED_{50} value of the combination if the interaction is additive. The observed combination ED_{50} (●) is not significantly ($p<0.05$; t-test) different from the theoretical additive ED_{50} (○), indicating that the interaction is additive. **B**. Systemically administered morphine (●) and clonidine (■) dose-dependently inhibited rotarod performance when administered alone or in combination at a constant morphine:clonidine dose ratio of 10:1 (○ morphine; □ clonidine). **B′**. Isobolographic analysis applied to the data from Figure 2B. The observed combination ED_{50} (●) is not significantly ($p<0.05$; t-test) different than the theoretical additive ED_{50} (○), indicating that the interaction is additive. Data pictured were obtained 15 minutes following intrathecal (Figures 2A, A′) and 20 minutes following systemic administration (Figures 2B, B′). Error bars represent ±SEM for each dose point (n=6–10 animals/dose). See Table 1 for ED_{50} values.

60 minutes and rotarod retention times were obtained 20 and 65 minutes post-injection. The tail flick and rotarod assays were performed in the same animals sequentially. The cardiovascular measures were obtained in a separate set of mice.

Antinociception

Antinociception was assessed using the warm water (52.5°C) tail immersion assay [40]. Mice were gently wrapped in a soft cloth such that their tails were exposed and three quarters of the length of each tail was dipped into the hot water. Tail flick latencies were obtained before and after drug administration. A maximum cut-off of 12 seconds was set in order to avoid tissue damage. A minimum of three mice were used for each dose. The results are expressed as a percent of the maximum possible effect (%MPE) according to the equation:

$$\%MPE = (Post-drug\ latency\ -\ Pre-drug\ latency)\ /(Cutoff\ -\ Pre-drug\ latency)\ x\ 100.$$

Sedation/Motor Impairment

Retention time on an accelerating rotorod was used as a model of motor coordination and/or sedation, since sedation will also cause the animals to fall. Animals were trained until retention times exceeded 240 seconds. A maximum cutoff of 5 min was used. The results are expressed as a percent of the maximum possible effect (%MPE) according to the equation:

$$\%MPE = (Pre-drug\ latency\ -\ Post-drug\ latency)\ /(Pre-drug\ latency)\ x\ 100.$$

Cardiovascular Measurements

Cardiovascular function was monitored in awake, freely moving mice trained one day prior to tolerate the presence of a pulse oximetry clip on the dorsal half of the neck (MouseOx, Starr Life Sciences Corp). Because albino ICR mice were used in this study, pulse oximetry of the carotid arteries was possible without shaving. Carotid distension and heart rate were recorded before and after drug or combination administration. Carotid distension (μm) is an indicator of carotid blood flow and was used as a surrogate for blood pressure. Maximum efficacy was set at 300 beats/minute for heart rate and 300 μm for carotid distension. Oxygen saturation remained between 97-100% regardless of treatment. The results are expressed as a percent of the maximum possible effect (%MPE) according to the equation:

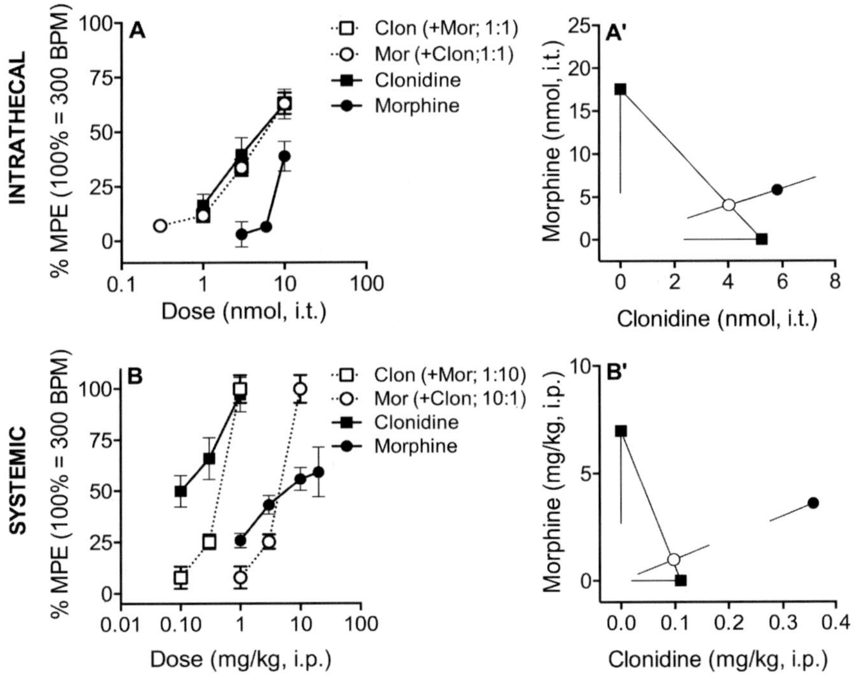

Figure 3. Effects of Morphine and Clonidine on Heart Rate. A. Heart rate was challenged by intrathecal morphine, clonidine or both. Morphine (●) and clonidine (■) inhibited heart rate in a dose-dependent manner. When the agonists were co-administered at a constant ratio of 1:1 (○ morphine; □ clonidine), no increases in potency or efficacy were observed. **A′**. Isobolographic analysis applied to the data from Figure 3A. The y-intercept represents the ED_{50} for morphine and the x-intercept represents the ED_{50} for clonidine. The lines directed from each ED_{50} value toward zero represent the respective lower 95% confidence limits of each ED_{50}. The line connecting these two points is the theoretical additive line. The unfilled circle on the theoretical additive line represents the calculated theoretical ED_{50} value of the combination if the interaction is additive. The observed combination ED_{50} (●) is not significantly ($p<0.05$; t-test) different from the theoretical additive ED_{50} (○), indicating that the interaction is additive. **B**. Systemically administered morphine (●) and clonidine (■) dose-dependently inhibited heart rate when administered alone or in combination at a constant morphine:clonidine dose ratio of 10:1 (○ morphine; □ clonidine). **B′**. Isobolographic analysis applied to the data from Figure 3B. The observed combination ED_{50} (●) is significantly ($p<0.05$; t-test) higher than the theoretical additive ED_{50} (○), indicating that the interaction is sub-additive. Data pictured were obtained 10 minutes following intrathecal (Figures 3A, A′) and 15 minutes following systemic administration (Figures 3B, B′). Error bars represent ±SEM for each dose point ($n = 6$–10 animals/dose). See Table 1 for ED_{50} values. *Note: 100% MPE was artificially set at 300 beats per minute (baseline ~800) to facilitate dose-response and isobolographic analysis.*

$$\%MPE = (Pre-drug\ value - Post-drug\ value) / (Pre-drug\ value)\ x\ 100.$$

Dose-Response Analysis

Individual dose points are expressed as means with standard error of the mean (SEM). ED_{50} values and confidence limits were calculated according to the graded dose-response method of Tallarida and Murray [41] on the linear portion of each dose-response curve. A minimum of three doses were used for each drug or combination of drugs.

Therapeutic Window

The therapeutic window (TW) was estimated using the ratio: TW = (ED_{50} value for sedation, heart rate or carotid distension)/(ED_{50} value for antinociception).

Isobolographic Analysis

Isobolographic analysis is the 'gold standard' for evaluating drug interactions [41,42]. Dose-response curves were constructed for each agonist administered alone, the ED_{50} values were calculated and used to determine an equieffective dose ratio between the agonists. This ratio was then maintained when both agonists were administered in combination, a third dose-response curve was constructed and an experimentally derived combination ED_{50} was calculated. To test for interactions between agonists, the ED_{50} values and standard error of all dose-response curves were arithmetically arranged around the ED_{50} value using the following equation:

$$(ln(10)\ x\ ED_{50})\ X\ (S.E.\ of\ log\ ED_{50})$$

[42]. Isobolographic analysis necessitates this manipulation. When testing an interaction between two drugs, a theoretical additive ED_{50} value is calculated for the combination based on the dose-response curves of each drug administered separately. This theoretical value is then compared by a *t*-test with the observed experimental ED_{50} value of the combination. These values are based on the total dose of both drugs. An interaction is considered synergistic if the experimental ED_{50} is significantly less ($p<0.05$) than the calculated theoretical additive ED_{50}.

Visualization of drug interactions can be facilitated and enhanced by graphical representation of isobolographic analysis (Figures 1–3, A′ and B′). This representation depicts the ED_{50} of each agent as the x- or y-intercept. For example, Figure 1A′ presents the ED_{50} of morphine as the y-intercept and the ED_{50} of clonidine as the x-intercept. The line connecting these two points

Table 1. Effect of Combination Therapy on Drug Potency.

Assay	Route	Time (min)	Morphine ED_{50} (±SEM)	Clonidine ED_{50} (±SEM)	Observed combination ED_{50} (±SEM)	Theoretical combination ED_{50} (±SEM)	γ	Interaction
Tail Flick	**Spinal (nmol)**	**10**	*~11 (±11)*	8.5 (±7.2)	0.14 (±0.12)	9.5 (±6.8)	0.02	**Synergistic**
		30	5.3 (±3.3)	2.5 (±1.4)	0.25 (±0.16)	3.4 (±1.5)	0.07	**Synergistic**
	Systemic (mg/kg)	**15**	*~16 (±7)*	1.0 (±0.7)	2.4 (±1.1)	6.9 (±3.2)	0.4	**Synergistic**
		60	*~7.8 (±4.6)*	1.0 (±0.7)	1.6 (± 0.8)	4.9 (±2.2)	0.3	**Synergistic**
Rotarod	**Spinal (nmol)**	**15**	*~20 (±11)*	4.1 (±1.9)	6.3 (±3.7)	6.8 (±2.9)	0.9	**Additive**
		35	*~30 (±10)*	*~9.4 (±6.3)*	*~50 (±60)*	14 (±7.4)	3.5	**Additive**
	Systemic (mg/kg)	**20**	*~18 (±6)*	1.1 (±0.6)	*5.3 (±2.8)*	7.5 (±2.6)	0.7	**Additive**
		65	*No efficacy*	2.4 (±1.2)	11 (±9)	*NA*	*NA*	**No interaction*
Heart Rate	**Spinal (nmol)**	**10**	*~18 (±12)*	5.2 (±2.4)	12 (±3)	8.1 (±3.1)	1.4	**Additive**
		30	*~14 (±8)*	5.3 (±2.1)	13 (±5)	7.6 (±2.5)	1.7	**Sub-additive**
	Systemic (mg/kg)	**15**	7.0 (±4.3)	0.11 (±0.09)	3.9 (±0.9)	1.1 (±0.7)	3.8	**Sub-additive**
		60	4.6 (±1.7)	0.27 (±0.09)	2.9 (±0.6)	1.9 (±0.5)	1.6	**Sub-additive**
Carotid Distension	**Spinal (nmol)**	**10**	*No efficacy*	5.4 (±3.1)	5.0 (±2.4)	*NA*	*NA*	**No interaction*
		30	*No efficacy*	*~10 (±8)*	*~11 (±7)*	*NA*	*NA*	**No interaction*
	Systemic (mg/kg)	**15**	*No efficacy*	0.21 (±0.09)	0.45 (±0.20)	*NA*	*NA*	**No interaction*
		60	*No efficacy*	0.68 (±0.59)	*No efficacy*	*NA*	*NA*	*NA*

Morphine and clonidine were administered in a dose-ratio of 1:1 for spinal and 10:1 for systemic administration; ~ indicates that the ED_{50} value was determined by extrapolation (in cases where maximum efficacy was between 30 and 50%); γ = Interaction index (an index of 1 = no interaction, index >1 = potentiation, index <1 = antagonism); * indicates that the ED_{50} value of clonidine alone was not significantly different from that of clonidine in the presence of morphine; NA = not available (it is not possible to calculate these values).

Table 2. Effect of Combination Therapy on Drug Efficacy.

Assay	Route	Time (min)	Morphine Max (±SEM)	Clonidine Max (±SEM)	Mor+ Clon Max (±SEM)
Tail Flick	Spinal	10	42 (±9)	57 (±13)	**99 (±0.9)**
		30	69 (±15)	84 (±9)	**100 (±0)**
	Systemic	15	33 (±11)	62 (±11)	**94 (±6.0)**
		60	48 (±13)	76 (±15)	**100 (±0)**
Rotarod	Spinal	15	46 (±10)	**78 (±5)**	73 (±5)
		35	34 (±11)	**48 (±12)**	43 (±15)
	Systemic	20	37 (±13)	**77 (±8)**	71 (±8)
		65	21 (±11)	**66 (±13)**	48 (±12)
Heart Rate	Spinal	10	39 (±7)	**63 (±7)**	**63 (±5)**
		30	47 (±4)	**73 (±9)**	63 (±6)
	Systemic	15	59 (±12)	97 (±8)	**100 (±7)**
		60	69 (±2)	92 (±14)	**113 (±7)**
Carotid Distension	Spinal	10	12 (±8)	58 (±8)	**62 (±6)**
		30	9.4 (±2.2)	**48 (±9)**	43 (±5)
	Systemic	15	7.3 (±3.1)	**88 (±8)**	72 (±18)
		60	9.5 (±4.5)	**63 (±19)**	27 (±9)

Max = maximum efficacy, the drug or drug combination that achieved the maximum efficacy is indicated in bold, BPM = beats per minute.

depicts the dose combinations expected to yield 50% efficacy if the interaction is purely additive and is called the theoretical additive line. The theoretical additive ED_{50} and its confidence interval are determined mathematically and plotted spanning this line. The observed ED_{50} for the combination is plotted at the corresponding x,y co-ordinates along with its 95% confidence interval for comparison to the theoretical additive ED_{50}.

Interaction Index

The magnitude of drug interactions can be expressed in terms of an Interaction Index (γ) [43]. The index is defined by the equation: $a/A + b/B = \gamma$, where A and B are the doses of drugs A and B alone that give a specified level of effect and (a,b) is the combination dose that produces this same level of effect. In the absence of a drug interaction, $\gamma = 1$. If the interaction is synergistic, $\gamma < 1$. The interaction index is used here as a quantitative measure to characterize the magnitude of the interactions afforded by a combination; smaller γ indicates a more profound synergistic interaction.

All dose-response and isobolographic analyses were performed with the FlashCalc pharmacological statistics software package generously supplied by Dr. Michael Ossipov. Figures were prepared using Graphpad Prism 6.0.

Results

Intrathecal co-administration of morphine and clonidine has a synergistic effect on antinociception

Intrathecal administration of either morphine or clonidine produced dose-dependent antinociception at 10 (Figure 1A, Table 1) and 30 minutes post-injection (Table 1) at a potency ratio of approximately 1:1 morphine:clonidine.

Co-administration of morphine and clonidine at a dose ratio equal to the potency ratio (1:1) resulted in an ~100-fold increase in potency, suggesting that the interaction is synergistic. If the interaction were additive, the potency of the combination would have increased by ~2-fold. The dose-response data from Figure 1A are presented in an isobologram in Figure 1A′. As shown in Figure 1A′, the ED_{50} of the combination (closed circle) is lower than the theoretical additive ED_{50} (open circle), indicating that this interaction is synergistic. Similar results were obtained at 10- and 30-minutes post-treatment (Table 1). The interaction index, γ, was 0.02 and 0.07 at these two time points, respectively. Since smaller γ values indicate increasing levels of synergism, these values indicate that the synergistic interaction between morphine and clonidine is profound.

When administered alone, neither morphine nor clonidine reached full efficacy (defined as ≥75%) 10 minutes following injection (Figure 1A, Table 2). In contrast, 100% efficacy was achieved by the combination (Table 2).

Systemic co-administration of morphine and clonidine has a synergistic effect on antinociception

Systemic (i.p.) administration of either morphine or clonidine produced dose-dependent antinociception 15 (Figure 1B, Table 1) and 60 minutes (Table 1) at a potency ratio of approximately 10:1 morphine:clonidine.

Co-administration of morphine and clonidine at a dose ratio equal to the potency ratio (10:1) resulted in an ~10-fold increase in potency, suggesting that the interaction is synergistic (Figure 1B, Table 1). As shown in Figure 1B′, the ED_{50} of the combination (closed circle) is lower than the theoretical additive ED_{50} (open circle), indicating that the interaction is synergistic. The interaction index, γ, was 0.4 and 0.3 at 15 and 60 minutes post-treatment, respectively (Table 1). Although synergistic, the interaction is less profound following systemic compared to intrathecal administration.

When administered alone, morphine failed to produce >50% efficacy at either time point (15 or 60 minutes). Clonidine reached full efficacy (defined as ≥75%) at 60 but not 15 minutes following injection (Figure 1B, Table 2). In contrast, >90% efficacy was achieved by the combination at both time points (Table 2).

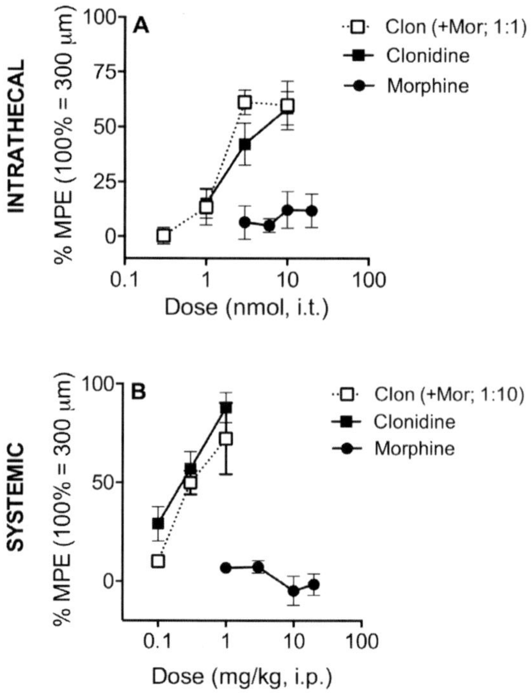

Figure 4. Effects of Morphine and Clonidine on Carotid Distension. Carotid distension was used as an indirect measure of blood pressure in awake, behaving animals. **A.** Carotid distension was challenged by intrathecal morphine, clonidine or both. While clonidine (■) reduced carotid distension in a dose-dependent manner, morphine (●) was ineffective. When the agonists were co-administered at a constant ratio of 1:1 (○ morphine; □ clonidine), the potency and efficacy of the combination was not different from that of clonidine given alone. **B.** Systemically administered clonidine (■), but not morphine (●), reduced carotid distension in a dose-dependent manner. Neither the potency nor the efficacy of the combination of morphine:clonidine at a dose ratio of 10:1 (○ morphine; □ clonidine) were different from clonidine given alone. Data pictured were obtained 10 minutes following intrathecal (Figure 4A) and 15 minutes following systemic administration (Figure 4B). Error bars represent ±SEM for each dose point ($n = 6$-10 animals/dose). See Table 1 for ED_{50} values. *Note: 100% MPE was artificially set at* 300 μm for carotid distension *(baseline ~700 μm) to facilitate dose-response and isobolographic analysis.*

Intrathecal co-administration of morphine and clonidine has an additive effect on sedation/motor impairment

Intrathecal administration of either morphine or clonidine produced dose-dependent sedation/motor impairment 15 and 35 minutes post-injection (Figure 2A, Table 1). Potency was not significantly altered following co-administration at a dose ratio of 1:1, indicating that the interaction was additive (Figure 2A, Table 1). The interaction index, γ, was 0.9 at 15 minutes and 3.5 at 35 minutes, consistent with the lack of synergism (Figure 2A, Table 1).

When administered alone, neither morphine nor clonidine produced greater than 50% sedation 35 minutes following injection and only clonidine was fully efficacious (≥75%) at 15 minutes (Figure 2A, Table 2). Maximum efficacy was not increased by co-administration at either time point (Table 2).

Systemic co-administration of morphine and clonidine has an additive effect on sedation/motor impairment

Systemic (i.p.) administration of either morphine or clonidine produced dose-dependent sedation/motor impairment 20 minutes post-injection (Figure 2B, Table 1) and only clonidine had efficacy (defined as >30% MPE) at 65 minutes (Tables 1,2). Co-administration at a ratio of 10:1 did not significantly alter drug potency. While isobolographic analysis was not performed 65 minutes post-injection because one drug lacked efficacy, the ED_{50} values of clonidine alone vs. the combination were not statistically different, suggesting that the relationship between morphine and clonidine at this time-point is additive (Table 1). Maximum efficacy was not significantly altered by co-administration (Table 2).

Intrathecal and systemic co-administration of morphine and clonidine have additive or sub-additive effects on heart rate

Intrathecal administration of either morphine or clonidine produced dose-dependent decreases in heart rate 10 and 30 minutes post-injection (Figure 3A, Table 1). Co-administration at a constant dose ratio 1:1 did not alter drug potency (Figure 3A, Table 1). As shown in Figure 3A′, at 10 minutes post-injection the ED_{50} of the combination is not significantly different from that of the theoretical additive ED_{50}, indicating that the combination has an additive effect on sedation. At 30 minutes post-injection, similar analysis revealed that the interaction was sub-additive (Table 1). The interaction indices were 1.4 and 1.7, consistent with the additive to sub-additive interactions (Table 1). Maximum efficacy was not significantly altered by drug co-administration (Table 2).

Systemic (i.p.) administration of either morphine or clonidine produced dose-dependent inhibition of heart rate 15 and 60 minutes post-injection (Figure 3B, Table 1). Co-administration at a ratio of 10:1 resulted in a sub-additive interaction at both time points (Figure 3B′, Table 1). The interaction indices were 3.8 and 1.6 at 15 and 60 minutes, respectively, consistent with a sub-additive interaction. Maximum efficacy was not significantly altered by co-administration (Table 2).

The maximum possible effect was set at 300 beats per minute (compared to pre-drug baseline of ~800 BPM) to facilitate isobolographic analysis. 100% MPE therefore corresponds to a decrease in BPM from 800 to 300.

Intrathecal and systemic co-administration of morphine and clonidine have no interaction on blood pressure

Carotid distension was used as an indirect measure of blood pressure in awake, behaving animals. Whereas intrathecal administration of clonidine produced dose-dependent decreases in carotid distension 10 and 30 minutes post-injection (Figure 4A, Table 1), morphine lacked efficacy in this measure. When co-administered at a constant ratio of 1:1, the ED_{50} value of clonidine was not statistically different from the ED_{50} value of the combination, suggesting there is no interaction (Figure 4A, Table 1). Similarly, the maximum efficacy achieved by clonidine was not affected by the presence of morphine (Figure 4A, Table 2). Isobolographic analysis was not performed because one drug lacked efficacy.

Consistent with the intrathecal results, while systemic administration of clonidine produced dose-dependent decreases in carotid distension, morphine lacked efficacy and had no effect on clonidine potency or efficacy (Figure 4B, Tables 1&2).

The maximum possible effect was set at 300 μm for carotid distension (compared to pre-drug baseline of ~700 μm) to facilitate isobolographic analysis. 100% MPE therefore corresponds to a decrease in carotid distension from 700 to 300 μm.

Table 3. Combination Therapy Improves Therapeutic Window.

			Therapeutic Window	Therapeutic Window	Therapeutic Window
Route	**Time-point**	**Drug(s)**	**Sedation/Antinociception**	**Heart Rate/Antinociception**	**Carotid Distension/ Antinociception**
Spinal	**10–15 min**	Clonidine	0.5	0.6	0.6
		Morphine	1.8	1.6	NA
		Clon+Mor	**45**	**86**	**36**
	30–35 min	Clonidine	3.8	2.1	4.0
		Morphine	5.7	2.6	NA
		Clon+Mor	**200**	**52**	**44**
Systemic	**15–20 min**	Clonidine	1.1	0.1	0.2
		Morphine	1.1	0.4	NA
		Clon+Mor	**2.2**	**1.6**	**2.0**
	60–65 min	Clonidine	2.4	0.3	0.7
		Morphine	*NA*	0.6	NA
		Clon+Mor	**6.8**	**1.8**	**NA**

Therapeutic Window is the ratio of the indicated ED_{50} values. Larger therapeutic windows are more advantageous therapeutically.

Effect of morphine and clonidine co-administration on therapeutic window

The data presented above demonstrate that co-administration of morphine and clonidine produces synergy in antinociception but not in the side effects of sedation/motor impairment or cardiovascular depression. We therefore examined the impact of co-administration on the therapeutic window (TW), a comparison of the amount of an agent required to produce the desired effect (i.e. antinociception) to the amount that produces the undesired effect (i.e. sedation, heart rate, carotid flow). Specifically, the TW is defined as the ED_{50} (undesired effect)/ED_{50} (desired effect). A TW >1 indicates that the desired effect can be achieved in the absence of the side effect and higher indices are more advantageous therapeutically.

In Table 3, the TW has been calculated for morphine and clonidine alone and in combination following intrathecal or systemic administration for each endpoint. Following intrathecal delivery, combination therapy increased the TW from between 0.5–5.7 to 36–200. These large increases in TW are the result of profound antinociceptive synergy in parallel with additive or sub-additive interactions in the undesired side effects. Systemic combination therapy resulted in more modest increases in TW compared to intrathecal delivery. This is due primarily to the magnitude of the synergistic interaction in the antinociceptive assay being greater for intrathecal vs. systemic administration.

Discussion

In this manuscript, the beneficial effects of adrenergic-opioid combination therapy on therapeutic window in the treatment of acute pain were determined. Significant increases in therapeutic window were observed following both intrathecal and systemic administration. The opening of the therapeutic window can be explained by the presence of a synergistic interaction in antinociception in the absence of similar potentiation in the side effects of sedation/motor impairment and cardiovascular depression. In addition to increasing the therapeutic window, combination therapy resulted in increased maximum antinociceptive efficacy. Clinically, these data suggest that improved analgesia can be obtained with combination therapy at doses that do not produce sedation or cardiovascular depression.

Intrathecal Morphine + Clonidine

This report confirmed prior observations that the prototypic α_2AR agonist clonidine synergizes with morphine when given spinally to mice, increasing the potency by 100-fold over either agent given alone. By contrast, the combination synergized in neither the rotarod test of sedation/motor impairment nor in measures of cardiovascular depression. The antinociceptive/sedative therapeutic window range was increased from 0.5–5.7 to 45–200 as a result of the mulitmodal vs. unimodal approach. Similarly the antinociceptive/cardiovascular therapeutic window range was increased from 0.6–4.0 to 36–86. As a result, maximum antinociceptive efficacy is obtained at doses where neither sedation/motor impairment nor cardiovascular depression is evident. This separation between antinoception/sedation or antinociception/cardiovascular depression was not observed when either drug was administered alone.

In addition to the increased therapeutic window, the maximum antinociceptive efficacy was significantly higher in the combination group than either drug administered alone. No similar increases in the maximum efficacy were observed in the sedative/motor or cardiovascular measures. Therefore, intrathecal combination therapy affords an increase in both analgesic efficacy and potency in the absence of similar increases in the undesired side effects examined in this study.

Systemic (i.p.) Morphine + Clonidine

Following systemic administration, synergy was observed for antinociception but not in the sedative/motor or cardiovascular side-effects. However, the magnitude of the synergistic effect on antinociception was modest, yielding interaction index values of 0.3–0.4 compared to the much lower, and therefore more profound, intrathecal values of 0.02–0.07. As a result, the therapeutic window was only marginally increased by the combination. Thus, to maximize the effect of the morphine-clonidine combination therapy on therapeutic window, intrathecal delivery is advantageous.

Systemic combination therapy resulted in significant increases in the maximum antinociceptive efficacy of the combination compared to either drug alone. Thus, systemic morphine-clonidine combination therapy may result in therapeutically important increases in analgesic efficacy even in the absence of a profound impact on therapeutic window.

Integration with pre-clinical and clinical literature

Although several studies have probed the cardiovascular interactions between α_2AR and OR agonists [4,34,44], the goal of the current study was to systematically compare antinociceptive, sedative/motor and cardiovascular interactions under identical conditions (e.g. mouse strain, sex, age, housing and experimental environment). Loomis and colleagues (1988) evaluated the effects of intrathecally co-administered sub-effective doses of morphine and clonidine on sensitivity to heat (tail flick assay) and mechanical (paw pressure test) stimuli and blood pressure (tail cuff); the drug combination produced robust antinociception but had no effect on blood pressure. Solomon and Gebhart (1988) evaluated both antinociceptive and cardiovascular tolerance and cross-tolerance to the two single drugs given intrathecally, but the drugs were never co-administered. Although both drugs produced antinociceptive tolerance, chronic clonidine produced cardiovascular tolerance but unmasked a dose-related hypotensive effect of morphine. An analogous interaction on hypotension was not observed in the present study, although the current study was limited to acute drug administration. Randich and colleagues (1992) observed that a single, acute, systemic dose of morphine produced long-lived antinociception accompanied by transient (10 min) hypotension and heart rate. In the current study, while neither intrathecal nor systemic morphine effected carotid distension, they did dose-dependently reduce heart rate. Puig and colleagues (1996) performed an isobolographic analysis of systemic co-administration of clonidine and morphine and observed synergistic inhibition of gastrointestinal transit at low doses; therefore, the results reported here cannot be generalized to include all side effects [38].

In humans, studies examining the interaction between opioids and epidural clonidine in acute, post-surgical or chronic pain largely agree with our observations. For example, studies on labor or post-cesarean pain have shown that either a) clonidine reduced the need for intravenous morphine, did not affect heart rate or sedation but decreased blood pressure [13], b) clonidine improved opioid analgesia and reduced opioid self-administration in the absence of clinically important changes in side-effects [45], c) clonidine improved opioid analgesia but increased sedation [37], or d) epidural clonidine lowered fentanyl requirements during surgical anesthesia and improved cardiovascular stability with no serious untoward effects [46]. Common amongst those studies is the improved analgesic efficacy in the absence of consistent increases in the sedative and cardiovascular side effects. Furthermore, epidural clonidine has been shown to benefit patients with intractable cancer pain, particularly those with a significant neuropathic component [47], and the combination of intrathecal morphine + clonidine is useful for the management of chronic pain after spinal cord injury [17,20].

The current data demonstrate that the combination of morphine and clonidine can yield therapeutic windows greater than those of either agent alone. Similar observations have been reported in the pre-clinical literature for the mixed opioid agonist and serotonin-norepinephrine reuptake-inhibiting effects of tramadol [48] and tapentadol [49]. In addition, the current study extends prior antinociception/cardiovascular studies [34,50] to include full dose-response and isobolographic analysis along with the assessment of sedative/motor effects.

Limitations and Future Directions

In the current study, sedative and cardiovascular side effects were selected for this study because they are common to both drug classes, can be a limiting factor in the therapeutic use of either drug and can be easily measured in awake, behaving mice. While sedation will result in motor impairment, factors in addition to sedation likely contribute to the treatment-related motor impairment observed in this study. Additional studies addressing other physiological effects such as the respiratory depression associated with systemic opioid agonists are necessary.

The current study was performed in acute assays in normal, drug-naive and pain-free animals. Clinically, multimodal therapies are employed in chronic pain patients that are unresponsive to other therapeutic interventions [10,18]. While opioid-adrenergic synergy has also been demonstrated in pre-clinical models of chronic neuropathic pain [51,52], the side-effect profiles were not simultaneously assessed. In addition, the impact of opioid tolerance [53,54] on opioid-adrenergic synergy is not clear; for example, studies have suggested that synergy is either decreased [53] or unaltered [54] in morphine-tolerant mice. Finally, it will be important to examine these interactions during chronic administration of the combination as the rate and incidence of tolerance may develop differently in the desired vs. undesired effects, thus altering therapeutic window. If synergy-enabled reductions in total dose translate into reductions in analgesic tolerance, an important additional benefit of multimodal therapy will be realized. However, this possibility remains to be tested.

Advantages of Multimodal Analgesic Pharmacology

The search for new analgesic agents is focused on the identification of novel drug targets and the development of highly selective compounds directed at subtypes or subunits of these targets. This quest has eclipsed the search for ways to optimize the therapeutic benefit of well-known agents with proven efficacy in patients. Recent pharmaceutical history shows that highly potent, highly selective agents, upon translation to human subjects, either lack sufficient efficacy or manifest intolerable side effects or toxicities. For example, NK-1 antagonists, COX-2 selective inhibitors and TRPV1 antagonists have all failed to meet expectations for one of the aforementioned reasons [55–57]. These examples suggest that the rationale underlying drug development strategies that use potency and selectively as primary criteria may be flawed. Many of the most successful analgesics historically are non-selective, including morphine and other clinically used opioids, tramadol (targets both opioid receptors and monoaminergic reuptake), cannabis, tricyclic anti-depressants and aspirin.

Building on the foundation of therapeutically validated compounds with known side-effect profiles in humans presents huge potential for development of combination therapies [58,59]. Examples of combination medications abound, such as local anesthetics with morphine for intrathecal infusion and opioid-acetaminophen combinations for oral administration. In addition to lowering the prevalence of adverse effects and improving analgesia, multimodal analgesia techniques may shorten hospitalization times, improve recovery and function, and decrease healthcare costs [60,61]. However, few of these combinations exploit well-characterized synergistic interactions such as the α_2AR-opioid interaction described in this paper. Furthermore, the impact of the combination on therapeutic window is rarely considered. A systematic search of therapeutically used agents for identification of synergistic pairs and exploitation of these pairs for therapeutic development would be of great value.

Acknowledgments

The authors thank Dr. M. Ossipov for the use of JFlashCalc.

Author Contributions

Conceived and designed the experiments: LSS CAF GLW. Performed the experiments: LSS JG KFK. Analyzed the data: LSS GLW. Wrote the paper: LSS CAF GLW.

References

1. Cousins MJ, Mather LE (1984) Intrathecal and epidural administration of opioids. Anesthesiology 61: 276–310.
2. Hylden JLK, Wilcox GL (1980) Intrathecal morphine in mice: a new technique. Eur J Pharmacol 67: 313–316.
3. American Pain Society. (2006) Pain Control in the Primary Care Setting. Glenview, IL: American Pain Society.
4. Randich A, Thurston CL, Ludwig PS, Robertson JD, Rasmussen C (1992) Intravenous morphine-induced activation of vagal afferents: peripheral, spinal, and CNS substrates mediating inhibition of spinal nociception and cardiovascular responses. J Neurophysiol 68: 1027–1045.
5. Reddy SVR, Maderdrut JL, Yaksh TL (1980) Spinal cord pharmacology of adrenergic agonist-mediated antinociception. J Pharmacol Exp Ther 213: 525–533.
6. Reddy SV, Yaksh TL (1980) Spinal noradrenergic terminal system mediates antinociception. 189: 391–401.
7. Yaksh TL, Reddy SV (1981) Studies in the primate on the analgetic effects associated with intrathecal actions of opiates, alpha-adrenergic agonists and baclofen. Anesthesiology 54: 451–467.
8. Kaalzow L (1974) Analgesia produced by clonidine in mice and rats. J Pharm Pharmacol 26: 361.
9. Eisenach JC, Lysak SZ, Viscomi CM (1989) Epidural clonidine analgesia following surgery: phase I. Anesthesiology 71: 640–646.
10. Eisenach JC, Rauck RL, Buzzanell C, Lysak SZ (1989) Epidural clonidine analgesia for intractable cancer pain: phase I. Anesthesiology 71: 647–652.
11. Mendez R, Eisenach JC, Kashtan K (1990) Epidural clonidine analgesia after cesarean section. Anesthesiology 73: 848–852.
12. Rauck RL, Eisenach JC, Jackson K, Young LD, Southern J (1993) Epidural clonidine treatment for refractory reflex sympathetic dystrophy. Anesthesiology 79: 1163–1169; discussion 1127A.
13. Eisenach JC, D'Angelo R, Taylor C, Hood DD (1994) An isobolographic study of epidural clonidine and fentanyl after cesarean section. Anesthesia & Analgesia 79: 285–290.
14. Eisenach JC, DuPen S, Dubios M, Miguel R, Allin D (1995) Epidural clonidine analgesia for intractable cancer pain. pain 61: 391–399.
15. Giovannoni MP, Ghelardini C, Vergelli C, Dal Piaz V (2009) Alpha2-agonists as analgesic agents. Med Res Rev 29: 339–368.
16. Bouaziz H, Hewitt C, Eisenach JC (1995) Subarachnoid neostigmine potentiation of alpha 2-adrenergic agonist analgesia. Dexmedetomidine versus Clonidine. Regional Anesthesia 20: 121–127.
17. Siddall PJ, Gray M, Rutkowski S, Cousins MJ (1994) Intrathecal morphine and clonidine in the management of spinal cord injury pain: a case report. Pain 59: 147–148.
18. Coombs DW, Saunders RL, Fratkin JD, Jensen LE, Murphy CA (1986) Continuous intrathecal hydromorphone and clonidine for intractable cancer pain. J Neurosurg 64: 890–894.
19. Plummer JL, Cmielewski PL, Gourlay GK, Owen H, Cousins MJ (1992) Antinociceptive and motor effects of intrathecal morphine combined with intrathecal clonidine, noradrenaline, carbachol or midazolam. Pain 49: 145–152.
20. Siddall PJ, Molloy AR, Walker S, Mather LE, Rutkowski SB, et al. (2000) The efficacy of intrathecal morphine and clonidine in the treatment of pain after spinal cord injury. Anesth Analg 91: 1493–1498.
21. Hassenbusch SJ, Gunes S, Wachsman S, Willis KD (2002) Intrathecal clonidine in the treatment of intractable pain: a phase I/II study. Pain Med 3: 85–91.
22. Kedlaya D, Reynolds L, Waldman S (2002) Epidural and intrathecal analgesia for cancer pain. Best Pract Res Clin Anaesthesiol 16: 651–665.
23. Uhle EI, Becker R, Gatscher S, Bertalanffy H (2000) Continuous intrathecal clonidine administration for the treatment of neuropathic pain. Stereotact Funct Neurosurg 75: 167–175.
24. Solomon RE, Brody MJ, Gebhart GF (1989) Pharmacological characterization of alpha adrenoceptors involved in the antinociceptive and cardiovascular effects of intrathecally administered clonidine. J Pharmacol Exp Ther 251: 27–38.
25. Walker SM, Goudas LC, Cousins MJ, Carr DB (2002) Combination spinal analgesic chemotherapy: a systematic review. Anesth Analg 95: 674–715.
26. Solomon RE, Gebhart GF (1994) Synergistic antinociceptive interactions among drugs administered to the spinal cord. Anesth Analg 78: 1164–1172.
27. Wilcox GL, Carlsson KH, Jochim A, Jurna I (1987) Mutual potentiation of antinociceptive effects of morphine and clonidine on motor and sensory responses in rat spinal cord. Brain Res 405: 84–93.
28. Ossipov MH, Harris S, Lloyd P, Messineo E (1990) An isobolographic analysis of the antinociceptive effect of systemically and intrathecally administered combinations of clonidine and opiates. J Pharmacol Exp Ther 255: 1107–1116.
29. Ossipov MH, Harris S, Lloyd P, Messineo E, Lin BS, et al. (1990) Antinociceptive interaction between opioids and medetomidine: systemic additivity and spinal synergy. Anesthesiology 73: 1227–1235.
30. Ossipov MH, Lozito R, Messineo E, Green J, Harris S, et al. (1990) Spinal antinociceptive synergy between clonidine and morphine, U69593, and DPDPE: isobolographic analysis. Life Sci 47: PL71–76.
31. Drasner K, Fields HL (1988) Synergy between the antinociceptive effects of intrathecal clonidine and systemic morphine in the rat. Pain 32: 309–312.
32. Monasky MS, Zinsmeister AR, Stevens CW, Yaksh TL (1990) Interaction of intrathecal morphine and ST-91 on antinociception in the rat: dose-response analysis, antagonism and clearance. J Pharmacol Exp Ther 254: 383–392.
33. Meert TF, De Kock M (1994) Potentiation of the analgesic properties of fentanyl-like opioids with alpha 2-adrenoceptor agonists in rats. Anesthesiology 81: 677–688.
34. Loomis CW, Milne B, Cervenko FW (1988) A study of the interaction between clonidine and morphine on analgesia and blood pressure during continuous intrathecal infusion in the rat. Neuropharmacology 27: 191–199.
35. Tajerian M, Millecamps M, Stone LS (2012) Morphine and clonidine synergize to ameliorate low back pain in mice. Pain Research and Treatment 2012: 150842.
36. Chabot-Dore AJ, Millecamps M, Stone LS (2013) The delta-opioid receptor is sufficient, but not necessary, for spinal opioid-adrenergic analgesic synergy. The Journal of pharmacology and experimental therapeutics 347: 773–780.
37. Paech MJ, Pavy TJ, Orlikowski CE, Yeo ST, Banks SL, et al. (2004) Postcesarean analgesia with spinal morphine, clonidine, or their combination. Anesth Analg 98: 1460–1466, table of contents.
38. Puig MM, Pol O, Warner W (1996) Interaction of morphine and clonidine on gastrointestinal transit in mice. Anesthesiology 85: 1403–1412.
39. Zimmermann M (1983) Ethical guidelines for investigations of experimental pain in conscious animals. Pain 16: 109–110.
40. Janssen PA, Niemegeers CJE, Dony JGH (1963) The inhibitory effect of fentanyl and other morphine-like analgesics on the warm water induced tail withdrawal reflex in rats. Arzneim Forsch 13: 502–507.
41. Tallarida RJ, Murray RB (1987) Manual of pharmacological calculations with computer programs. Springer Verlag:New York: 26–31.
42. Tallarida RJ (1992) Statistical analysis of drug combinations for synergism [published erratum appears in Pain 1993 Jun;53(3):365] [Review]. Pain 49: 93–97.
43. Tallarida RJ (2002) The interaction index: a measure of drug synergism. Pain 98: 163–168.
44. Solomon RE, Gebhart GF (1988) Intrathecal morphine and clonidine: antinociceptive tolerance and cross-tolerance and effects on blood pressure. J Pharmacol Exp Ther 245: 444–454.
45. Paech MJ, Banks SL, Gurrin LC, Yeo ST, Pavy TJ (2002) A randomized, double-blinded trial of subarachnoid bupivacaine and fentanyl, with or without clonidine, for combined spinal/epidural analgesia during labor. Anesth Analg 95: 1396–1401, table of contents.
46. Murga G, Samso E, Valles J, Casanovas P, Puig MM (1994) The effect of clonidine on intra-operative requirements of fentanyl during combined epidural/general anaesthesia. Anaesthesia 49: 999–1002.
47. Eisenach JC, DuPen S, Dubois M, Miguel R, Allin D (1995) Epidural clonidine analgesia for intractable cancer pain. The Epidural Clonidine Study Group. Pain 61: 391–399.
48. Raffa RB, Friderichs E, Reimann W, Shank RP, Codd EE, et al. (1993) Complementary and synergistic antinociceptive interaction between the enantiomers of tramadol. J Pharmacol Exp Ther 267: 331–340.
49. Meske DS, Xie JY, Oyarzo J, Badghisi H, Ossipov MH, et al. (2013) Opioid and noradrenergic contributions of tapentadol in experimental neuropathic pain. Neuroscience Letters.
50. Loomis CW, Cervenko FW, Jhamandas K, Sutak M, Milne B (1985) Analgesia and autonomic function following intrathecal administration of morphine and norepinephrine to the rat. Can J Physiol Pharmacol 63: 656–662.
51. Fairbanks CA, Nguyen HO, Grocholski BM, Wilcox GL (2000) Moxonidine, a selective imidazoline-alpha2 -adrenergic receptor agonist, produces spinal synergistic antihyperalgesia with morphine in nerve-injured mice. Anesthesiology 93: 765–773.
52. Ossipov MH, Lopez Y, Bian D, Nichols ML, Porreca F (1997) Synergistic antinociceptive interactions of morphine and clonidine in rats with nerve-ligation injury. Anesthesiol 86: 1–9.
53. Roerig SC (1995) Decreased spinal morphine/clonidine antinociceptive synergism in morphine-tolerant mice. Life Sciences 56: PL115–122.

54. Fairbanks CA, Wilcox GL (1999) Spinal antinociceptive synergism between morphine and clonidine persists in mice made acutely or chronically tolerant to morphine. J Pharmacol Exp Ther 288: 1107–1116.
55. Solomon SD, McMurray JJ, Pfeffer MA, Wittes J, Fowler R, et al. (2005) Cardiovascular risk associated with celecoxib in a clinical trial for colorectal adenoma prevention. N Engl J Med 352: 1071–1080.
56. Nussmeier NA, Whelton AA, Brown MT, Langford RM, Hoeft A, et al. (2005) Complications of the COX-2 inhibitors parecoxib and valdecoxib after cardiac surgery. N Engl J Med 352: 1081–1091.
57. Hill R (2000) NK1 (substance P) receptor antagonists–why are they not analgesic in humans? Trends Pharmacol Sci 21: 244–246.
58. Chaparro LE, Wiffen PJ, Moore RA, Gilron I (2012) Combination pharmacotherapy for the treatment of neuropathic pain in adults. The Cochrane database of systematic reviews 7: CD008943.
59. Gilron I, Jensen TS, Dickenson AH (2013) Combination pharmacotherapy for management of chronic pain: from bench to bedside. Lancet neurology 12: 1084–1095.
60. Reuben SS, Buvanendran A (2007) Preventing the development of chronic pain after orthopaedic surgery with preventive multimodal analgesic techniques. J Bone Joint Surg Am 89: 1343–1358.
61. Reuben SS, Buvanendran A, Kroin JS, Raghunathan K (2006) The analgesic efficacy of celecoxib, pregabalin, and their combination for spinal fusion surgery. Anesth Analg 103: 1271–1277.

ecided that, an acute onset of febrile painful typical MSK illness n a naïve subject during the epidemic period (with several ommunities suffering from similar illness) was sufficient for the linical diagnosis. However, the subjects under the study were arefully screened for common community infections (in particular nalaria and dengue) and subjected to serological testing of anti HIKV antibodies. All cases (survey) were clinically examined nd empirically classified as CHIKV by AC and other team octors, as per protocol. Typical cases were characterized by a hort duration (<3 days) of high fever accompanied by severe ebilitating polyarthralgias and musculoskeletal aches and pains asting less than 10 days. Subjects with milder intensity of CHIKV ke illness (and/or other symptoms like fatigue, headaches, skin sions) and lasting up to seven days were labeled 'probable' and ere observed further. All individuals who were asymptomatic but rovided a typical prior history of acute CHIKV illness suffered uring the epidemic were included if the first evaluation (clinical nd laboratory) was carried out within the study window period our weeks) and labeled 'recovered'. All cases which tested eropositive for anti CHIKV antibody (IgM and/or IgG) were lassified as 'definite cases'.

Based on the time point of the first clinical examination (blood ollected simultaneously) following the onset of the illness (fever), ases were empirically classified into acute (0–5 days), subacute (6–4 days) and extended phase (15–30 days) illness.

lood Samples

Blood samples were aseptically collected and suitably transport-d (road) in ice packs to the Center for Rheumatic Diseases: esearch & Diagnostic (CRD: R & D) Lab, Pune within 6–8 hours f collection. Serum was separated immediately and stored at − 0°C. Pune city was 156 kms from the Bavi survey site. Routine ematology and immunology tests were carried out within 24 ours of blood collection. Peripheral blood smears were examined exclude malarial parasite. Acute phase reactants included rythrocyte sedimentation rate (ESR, Westergren, reported as mm ll at end of 1st hour) and C - reactive protein (CRP, using ephelometry; cut off value 5 mg/L). The autoantibody profile ncluded Rheumatoid Factor (RF, estimated by nephelometry; cut ff value 40 IU/ml), anti-Cyclic Citrullinated Peptide (anti CCP, ommercially available second generation ELISA, Euroimmun, ermany; cut off value of ≥5 RU/ml) and Antinuclear Antibody ANA, using qualitative enzyme immunoassay).

nti CHIKV Antibodies

Specific IgM and IgG antibodies to CHIKV were tested by mmunochromatography [10] and indirect immunofluorescence espectively. Due to limited budget grant, it was decided to test for nti CHIKV antibody IgG in all the acute phase subjects and hose blood samples available at more than two follow-up visits. In he current study cohort, IgG was tested in 58 subjects [42 ymptomatic (acute phase = 23, subacute phase = 3, extended ymptomatic phase = 16) and 16 recovered subjects]. Anti-dengue ntibodies (IgG and IgM) were also tested in all samples using On-ite lateral flow chromatographic immunoassay.

erum Cytokines

In the study, Interferon (IFN) –α, -β and -γ, Tumor Necrosis actor - α (TNF-α), Interleukin (IL) −1β, IL-6, IL-13, Interferon amma-Induced Protein-10 (CXCL-10/IP-10), Monocyte Che-noattractant Protein-1 (MCP-1), IL –4 and IL-10 were measured sing development kits (R&D Systems, USA). The DuoSeT LISA Development kit (R&D Systems Inc., USA) contained the asic components required for the development of sandwich ELISAs to measure natural and recombinant cytokines. The assay procedure was similar for all cytokines. The working concentrations of capture antibody, detection antibody and standards for each of the individual components was as per the literature provided by the manufacturer. Due to limited study grant budget IFN-α, IFN-β, IL-1β, MCP-1, IL-4 and IL-10 were measured 31 in symptomatic cases (acute phase = 23; subacute phase = 4; extended symptomatic phase = 4) and in 80 healthy controls.

Based on standard literature, cytokines were broadly classified into Th1 (IFN –α, -β and -γ, TNF-α, IL- 1β, CXCL-10/IP-10, MCP-1) and Th2 (IL-6, IL –4, IL-10, IL-13) phenotype.

Study Cohort

The current study cohort for cytokine assay was made up of 132 cases (110 symptomatic and 22 recovered) who were first evaluated (clinical and laboratory) during the epidemic survey within 4 weeks of onset of fever (Fig. 1) The male:female ratio in the symptomatic and recovered groups was 1:1.5 and 1:3 respectively. The median age was 36 years in both groups.

The study cohort was drawn from 225 community cases (44% survey cases) who consented to donate blood for laboratory investigations and a selection was made on first come first serve basis (Fig. 1).

Several cases were evaluated at regular intervals and followed up for periods ranging from 6–22 months as per the survey protocol. The follow up data is not included in the current study report.

Survey Controls

49 subjects in the village who did not recall having had fever or any symptoms suggestive of CHIKV infection (during the CHIKV epidemic) also consented to give blood samples during the survey.

Healthy Controls

Coincidentally, Bavi village was close to our rural project site (Bhigwan) for an ongoing WHO ILAR (International League of Associations for Rheumatology) COPCORD (Community Oriented Program for Control of Rheumatic Diseases) since 1996 [11]. Blood samples (N = 80) collected from consenting healthy villagers (without any symptomatic chronic illness and in particular arthritis) examined during a COPCORD activity in 2005 (a year prior to the CHIKV epidemic of 2006) and stored at −80°C in CRD lab were used as healthy controls. The male : female ratio was 1:1 and the median age was 41 years. These samples tested negative for dengue and CHIKV antibodies.

Statistics

The survey sample size was not based on any statistical (power of the study) calculation. SPSS version 12.0 (USA) was used for all statistical calculations. The differences in serum cytokines between the groups was compared by a non-parametric analysis with Kruskal – Wallis test with significance at $p<0.05$. Standard Pearson's correlation coefficient was calculated and the strength (correlation) was classified as weak (0.1–0.3), moderate (0.4–0.6), strong (0.7–0.9) and perfect (1.0). Linear regression analysis was performed to determine predictors of resolution of symptoms within one month in the study cohort.

Results

Fig. 1 provides an overview of the survey subjects screened, cases detected, cases with blood sample collection and distribution of various subject groups characterized by symptomatic status and illness duration at the time of initial evaluation. As per the study

Cytokines in Acute Chikungunya

Anuradha Venugopalan*, Ravi P. Ghorpade, Arvind Chopra

Center for Rheumatic Diseases, Pune, India

Abstract

Introduction: Acute chikungunya (CHIKV) is predominantly an acute onset of excruciatingly painful, self-li musculoskeletal (MSK) arbovirus illness and this was further reported by us during the 2006 Indian epidemic [Chopr Epidemiol Infect 2012]. Selected serum cytokines profile in subjects within one month of onset of illness is being pre

Methods: Out of 509 clinical CHIKV cases (43% population) identified during a rural population survey, 225 s consented blood investigations. 132 examined within 30 days of febrile onset are the study cohort. Anti-CHIKV IgM a antibodies tested by immunochromatography and indirect immunofluorescence respectively. Interferons (IFN)-α, -β Interferon Gamma-Induced Protein-10 (CXCL-10/IP-10), Tumor Necrosis Factor-α (TNF-α), Interleukin-1β (IL-1β), Interl (IL-6), Interleukin-13 (IL-13), Monocyte Chemoattractant Protein-1 (MCP-1), Interleukin–4 (IL-4) and Interleukin–10 performed by ELISA. Samples collected from neighboring community a year prior to the epidemic used as healthy c

Results: Seropositivity for anti-CHIKV IgM and IgG was 65% and 52% respectively. IFN-α, IFN-β, IFN-γ, CXCL10/IP-10 1β showed intense response in early acute phase. Cytokines (particularly TNF-α, MCP-1, IL-4, IL-6 and IL-10) was maxir extended symptomatic phase and remained elevated in recovered subjects. Higher ($p<0.05$) IFN and IL-4 seen in p seropositive for anti-CHIKV IgG. Elderly cases (≥65 years) showed elevated cytokines (except IFN) and anti-CHIKV ant near similar to younger subjects. Significant correlations ($p<0.05$) found between cytokines and clinical features (f low back ache, myalgia) and anti-CHIKV antibodies.

Conclusion: An intense cytokine milieu was evident in the early and immediate persistent symptomatic phase recovered subjects. Early persistent IgM and lower IgG to anti-CHKV and intense Th2 cytokine phenotype seem associated with delay in resolution of MSK symptoms. Intriguingly, maximum TNF-α, IL-6 and IL-13 with low anti-CHI response found in subjects recovered from CHIKV within one month of illness.

Editor: Dirk Homann, Mount Sinai School of Medicine, United States of America

Funding: This project was funded by Indian Council of Medical Research (Government of India, 5/8/7/20/2006-ECD-I) and Arthritis Research Care Fo (CRD, Pune). The funders had no role in study design, data collection and analysis, decision to publish, or preparation of the manuscript.

Competing Interests: The authors have declared that no competing interests exist.

* Email: venugopalan_anuradha@hotmail.com

Introduction

Chikungunya (CHIKV), an arbovirus belonging to the family *Togaviridae*, is transmitted by mosquito (*Aedes aegypti* and *A. albopictus*) and causes an acute onset of febrile excruciatingly painful musculoskeletal (MSK) illness which is predominantly selflimiting. A reemergence of an African strain of the CHIKV in 2006 caused a widespread unprecedented epidemic in South Asia and several neighboring regions and islands [1–7]. Inundated by several hundred clinical referrals to the rheumatology outpatient, we reported a unique spectrum of arthritis and rheumatism in naïve patients following the CHIKV illness [8]. We carried out a rural community survey during the epidemic and reported the clinical profile of acute CHIKV and its MSK sequel [1]. We were intrigued by the sheer intensity of musculoskeletal pain (MSK) and polyarthralgias at the onset of illness but the large majority of our cases recovered within three weeks. However, about one third of cases continued to suffer from persistent MSK pain and arthritis beyond one month of onset of illness. This was much more than what was reported from earlier epidemics [9]. To explore this further, we carried out a detail laboratory evaluation of the rural community survey subjects which included selected cytokine assay. The purpose was to unravel some of the immune p correlations and patterns of cytokine upregulation. In we primarily focus on the cytokine profile of the cases examined within four weeks of the onset of CHIKV il

Methods

The protocol was approved by the ethic committe Pune. All eligible patients were provided a study i brochure and signed an informed consent form (local prior to enrollment.

The principal study [1,2] was designed as a house to h population survey during the Indian epidemic of CHIK in Bavi (a village in district Sholapur, state of Maharas India). The currentstudy design used was a cross section of cytokine assay in subjects diagnosed with CH evaluated within four weeks (current study period) of of febrile illness.

Definition and Classifications

For the study an epidemic based definition, decided a the rheumatologist (AC), was used to diagnose CHIK

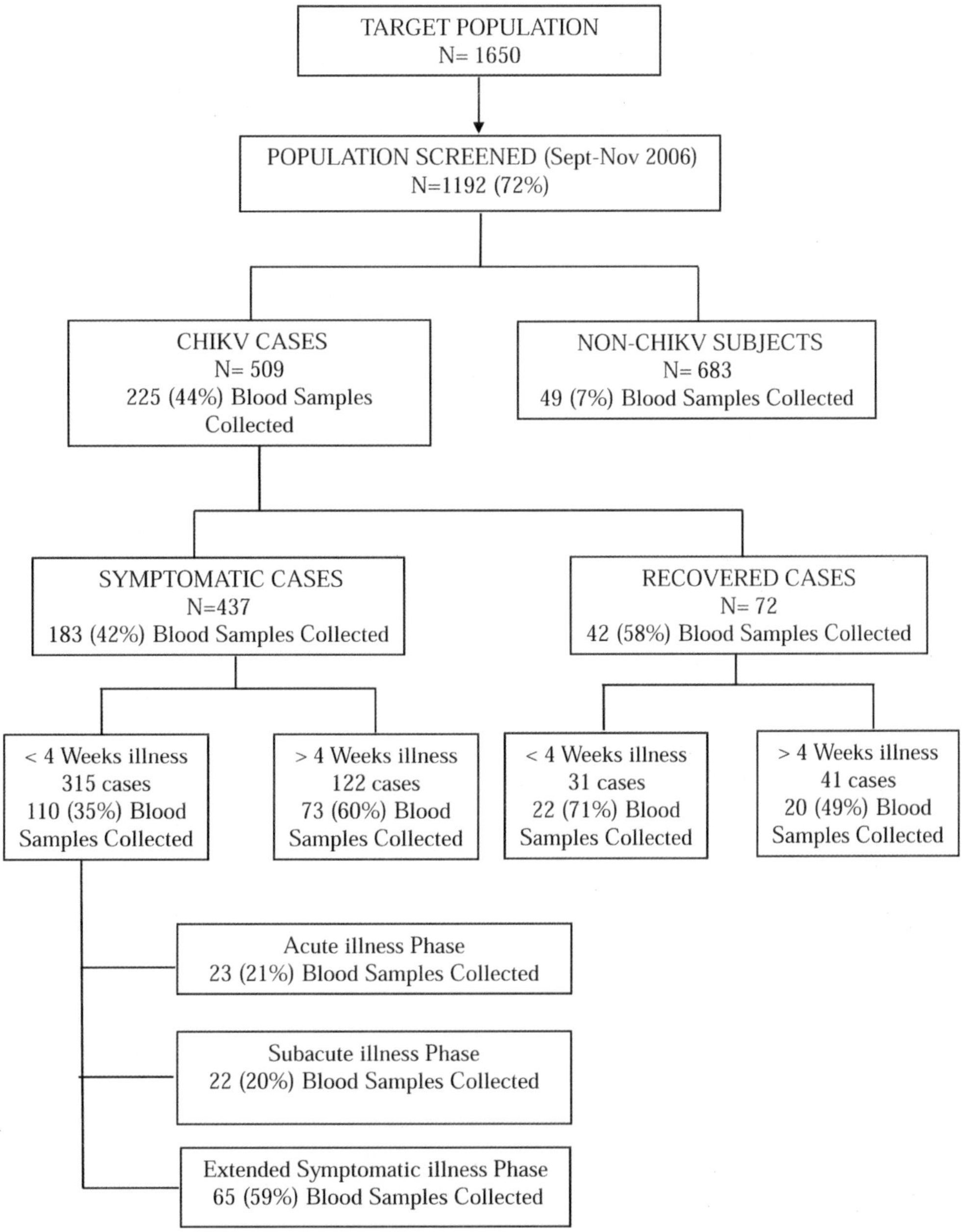

Figure 1. Number of cases identified and blood samples collected during survey and at subsequent follow-up period.

protocol, all cases in the current study cohort were clinically classifiable as typical or definite (see above).

1 Anti CHIKV antibodies

The serological profile of the study cohort is shown in Table 1. 51% symptomatic and 32% recovered subjects tested seropositive for specific anti-CHIKV IgM antibodies; corresponding positivity for anti-CHIKV IgG antibody was in 40% symptomatic and 50% recovered subjects. 4% and 8% survey controls (without history of CHIKV) tested positive for anti-CHIKV IgM and IgG antibody respectively. The proportion of cases with seropositive IgM was observed to increase with higher duration of illness; 17% acute, 55% sub acute and 62% extended symptoms. In contrast, the proportion of cases with seropositive IgG was much lesser with increased duration; 52% acute, 100% sub acute and 13% extended symptoms. 32% and 50% of recovered cases in the study cohort were seropositive for anti CHIKV IgM and IgG antibody respectively.

2 Acute Phase Reactants

Though not strictly fasting, the mean ESR was 75 mm fall at the end of 1st hour (range 5–89). 16 (14.5%) cases in the study cohort were seropositive for CRP with a median value of 12 mg/L (range 6–48). A higher proportion of cases (26.1%) showed seropositive CRP in the acute phase illness as compared to subacute and extended duration (Table 1). 18.2% recovered cases were seropositive for CRP.

Table 1. Serological profile (frequency of positive result) of symptomatic cases (N = 110) with recovered cases (N = 22) of CHIKV with illness within one month duration.

Test	Acute (N = 23)*	Subacute (N = 22)*	Extended Symptomatic (N = 65)*	Total Symptomatic (N = 110)*	Recovered (N = 22)*
	N (%)	N (%)	N (%)	N (%)	N (%)
CHIKV IgM +	4 (17%)	12 (55%)	40 (62%)	56 (51%)	7 (32%)
CHIKV IgG+	12 (52%)	3 (100%)	2 (13%)	17 (40%)	8 (50%)
CHIKV IgM+IgG−	1 (4%)	0	10 (63%)	11 (26%)	2 (13%)
CHIKV IgM−IgG+	9 (39%)	1 (33%)	0	10 (24%)	4 (25%)
CHIKV IgM+IgG+	3 (13%)	2 (67%)	2 (13%)	7 (17%)	4 (25%)
CHIKV IgM−IgG−	10 (43%)	0	4 (25%)	14 (33%)	6 (38%)
CRP (≥6 mg/L)	6 (26.1%)	2 (9.1%)	8 (12.3%)	16 (14.5%)	4 (18.2%)
RF (≥40 IU/ml)	2 (8.7%)	0	3 (4.6%)	5 (4.5%)	0
ANA	1 (4.3%)	1 (4.5%)	3 (4.6%)	5 (4.5%)	2 (9.1%)

CRP = C-reactive Protein; RF = Rheumatoid Factor; ANA = Antinuclear Antibody.
*Note : Anti CHIKV IgM was tested in all the 110 symptomatic and 22 recovered subjects; Anti CHIKV IgG was only tested in 42 symptomatic subjects (Acute = 23; subacute = 3 and extended symptomatic = 16) and 16 recovered subjects; CRP, RF and ANA was tested in all subjects.

3 Serum Cytokines

Fig. 2 shows the scatter distribution of various cytokines assay in the study cohort and healthy controls. Interestingly, several healthy control cases showed strikingly high assay of IFN-γ, TNF-α and IL-6. However, the serum cytokines assay (median) was significantly higher ($p<0.05$) in the study cohort (symptomatic and recovered) as compared to that observed in the healthy controls (Fig. 2). Except for IFN-γ, the serum assays (median) for TNF-α, IL-6, IL-13, CXCL-10/IP-10, were higher in the recovered group (Fig. 2) as compared to healthy control [IL-6 ($p = 0.01$), IL-13 ($p = 0.06$)]; assay for other cytokines could not be carried out in this group.

Table 2 shows serum cytokine assay in the acute, subacute and extended symptomatic sub-groups. Compared to healthy controls (Fig. 2), all cytokines were elevated several folds in each of the subgroups. In the symptomatic group, maximum elevation for IFN (α, β, γ), CXCL-10/IP-10, IL-1β and IL-13 was observed in the acute phase illness and TNF-α, MCP-1, IL-6 and IL-10 in patients with extended symptoms. It was observed that IL-4 (marker for Th2 cytokine response) was maximal in the subacute illness group (7–14 days post onset). However, on comparison across board, IL-4, TNF-α, CXCL-10/IP-10, IL-6 and IL-13 was maximally elevated in the recovered group.

4 Serum Cytokine Correlations

Table 3 and Table 4 show significant ($p<0.05$) correlations (positive and negative) between cytokines and selected clinical and laboratory features and specific anti CHIKV antibodies.

4.1 Acute phase. Moderate to perfect positive correlations were found between several cytokines. Each of the interferon subtypes showed moderate positive correlation with chemokine CXL-10/IP-10. IL-4 showed moderate positive correlation with anti CHIKV IgM. A moderate negative correlation was seen between IL-1β and anti CHIKV IgG antibody. As is well known, a significant moderate positive correlation was demonstrated between IL-6 and CRP, and TNF-α and IL-6. A moderate positive correlation was also observed between myalgias and the pro-inflammatory cytokine TNF-α. Several pro-inflammatory cytokines (CXCL-10/IP-10, MCP-1 and TNF-α) individually showed moderate negative correlation with blood hemoglobin and cell counts (leucocytes, platelets). Inflammation leads to increased iron utilization and TNF-α and pro-inflammatory cytokines contribute to chronic anemia [12]. Significant moderate to strong negative correlations was observed between several Th1 cytokines (IF and CXCL-10/IP-10) and Th2 cytokines (MCP-1, IL-10 and IL-6) suggesting counter check immune inflammation mechanisms.

4.2 Subacute phase. There were several interesting departures from the correlation pattern seen in the acute phase. In contrast, leukocyte and platelet counts gained positive correlations (CXCL-10/IP-10 and IL-6). TNF-α and IL-13 showed moderate positive correlation with headache. A strong correlations was observed for serum anti CHIKV IgG response and some cytokines (CXCL-10/IP-10 and IL-6).

4.3 Extended symptomatic phase. Several moderate to strong correlations seen with the cytokines in the sub acute illness were observed in this group especially with reference to anti CHIKV IgG antibody response. The correlation between TNF-α and IL-6 was further strengthened (0.60). However, the overall correlation pattern appeared much different from that seen in the acute phase and in particular with loss of several negative correlations (Table 3 and Table 4).

4.4 Recovered group. In the recovered group, IFN-γ correlated positively with a history of low backache and with TNF-α. TNF-α showed a moderate positive correlation with blood hemoglobin and we suspect that the improved hemoglobin level is due to recovery from illness. As stated earlier, for reasons not well understood several cytokines including TNF-α persisted high in the recovered group (Table 2). A moderate negative correlation was also seen between blood hemoglobin and age.

4.5 Study cohort (symptomatic and recovered). Several of the moderate, strong positive and negative correlations observed in the acute phase remained more or less unchanged when the total study cohort was considered. Some positive clinical correlations (weak to moderate) of interest need to be mentioned- IFN-γ and pain intensity, IFN-β, IL-1β individually and fatigue, TNF-α and headache, IL-4 and myalgia, IL-6 and skin rash. A moderately negative correlation was seen between IFN-α and myalgias. A moderate correlation between MCP-1 and leukocyte and platelet count was only seen in the study cohort. In contrast to

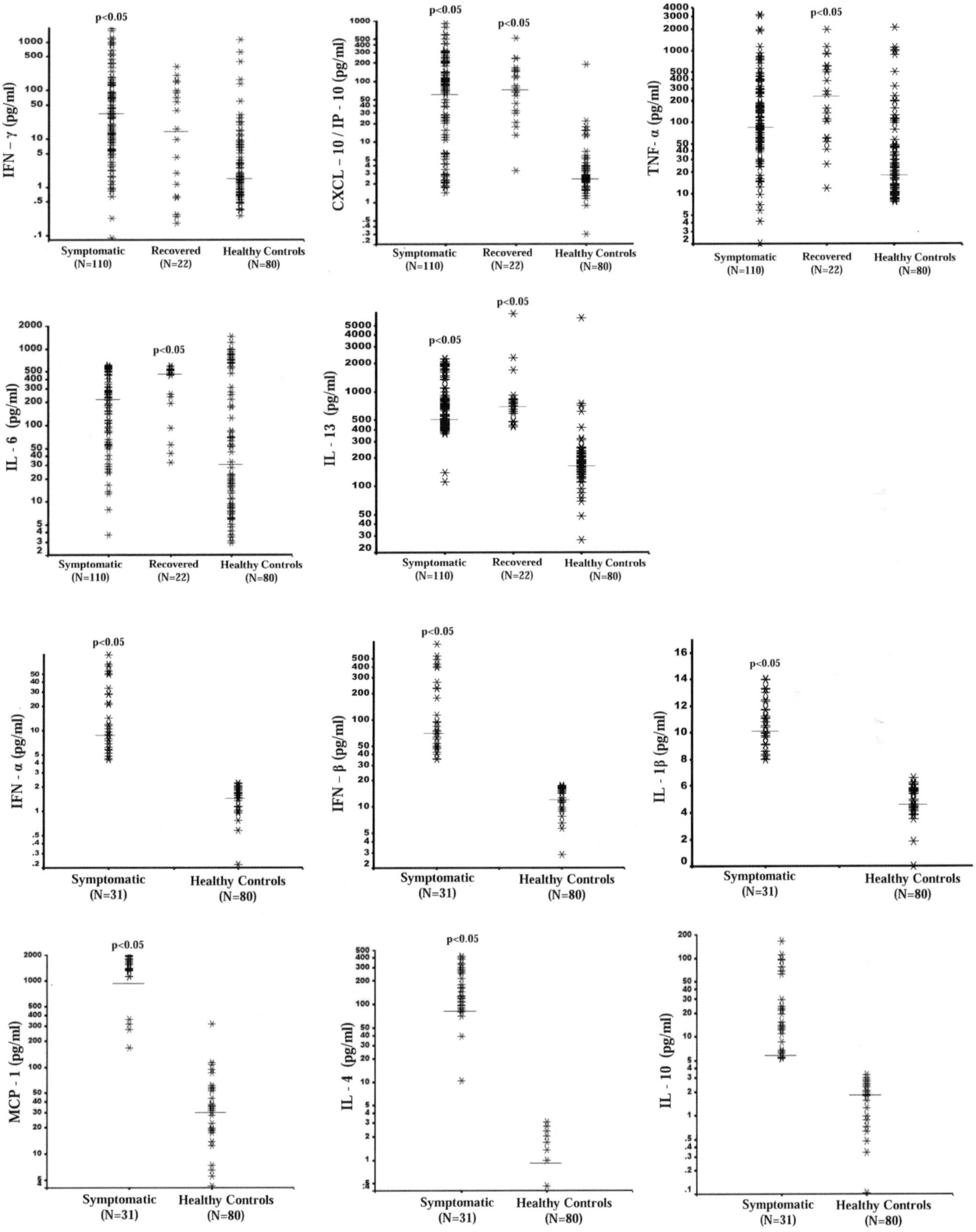

Figure 2. Selected Serum cytokine profile at of CHIKV cases (Symptomatic N = 110; Recovered N = 22) with CHIKV illness duration of 30 days compared with Healthy Controls (N = 80). *(Horizontal bars indicate medians of each category.).* **Footnote to Figure 2 :** IFN-Interferon; TNF = Tumor Necrosis Factor; CXCL-10/IP-10 = Interferon Gamma-Induced Protein-10; IL = Interleukin; MCP = Monocyte Chemoattractant Protein.

Statistical analyses were performed using non-parametric Kruskal Wallis test. 'p' values indicate significant difference between the corresponding group when compared with healthy control group. No significant ($p<0.05$) differences were observed between the symptomatic (N = 110) and recovered groups (N = 22) for any of the cytokines.

positive correlations observed in the subgroups, significant moderate negative correlations were observed between anti CHIKV IgM antibody response and each of three cytokines individually - IFN- α, IFN-β and IL-1β. Both IL-6 and IL-13, showed significant but weak positive correlation with several Th1 cytokines (IFN -γ, CXCL-10/IP-10, and TNF-α).

5 Cytokine Responses and Anti-CHIKV Antibody Seropositivity

Cytokine responses were compared between the two groups - seropositive and seronegative anti-CHIKV IgM and IgG antibodies (Table S1, Table S2, Table S3, Table S4, Table S5, Table S6, Table S7 and Table S8 in File S1).

Table 2. Cytokine profile of cases with CHIKV illness within one month duration (N = 110).

Cytokine	Acute Phase	Subacute Phase	Extended Symptomatic Phase	Total Symptomatic	Recovered	Healthy Controls
(pg/ml)	n = 23	n = 22#	n = 65#	n = 110	n = 22	n = 80
	14.16	5.71	4.68	9.61		1.58
IFN-α	[23.51]	[0.26]	[0.40]	[22.32]	ND	[0.50]
	(8.90–4.90)	(5.37–5.82)	(4.40–5.16)	(5.84–28.42)		(1.15–1.90)
	112.57	46.24	38.11	76.00		13.36
IFN-β	[191.88]	[2.57]	[3.43]	[181.64]	ND	[3.92]
	(70.10–390.40)	(43.11–47.82)	(35.28–41.70)	(48.26–227.99)		(9.82–16.25)
	85.24	29.33	26.84	37.70	15.82	1.72
IFN-γ	[476.59]	[201.56]	[329.49]	[348.42]	[86.18]	[153.13]
	(30.61–416.17)	(10.02–76.40)	(8.34–127.36)	(9.62–133.69)	(0.64–97.57)	(0.88–8.22)
	71.44	61.81	66.15	65.65	79.48	2.65
CXCL-10/IP-10	[277.41]	[118.57]	[93.85]	[161.87]	[111.97]	[21.44]
	(21.76–415.95)	(6.09–97.82)	(5.98–99.86)	(6.67–107.23)	(31.79–149.04)	(2.06–3.96)
	11.15	8.56	8.19	10.44		4.92
IL-1β	[1.49]	[0.32]	[0.18]	[1.82]	ND	[1.34]
	(10.02–12.44)	(8.41–8.99)	(8.02–8.36)	(9.11–11.80)		(4.19–5.70)
	90.99	94.30	107.54	97.20	257.88	20.65
TNF-α	[26.12]	[60.38]	[231.76]	[355.80]	[475.71]	[328.60]
	(18.01–188.33)	(4.2–1959.1)	(57.79–276.20)	(53.05–229.05)	(60.69–610.03)	(11.73–50.51)
	1576.40	1218.88	1869.23	1605.09		32.23
MCP-1	[541.83]	[584.95]	[776.26]	[570.59]	ND	[76.45]
	(1333.64–1892.25)	(514.56–1608.27)	(711.79–1955.56)	(1254.59–1892.25)		(18.31–58.73)
	119.58	392.57	170.53	137.94		1.00
IL-4	[89.36]	[34.10]	[24.26]	[111.85]	ND	[0.61]
	(88.98–249.31)	(347.36–409.73)	(162.00–204.77)	(96.83–273.78)		(1.00–1.69)
	172.39	233.74	250.93	235.07	501.16	33.40
IL-6	[230.68]	[142.59]	[197.89]	[194.47]	[203.08]	[354.81]
	(29.19–513.40)	(103.16–278.85)	(86.60–498.81)	(82.21–456.99)	(224.57–557.53)	(8.46–472.96)
	13.12	46.12	72.97	17.44		1.98
IL-10	[43.88]	[22.11]	[11.87]	[41.47]	ND	[0.87]
	(6.46–22.05)	(25.84–66.39)	(68.89–89.82)	(8.17–68.90)		(1.91–2.55)
	581.34	449.69	576.09	558.63	751.61	177.77
IL-13	[46.63]	[345.68]	[939.43]	[784.39]	[1315.41]	[688.76]
	(420.15–780.05)	(427.82–830.07)	(461.38–1093.22)	(440.37–856.74)	(606.44–835.81)	(142.29–212.07)

Values expressed as median [standard deviation](interquartile range) pg/ml.

IFN-Interferon; TNF = Tumor Necrosis Factor; CXCL-10/IP-10 = Interferon Gamma-Induced Protein 10; IL = Interleukin; MCP = Monocyte Chemoattractant Protein. #**Note**: IFN-α, IFN-β, IL-1β, MCP-1, IL-4 and IL-10 were tested in 4 subjects each of subacute phase and extended symptomatic phase. All other cytokines were tested in 23, 22 and 65 subjects of acute, subacute and extended symptomatic phase respectively. Statistical analyses were performed using non-parametric Kruskal Wallis test for significant differences within subgroups in the symptomatic group and for differences within total symptomatic group and recovered group versus healthy controls.

Table 3. Significant positive correlations between cytokines and selected clinical and laboratory variables.

Cytokine	Acute Phase	Subacute Phase	Extended Symptomatic Phase	Recovered	Total
(pg/ml)	n = 23	n = 22	n = 65	n = 22	N = 132
	IFN-β (1.00)				IFN-β (1.00)
IFN-α	IL-1β (0.94)	ND	ND	ND	IL-1β (0.90)
	CXCL-10/IP-10 (0.59)				CXCL-10/IP-10 (0.51)
IFN-β	CXCL-10/IP-10 (0.50)	ND	ND	ND	CXCL-10/IP-10 (0.52)
					Fatigue (0.42)
					Pain Intensity (0.23)
	CXCL-10/IP-10 (0.45)	–	Platelet Count (0.35)	Low Backache (0.48)	CXCL-10/IP-10 (0.18)
IFN-γ	MCP-1 (0.65)		CXCL-10/IP-10 (0.25)	TNF-α (0.51	MCP-1 (0.74)
					IL-6 (0.31)
					IL-13 (0.18)
		CHIKV-G (0.83)			TNF-α (0.24)
CXCL-10/IP-10	IL-6 (0.57)	Platelet Count (0.52)	CHIKV-G (0.58)	–	IL-10 (0.37)
		IL-6 (0.62)			IL-6 (0.39)
					IL-13 (0.45)
					Fatigue (0.47)
IL-1β	CXCL-10/IP-10 (0.61)	ND	ND	ND	CRP (0.37)
					CXCL-10/IP-10 (0.41)
					Headache (0.20)
TNF-α	IL-6 (0.48)	Headache (0.48)	IL-6 (0.60)	Hemoglobin (0.44)	IL-6 (0.61)
					IL-13 (0.23)
					Platelet Count (0.41)
MCP-1	–	ND	ND	ND	TLC (0.37)
					♀ Gender (0.38)
IL-4	CHIKV-M (0.58)	ND	ND	ND	Myalgia (0.47)
					IL-10 (0.85)
IL-6	CRP (0.54)	CHIKV-G (0.72)	CHIKV-G (0.53)	–	Skin Rash (0.19)
	♀ Gender (0.48)	TLC (0.51)			IL-13 (0.26)
IL-13	–	Headache (0.52)	CRP (0.28)	–	–

(*Pearson correlation co-efficient in parenthesis.*).
IFN-Interferon; TNF = Tumor Necrosis Factor; CXCL-10/IP-10 = Interferon Gamma-Induced Protein-10; IL = Interleukin; MCP = Monocyte Chemoattractant Protein. ND = Not Done; TLC = Total Leucocyte Count; CRP = C-reactive protein; ♀ = Female.

5.1 Acute phase. An intense IFN-α/−β, IL1β, CXCL-10/IP-10, TNF-α and IL-6 response was seen in the seronegative group (often $p<0.05$) as compared to seropositive groups and may suggest a blunted Th1 response once the specific antibodies appear. (Table S1, Table S2 and Table S3 in File S1). Significantly elevated ($p<0.05$) IL-4 and IL-10 in the seropositive group suggested B cell activation.

5.2 Subacute phase. The results were similar to those observed in acute phase except that the assays though elevated were comparatively reduced (Table S4 in File S1). There was no significant difference in IL-4 and IL-10 between the two groups and this may be attributed to a non-selected cytokine response once a robust IgM response is obtained.

5.3 Extended symptomatic phase. Overall the observations were similar except for a further reduction in cytokine assays in both groups (Table S5 in File S1). There was an increase in IL-10 in the seropositive IgM group as compared to acute and subacute illness. IL-10 is a potent inhibitor of Th1 cytokine response and in this study it may reflect a host attempt towards recovery from illness.

5.4 Recovered group. In the recovered group, there were no differences between seropositive and seronegative IgM groups for cytokine assay except for IFN-γ (increased in seronegative IgM group) (Table S6 in File S1).

5.5 Study cohort (Antibody response. Overall the results were similar to those obtained in individual subset groups (Table S1, Table S4 and Table S5 in File S1) with respect to anti CHIKV IgM response in the symptomatic group (Table S7 in File S1); significantly elevated IL-4 and IL-10 was observed with seropositive IgM. When IgM positive cases were compared with IgG positive cases in the symptomatic group, IFN-α, IFN-β and IL-1β responses was significantly higher among the IgG positive group (Table S8 in File S1). Though not significant ($p = 0.07$), a much higher IL-6 response in the IgM group (Table S8 in File S1) as compared to IgG may suggest an ongoing intense inflammation with a failure to mount (switch) an IgG response. The persistent early elevation of MCP-1 and IL-13 observed in both, seropositive

Table 4. Significant negative correlations between cytokines and selected clinical and laboratory variables.

Cytokine	Acute Phase	Subacute Phase	Extended Symptomatic Phase	Recovered	Total
(pg/ml)	n = 23	n = 22	n = 65	n = 22	N = 132
IFN-α	IL-4 (−0.73)	ND	ND	ND	CHIKV-M (−0.51)
	IL-10 (−0.44)				Myalgia (−0.37)
					IL-4 (−0.69)
					IL-10 (−0.51)
IFN-β	IL-4 (−0.73)	ND	ND	ND	Myalgia (−0.37)
	IL-10 (−0.44)				CHIKV-M (−0.50)
					IL-4 (−0.68)
					IL-10 (−0.51)
IFN-γ	–	–	Headache (−0.27)	–	–
CXCL-10/IP-10	TLC (−0.51)	–	–	–	–
	MCP-1 (−0.54)				
	IL-4 (−0.52)				
IL-1β	IL-4 (−0.86)	ND	ND	ND	CHIKV-M (−0.69)
	IL-10 (−0.56)				IL-4 (−0.77)
	CHIKV-G (−0.49)				IL-10 (−0.62)
TNF-α	Hemoglobin (−0.47)	TLC (−0.56)	–	Age ≥45 years (−0.49)	–
	Myalgia (−0.48)				
MCP-1	Platelet Count (−0.54)	–	–	–	–
	♀ Gender (−0.51)				
	IL-6 (−0.45)				
IL-4	IL-6 (−0.42)	ND	ND	ND	–
IL-10	IL-6 (−0.45)	ND	ND	ND	–

(Pearson correlation co-efficient in parenthesis.).
IFN-Interferon; TNF = Tumor Necrosis Factor; CXCL-10/IP-10 = Interferon Gamma-Induced Protein-10; IL = Interleukin; MCP = Monocyte Chemoattractant Protein.
ND = Not Done; TLC = Total Leucocyte Count; CRP = C-reactive protein; ♀ = Female.

and seronegative groups of subjects with varying illness duration and recovered individuals does not support any role for these cytokines in antibody production.

Finally, the cytokine repertoire was compared between subjects of seropositive and seronegative groups for specific anti CHIKV antibodies (IgM/IgG) (Table S10 in File S1). Consistent with earlier observations (Table S1, Table S2 and Table S8 in File S1), IFN-α, -β and IL-10 were significantly elevated in seronegative group while IL-4 and IL-10 were significantly elevated in seropositive group. Figure S1 shows the scatter plot for cytokines in cases with serologically confirmed diagnosis of CHIKV.

6 Regressions

We further performed a step-wise linear regression using several clinical and lab variables in order to determine predictors of 'failure to remission of musculoskeletal symptoms within one month of onset of illness'. Anti CHIKV IgG antibody was not included among the independent variables. IL-6, CXCL-10/IP-10, CRP and presence of knee pain and myalgia were found to significantly predict persistence of post CHIKV musculoskeletal pain.

7 Age and Response

The cytokine and anti CHIKV antibody response was classified as per age groups (Table S9 in File S1). We observed that 69% in the age group of less than 20 years, 53% in age group 21–44 years, 65% in age group 45–65 years and 42% of more than 65 years belonged to the extended symptomatic subgroup in the study cohort. Though the number of cases more than 65 years age was less (12 symptomatic), overall the responses were near similar to young age groups. Also, we observed a somewhat lower response for IFN-γ. The CHIKV IgG antibody response in elderly appeared robust.

Discussion

This report describes the serological cytokine phenotype of acute CHIKV based on a rural community survey carried out during the major CHIKV epidemic in India in 2006. An intensely up regulated Th1 (IFN −α, -β and -γ, TNF-α, IL −1β, CXCL-10/IP-10, and MCP-1) and Th2 (IL-4, IL-6, IL-10 and IL-13) cytokines was demonstrated both in the symptomatic and recovered subjects within four weeks of onset of illness. While the Th1 cytokines were found maximal during the acute phase (< 6 days), Th2 cytokines appeared to peak in subjects with extended symptomatic phase (15–30 days). Though several cytokines

Table 5. Comparison of the cytokine profile in CHIKV cases with healthy controls in different studies reported.

Cytokine/Chemokine	Current Study (HC = 80)			Ng et al 2009 (HC = 9)	Kelvin et al 2011 (HC = 10)	Chaaithanya et al 2011 (HC = 6)	El-Gabalawy et al 2012 (HC = 200)
	Acute (n = 23)	**Subacute (n = 22)**	**Extended Symptomatic (n = 65)**	**2–19 days (n = 10)**	**Acute (n = 35)**	**Acute (n = 6)**	**RA (n = 105)**
IFN-α	8.9	3.6	3.0	1.5	ND	ND	2.8
IFN-β	8.4	3.5	2.9	ND	ND	ND	ND
IFN-γ	50.1	17.2	15.8	+	0.9	ND	2.7
CXCL-10/IP-10	26.9	23.3	25.0	1000	2.3	33.9	1.2
IL1-β	2.3	1.7	1.7	+	0.82	ND	4.9
TNF-α	4.4	4.6	5.2	+	1.5	ND	3.7
MCP-1	49.0	37.9	33.2	ND	ND	1.9	1.1
IL-4	108.7	392.6	170.5	+	0.07	ND	6.5
IL-6	3.8	7.0	7.5	4.0	2.0	196.7	9.3
IL-10	6.4	23.1	38.5	1.5	0.4	1.9	3.3
IL-13	3.3	2.5	3.2	+	ND	ND	10

Values expressed as ratio of medians of cases to controls.

IFN-Interferon; TNF = Tumor Necrosis Factor; CXCL-10/IP-10 = Interferon Gamma-Induced Protein-10; IL = Interleukin; MCP = Monocyte Chemoattractant Protein. HC = Healthy controls; ND = Not Done;+ = Higher than Healthy controls; **Note**: In the current study, IFN-α, IFN-β, IL-1β, MCP-1, IL-4 and IL-10 were tested in 4 subjects of sub-acute phase and of extended symptomatic phase. All other cytokines were tested in 23, 22 and 65 subjects of acute, sub-acute and extended symptomatic phase respectively.

remained persistently elevated in the asymptomatic subjects during the study period, the level was lower than that observed in symptomatic subjects. The cytokine repertoire phenotype in serologically confirmed cases of CHIKV (Table S10 in File S1, Figure S1) was almost similar to that observed in study cohort (Table 2, Figure 2). Several significant ($p<0.05$) and robust (moderate to strong) correlates of cytokines pertaining to clinical (pain, myalgias, fatigue, headaches), laboratory (blood hemoglobin, leukocyte and platelet counts, CRP) and antibody (anti CHIKV IgM and IgG) parameters were described. Increased ESR at initial evaluation and persistently elevated CRP (Table 1) indicated an intense systemic inflammatory response by the CHIKV virus that spilled over beyond the acute illness phase.

The detail clinical and immunological profile of CHIKV in our rural survey has been reported earlier [1,2]. However, some observations may be relevant to the current cytokine phenotype. It is prudent to state that this study was designed a-priori to the rural population survey. The survey was prompted by several clinically important observations of post CHIKV arthritis and rheumatism made by us from a popular rheumatology outpatient clinic [8]. The survey team headed by a rheumatologist (AC) and microbiologist (AV) worked in field conditions to complete the survey and collect blood samples. Thus a large spectrum of data of patients with varying duration of illness beginning with the very acute phase was captured. Overall, unlike several published studies with retrospective design, the current cross-sectional and prospective design study pertain to real life scenario in acute CHIKV.

It is uncommon to detect IgM within 4 days of illness [13] and unusual to demonstrate IgG in acute phase [14]**.** In the current acute illness subjects, 17% showed anti IgM and 52% showed IgG antibodies to CHIKV. We have earlier validated the current study technique of IgM detection by comparing it with standard Mac ELISA [1]. 51% and 40% patients in the current cohort were seropositive for anti CHIKV IgM and IgG antibodies. The phase of viraemia is generally over within a week of onset of illness [15,5]. During the Indian epidemic (2006), 37.3% cases were reported positive for anti-CHIKV IgM antibody [13]. 35.7%, 4.9% and 0.4% of the sera samples respectively collected from 473 cases, predominantly rural, tested positive for anti-CHIKV IgM, anti-dengue IgM, and anti-CHIKV plus anti-dengue IgM response respectively in another Indian study during the epidemic [3]. 48.6%, 55.4%, 21.5% and 62.5% blood samples respectively tested positive for CHIKV using RT-PCR (reverse transcriptase-polymerase chain reaction), RT-LAMP (reverse transcriptase light isothermal loop amplification), IgM (ELISA) and virus isolation technique respectively in 296 clinically suspected patients referred to a tertiary medical center; time of collection of blood sample with respect to onset of illness was not described [16]. We could not find published data on serum anti CHIKV IgG antibodies during the early phase of illness. The very early switch from only IgM to IgM and IgG response to CHIKV shown in the current study is intriguing and not described to the best of our knowledge. It is likely that this early antibody response was preceded by an intense early Th2 cytokine up regulation (Table 2). However, a large number of patients with typical acute illness and intense Th1 and Th2 cytokine response did not test seropositive for anti CHIKV antibodies and needs to be investigated further. Our regression model to predict early clinical remission of the musculoskeltal symptoms did not identify anti CHIKV IgM response as a predictor of extended symptomatic phase (delay resolution). 50% recovered cases were seropositive for anti CHIKV IgG antibody (Table 1). Only 13% extended symptomatic patients tested seropositive for anti CHIKV IgG and this suggests the lack of specific IgG response with 'prolonged/extended symptoms (MSK)' in CHIKV. Overall, the cytokine rise in the current study (except IL-4 and IL-10) was much more in subjects seronegative for specific anti CHIKV antibodies (Tables in File S1) and suggests an immune host response to control the illness. A recent study, using mouse model, demonstrated an essential role for B cells and specific antibodies in controlling CHIKV infection [17].

We demonstrated an early intense interferon response (IFN-α, -β, -γ) which persisted in patients with extended symptoms. Persistent interferon response is likely to be associated with a failure to eradicate virus by the host at least during the current study period of four week post illness onset. As shown in Table 3, significant positive correlation was observed between IFN-β and fatigue, IFN-γ and low backache and IFN-γ and pain intensity; IFN-α and –β both showed inverse correlation with myalgia. Both Th1 and Th2 cytokines were intensely elevated (Table 2, Fig. 2) during all illness phases and recovered group with varying intensity. Interestingly, both Th1 and Th2 cytokines demonstrated a highly intense or maximum response in the subgroup with persistent musculoskeletal symptoms beyond 14 days of illness; only exception being a conspicuous drop in IL-4 assay. Another added feature was a relatively low IgG (anti CHIKV) antibody response (Table 1). All this perhaps indicates a somewhat failed host response to curb the virus in a landscape marked by heightened activation of T cells and macrophages and lesser intense B cell activation. The strong negative correlations (Table 4) of the Th2 cytokines (IL 4 and IL 6) with those of interferon response (Th1 proinflammatory cytokines) probably show an attempt by the cellular, humoral and immune events to curtail the Th1 cytokine reactivity and stop the progression of virus in the host.

Rapid induction of type I interferon (IFN) expression is critical to stimulating a robust innate immune response against viral infection and requires the activation of multiple transcriptional proteins following engagement and signaling through Toll-like receptor-dependent and independent pathways [18]. Alpha viruses, like several other viruses are potent inducers of interferon which in turn inhibits viral replication. Gifford and Heller [19] reported for the first time during the 1954–1964 CHIKV epidemic in Asia and South India, that chick embryo fibroblasts infected with CHIKV produced detectable levels of type 1 interferon three hours after infection. Macrophages, a major source of interferon, are readily infected by CHIKV and play a pivotal role in several cellular responses shown in experimental studies [20,21] and in both Th1 and Th2 cytokine response. Based on the observation of a sharp decline in viraemia before the appearance of high-affinity neutralizing antibodies, it was hypothesized that type 1 IFNs mediate antiviral response [22]. Type II IFN (IFN-γ) produced in early CHIKV infection further promotes the transition from innate to adaptive immunity [22]. An earlier study had shown that CHIKV-specific CD4+ T cells induced by CHIKV infection were the major producers of IFN- γ and that Th1 cells were probably responsible for a skewed production of IgG2 antibodies by B cells in response to IFN- γ [23]. IFN-gamma is made exclusively by natural killer and T cells and has important immunoregulatory functions including intense stimulation of macrophages, monocytes, fibroblasts and dendritic cells.

Pro-inflammatory mediators including TNF-α, MCP-1, IFN- γ, IFN- α/β and IL-6 have been identified in primates and humans infected with CHIKV and in other alphaviral arthritides [24,25,26]. Immunological studies on muscle biopsies from CHIKV infected patients with myositis syndrome showed presence of viral antigens located exclusively inside skeletal muscle progenitor cells and not in muscle fibres [27]. Though pathophysiologically, the intense and conjoint upregulation of Th1 and Th2 cytokines definitely contribute to the severe but self limiting profile of painful inflammatory pattern of the musculoskeletal illness in CHIKV, the literature is silent on the individual contribution of cytokines towards the clinical phenotype. In this report (Table 2 and tables S1–S8 in File S1) we have attempted to describe interesting and plausible clinical, laboratory and serological (antibody) correlations of the up-regulated cytokines.

To the best of our knowledge, this is the first report to describe IL-13 responses in acute CHIKV. While IFN – γ, TNF- α and CXCL-10/IP-10 are pro-inflammatory and a hallmark of Th1 response, IL-13 (strikingly homologous to IL-4) is a signature cytokine of the Th2 response and several subjects in the current study belonging to different symptomatic subgroups and recovered group showed intense elevation (Fig. 2). IL-13 is considered to an important immunomodulatory cytokine which also induces B cell proliferation and IgE switching. IL-13 was reported to play an important role in the hypersensitive and allergy responses in the respiratory tract and gut (nematode infestations) and is implicated with fibrosis in scleroderma [28]. In the current study, there were no differences in the IL-13 assay results obtained in the acute, sub acute and convalescent cases. We are not able to find a satisfactory explanation for persistent heightened IL-13 response in the study. We speculate that IL-13 may be associated with persistent arthritis in CHIKV.

Several other researchers have published data on cytokines in CHIKV [29,30,31,32]. We have chosen some of the studies for comparison (Table 5). It is prudent to add that precise comparison is not appropriate for several reasons pertaining to small sample size, timing of blood collection and assay methods. Our focus was on cytokines in acute illness and persistence of musculoskeletal symptoms from 14–30 days after onset of illness (extended symptomatic group). Increased IL-1, IL-10 and IFN-γ assay reported suggests an early engagement of adaptive immunity [33]. On comparison, discrepant results were observed in the study reported by Kelvin et al (2011) where the median levels of IL-4 and IL-10 was lower in the acute cases than in the healthy controls. Increased levels (1.5 times higher than controls) of IL-2R was reported in acute CHIKV cases [25,31]. Also, Chaaithanya et al (2011) have also reported high levels of IL-1 receptor antagonist in acute CHIKV cases. Increased levels of several other cytokines (IFN-α, CXCL-9, CCL2, IL-8 and IL-17 have been reported [25,30,31].

In Table 5, we have compared studies by computing a ratio of median value of cytokine obtained in illness to that in healthy subjects (control). We used published data and we chose acute or early illness. The ratio of several cytokines in the current study was several fold higher than that calculated for other studies. To provide an interesting perspective to the intense cytokine phenotype in the current study (Table 5) we also included a similar cytokine assay ratio profile from a study of patients suffering from Rheumatoid Arthritis (RA) [34] which is a prototype of an intense immune inflammatory disorder. However, unlike CHIKV, RA is a chronic disorder and an upregulation of immune cytokine response is reported several years prior to onset of the clinical disease [35]. Infrequently, CHIKV can lead to chronic persistent painful MSK illness and arthritis and was the subject of our earlier publications [1,8].

The current study had several limitations. Compared to the large number of clinically identified cases, much lesser number of cases consented to donate blood samples. Cases identified during the survey had varying period of illness and in several the clinical diagnosis was based on historical narration. We did not use concurrent controls but chose blood samples collected a year earlier to CHIKV epidemic to avoid sub-clinical illness during the epidemic (see methods section). Despite the fact, that we made frequent visits to the study village during the epidemic period, we managed to collect blood samples of only 23 acute cases. Anti CHIKV IgG assay was only carried out in limited number of cases. We faced several difficult logistic issues including prolonged and cumbersome travel between our center (CRD) and the village. We were unable to carry out tests for viral RNA detection and viral load. However, the relevance of the study was increased by the fact that a well defined rural population was meticulously screened during the epidemic as per a strict protocol. A large number of clinical cases were evaluated by a an investigation team (CRD) that has been engaged in epidemiological studies in the region since 1996.

We have followed our survey cases for periods ranging from 12–24 months and repeatedly collected blood samples for cytokines assay and other relevant autoantibodies (rheumatic diseases) in a prospective study. Our principal focus was on persistent chronic arthritis and a separate report will describe the results. Meanwhile, we have published two studies [1,36] to demonstrate persistence of IL-6 upto 18 months of follow-up of cases with chronic musculoskeletal symptoms and minimal or nil effect of chloroquin on selected Th1 and Th 2 cytokines in a 24 week randomized blind control drug trial study.

This is the first comprehensive clinical report on the pathophysiology of acute CHIKV based on Th1 and Th2 cytokines and anti CHIKV antibodies based on a rural population survey during the 2006 Indian epidemic. An early and intense up regulation of number of pro-inflammatory and anti inflammatory cytokines was demonstrated during the early period in subjects with a typical self limiting illness. However, this phenomenon, albeit a lesser intensity, was also evident in cases with extended symptoms and in asymptomatic individuals. An early specific IgM and IgG antibody response to CHIKV was also seen in a significant number of cases. Early persistent IgM and lower IgG to anti CHKV and intense Th2 cytokine phenotype seem to be associated with delay in resolution and prolonged MSK symptoms. Interestingly, maximum assay of TNF-α, IL-6 and IL-13 with low anti CHIKV IgM response were found in subjects recovered from CHIKV within one month of illness onset. Though we are able to provide reasonable explanation on the likely associations of several upregulated cytokines (Th1 and Th2) with the clinical phenotype and specific anti CHIKV antibody response (IgM and IgG), a more comprehensive work-up of virus markers, cytokines and immune responses (cellular and humoral) would be required to establish concrete causal and contributory relationships.

Supporting Information

Figure S1 Scatter graphs of cytokines of anti CHIKV seropositive (IgM and/or IgG) versus seronegative (IgM and IgG) in symptomatic cases. Footnote to Supplementary Figure 1: IFN-Interferon; TNF = Tumor Necrosis Factor; CXCL-10/IP-10 = Interferon Gamma-Induced Protein 10; IL = Interleukin; MCP = Monocyte Chemoattractant Protein. Statistical analysis was performed using non-parametric Kruskal Wallis test. Significant differences between the two groups was observed in IFN-α, IFN-β, IL-1β, IL-4 and IL-10.

File S1 Supporting tables. Table S1, Comparison of cytokine profile of CHIKV IgM negative versus IgM positive in acute Cases (N = 23). **Table S2**, Comparison of cytokine profile of CHIKV IgG negative versus IgG positive in acute cases (N = 23). **Table S3**, Comparison of cytokine profile of CHIKV IgM &/or IgG negative versus IgM &/or IgG positive in acute cases (N = 23).

Table S4, Comparison of cytokine profile of CHIKV IgM negative versus IgM positive in subacute cases. **Table S5**, Comparison of cytokine profile of CHIKV IgM negative versus IgM positive in extended subacute cases. **Table S6**, Comparison of cytokine profile of CHIKV IgM negative versus IgM positive in recovered cases (N = 22). **Table S7**, Comparison of cytokine profile of CHIKV IgM negative versus IgM positive in symptomatic cases. **Table S8**, Comparison of cytokine profile of CHIKV IgM positive versus IgG positive in symptomatic cases. **Table S9**, Comparison of serological profile (frequency of positive result) and cytokine profile (medians) of symptomatic cases (N = 110) and recovered cases (N = 22) of CHIKV with illness within one month duration between age groups. **Table S10**, Comparison of cytokine profile of anti CHIKV seropositive (IgM and/or IgG) versus seronegative (IgM and IgG) in symptomatic cases.

Acknowledgments

We gratefully acknowledge the efforts of the clinical Staff team, which includes Dr Meenaz Modak and Dr Harbeer Ahedi who assisted in examining the patients; Ms Manjit Saluja for co-ordinating the study; Ms Amruta, Ms Poonam and Ms Tanvira for helping with data collection and for their assistance in blood sample collection and processing. Finally, we thank the participants and healthy volunteers for their participation in the study.

Author Contributions

Conceived and designed the experiments: AC AV. Performed the experiments: AV RPG. Analyzed the data: AC AV RPG. Wrote the paper: AC AV RPG.

References

1. Chopra A, Anuradha V, Ghorpade R, Saluja M (2012) Acute Chikungunya (CHIKV) and persistent musculoskeletal pain following the 2006 Indian epidemic: A two year prospective rural community study. Epidemiol Infect 140(5): 842–50.
2. Chopra A, Anuradha V (2011) Persistent rheumatic musculoskeletal pain and disorders at one year post-chikungunya epidemic in south Maharashtra - a rural community base observational study with special focus on naïve persistent rheumatic musculoskeletal cases and selected cytokine expression. Indian J R-heumatol 6(1): 5–11.
3. Yergolkar PN, Tandale BV, Arankalle VA, Sathe PS, Sudeep AB, et al. (2006) Chikungunya outbreaks caused by African genotype, India. Emerg Infect Dis 12(10): 1580–1583.
4. Hapuarachchi HAC, Bandara KBAT, Hapugoda MD, Williams S, Abeyewickreme W (2008) Laboratory confirmation of dengue and chikungunya co-infection. Ceylon Med J 53: 104.
5. Pialoux G, Gauzere BA, Jaureguiberry S, Strobel M (2007) Chikungunya, an epidemic arbovirosis. Lancet Infect Dis 7: 319–27.
6. Noridah O, Paranthaman V, Naya SK, Masliza M, Ranjit K, et al. (2007) Outbreak of Chikungunya due to virus of Central/East African genotype in Malaysia. Med J Malaysia 62: 323–328.
7. Leo YS, Chow ALP, Tan LK, Lye DC, Lin L, et al. (2009) Chikungunya outbreak, Singapore, 2008. Emerg Infect Dis 15: 836–837.
8. Chopra A, Anuradha V, Lagoo-Joshi V, Kunjir V, Salvi S, et al. (2008) Chikungunya virus aches and pains: An emerging challenge. Arthritis Rheum 58(9): 2921–2922.
9. Brighton SW, Porzesky OW, De La Harpe AL (1983) Chikungunya virus infection. A retrospective study of 107 cases. South African Med J 63: 313–315.
10. CTK Biotech website. Available: http://ctkbiotech.com/ctk-product/chikungunya-igm-combo-rapid-test/. Accessed 2014 Oct 04.
11. Chopra A (2009) Community rheumatology in India-A COPCORD driven perspective. Indian J Rheumatol 4(3): 119–126.
12. Morceau F, Dicato M, Diederich M (2009) Pro-inflammatory cytokine-mediated anemia: Regarding molecular mechanisms of erythropoiesis. Mediators Inflamm 2009: 405016. doi:10.1155/2009/405016.
13. Kalantri SP, Joshi R, Riley LW (2006) Chikungunya epidemic: An Indian perspective. Natl Med J India 19: 315–322.
14. Kam YW, Ong EKS, Renia L, Tong JC, Ng LFP (2009) Immuno-biology of Chikungunya and implications for disease intervention. Microbes and Infection 11: 1186–1196.
15. Broom AK, Smith DW, Hall RA, Johansen CA, Mackenzie JS (2003) Arbovirus infections, In: Manson's Tropical Diseases. Cook G and Zumla A editors. 21st edition. London: Saunders. 737–738.
16. Lakshmi V, Neeraja M, Subbalaxmi MVS, Patida MM, Dash PK, et al. (2008) Clinical features and molecular diagnosis of Chikungunya fever from South India. Clin Infect Dis 46: 1436–1442.
17. Lum FM, Teo TH, Lee WW, Kam YW, Rénia L, et al. (2013) An essential role of antibodies in the control of Chikungunya virus infection. J Immunol 190: 6295–6302.
18. Hiscott J (2007) Triggering the innate antiviral response through IRF-3 activation. J Biol Chem 282: 15325–15329.
19. Gifford GE, Heller E (1963) Effect of actinomycin D on interferon production by 'active' and 'inactive' chikungunya virus in chick cells. Nature 200: 50–51.
20. Couderc T, Chrétien F, Schilte C, Disson O, Brigitte M, et al. (2008) Mouse model for chikungunya: young age and inefficient type-1 interferon signaling are risk factors for severe disease. PLoS Pathog 4(2)e 29: 0001–0012.
21. Ziegler SA, Lu L, Travassos RA, Xiao SY, Tesh RB (2008) An animal model for studying pathogenesis of Chikungunya virus infection. Am J Trop Med 79(1): 133–139.
22. Schilte C, Couderc T, Chretien F, Sourisseau M, Gangneux N, et al. (2010) Type I IFN controls chikungunya virus via its action on nonhematopoietic cells. J Exp Med 207(2): 429–442.
23. Barr TA, Brown S, Mastroeni P, Gray D (2009) B cell intrinsic MyD88 signals drive IFN-gamma production from T cells and control switching to IgG2c. J Immunol 183: 1005–1012.
24. Labadie K, Larcher T, Joubert C, Mannioui A, Delache B, et al. (2010) Chikungunya disease in nonhuman primates involves long-term viral persistence in macrophages. J Clin Invest 120: 894–906.
25. Ng LFP, Chow A, Sun YJ, Kwek DJC, Lim PL, et al. (2009) IL-1b, IL-6, and RANTES as biomarkers of Chikungunya severity. PLoS ONE 4(1): e4261. doi:10.1371/journal.pone.0004261.
26. Suhrbier A, Mahanlingam S (2009) The immunobiology of viral arthritides. Pharmacol Ther 124: 301–308.
27. Ozden S, Huerre M, Riviere JP, Coffey LL, Afonso PV, et al. (2007) Human muscle satellite cells as targets of Chikungunya virus infection. PLoS ONE 2(6): e527.doi:10.1371/journal.pone.0000527.
28. Aliprantis AO, Wang J, Fathman JW, Lemaire R, Dorfman DM, et al. (2007) Transcription factor T-beta regulates skin sclerosis through its function in innate immunity and vial IL-13. Proc Natl Acad Sci USA 104(8): 2827–2830.
29. Chow A, Her Z, Ong EKS, Chen J, Dimatatac F, et al. (2011) Persistent arthralgia induce by Chikungunya virus infection is associated with Interleukin – 6 and granulocyte macrophage colony stimulating factor. J Infect Dis 203: 149–157.
30. Kelvin AA, Banner D, Silvi G, Moro ML, Spataro N, et al. (2011) Inflammatory cytokine expression is associated with Chikungunya virus resolution and symptom severity. PLoS Negl Trop Dis 5(8): e1279, doi:10.1371/journl.pntd.0001279.
31. Chaaithanya IK, Muruganandam N, Sundaram SG, Kawalekar O, Sugunan AP, et al. (2011) Role of proinflammatory cytokines and chemokines in chronic arthropathy in CHIKV infection. Viral Immunol 24(4): 265–271.
32. Dupuis-Maguiraga L, Noret M, Brun S, Le Grand R, Gras G, et al. (2012) Chikungunya disease: Infection-associated markers from the acute to the chronic phase of arbovirus-induced arthralgia. PLoS Negl Trop Dis 6(3): e1446. doi:10.1371/journal.pntd.0001446.
33. Wauquier N, Becquart P, Nkoghe D, Padilla C, Ndjoyi-Mbiguino A, et al. (2011) The acute phase of Chikungunya virus infection in humans is associated with strong innate immunity and T CD8 cell activation. J Infect Dis 204 (1): 115–123.
34. El-Gabalawy HS, Robinson DB, Smolik I, Hart D, Elias B, et al. (2012) Familial clustering of the serum cytokine profile in the relatives of rheumatoid arthritis patients. Arthritis Rheum 64(6): 1720–1729.
35. Kokkonen H, Soderstrom I, Rocklov J, Hallmans G, Lejon K, et al. (2010) Up-regulation of cytokines and chemokines predates the onset of rheumatoid arthritis. Arthritis Rheum 62(2): 383–391.
36. Chopra A, Saluja M, Anuradha V (2013) Chloroquine effectiveness and inflammatory cytokine response in early persistent post Chikungunya musculoskeletal pain and arthritis. Arthritis Rheum 66(2): 319–326.

The Andersen Aerobic Fitness Test: Reliability and Validity in 10-Year-Old Children

Eivind Aadland[1]*, Torkil Terum[2], Asgeir Mamen[2,3], Lars Bo Andersen[4,5], Geir Kåre Resaland[2,6]

1 Sogn og Fjordane University College, Faculty of Health Studies, Førde, Norway, **2** Sogn og Fjordane University College, Faculty of Teacher Education and Sports, Sogndal, Norway, **3** University College of Health Sciences – Campus Kristiania, Oslo, Norway, **4** Department of Sports Medicine, Norwegian School of Sport Sciences, Oslo, Norway, **5** Department of Sport Sciences and Clinical Biomechanics, University of Southern Denmark, Odense, Denmark, **6** Sogn og Fjordane Center for Health Research, Førde Central Hospital, Førde, Norway

Abstract

Background: High aerobic fitness is consistently associated with a favorable metabolic risk profile in children. Direct measurement of peak oxygen consumption (VO_{2peak}) is often not feasible, thus indirect tests such as the Andersen test are required in many settings. The present study seeks to determine the reliability and validity of the Andersen test in 10-year-old children.

Methods: A total of 118 10-year-old children (67 boys and 51 girls) were recruited from one school and performed four VO_{2peak} tests over three weeks: three Andersen tests (indirect) and one continuous progressive treadmill test (direct). Of these, 104 children provided valid data on all Andersen tests and 103 children also provided valid data on the direct treadmill test. Reliability and validity were assessed using Bland Altman plots and linear regression analysis.

Results: Bias (mean change) and random error (limits of agreement) were 26.7±125.2 m for test 2 vs. test 1 ($p<.001$ for mean difference) and 3.9±88.8 m for test 3 vs. test 2 ($p=.514$ for mean difference). The equation to estimate VO_{2peak} suggested by Andersen et al. (2008) showed a poor fit in the present sample; thus, we suggest a new equation: $VO_{2peak}=23.262+0.050*\text{Andersen distance}-3.858*\text{gender}-0.376*\text{body weight}$ ($R^2=0.61$, standard error of the estimate = 5.69, $p<.001$, boys = 0, girls = 1).

Conclusions: The Andersen test provided reliable and valid data on a group level. However, a substantial degree of individual variability was found for estimates of VO_{2peak}. Researchers should be aware of the amount of noise in indirect tests that estimate aerobic fitness.

Editor: Neil M. Johannsen, Louisiana State University, United States of America

Funding: The authors have no support or funding to report.

Competing Interests: The authors have declared that no competing interests exist.

* Email: eivind.aadland@hisf.no

Introduction

High aerobic fitness is consistently associated with a favorable metabolic risk profile in children [1,2]. In adults, the relationship between aerobic fitness and health becomes evident through increased incidence of cardiovascular disease and mortality in those having a poor fitness level compared to their more fit peers [3,4]. In order to inform the society regarding targets for public health management in childhood and to determine effective interventions in this population, being able to measure aerobic fitness in a valid and reliable way in relatively large groups of children (e.g. a school setting) is a prerequisite.

The most-used criterion measure for maximal aerobic fitness is maximal (peak) oxygen consumption measured to voluntary exhaustion during an incremental treadmill or bicycle protocol. However, such testing is time-consuming and requires expensive equipment and highly trained test personnel, and would therefore not be feasible for testing large samples of children (e.g. school classes). Therefore, both maximal and submaximal performance measures have been developed to estimate VO_{2max} for use with different groups in various settings [5]. A highly used test in children is the 20 m multistage shuttle run test (MSRT) [6,7]. However, recent external validation studies have shown that current equations to estimate VO_{2peak} in children 8–13 years old may be questionable [8,9] due to biased estimates and large individual errors. In addition, the MSRT test protocol has some drawbacks, especially when applied for children. Therefore, an alternative test was proposed by Andersen et al. [10] and is now included as a measure of aerobic fitness in several large studies [11–13]. The Andersen test is an intermittent running test (15 seconds working, 15 seconds resting) using a 20 m lane, where children aim to cover as long a distance as possible during 10 minutes. Compared to the MSRT, the Andersen test may have several advantages: 1) it relates closer to children's usual running pattern (i.e. intermittent vs. continuous activity), 2) it does not stigmatize children having poor fitness and therefore does not exclude them early from the test (i.e. all children finish the test at their own maximal pace independent of fitness level), and 3) it does not require any equipment besides a stopwatch, measuring tape, and a whistle. However, besides the original study by Andersen et al. [10] and a small study by Ahler et al. [14] (in children 6–9 years old), the measurement properties of the Andersen test have not been thoroughly examined.

The present study seeks to determine the reliability and criterion validity of the Andersen test in a relatively large sample (n>100) of 10-year-old children. Reliability was assessed using three admissions of the Andersen test over three weeks. Validity was assessed using VO_{2peak} determined from a maximally graded treadmill protocol as the criterion measure.

Materials and Methods

Ethics statement

Children and their parents were given thorough oral and written information regarding the study protocol. Each child orally agreed to participate in the study, and written informed consent was obtained from each child's parent(s)/guardian(s) prior to the child's inclusion in the study. The study met the standards of the Declaration of Helsinki and was approved by the Regional Committee for Medical Research Ethics (REC West) in Norway.

Subjects

All 121 children in fifth grade (10-year olds) at one school in the western part of Norway over two consecutive school years were invited to participate in the study. A total of 118 children (67 boys and 51 girls; 58 during 2012–2013 and 60 during 2013–2014) were included in the study. Three children were excluded from the study (one child performed the testing, but were excluded for being severely short of growth; two children did not perform the testing for medical reasons (one for having heart problems and one for having a skeletal disease).

Study protocol

Children performed three Andersen tests (weeks 1, 3, and 4), and performed one incremental treadmill test to exhaustion (week 2) to measure their peak oxygen consumption (VO_{2peak}) within three weeks. Children were instructed not to eat during the last two hours prior to testing and to engage in normal physical activity the day before the test and the day of testing.

The Andersen test was performed according to standard procedures [10]. Two parallel lines 20 m apart were marked in a gym hall with a wooden floor. The children were informed about the procedures and performed a collective five-minute warm-up before the test. The test has a total duration of 10 minutes, where children run from one end line to another in a to-and-fro movement intermittently, with 15-second work periods and 15-second breaks signaled by the test leader's blowing a whistle. When the children finished one 15-second period of work, they were instructed to stop as fast as possible and to take one to three steps back, depending on how fast they were able to stop. Each time the children turned around at an end line, they had to touch with one finger the floor behind the end line. The goal was to cover the longest possible distance during the 10-minute run. Verbal encouragement was highly standardized across all tests. It was kept to a minimum during the first half of the test and increased gradually and consistently toward the test's final part. The distance covered (number of laps performed) was recorded by adult test assistants who counted for one or two children each. Each of the two classes was split into three subgroups for testing (according to how their classes were usually divided in school), leaving approximately 20 children per test. The gym hall was 18.1 m wide, giving each child a lane of about 1 m.

Peak oxygen consumption was measured to exhaustion using an incremental treadmill test. The treadmill's inclination (Woodway PPS 55, Woodway GmbH, Weil am Rhine, Germany) was constant at 5.3% during the whole test. Children started to walk at 5 km/h for 5 minutes. Thereafter the speed increased by 1 km/h each minute until the children were exhausted. Oxygen consumption was measured using the Moxus Modular Metabolic System (AEI Technologies Inc., Pittsburgh, USA). A two-point gas calibration according to known concentrations and calibration according to atmospheric pressure were performed each test day. Volume calibration of the breathing valve (Hans Rudolph model 2700, Hans Rudolph Inc., Shawnee, Kansas, USA) was performed between each test using a 3-l syringe (Series 5530, Hans Rudolph, Kansas, USA). The oxygen analyzer has shown to be reliable and valid compared to the Douglas-bag technique [15]. To prevent injuries in case of falls during the test, children performed the test with a safety rope connected to a chest-belt system from Cosmos (h/p/cosmos sports & medical GmbH, Nussdorf-Traunstein, Germany). Throughout the test, a test assistant was in charge of the subject's safety by tightly holding the safety rope. If the subject stumbled, the test assistant could pull the rope, thereby raising the subject and preventing a fall. The child and parent(s)/guardian(s) were informed of test procedures before testing, and the child's parent(s)/guardian(s) were allowed and encouraged to observe the testing.

After each test, test leader and associates discussed several subjective criteria to verify a near maximal performance: hyperpnoea, unsteady running pattern, and verbal and body language clearly indicating that the child wanted to stop testing despite repeated strong verbal encouragement. Additionally, the respiratory exchange ratio (RER) and maximal heart rate (HR_{peak}) (Polar S610i HR monitor, Polar Electro OY, Kempele, Finland) were noted. The reliability of VO_{2peak} tested directly in children is shown to be approximately 4%, which compares favorably with the reliability of testing of adults' VO_{2max} [16].

The VO_{2peak} is presented as absolute (l/min) and relative values (ml/kg/min), each of which is defined as the highest value of two successive 30-second measurements. Height and body weight were measured without shoes and socks before the children started the VO_{2peak} test. Height was measured to the nearest 0.1 cm using a wall-mounted stadiometer. Body weight was measured to the nearest 0.1 kg (subtracting 0.2 kg for light clothes) using an electronic scale (Seca 770, SECA GmbH, Hamburg, Germany). Body weight was used as a continuous variable in the statistical analyses. For the purpose of reporting of descriptive statistics, children were also categorized as normal weight, overweight, or obese according to the criteria set by Cole et al. [17].

Statistical analyses

The anthropometric subject characteristics and data on VO_{2peak} and the Andersen test are presented as the mean values and standard deviation (SD).

Reliability of the Andersen test was assessed by determining a) bias (learning effect) and b) random errors over the three tests. Bias was determined using a linear mixed model that included a random intercept for subjects. Test number was included as a fixed-effect factor variable. The effect of gender was tested by adding the main effect and an interaction term (gender*test number) to the model. Effects are reported as effects estimates and 95% confidence intervals (CI). Random error was determined using Pearson correlation (r), intraclass correlation coefficient ($ICC_{3,1}$), and Bland Altman plots. The Bland Altman plots show the difference between two subsequent tests as a function of the mean of the two tests [18]. Because the data were deemed to be homoscedastic, the limits of agreement (LoA) were calculated according to Hopkins [19] (LoA = SD of the differences*1.96).

Validity of the Andersen test was assessed using Pearson's r, linear regression, and Bland Altman plots in three steps: 1) We applied the suggested equation (VO_{2max} = 18.38+0.033*Andersen distance −5.92*gender [boys = 0; girls = 1]) from Andersen et al. [10] to predict VO_{2peak} in our sample. 2) To develop a new equation to predict VO_{2peak} from the Andersen test, we initially split our sample in two to perform a validation of our equation in an independent dataset. The children included during 2012–2013 served as the training dataset (n = 52) from which the equation was developed, whereas the group included during 2013–2014 served as the testing dataset (n = 51) Three variables were included in the model (VO_{2peak} = a+b*Andersen distance+c*gender+d*body weight, [boys = 0; girls = 1]). The predicted and measured VO_{2peak} were then compared using linear regression and a Bland Altman plot. Means were compared using a one-sample t-test. 3) Finally, we calculated a new equation based on the whole sample (n = 103) using the following model (VO_{2peak} = a+b*Andersen distance+ c*gender+d*body weight, [boys = 0; girls = 1]). The final model is reported as regression coefficients with 95% bootstrapped CIs. The better of the Andersen tests 1 and 2 was used in all analyses of validity.

All analyses were performed using IBM SPSS v. 20 (IBM Corporation, Software Group, Somers, New York, USA). A p-value<.05 indicated statistically significant findings.

Results

Children's characteristics

Except for a significantly higher VO_{2peak} in boys than in girls (p<.001), there were no significant differences between genders or the two subsamples included (p>.095) (table 1). Of the total sample included (n = 118), 113, 112, and 112 children provided valid data for the Andersen test numbers 1, 2, and 3, respectively. A total of 104 children provided valid data on all Andersen tests and were included in analyses of reliability. Reasons for not undertaking the test were sickness or being out of school (n = 3, 4, and 4 at tests 1, 2, and 3, respectively), whereas reasons for not providing a valid test were falls and complaints about being uncomfortable (nausea or musculoskeletal pain) (3, 2, and 2 at tests 1, 2, and 3, respectively). Of the children reporting musculoskeletal pain, the pain for two individuals was directly related to the test performed (one fell and hit his knee in the floor; one suffered an acute ankle sprain). A total of 113 children provided valid data on directly measured VO_{2peak} on the graded treadmill protocol (two children did not perform the test, one child was excluded for not performing a maximal test, and two children were excluded due to technical errors). Of these, 103 children provided valid data on Andersen test numbers 1 and 2 (the better of performance 1 or 2 was used for the purpose of analyzing validity); thus, 103 children were included in the analyses of validity.

Maximal heart rate and respiratory exchange ratio on the VO_{2peak} test were (mean (SD)) 201 (8.9) beats/minute and 1.07 (0.07), respectively.

Reliability

Running distance on the Andersen test across the three tests is shown in table 2. Running distance increased significantly from test 1 to test 2 (mean (95% CI) 26.7 (14.8 to 38.6) m or 3.0 (1.6 to 4.3)%, p<.001), whereas no difference was found between test 2 to test 3 (3.9 (−8 to 15.8) m, p = .514). Boys ran 59.2 (20.5 to 97.9) m farther than girls did (p = .003). However, the initial increase and thereafter a plateau in performance were similar between genders (p for gender*test number = .189). Overall, 19 (18%), 38 (37%), and 47 (45%) children achieved their longest running distance (personal best) on tests 1, 2, and 3, respectively.

The relationship between all Andersen tests was high and similar between genders (test 1 vs. 2: r = 0.82; test 1 vs. 3: r = 0.79; test 2 vs. 3: r = 0.92, best of tests 1 and 2 vs. overall best: r = 0.97, all p<.001) having an overall $ICC_{3,1}$ = 0.84 (CI 0.78 to 0.88). Still, the Bland Altman plots (figure 1) reveal some individual variability in distance covered between test 1 and test 2 (bias ± LoA = 26.7±125.2 m (LoA = 13.9% of test 1 mean)), but smaller for test 2 vs. test 3 (3.9±88.8 m (LoA = 9.6% of test 2 mean)).

Validity and prediction equation

The bivariate relationships between the Andersen tests and VO_{2peak} were r = 0.63, r = 0.70, r = 0.68, r = 0.72, and r = 0.73 for Andersen tests 1, 2, and 3, the best of tests 1 and 2, and the overall best test vs. VO_{2peak}, respectively (n = 100, i.e. those having valid data on all of these measurements).

The equation to predict VO_{2peak} suggested by Andersen et al. [10] was clearly inadequate to predict VO_{2peak} in the present sample (slope for mean vs. differences of measured vs. predicted VO_{2peak}: p<.001). Figure 2 shows that the Andersen et al. equation severely and systematically underestimates VO_{2peak} (mean ± SD 46.9 (4.8) vs. 54.5 (9.0) ml/kg/min, p<.001), especially for children having above median VO_{2peak} values. Thus, a new equation would be required to better fit our data.

To develop a new equation to predict VO_{2peak} from the Andersen test, we initially split our sample in two groups (a training dataset including 52 children and a testing dataset including 51 children) to perform a validation of our equation in an independent dataset. The equation developed was as follows (regression coefficients and 95% CI): VO_{2peak} = 22.887 (−0.591 to 46.365)+0.052 (0.033 to 0.071)*Andersen distance −5.632 (−8.774 to −2.491)*gender −0.386 (−0.598 to −0.174)*body weight (R^2 = 0.71, standard error of the estimate (SEE) = 5.37, p<.001, boys = 0, girls = 1). Predicted vs. measured VO_{2peak} yielded R^2 = 0.46 and SEE = 6.06. Mean values were close to identical between predicted and measured VO_{2peak} (53.6 (7.0) vs. 53.1 (8.2) ml/kg/min, p = .514). Limits of agreement between the predicted and measured values were±12.1 ml/kg/min (±22% of mean VO_{2peak}), indicating a relatively large degree of uncertainty on individual-level predictions (figure 3).

As the derived equation performed sufficiently in the independent testing set, we established a new equation based on the whole sample (regression coefficients and 95% bootstrapped CI): VO_{2peak} = 23.262 (4.934 to 39.694)+0.050 (0.038 to 0.063)*Andersen distance −3.858 (−6.106 to −1.539)*gender −0.376 (−0.509 to −0.248)*body weight (R^2 = 0.61, SEE = 5.69, p<.001, boys = 0, girls = 1, n = 103).

Discussion

The present study's main finding was that the Andersen test is a reliable and valid tool for determination of aerobic fitness on a group level. However, a substantial degree of individual variability should be expected for estimates of VO_{2peak} based on the Andersen test. Moreover, at least two Andersen tests should be performed to obtain valid results.

We detected an increased running distance of 3% from test 1 to test 2. This increase is in contrast to previous studies showing no significant bias over subsequent tests examining the Andersen test [10,14] and the MSRT [20–23] in children and youth. Our

Table 1. Children's characteristics (mean (SD)).

	Overall	Boys	Girls	Year 1	Year 2
Number (%)	118	67 (57)	51 (43)	58 (49)	60 (51)
Age (years)	10.3 (0.3)	10.3 (0.3)	10.3 (0.3)	10.3 (0.3)	10.2 (0.3)
Height (cm)	143.4 (5.8)	143.9 (6.2)	142.7 (5.1)	143.5 (5.5)	143.3 (6.0)
Body weight (kg)	38.0 (8.4)	38.3 (9.5)	37.6 (6.8)	38.2 (9.0)	37.7 (8.0)
Body mass index (kg/m^2)	18.4 (3.2)	18.3 (3.6)	18.4 (2.7)	18.4 (3.3)	18.3 (3.2)
% overweight/obese	20.3	20.9	19.6	22.4	18.3
Waist circumference (cm)	64.3 (8.6)	64.9 (9.5)	63.6 (7.3)	63.9 (8.6)	64.7 (8.8)
VO_{2peak} (l/min)*	2.00 (0.34)	2.10 (0.35)	1.88 (0.29)	2.06 (0.33)	1.96 (0.35)
VO_{2peak} (ml/kg/min)*	54.0 (9.0)	56.6 (9.1)	50.5 (7.5)	55.4 (9.5)	52.6 (8.2)

*overall n = 113; n = 66 for boys and 47 for girls; n = 57 for first year and 56 for second year.

estimate shows that one should expect the distance ran to increase 15–39 meters (1.6–4.3%) from the first to the second test admission on a group level. This improvement equals an increased VO_{2peak} of 1.3 (95% CI 0.7 to 1.9) ml/kg/min, when the suggested equation from the present study is used to estimate it. There was no further increase in distance ran to the third test admission. These results indicate that one familiarization trial prior to the test admission, or using the better of two tests, would be recommended to avoid any learning effect that might invalidate the test results. This finding is in line with findings from a study examining three admissions of the MSRT in adults [24]. Still, the bias may be interpreted as relatively minor, and might also be adjusted based on the current findings.

However, if the test is used to evaluate the aerobic fitness of individual children (e.g. evaluation of children in a practical school setting or if regression analysis is run on the subject level), some variation from test to test must be expected. Despite the high correlation found between test 2 and test 3 (r = 0.92), individual differences would be expected to be from −85 to 93 m (±10% of the mean performance) between these tests. However, using the better result of two tests will provide researchers with a precise estimate of the Andersen test's performance (r = 0.97 with the overall best test).

As reliability is a premise for validity, variation in test performance over time will weaken the "real" relationship with VO_{2peak}, as noise in the predictor (x-variable) induces regression dilution bias [25]. The amount of random error decreased over time (test 2 vs. test 1 compared to test 3 vs. test 2) in the present study. Thus, the use of a second or third test, or the best of two or more tests, will increase both reliability and validity of the test. Although a marginally increased fit was found in the present study using the best Andersen test compared to one single test (results

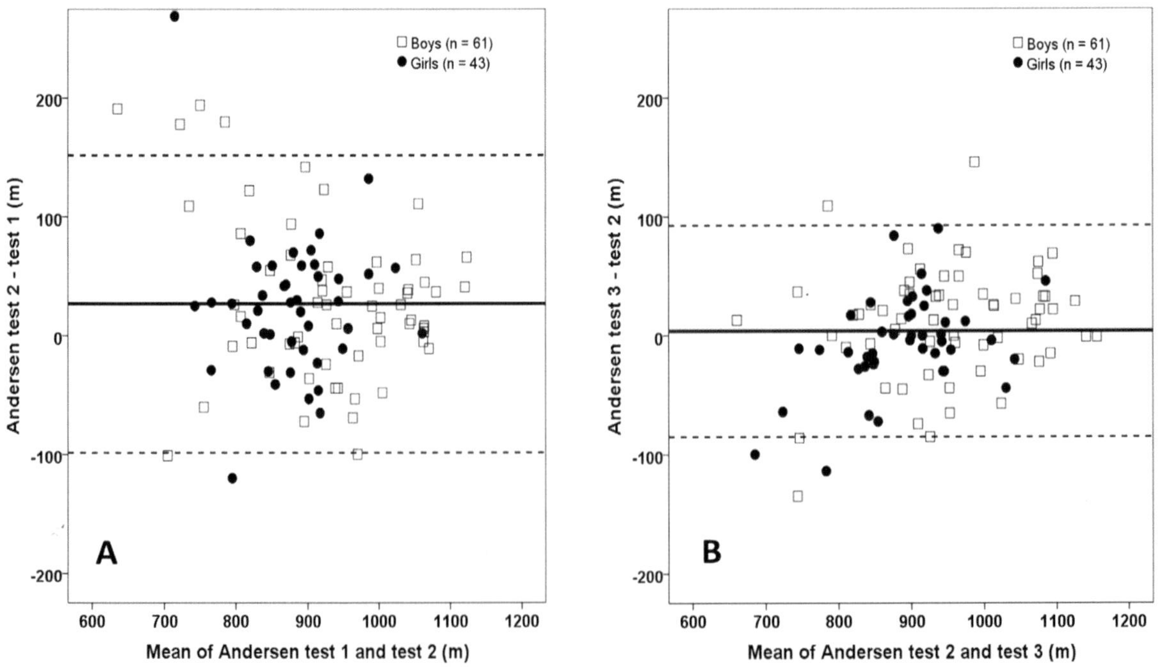

Figure 1. Bland Altman plots showing differences between test 1 and test 2 (A) and between test 2 and test 3 (B) as a function of the mean of the two corresponding tests. The solid line is the mean difference; dotted line is limits of agreement (bias±1.96*SD of the difference).

Table 2. Running distance (m) on the three Andersen tests (mean (SD)).

Test number	Overall (n = 104)	Boys (n = 61)	Girls (n = 43)	Year 1 (n = 51)	Year 2 (n = 53)
1	897 (111)	918 (126)	867 (79)	923 (102)	871 (115)
2	923 (99)	946 (108)	891 (74)	957 (104)	891 (84)
3	927 (112)	957 (117)	885 (92)	968 (106)	888 (105)
Better of 1 and 2	935 (93)	958 (102)	902 (69)	965 (95)	906 (83)
Overall best	947 (98)	974 (104)	909 (73)	978 (100)	919 (86)

not shown), others have shown clear improvement in predictive ability for VO_{2peak} using the overall best test [20]. Nevertheless, although each researcher must ultimately decide whether a measurement tool is reliable, given the purpose of the study [19,26], we believe the Andersen test, given the use of a familiarization trial or the best of two or more scores, provides reliable data regarding a child's level of aerobic fitness.

Estimation of VO_{2peak} based on the equation suggested by Andersen et al. [10] yielded a poor fit in our sample due to a lower slope than that of the present study. This picture is very similar to that of studies that externally validated various equations for the MSRT [8,9]. Although such systematic differences between measured and predicted VO_{2peak} possibly could be explained by many factors, there are few clear answers. An obvious reason for a biased equation (slope) is inherent (random) variation in the

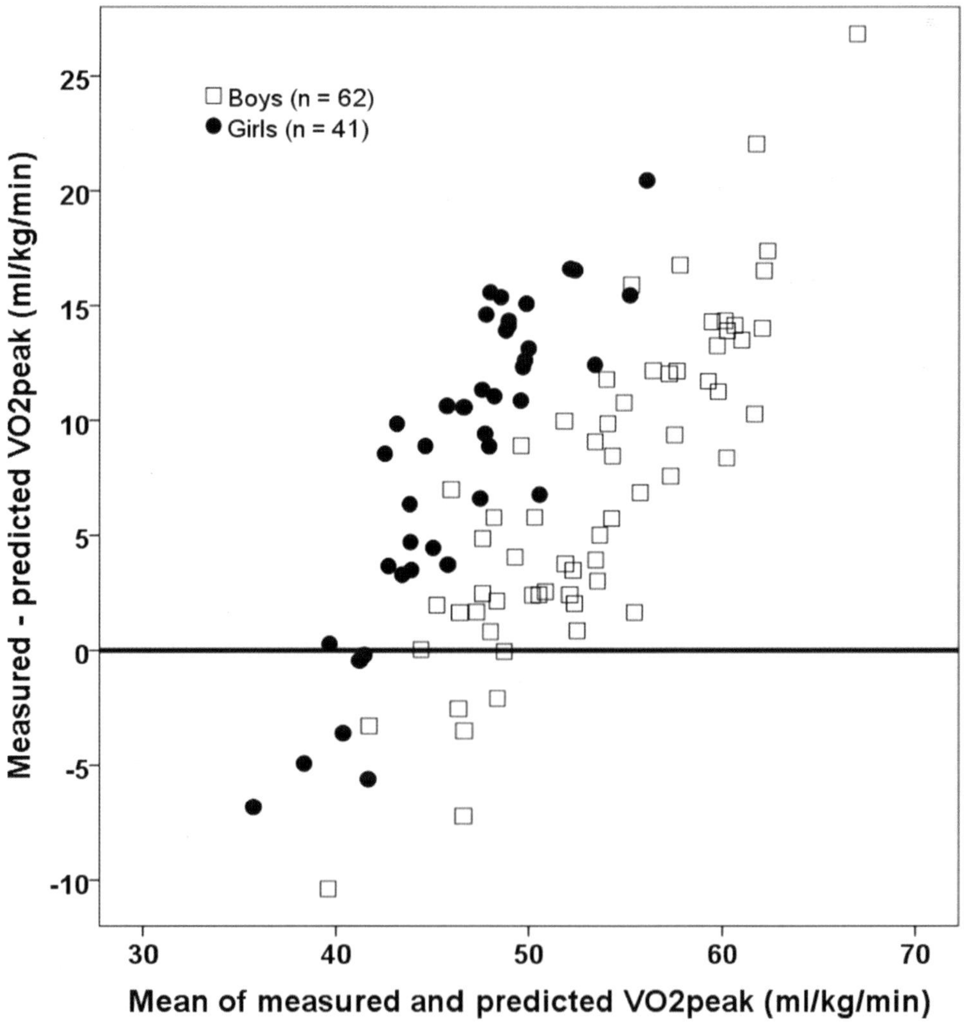

Figure 2. Bland Altman plots showing differences between measured VO_{2peak} and predicted VO_{2peak} from Andersen et al. (VO_{2peak} = 18.38+0.033*Andersen test –5.92*gender) as a function of the mean of the two values.

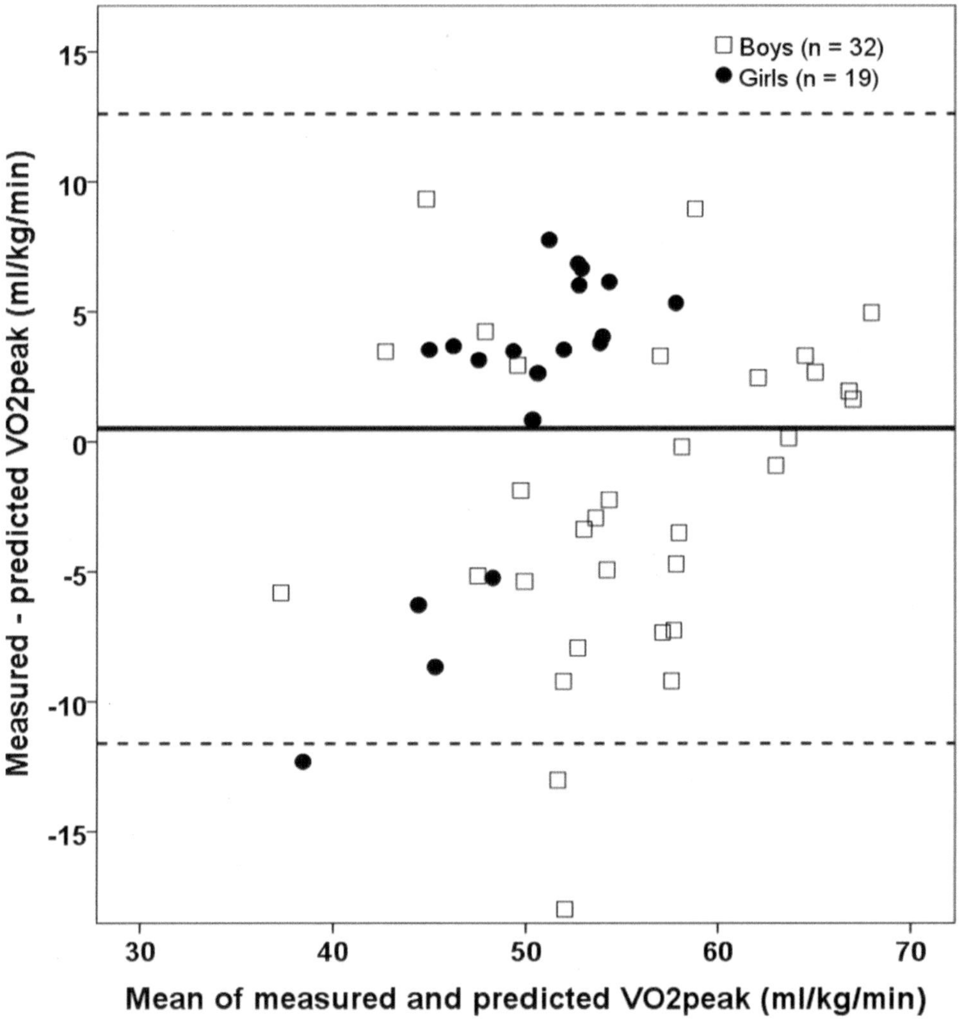

Figure 3. Bland Altman plots showing differences between measured VO_{2peak} and predicted VO_{2peak} as a function of the mean of the two values in class 2 (testing dataset) based on the regression equation derived from class 1 (training dataset) (VO_{2peak} = 22.887+0.052*Andersen test –5.632*gender –0.386*body weight). The solid line is the mean difference; dotted line is limits of agreement (bias±1.96*SD of the difference).

examined relationship from study to study, especially when the dataset upon which the equation is based (or the equation is tested) is small. In the present study, regression coefficients from 0.022 to 0.054 (CIs 0.004 to 0.080) (results not shown) were found across the three Andersen tests in the two classes, despite a more or less identical setting across all tests (children from the same population, same procedures, same testers). The bias could also be caused by a confounding variable that may change across samples, time, places, and testers (i.e. the model is underfitted and fails to account for an important variable). Equations for the MSRT vary in their included variables – some include age, gender, and a measure of body fat [8,9]. Andersen et al. [10] did not include body fat or weight in their original equation to estimate VO_{2peak}, however, body weight was a highly significant predictor in the present study. Moreover, body weight was significantly ($p<.001$) related to the difference between measured VO_{2peak} and VO_{2peak} predicted from Andersen et al. (result not shown), which may indicate that the original model was underfitted.

To create a new equation, we performed an external validation within our sample (using a training dataset and an independent test dataset) prior to establishing the final equation [27]. The procedure showed no bias, and no significantly different slope between the predicted and measured VO_{2peak} in the test dataset. This lack of both slope difference and bias indicated that the equation was sufficiently stable for estimating VO_{2peak} in an independent sample. However, consistent with previous studies [8,9], we found quite large limits of agreement for estimates on an individual level. Our results showed that one must expect individual deviations in VO_{2peak} of ±12 ml/kg/min (±22% of mean VO_{2peak}) based on the Andersen test, gender, and body weight. This level of deviation limits the usefulness of the Andersen test to estimate VO_{2peak} on an individual basis. Batista et al. [9] and Melo et al. [8], who found LoAs of similar size for estimating VO_{2peak} from the MSRT in external validation studies, both concluded that the test is unsuitable to estimate VO_{2peak} on an individual level. We do not believe such tests are unsuitable for individual predictions; however, we agree that researchers should be aware of the amount of noise in these indirect tests, because it may greatly dilute any relationship between aerobic fitness and health [25]. Thus, future studies should directly compare the use

of direct and indirect measures of aerobic fitness regarding their ability to predict health outcomes.

Strengths and limitations

The present study has two main strengths. First, we included a relatively large sample of children, which made it possible to perform an external validation of our equation for VO_{2peak} and to arrive at relatively stable estimates for VO_{2peak}, compared to many other studies that are based on small sample sizes. Second, we included three admissions of the Andersen test, an approach which allowed us to evaluate the performance difference between test 2 and test 3. None of the previous studies of the Andersen test included more than two admissions [10,14].

Limitations of the study are related to the sample included. One could argue that our test dataset was not fully independent, as the children composing both the training and test datasets came from the same school and performed the tests in the same gym hall, led by the same testers [27]. Thus, the equation could be expected to perform worse in other contexts, and further external validation studies are desired. Moreover, our sample was restricted to 10-year-old children. Although Andersen et al. [10] did not find any age-specific relationship with directly measured VO_{2peak} in their original study, running economy improves with age [28]; thus, the equation suggested to estimate VO_{2peak} in the present study may not be valid in other age groups.

Conclusions

We conclude that the Andersen test provided reliable and valid data on a group level for 10-year-old children. However, a substantial degree of individual variability was found for estimates of VO_{2peak} based on the Andersen test. Researchers should be aware of the amount of noise in the Andersen test and in other indirect tests to estimate aerobic fitness, because "real" relationships between aerobic fitness and health are diluted and increase the probability of performing type II errors. In any case, we recommend that a familiarization trial or several Andersen tests be performed to increase the precision of the measurement.

Acknowledgments

We thank all children and teachers at the participating school for their excellent cooperation during the data collection. We also thank students at Sogn og Fjordane University College for their assistance during the test sessions.

Author Contributions

Conceived and designed the experiments: EA TT AM LBA GKR. Performed the experiments: TT AM GKR. Analyzed the data: EA. Wrote the paper: EA TT AM LBA GKR.

References

1. Andersen LB, Sardinha LB, Froberg K, Riddoch CJ, Page AS, et al. (2008) Fitness, fatness and clustering of cardiovascular risk factors in children from Denmark, Estonia and Portugal: the European Youth Heart Study. Int J Pediatr Obes 3 Suppl 1: 58–66.
2. Anderssen SA, Cooper AR, Riddoch C, Sardinha LB, Harro M, et al. (2007) Low cardiorespiratory fitness is a strong predictor for clustering of cardiovascular disease risk factors in children independent of country, age and sex. Eur J Cardiovasc Prev Rehabil 14: 526–531.
3. Fogelholm M (2010) Physical activity, fitness and fatness: relations to mortality, morbidity and disease risk factors. A systematic review. Obes rev 11: 202–221.
4. Myers J, Prakash M, Froelicher V, Do D, Partington S, et al. (2002) Exercise capacity and mortality among men referred for exercise testing. N Engl J Med 436: 793–801.
5. Jorgensen T, Andersen LB, Froberg K, Maeder U, Smith LV, et al. (2009) Position statement: Testing physical condition in a population - how good are the methods? Eur J Sport Sci 9: 257–267.
6. Leger LA, Lambert J (1982) A maximal multistage 20-m shuttle run test to predict VO_{2max}. Eur J Appl Physiol Occup Physiol 49: 1–12.
7. Leger LA, Mercier D, Gadoury C, Lambert J (1988) The multistage 20 metre shuttle run test for aerobic fitness. J Sports Sci 6: 93–101.
8. Melo X, Santa-Clara H, Almeida JP, Carnero EA, Sardinha LB, et al. (2011) Comparing several equations that predict peak VO_2 using the 20-m multistage-shuttle run-test in 8–10-year-old children. Eur J Appl Physiol 111: 839–849.
9. Batista MB, Cyrino ES, Arruda M, Dourado AC, Coelho-E-Silva MJ, et al. (2013) Validity of equations for estimating VO_{2peak} from the 20-m shuttle run test in adolescents aged 11–13 years. J Strength Cond Res 27: 2774–2781.
10. Andersen LB, Andersen TE, Andersen E, Anderssen SA (2008) An intermittent running test to estimate maximal oxygen uptake: the Andersen test. J Sports Med Phys Fitness 48: 434–437.
11. Damsgaard CT, Dalskov SM, Petersen RA, Sorensen LB, Molgaard C, et al. (2012) Design of the OPUS School Meal Study: A randomised controlled trial assessing the impact of serving school meals based on the New Nordic Diet. Scand J Public Health 40: 693–703.
12. Toftager M, Christiansen LB, Kristensen PL, Troelsen J (2011) SPACE for physical activity - a multicomponent intervention study: study design and baseline findings from a cluster randomized controlled trial. BMC Public Health 11: 777.
13. Wedderkopp N, Jespersen E, Franz C, Klakk H, Heidemann M, et al. (2012) Study protocol. The Childhood Health, Activity, and Motor Performance School Study Denmark (The CHAMPS-study DK). BMC Pediatrics 12: 128.
14. Ahler T, Bendiksen M, Krustrup P, Wedderkopp N (2012) Aerobic fitness testing in 6- to 9-year-old children: reliability and validity of a modified Yo-Yo IR1 test and the Andersen test. Eur J Appl Physiol 112: 871–876.
15. Medbø JI, Mamen A, Beltrami FG (2012) Examination of the Moxus Modular Metabolic System by the Douglas-bag technique. Appl Physiol Nutr Metab 37: 860–871.
16. Welsman J, Bywater K, Farr C, Welford D, Armstrong N (2005) Reliability of peak VO_2 and maximal cardiac output assessed using thoracic bioimpedance in children. Eur J Appl Physiol 94: 228–234.
17. Cole TJ, Bellizzi MC, Flegal KM, Dietz WH (2000) Establishing a standard definition for child overweight and obesity worldwide: international survey. BMJ 320: 1240–1243.
18. Bland JM, Altman DG (1986) Statistical methods for assessing agreement between two methods of clinical measurement. Lancet 1: 307–310.
19. Hopkins WG (2000) Measures of reliability in sports medicine and science. Sports Med 30: 1–15.
20. McVeigh SK, Payne AC, Scott S (1995) The reliability and validity of the 20-meter shuttle test as a predictor of peak oxygen uptake in Edinburgh school children, age 13 to 14 years. Pediatr Exerc Sci 7: 69–79.
21. Liu NYS, Plowman SA, Looney MA (1992) The reliability and validity of the 20-meter shuttle test in american students 12 to 15 years old. Res Q Exerc Sport 63: 360–365.
22. Ortega FB, Artero EG, Ruiz JR, Vicente-Rodriguez G, Bergman P, et al. (2008) Reliability of health-related physical fitness tests in European adolescents. The HELENA Study. Int J Obes 32: S49–S57.
23. Pitetti KH, Fernhall B, Figoni S (2002) Comparing two regression formulas that predict VO_{2peak} using the 20-m shuttle run for children and adolescents. Pediatr Exerc Sci 14: 125–134.
24. Lamb KL, Rogers L (2007) A re-appraisal of the reliability of the 20 m multi-stage shuttle run test. Eur J Appl Physiol 100: 287–292.
25. Hutcheon JA, Chiolero A, Hanley JA (2010) Random measurement error and regression dilution bias. BMJ 340: 1402–1406.
26. Atkinson G, Nevill AM (1998) Statistical methods for assessing measurement error (reliability) in variables relevant to sports medicine. Sports Med 26: 217–238.
27. Steyerberg EW (2009) Clinical prediction models: a practical approach to development, validation and updating. New York: Springer Science+Business Media.
28. Rowland T (2005) Children's exercise physiology. USA: Human Kinetics.

The Impact of Prophylactic Dexamethasone on Nausea and Vomiting after Thyroidectomy

Zhenhong Zou[1¶], Yuming Jiang[1¶], Mingjia Xiao[2], Ruiyao Zhou[3*]

1 Department of General Surgery, Nanfang Hospital, Southern Medical University, Guangzhou City, Guangdong Province, China, **2** Department of Hepatobiliary Surgery, Wuxi People's Hospital of Nanjing Medical University, Wuxi, Jiangsu Province, China, **3** Department of General Surgery, The Third Affiliated Hospital of Wenzhou Medical University, Ruian City, Zhejiang Province, China

Abstract

Background: We carried out a systematic review and meta-analysis to evaluate the impact of prophylactic dexamethasone on post-operative nausea and vomiting (PONV), post-operative pain, and complications in patients undergoing thyroidectomy.

Methods: We searched Pubmed, Embase, and Cochrane Library databases for randomized controlled trials (RCTs) that evaluated the prophylactic effect of dexamethasone versus placebo with or without other antiemetics for PONV in patients undergoing thyroidectomy. Meta-analyses were performed using RevMan 5.0 software.

Results: Thirteen RCTs that considered high quality evidence including 2,180 patients were analyzed. The meta-analysis demonstrated a significant decrease in the incidence of PONV (RR 0.52, 95% CI 0.43 to 0.63, $P<0.00001$), the need for rescue anti-emetics (RR 0.42, 95% CI 0.30 to 0.57, $P<0.00001$), post-operative pain scores (WMD −1.17, 95% CI −1.91 to −0.44, $P=0.002$), and the need for rescue analgesics (RR 0.65, 95% CI 0.50–0.83, $P=0.0008$) in patients receiving dexamethasone compared to placebo, with or without concomitant antiemetics. Dexamethasone 8–10 mg had a significantly greater effect for reducing the incidence of PONV than dexamethasone 1.25–5 mg. Dexamethasone was as effective as other anti-emetics for reducing PONV (RR 1.25, 95% CI 0.86–1.81, $P=0.24$). A significantly higher level of blood glucose during the immediate post-operative period in patients receiving dexamethasone compared to controls was the only adverse event.

Conclusions: Prophylactic dexamethasone 8–10 mg administered intravenously before induction of anesthesia should be recommended as a safe and effective strategy for reducing the incidence of PONV, the need for rescue anti-emetics, post-operative pain, and the need for rescue analgesia in thyroidectomy patients, except those that are pregnant, have diabetes mellitus, hyperglycemia, or contraindications for dexamethasone. More high quality trials are warranted to define the benefits and risks of prophylactic dexamethasone in potential patients with a high risk for PONV.

Editor: Richard E. Burney, University of Michigan, United States of America

Funding: The authors have no support or funding to report.

Competing Interests: The authors have declared that no competing interests exist.

* Email: doctor_zry@126.com

¶ These authors are co-first authors on this work.

Introduction

Post-operative nausea and vomiting (PONV) is a common and distressing complication associated with surgery. The overall incidence of PONV ranges from 20 to 30% in general surgery and up to 80% in high-risk surgical patients when no prophylactic anti-emetic is given [1,2]. For patients undergoing thyroidectomy, PONV is a risk factor for post-operative bleeding [3,4], and prophylactic anti-emetics may be beneficial.

Previous studies have shown that prophylactic dexamethasone has anti-emetic and analgesic effects. Glucocorticoids are anti-inflammatory and immunosuppressive agents, and dexamethasone may exert its therapeutic actions through central inhibition of prostaglandin synthesis, by decreasing serotonin turnover in the central nervous system, and by influencing the systemic inflammatory response in favor of anti-inflammatory mediators [5–9].

A systematic review demonstrated that prophylactic dexamethasone was safe and effective for reducing the incidence of PONV and post-operative pain in patients undergoing laparoscopic cholecystectomy compared to placebo [10]. In patients undergoing thyroidectomy, a previous meta-analysis demonstrated a significant reduction of PONV in patients treated with a single dose of dexamethasone versus placebo [11]. However, the relatively small sample size included in this review precluded the authors from drawing definitive conclusions, and the optimal dose and timing of dexamethasone administration, and efficacy of combining dexamethasone with other anti-emetics, remains unclear.

The objective of the current study was to confirm, and continue to investigate the impact of prophylactic corticosteroid administration on PONV, post-operative pain, and complications following thyroidectomy.

Methods

This systematic review and meta-analysis is reported in accordance with the recommendations of the PRISMA statement [12].

2.1 Outcome measures

2.1.1 Primary outcome measure

1. Incidence of PONV during the immediate 24 h post-operative period, dichotomized as no nausea versus others; this was evaluated according to a 3-point ordinal scale: no nausea; nausea; retching and/or vomiting

2.1.2 Secondary outcome measures

1. Post-operative pain scores
2. Need for rescue anti-emetic or analgesic agent(s)
3. Incidence of steroid-related complications, including hyperglycemia, wound infection, delayed wound healing, headaches, dizziness, facial flushing, constipation, and abdominal pain

2.2 Data collection and analysis

2.2.1 Searches. We searched PubMed, Embase, and Cochrane Library databases from their inception to October 1, 2013 using Cochrane Highly Sensitive Search Strategies to identify randomized controlled trials (RCTs) for potential inclusion in our review [13]. We used the following MeSH terms and keywords: thyroid surgery OR thyroidectomy AND corticosteroid, glucocorticoid, steroid, OR dexamethasone. The search strategy is summarized in Table S1. Authors' names were entered as search terms in the PubMed database to check for additional studies. Trials were also identified using the "related articles" function in PubMed. We hand-searched reference lists from articles identified by the electronic search and from previous meta-analyses. This process was performed iteratively until no additional articles could be identified.

2.2.2 Inclusion and Exclusion Criteria. We included RCTs that: evaluated the prophylactic effect of dexamethasone versus placebo without other anti-emetics, dexamethasone versus placebo plus concomitant administration of a different anti-emetic, dexamethasone versus a different anti-emetic, and comparisons using different doses of dexamethasone for PONV in patients

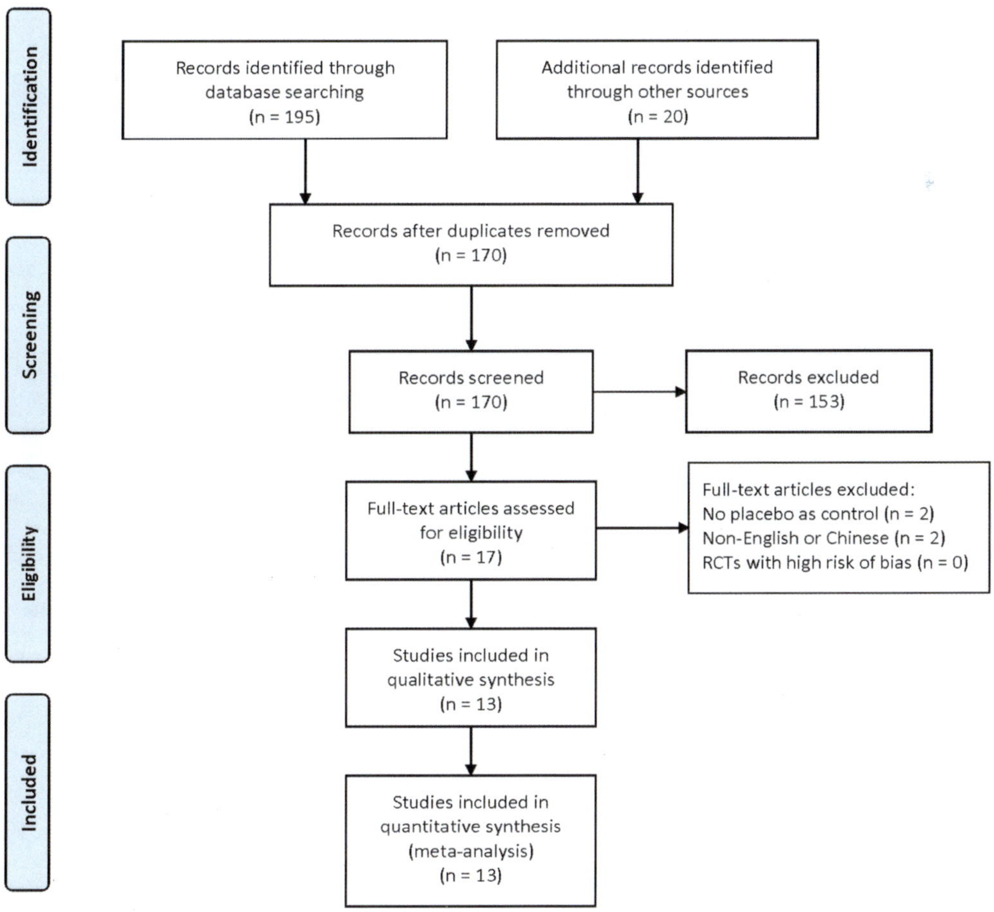

Figure 1. Flow chart for selecting the trials. On the basis of the search strategy, 195 articles were identified by the initial search, and 17 required further assessment. Finally, 13 articles were included in this review.

Table 1. Characteristics of trials included in the meta-analysis.

Study	Sample size	Interventions	Studies divided
Wang 1999 [18]	120	D 10 mg vs. Droperidol 1.25 mg vs. Placebo, all IV at 1 minute before induction	Wang 1999 D 10: D 10 mg vs. Placebo; Wang 1999: D 10 mg vs. Droperidol 1.25 mg
Wang 2000 [19]	225	D 10 mg vs. D 5 mg vs. D 2.5 mg vs. D 1.25 mg vs. Placebo, all IV immediately after induction	Wang 2000 D 10: D 10 mg vs. Placebo; Wang 2000 D 5: D 5 mg vs. Placebo; Wang 2000 D 2.5: D 2.5 mg vs. Placebo; Wang 2000 D 1.25: D 1.25 mg vs. Placebo
Lee 2001 [20]	135	D 8 mg vs. D 5 mg vs. Placebo, all IV before anesthesia	Lee 2001 D 8: D 10 mg vs. Placebo; Lee 2001 D 5: D 5 mg vs. Placebo
Fujji 2007 [21]	75	D 8 mg vs. D 4 mg vs. Placebo, all IV at the end of surgery	Fujji 2007 D8: D 8 mg vs. Placebo; Fujji 2007 D4: D 4 mg vs. Placebo
Worni 2008 [22]	70	D 8 mg vs. Placebo, both IV at 45 minutes before anesthesia	Worni 2008 D8: D 8 mg vs. Placebo
Feroci 2010 [23]	102	D 8 mg vs. Placebo, both IV at 20 minutes before induction	Feroci 2010 D8: D 8 mg vs. Placebo
Doksrod 2012 [24]	120	D 0.3 mg/kg vs. D 0.15 mg/kg vs. Placebo, all IV within 10 min after induction	Doksrod 2012 D18: D 0.3 mg/kg vs. Placebo; Doksrod 2012 D9: D 0.15 mg/kg vs. Placebo
Song 2013 [25]	123	D 10 mg vs. Ramosetron 0.3 mg vs. Placebo, both IV immediately after anesthesia	Song 2013 D 10: D10: D 10 mg vs. Placebo; Song 2013: D 10 mg vs. Ramosetron 0.3 mg
Barros 2013 [26]	40	D 4 mg vs. Placebo, both IV immediately after induction	Barros 2013 D4: D 4 mg vs. Placebo
Schietroma 2013 [27]	328	D 8 mg vs. Placebo, both IV at 90 minutes before skin incision	Schietroma 2013 D8: D 8 mg vs. Placebo
Zhou 2012 [28]	150	D 8 mg + T 5 mg vs. D 8 mg vs. T 5 mg, all IV immediately before induction	Zhou 2012 Tropisetron: D 8 mg + T 5 mg vs.T 5 mg; Zhou 2012: D 8 mg vs. T 5 mg
Bononi 2010 [29]	562	D 4 mg +O 4 mg vs. O 4 mg, D IV at induction and ondansetron IV at 15 minutes before tracheal extubation	Bononi 2010 Ondansetron: D 4 mg +O 4 mg vs. O 4 mg
Fujji 2000 [30]	130	D 8 mg + G 40 ug/kg vs. G 40 ug/kg, both IV immediately before induction	Fujji 2000 Granisetron: D 8 mg + G 40 ug/kg vs. G 40 ug/kg

IV: intravenous; ASA, American Society of Anesthesiologists; D: dexamethasone; T: tropisetron; O: ondansetron; G: Granisetron.

undergoing thyroidectomy. The included trials reported at least one of our outcome measures, and clearly reported patient inclusion and exclusion criteria, anesthetic technique, protocols for administration of the experimental drugs, and a definition and evaluation of nausea and vomiting. Studies were excluded if they were not RCTs, included patients who were undergoing other surgical procedures concomitantly, reported insufficient data, or were duplicate studies.

2.2.3 Selection of studies. Two reviewers (ZH Zou and YM Jiang) independently examined titles and abstracts to select eligible RCTs. We removed records that were ongoing or unpublished studies, or were published as abstracts or conference proceedings. Where datasets were overlapping or duplicated, only the most recent information was included. We retrieved the full text of potentially relevant studies. Two reviewers (ZH Zou and YM Jiang) independently examined the full text records to determine which studies met the inclusion criteria. We resolved disagreements about selection of studies by discussion and consensus.

2.2.4 Data extraction and management. Two reviewers (ZH Zou and YM Jiang) independently extracted data from eligible RCTs including details describing study population, interventions, and outcomes. We resolved disagreements about data extraction by discussion and consensus.

2.2.5 Assessment of quality of evidence in included studies. Two reviewers (ZH Zou and YM Jiang) independently assessed RCT quality and risk of bias using tools provided by the Cochrane Collaboration [14]. The reviewers examined six domains including sequence generation, allocation concealment, double-blind evaluation (blinding), complete outcome data, selective outcome reporting, and baseline comparability of groups. The risk of bias was categorized as low, high, or unclear. RCTs with high risk of bias in at least three of six domains were not included in the meta-analysis. Baseline comparability of groups was assessed using seven matching criteria: age, sex, history of motion sickness, previous post-operative emesis, anesthetic technique, operation type (partial or total thyroidectomy), and duration of surgery. Baseline incomparability was defined as non-matching in at least three of the seven criteria. We resolved disagreements about quality of evidence by discussion and consensus.

2.2.6 Statistical analysis. Statistical analyses were performed using RevMan (ver. 5.0; The Cochrane Collaboration, Oxford, UK) software and STATA (ver. 11.2; STATA Corpora-

Table 2. Details of anesthetic technique, and rescue analgesics and anti-emetics in the included trials.

Study	Anesthetic technique	Rescue analgesics	Rescue antiemetics
Wang 1999 [18]	Propofol 2.0–2.5 mg/kg, glycopyrrolate 0.2 mg, fentanyl 2.0 ug/kg IV maintained with 1.0%–2.5% isoflurane in oxygen	Diclofenac 75 mg IM q12h	Ondansetron 4 mg IV
Wang 2000 [19]	Propofol 2.0–2.5 mg/kg, glycopyrrolate 0.2 mg, fentanyl 2.0 ug/kg IV maintained with 1.0%–2.5% isoflurane in oxygen	Diclofenac 75 mg IM q12h	Ondansetron 4 mg IV
Lee 2001 [20]	Glycopyrrolate 0.2 mg, fentanyl 2 ug/kg, thiopental 5 mg/kg IV maintained with desflurane in oxygen	Ketorolac 15 mg IV q6h	Droperidol 1.25 mg IV
Fujji 2007 [21]	Propofol 2 mg/kg, fentanyl 2 ug/kg, vecuronium 0.1 mg/kg IV maintained with 1–3% sevoflurane in oxygen	Indomethacin 50 mg rectally	Ranitidine 150 mg orally
Worni 2008 [22]	Propofol/thiopental, atracurium, isoflurane, or sevoflurane and fentanyl 5–10 ug/kg	Acetaminophen 4 g/day; second-line metamizole 1g or morphine	Ondansetron 4 mg IV; second-line droperidol 0.625 mg IV
Feroci 2010 [23]	Propofol 2 mg/kg, fentanyl 2 ug/kg, vecuronium 0.1 mg/kg IV maintained with sevoflurane in oxygen	Paracetamol 1000 mg IV q8 h; second-line ketorolac 30 mg IV q12h	Metoclopramide 10 mg IV; second-line ondansetron 4 mg IV
Doksrod 2012 [24]	Propofol, fentanyl, vecuronium IV maintained with desflurane (4–8%) and itrous oxide (60%) in oxygen	Oxycodone 5 mg orally; second-line metamizole or morphine 2.5 mg IV	Metoclopramide 20 mg IV; second-line ondansetron 4 mg IV
Song 2013 [25]	Remifentanil 1 ug/kg, propofol 1–2 mg/kg, rocuroniumin 0.9 mg/kg IV, maintained with desflurane in oxygen–air mixture	Ketorolac 30 mg IV	Metoclopramide 10 mg IV
Barros 2013 [26]	Propofol, fentanyl 2.0 ug/kg, cisatracurium 0.15 mg/kg, maintained with sevoflurane in oxygen	Ketorolac 30 mg or parecoxib 40 mg IV	Ondansetron 4 mg IV
Schietroma 2013 [27]	Sodium thiopental 5 mg/kg,atracurium besylate 0.5 mg/kg, maintained with oxygen in air, sevoflurane, and remifentanil hydrochloride	Ketorolac tromethamine 30 mg IV q6h	Ondansetron hydrochloride 4 mg IV
Zhou 2012 [28]	Propofol 1.5–2.5 mg/kg, midazolam 0.1–0.2 mg/kg, fentanyl 1.0–2.0 ug/kg, maintained with 1.0–3.0% sevoflurane in oxygen	Pethidine 25 mg IV	Metoclopramide 10 mg IV; second-line tropisetron 5 mg IV
Bononi 2010 [29]	Not stated[a]	Not stated	Not stated
Fujji 2000 [30]	Thiopentone 5 mg/kg, fentanyl 2 ug/kg, vecuronium 0.2 mg/kg maintained with isoflurane (1.0%–3.0%) and nitrous oxide (66%) in oxygen	Indomethacin 50mg rectally for moderae pain and buprenorphiine 0.2 mg IM for severe pain	Domperidone retally

IV, intravenous; IM, intramuscular; [a]no difference.

Table 3. Quality of evidence in included studies.

Included studies	Country	Sequence generation	Allocation concealment	Double blinding	Complete outcome data	No selective reporting	Baseline comparability	Risk of bias
Wang 1999 [18]	China	Adequate	Unclear	Yes	Yes	Yes	Yes	Low
Wang 2000 [19]	China	Adequate	Unclear	Yes	Yes	Yes	Yes	Low
Lee 2001 [20]	China	Adequate	Adequate	Yes	Yes	Yes	Yes	Low
Fujii 2007 [21]	Japan	Adequate	Adequate	Yes	Yes	Yes	Yes	Low
Worni 2008 [22]	Switzerland	Adequate	Adequate	Yes	Yes	Yes	Yes	Low
Feroci 2011 [23]	Italy	Adequate	Adequate	Yes	Yes	Yes	Yes	Low
Doksrod 2012 [24]	Norway	Adequate	Adequate	Yes	Yes	Yes	Yes	Low
Song 2013 [25]	Korea	Adequate	Adequate	Unclear	Yes	Yes	Yes	Low
Barros 2013 [26]	Portugal	Adequate	Adequate	Yes	Yes	Yes	Yes	Low
Schietroma 2013 [27]	Italy	Adequate	Adequate	Yes	Yes	Yes	Yes	Low
Zhou 2012 [28]	China	Adequate	Adequate	Unclear	Yes	Yes	Yes	Low
Bononi 2010 [29]	Italy	Adequate	Adequate	Unclear	Yes	Yes	Yes	Low
Fujii 2000 [30]	Japan	Adequate	Adequate	Yes	Yes	Yes	Yes	Low

tion, College Station, TX, USA) software. Weighted mean differences (WMDs) with 95% confidence intervals (CIs) were calculated for continuous variables, and risk ratios (RRs) with 95% CIs were calculated for dichotomous variables. A random-effects model was used to pool studies with significant heterogeneity, as determined by the chi-squared test ($P \leq 0.10$) and the inconsistency index ($I^2 \geq 50\%$). Potential sources of statistical heterogeneity were explored by carrying out subgroup and sensitivity analyses. Subgroup analyses were performed by stratifying patients according to dose of corticosteroid and timing of dexamethasone administration; sensitivity analyses explored the impact of excluding outlying results. The presence of publication bias was comprehensively assessed using Begg's funnel plot and Begg's rank correlation test of asymmetry. Publication bias was thought to be present when the continuity-corrected $Pr>|z|$ value was ≤ 0.1 [15]. The GRADE system was used to summarize the overall quality of evidence [16,17].

Results

3.1 Trial identification

The searches identified 195 articles. We screened titles and abstracts, and 17 were identified as potentially eligible for inclusion. We retrieved the full text articles. After analyzing the full text articles, 4 studies were excluded and 13 RCTs [18–30] were found eligible for inclusion according to our criteria for considering studies in this review (Fig. 1).

3.2 Characteristics of included studies

The characteristics of the included studies are shown in Table 1. The 13 eligible RCTs included 2,180 patients who underwent general anesthesia for thyroidectomy. The majority of RCTs included patients classified as American Society of Anesthesiologists (ASA) class I or II. Exclusion criteria were: pregnant women, patients with insulin-dependent diabetes mellitus, obesity, and patients with a high risk for PONV. Dexamethasone was administered intravenously in a single or combination dose ranging from 1.25–18 mg. Timing of administration varied from 90 minutes before skin incision to the end of surgery. Controls included placebo, droperidol, granisetron, ondansetron, tropisetron or a combination of these medications. Confounders such as anesthetic technique and rescue analgesics and anti-emetics were standardized within studies (Table 2). Risk of bias was low across all RCTs (Table 3).

3.3 Treatment effects

3.3.1 Primary outcome. *Incidence of PONV: Dexamethasone versus placebo, with or without concomitant anti-emetics* - Data reporting on the incidence of PONV in thyroidectomy patients treated with dexamethasone versus placebo with or without concomitant anti-emetics are described in 11 RCTs [18–25,28–30]. The meta-analysis demonstrated a significant decrease in the incidence of PONV in patients receiving dexamethasone compared to placebo, with or without concomitant anti-emetics (RR 0.52, 95% CI 0.43 to 0.63, $P<0.00001$; Fig. 2). There was evidence of significant heterogeneity between studies ($P=0.003$, $I^2=56\%$). The dose-response gradient may have caused most of the variation between RCTs (Fig. 3; Fig.S1).

Incidence of PONV: Dexamethasone versus a different anti-emetic - Data reporting on the incidence of PONV in thyroidectomy patients treated with dexamethasone versus a different anti-emetic, including droperidol, granisetron, or tropisetron, are described in three RCTs [18,25,28]. The meta-analysis demonstrated no significant difference in the incidence of PONV in

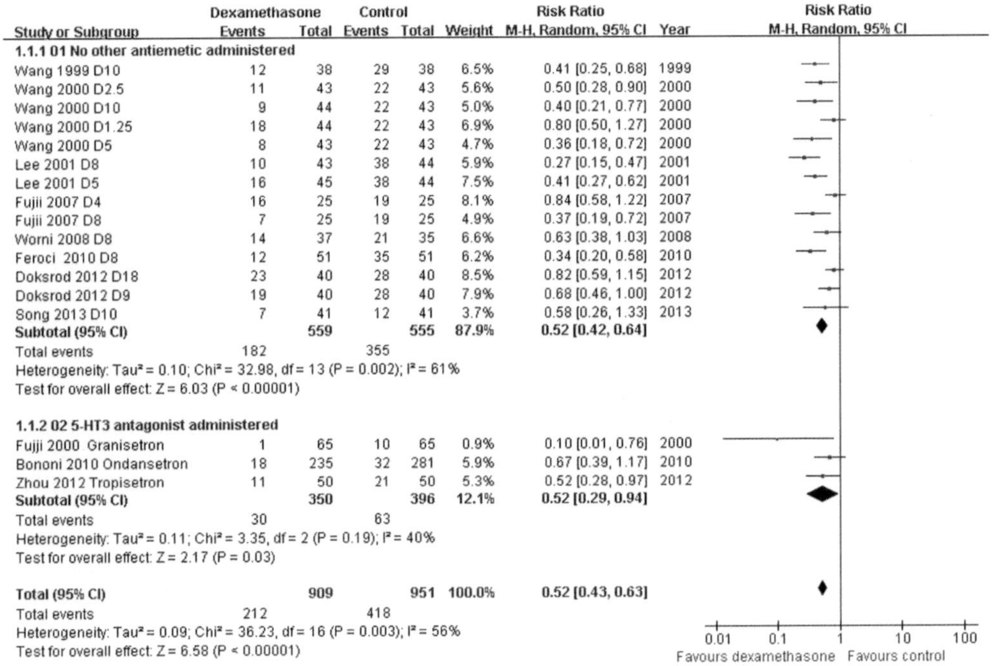

Figure 2. Incidence of PONV grouped by concomitant anti-emetics. Eleven studies described the incidence of PONV in thyroidectomy patients treated with dexamethasone versus placebo with or without concomitant anti-emetics (RR 0.52, 95% CI 0.43 to 0.63, $P<0.00001$). There was evidence of significant heterogeneity between studies ($P=0.003$, $I^2=56\%$).

patients receiving dexamethasone compared to these different anti-emetics (RR 1.25, 95% CI 0.86–1.81, $P=0.24$; Fig. 4). There was no evidence of significant heterogeneity between RCTs ($P=0.27$, $I^2=23\%$).

3.3.2 Secondary outcomes. *Postoperative pain scores and need for rescue analgesia: Dexamethasone versus placebo with or without concomitant anti-emetics* - Data reporting on post-operative pain scores in thyroidectomy patients treated with dexamethasone versus placebo with or without concomitant anti-emetics are described in six RCTs [18,20,22,23,25,26]. Pain scores were evaluated based on visual analogue scales (VAS) completed by patients 24 h post-operatively. Four RCTs [22,23,25,26] reported data as means ± standard deviations (SDs); two RCTs [18,20] reported data as medians (range) converted to estimated means and SDs [31]. The meta-analysis demonstrated a significantly lower post-operative VAS score in patients receiving dexamethasone compared to placebo, with or without concomitant anti-emetics (WMD −1.17, 95% CI −1.91 to −0.44, $P=0.002$; Fig. 5). There was evidence of significant heterogeneity between RCTs ($P<0.00001$, $I^2=94\%$). The doses of dexamethasone may have caused most of the variation between RCTs. The need for rescue analgesia was significantly less frequent in the patients that received dexamethasone (RR 0.65, 95% CI 0.50–0.83, $P=0.0008$; Fig. 6); there was no evidence of significant heterogeneity between RCTs ($P=0.25$, $I^2=25\%$).

Need for rescue anti-emetic: Dexamethasone versus placebo with or without concomitant antiemetics - Data reporting on the need for rescue anti-emetics in thyroidectomy patients treated with dexamethasone versus placebo with or without concomitant anti-emetics are described in six studies [19,25–28,30]. The meta-analysis demonstrated a significant decrease in the need for rescue anti-emetics in patients receiving dexamethasone compared to placebo, with or without concomitant anti-emetics (RR 0.42, 95% CI 0.30 to 0.57, $P<0.00001$; Fig. 7). There was no evidence of significant heterogeneity between RCTs ($P=0.43$, $I^2=0\%$).

Incidence of adverse events: Dexamethasone versus placebo with or without concomitant anti-emetics - Data reporting on blood glucose levels in thyroidectomy patients treated with dexamethasone are described in two RCTs. A significantly higher level of blood glucose was observed in patients receiving dexamethasone compared to controls during the first 8 hours post-operatively [23,24]. No statistical differences in symptomatic transient hypocalcemia and asymptomatic transient hypocalcemia were present [23]. One RCT [27] reported that dexamethasone administration prevented recurrent laryngeal nerve palsy; however, this effect was not described elsewhere [23]. There were no significant differences in the incidences of extrapyramidal signs including headache, dizziness, constipation, and muscle pain, and other adverse events such as wound infection and delayed wound healing, in patients receiving dexamethasone compared to controls.

3.4 Subgroup analyses

Incidence of PONV: Dose of dexamethasone. Subgroup analyses stratified by dose of dexamethasone (range, 1.25 mg to 18 mg) demonstrated that dexamethasone 4–5 mg and 8–10 mg significantly reduced the incidence of PONV compared to controls (1.25–5 mg: RR 0.59, 95% CI 0.44 to 0.79; 8–10 mg: RR 0.45, 95% CI 0.35–0.57), while dexamethasone 18 mg did not (RR 0.82, 95% CI 0.59–1.15) (Fig. 3). Dexamethasone 8–10 mg had a significantly greater effect for reducing the incidence of PONV than dexamethasone 1.25–5 mg (1.25–5 mg RR 0.40, 95% CI 0.28 to 0.55; 8–10 mg: RR 0.23, 95% CI 0.18–0.31; P = 0.02; Fig. S1).

Incidence of PONV: Timing of dexamethasone administration. The RCTs included in this review varied with regard to timing of dexamethasone administration. Some patients

Study or Subgroup	Dexamethasone Events	Dexamethasone Total	Control Events	Control Total	Weight	Risk Ratio M-H, Random, 95% CI	Year
1.2.1 Dexamethasone 18mg							
Doksrod 2012 D18	23	40	28	40	8.5%	0.82 [0.59, 1.15]	2012
Subtotal (95% CI)		**40**		**40**	**8.5%**	**0.82 [0.59, 1.15]**	
Total events	23		28				
Heterogeneity: Not applicable							
Test for overall effect: Z = 1.15 (P = 0.25)							
1.2.2 Dexamethasone 8-10mg							
Wang 1999 D10	12	38	29	38	6.5%	0.41 [0.25, 0.68]	1999
Fujii 2000 Granisetron	1	65	10	65	0.9%	0.10 [0.01, 0.76]	2000
Wang 2000 D10	9	44	22	43	5.0%	0.40 [0.21, 0.77]	2000
Lee 2001 D8	10	43	38	44	5.9%	0.27 [0.15, 0.47]	2001
Fujii 2007 D8	7	25	19	25	4.9%	0.37 [0.19, 0.72]	2007
Worni 2008 D8	14	37	21	35	6.6%	0.63 [0.38, 1.03]	2008
Feroci 2010 D8	12	51	35	51	6.2%	0.34 [0.20, 0.58]	2010
Doksrod 2012 D9	19	40	28	40	7.9%	0.68 [0.46, 1.00]	2012
Zhou 2012 Tropisetron	11	50	21	50	5.3%	0.52 [0.28, 0.97]	2012
Song 2013 D10	7	41	12	41	3.7%	0.58 [0.26, 1.33]	2013
Subtotal (95% CI)		**434**		**432**	**52.7%**	**0.45 [0.35, 0.57]**	
Total events	102		235				
Heterogeneity: Tau² = 0.05; Chi² = 14.29, df = 9 (P = 0.11); I² = 37%							
Test for overall effect: Z = 6.64 (P < 0.00001)							
1.2.3 Dexamethasone 4-5mg							
Wang 2000 D5	8	43	22	43	4.7%	0.36 [0.18, 0.72]	2000
Lee 2001 D5	16	45	38	44	7.5%	0.41 [0.27, 0.62]	2001
Fujii 2007 D4	16	25	19	25	8.1%	0.84 [0.58, 1.22]	2007
Bononi 2010 Ondansetron	18	235	32	281	5.9%	0.67 [0.39, 1.17]	2010
Subtotal (95% CI)		**348**		**393**	**26.2%**	**0.56 [0.37, 0.85]**	
Total events	58		111				
Heterogeneity: Tau² = 0.12; Chi² = 9.02, df = 3 (P = 0.03); I² = 67%							
Test for overall effect: Z = 2.72 (P = 0.006)							
1.2.5 Dexamethasone 1.5-2.5mg							
Wang 2000 D1.25	18	44	22	43	6.9%	0.80 [0.50, 1.27]	2000
Wang 2000 D2.5	11	43	22	43	5.6%	0.50 [0.28, 0.90]	2000
Subtotal (95% CI)		**87**		**86**	**12.5%**	**0.66 [0.41, 1.04]**	
Total events	29		44				
Heterogeneity: Tau² = 0.04; Chi² = 1.54, df = 1 (P = 0.21); I² = 35%							
Test for overall effect: Z = 1.81 (P = 0.07)							
Total (95% CI)		**909**		**951**	**100.0%**	**0.52 [0.43, 0.63]**	
Total events	212		418				
Heterogeneity: Tau² = 0.09; Chi² = 36.23, df = 16 (P = 0.003); I² = 56%							
Test for overall effect: Z = 6.58 (P < 0.00001)							

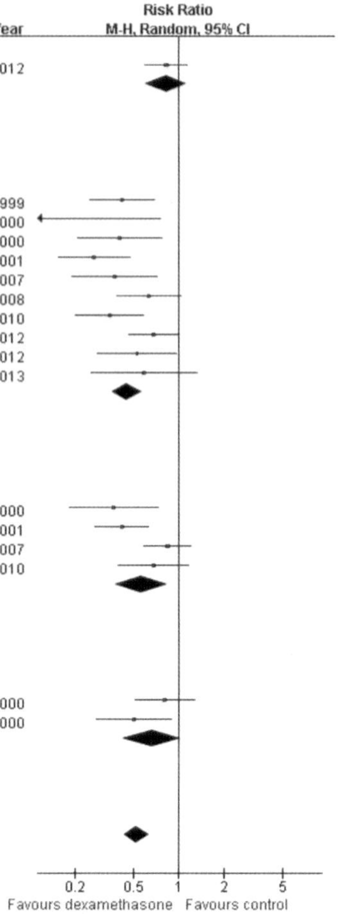

Figure 3. PONV according to dexamethasone dose. Higher dexamethasone doses (8–10 mg) were significantly more effective than lower dexamethasone doses (1.25–5 mg) ($P = 0.02$).

Study or Subgroup	Dexamethasone Events	Dexamethasone Total	antiemetic Events	antiemetic Total	Weight	Risk Ratio M-H, Fixed, 95% CI	Year
1.3.1 Dexamethasone 10mg vs. Droperidol							
Wang 1999	14	40	14	38	43.0%	0.95 [0.53, 1.72]	1999
Subtotal (95% CI)		**40**		**38**	**43.0%**	**0.95 [0.53, 1.72]**	
Total events	14		14				
Heterogeneity: Not applicable							
Test for overall effect: Z = 0.17 (P = 0.87)							
1.3.2 Dexamethasone 8mg vs. Tropisetron							
Zhou 2012	21	50	17	50	51.0%	1.24 [0.75, 2.05]	2012
Subtotal (95% CI)		**50**		**50**	**51.0%**	**1.24 [0.75, 2.05]**	
Total events	21		17				
Heterogeneity: Not applicable							
Test for overall effect: Z = 0.82 (P = 0.41)							
1.3.3 Dexamethasone 10mg vs. Ramosetron							
Song 2013	7	41	2	41	6.0%	3.50 [0.77, 15.85]	2013
Subtotal (95% CI)		**41**		**41**	**6.0%**	**3.50 [0.77, 15.85]**	
Total events	7		2				
Heterogeneity: Not applicable							
Test for overall effect: Z = 1.63 (P = 0.10)							
Total (95% CI)		**131**		**129**	**100.0%**	**1.25 [0.86, 1.81]**	
Total events	42		33				
Heterogeneity: Chi² = 2.61, df = 2 (P = 0.27); I² = 23%							
Test for overall effect: Z = 1.17 (P = 0.24)							
Test for subgroup differences: Not applicable							

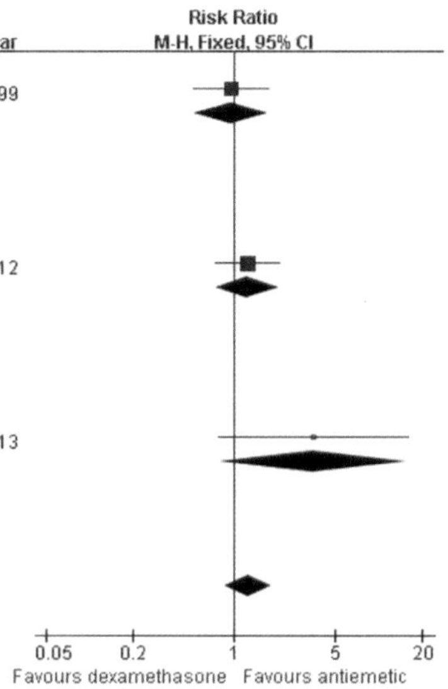

Figure 4. Comparison of dexamethasone with other anti-emetics. Three studies described the incidence of PONV in thyroidectomy patients treated with dexamethasone versus other anti-emetics (RR 1.25, 95% CI 0.86–1.81, $P = 0.24$). There was no evidence of significant heterogeneity between RCTs ($P = 0.27$, $I^2 = 23\%$).

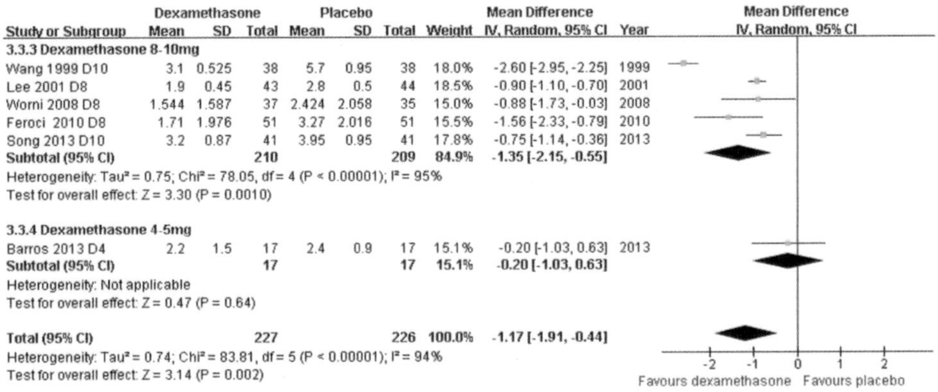

Figure 5. VAS post-operative pain score grouped by dexamethasone dose. Six studies described post-operative pain scores in thyroidectomy patients treated with dexamethasone versus placebo with or without concomitant anti-emetics (WMD −1.17, 95% CI −1.91 to −0.44, $P = 0.002$). There was evidence of significant heterogeneity between RCTs ($P < 0.00001$, $I^2 = 94\%$).

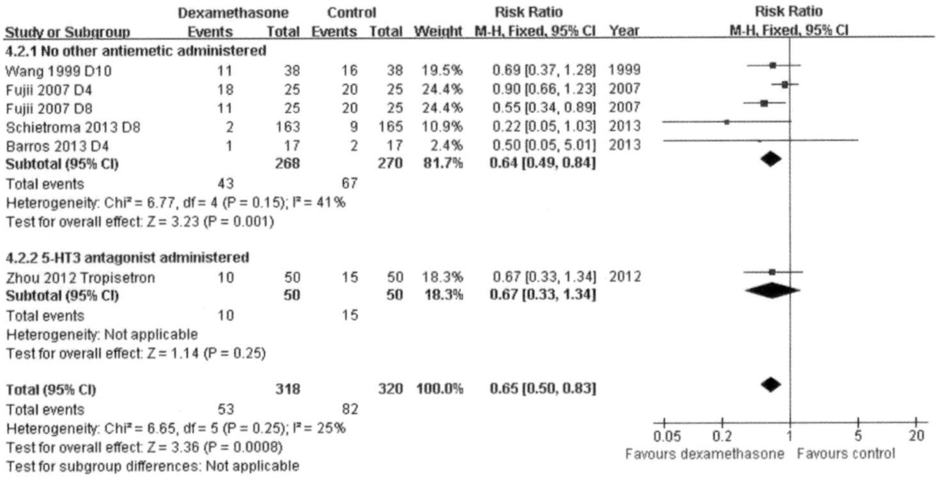

Figure 6. Need for rescue analgesics grouped by concomitant anti-emetics. Six studies described the need for rescue analgesics in thyroidectomy patients treated with dexamethasone versus placebo with or without concomitant anti-emetics (RR 0.65, 95% CI 0.50–0.83, $P = 0.0008$). There was no evidence of significant heterogeneity between RCTs ($P = 0.25$, $I^2 = 25\%$).

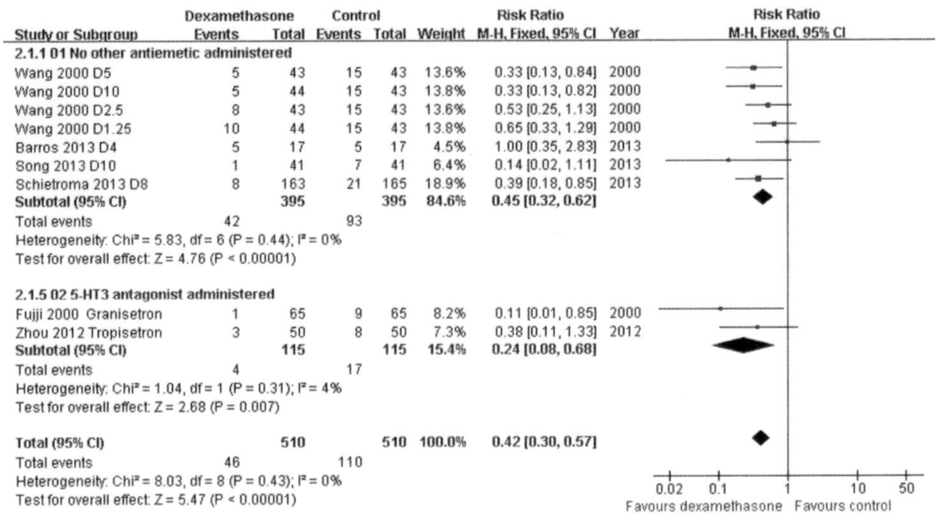

Figure 7. Need for rescue antiemetics grouped by concomitant antiemetics. Six studies described the need for rescue antiemetics in thyroidectomy patients treated with dexamethasone versus placebo with or without concomitant antiemetics (RR 0.42, 95% CI 0.30 to 0.57, $P < 0.00001$). There was no evidence of significant heterogeneity between RCTs ($P = 0.43$, $I^2 = 0\%$).

Table 4. GRADE evidence.

Outcomes	Illustrative comparative risks* (95% CI)		Relative effect (95% CI)	No of Participants (studies)	Quality of the evidence (GRADE)
	Assumed risk	Corresponding risk			
	Placebo	Dexamethasone			
Dexamethasone versus placebo (in addition to other antiemetics): PONV	**440 per 1000**	**229 per 1000** (189 to 277)	**RR 0.52** (0.43 to 0.63)	1860 (17 studies)	⊕⊕⊕⊕ **high**[1]
Dexamethasone versus placebo (in addition to other antiemetics): rescue antiemetics	**216 per 1000**	**91 per 1000** (65 to 123)	**RR 0.42** (0.3 to 0.57)	1020 (9 studies)	⊕⊕⊕ **high**
Dexamethasone comparison of doses: PONV	**440 per 1000**	**229 per 1000** (189 to 277)	**RR 0.52** (0.43 to 0.63)	1860 (17 studies)	⊕⊕⊕⊕ **high**[2]
Dexamethasone versus placebo: VAS pain score		The mean dexamethasone versus placebo: vas pain score in the intervention groups was **1.17 lower** (1.91 to 0.44 lower)		453 (6 studies)	⊕⊕⊕⊖ **moderate**[3]
Dexamethasone versus placebo (in addtion to other antiemetics): resuce analgesic	**256 per 1000**	**167 per 1000** (128 to 213)	**RR 0.65** (0.5 to 0.83)	638 (6 studies)	⊕⊕⊕⊖ **moderate**[4]
Dexamethasone versus a different antiemetic: PONV	**256 per 1000**	**320 per 1000** (220 to 463)	**RR 1.25** (0.86 to 1.81)	260 (3 studies)	⊕⊕⊕⊕ **high**

*The basis for the **assumed risk** (e.g. the median control group risk across studies) is provided in footnotes. The **corresponding risk** (and its 95% confidence interval) is based on the assumed risk in the comparison group and the **relative effect** of the intervention (and its 95% CI). **CI:** Confidence interval; **RR:** Risk ratio.
GRADE Working Group grades of evidence. **High quality:** Further research is very unlikely to change our confidence in the estimate of effect. **Moderate quality:** Further research is likely to have an important impact on our confidence in the estimate of effect and may change the estimate. **Low quality:** Further research is very likely to have an important impact on our confidence in the estimate of effect and is likely to change the estimate. **Very low quality:** We are very uncertain about the estimate.
[1]Although the PONV results demonstrated significant heterogeneity ($P=0.003$, $I^2=56\%$), it was partly explained by the dose of dexamethasone. [2]Downgraded by not comparing higher dose with lower dose directly, but upgraded by the dose-response gradient. [3]Although there was significant heterogeneity ($P<0.00001$, $I^2=94\%$), it was partly explained by the dose of dexamethasone. [4]Publication bias as $Pr>|z|=0.06$.
PONV: post-operative nausea and vomiting; VAS: visual analogue scales.
Patient or population: patients undergoing thyroidectomy. **Settings:** evidence from China, Japan, Korea, Italy, Switzerland, Norway, Portugal. **Intervention:** dexamethasone. **Comparison:** placebo.

received dexamethasone 90 minutes before skin incision, while others received dexamethasone postoperatively. Wang et al [32] demonstrated that dexamethasone administered before anesthesia was more effective in decreasing early PONV compared to dexamethasone administered after anesthesia. These observations are in accordance with data showing that the onset time of dexamethasone on anti-emesis is approximately 2 hours. In the current study, subgroup analysis stratified by the timing of dexamethasone administration showed that dexamethasone was most effective in preventing PONV when administered before rather than after induction of anesthesia ($P=0.0002$; Fig. S2).

3.5 Sensitivity analysis

To explore the effects of individual RCTs on the pooled OR estimates, we performed a sensitivity analysis omitting one study at a time. No single RCT significantly affected the overall results of the meta-analysis.

3.6 Publication bias

Visual inspection of a Funnel plot, Egger's test, and Begg's rank correlation test revealed no significant publication bias (Begg's rank correlation test, continuity-corrected $Pr>|z|>0.1$), except for RCTs reporting on the need for rescue anti-emetic in patients receiving dexamethasone versus placebo, with or without concomitant antiemetics ($Pr>|z|=0.06$), (Table S2).

3.7 Quality of evidence

Quality of available evidence from RCTs, which was downgraded by inconsistency (heterogeneity between studies), indirectness (variations in study setting), or publication bias, and upgraded by dose-response gradient, varied from moderate to high (Table 4).

Discussion

PONV is a common and distressing complication for patients undergoing thyroidectomy; therefore, prophylactic anti-emetics may be beneficial. An optimal anti-emetic regimen should be capable of decreasing the incidence of PONV without increasing the risk for adverse events. However, most of the currently used anti-emetics, including anti-histamines, butyrophenones, and dopamine receptor antagonists cause occasional undesirable adverse events, such as excessive sedation, hypotension, dry mouth, dysphoria, hallucinations, and extrapyramidal signs [33]. 5-HT3 antagonists are effective for preventing and treating PONV in patients undergoing various types of surgery [34]. However, the use of prophylactic anti-emetic therapy with 5-HT3 antagonists has been criticized for being too expensive [35].

Our meta-analysis of 13 RCTs demonstrated that prophylactic dexamethasone is effective in reducing the incidence of PONV, post-operative pain scores, and the need for rescue analgesia and anti-emetics compared to placebo administered with or without contaminant anti-emetics in patients undergoing thyroidectomy. In addition, our findings showed that dexamethasone is as effective as other anti-emetics for reducing PONV in this patient population. However, the benefits of administering dexamethasone as a more cost-effective anti-emetic and efficacious analgesic drug[35] should be weighed against the potential side effects. Our study indicated that dexamethasone administration is associated with an increase in blood glucose during the immediate post-operative period, but with no other serious adverse events.

For optimal dose and timing of dexamethasone administration, subgroup analyses showed that higher doses of dexamethasone (8–10 mg) are more effective than lower doses (1.5–5 mg), and dexamethasone is most effective in preventing PONV when administered before rather than after induction of anesthesia.

In terms of populations eligible for treatment, the RCTs in the current study mostly included healthy patients, and excluded pregnant women, patients with insulin-dependent diabetes mellitus, those who were obese, and patients with a high risk for PONV. As such, the impact of prophylactic dexamethasone on outcomes in high-risk patients is not known. A larger sample size and well-performed RCTs including high risk patients are required for further investigations.

This review has several limitations. First, data reporting on the effects of prophylactic dexamethasone on post-operative pain scores and need for rescue analgesics in thyroidectomy patients were limited by substantial heterogeneity and publication bias, respectively. Second, the studies in this systematic review included patients across various age groups receiving dexamethasone according to very different protocols.

Conclusion

The present meta-analysis shows that prophylactic dexamethasone is safe and effective for reducing the incidence of PONV, post-operative pain, and the need for rescue analgesia and anti-emetics in thyroidectomy patients. Prophylactic dexamethasone 8–10 mg administered before induction of anesthesia should be recommended for patients undergoing thyroidectomy except for those that are pregnant, have diabetes mellitus, hyperglycaemia or contraindications for corticosteroids. More high quality trials are warranted to define the benefits and risks of prophylactic dexamethasone in potential patients with high risk for PONV.

Supporting Information

Figure S1 Incidence of PONV stratified according to dexamethasone dose: 8–10 mg and 1.25–5 mg.

Figure S2 Incidence of PONV stratified by timing of dexamethasone administration.

Table S1 Search strategy from its inception to October 1, 2013.

Table S2 Begg's rank correlation test for publication bias.

Checklist S1 PRISMA 2009 Checklist.

Author Contributions

Conceived and designed the experiments: RZ ZZ MX. Performed the experiments: ZZ YJ. Analyzed the data: ZZ YJ. Contributed reagents/materials/analysis tools: ZZ YJ. Contributed to the writing of the manuscript: RZ MX.

References

1. Sonner JM, Hynson JM, Clark O, Katz JA (1997) Nausea and vomiting following thyroid and parathyroid surgery. J Clin Anesth 9(5): 398–402.
2. Kranke P, Eberhart LH (2011) Possibilities and limitations in the pharmacological management of postoperative nausea and vomiting. Eur J Anaesthesiol 28: 758–765.
3. Matory YL, Spiro RH (1993) Wound bleeding after head and neck surgery. J Surg Oncol 53(1): 17–19.
4. Schwartz AE, Clark OH, Ituarte P, Lo Gerfo P (1998) Therapeutic controversy: thyroid surgery–the choice. J Clin Endocrinol Metab 83(4): 1097–1105.
5. Fredrikson M, Hursti T, Fürst CJ, Steineck G, Börjeson S, et al. (1992) Nausea in cancer chemotherapy is inversely related to urinary cortisol excretion. Br J Cancer 65: 779–780.
6. Aapro MS, Plezia PM, Alberts DS, Graham V, Jones SE, et al. (1984) Double-blind crossover study of the antiemetic efficacy of high-dose dexamethasone versus high-dose metoclopramide. J Clin Oncol 2: 466–471.
7. Sapolsky RM, Romero LM, Munck AU (2000) How do glucocorticoids influence stress responses? Integrating permissive, suppressive, stimulatory, and preparative actions. Endocr Rev 21: 55–89.
8. Hargreaves KM, Costello A (1990) Glucocorticoids suppress levels of immunoreactive bradykinin in inflamed tissue as evaluated by microdialysis probes. Clin Pharmacol Ther 48: 168–178.
9. Hong D, Byers MR, Oswald RJ (1993) Dexamethasone treatment reduces sensory neuropeptides and nerve sprouting reactions in injured teeth. Pain 55: 171–181.
10. Karanicolas PJ1, Smith SE, Kanbur B, Davies E, Guyatt GH (2008) The Impact of Prophylactic Dexamethasone on Nausea and Vomiting After Laparoscopic Cholecystectomy A Systematic Review and Meta-Analysis. Ann Surg 248(5): 751–762.
11. Chen CC, Siddiqui FJ, Chen TL, Chan ES, Tam KW (2012) Dexamethasone for prevention of postoperative nausea and vomiting in patients undergoing thyroidectomy: meta-analysis of randomized controlled trials. World J Surg 36: 61–68.
12. Moher D, Liberati A, Tetzlaff J, Altman DG, PRISMA Group (2010) Preferred reporting items for systematic reviews and meta-analyses: the PRISMA statement. Int J Surg 8: 336–341.
13. Lefebvre C, Manheimer E, Glanville J (2011) Chapter 6: searching for studies. In: Higgins JPT, Green S (editors). Cochrane Handbook for Systematic Reviews of Interventions Version 5.1.0 [updated March 2011]. The Cochrane Collaboration, 2011. Available: www.cochrane-handbook.org.
14. Higgins JPT, Altman DG, Sterne JAC (2011) Chapter 8: assessing risk of bias in included studies. In: Higgins JPT, Green S (editors). Cochrane Handbook for Systematic Reviews of Interventions Version 5.1.0 [updated March 2011]. The Cochrane Collaboration, 2011. Available: www.cochrane-handbook.org.
15. Begg CB, Mazumdar M (1994) Operating characteristics of a rank correlation test for publication bias. Biometrics 50(4): 1088–1101.
16. Atkins D, Best D, Briss PA, Eccles M, Falck-Ytter Y, et al GRADE Working Group (2004) Grading quality of evidence and strength of recommendations. BMJ 328: 1490–1494.
17. Guyatt G, Gutterman D, Baumann MH, Addrizzo-Harris D, Hylek EM, et al. (2006) Grading strength of recommendations and quality of evidence in clinical guidelines. Chest 129: 174–181.
18. Wang JJ, Ho ST, Lee SC, Liu YC, Liu YH, et al. (1999) The prophylactic effect of dexamethasone on postoperative nausea and vomiting in women undergoing

thyroidectomy: a comparison of droperidol with saline. Anesth Analg 89: 200–203.
19. Wang JJ, Ho ST, Lee SC, Liu YC, Ho CM (2000) The use of dexamethasone for preventing postoperative nausea and vomiting in females undergoing thyroidectomy: a dose-ranging study. Anesth Analg 91: 1404–1407.
20. Lee Y, Lin PC, Lai HY, Huang SJ, Lin YS, et al. (2001) Prevention of PONV with dexamethasone in female patients undergoing desflurane anesthesia for thyroidectomy. Acta Anaesthesiol Sin 39: 151–156.
21. Fujii Y, Nakayama M (2007) Efficacy of dexamethasone for reducing postoperative nausea and vomiting and analgesic requirements after thyroidectomy. Otolaryngol Head Neck Surg 136: 274–277.
22. Worni M, Schudel HH, Seifert E, Inglin R, Hagemann M, et al. (2008) Randomized controlled trial on single dose steroid before thyroidectomy for benign disease to improve postoperative nausea, pain, and vocal function. Ann Surg 248: 1060–1066.
23. Feroci F, Rettori M, Borrelli A, Lenzi E, Ottaviano A, et al. (2011) Dexamethasone prophylaxis before thyroidectomy to reduce postoperative nausea, pain, and vocal dysfunction: a randomized clinical controlled trial. Head Neck 2011; 33: 840–846.
24. Doksrød S, Sagen Ø, Nøstdahl T, Ræder J (2012) Dexamethasone does not reduce pain or analgesic consumption after thyroid surgery; a prospective, randomized trial. Acta Anaesthesiol Scand 56: 513–519.
25. Song YK, Lee C (2013) Effects of ramosetron and dexamethasone on postoperative nausea, vomiting, pain, and shivering in female patients undergoing thyroid surgery. J Anesth 27: 29–34.
26. Barros A, Vale CP, Oliveira FC, Ventura C, Assunção J, et al. (2013) Dexamethasone effect on postoperative pain and tramadol requirement after thyroidectomy. Pharmacology 91: 153–157.
27. Schietroma M, Cecilia EM, Carlei F, Sista F, De Santis G, et al. (2013) Dexamethasone for the prevention of recurrent laryngeal nerve palsy and other complications after thyroid surgery: a randomized double-blind placebo-controlled trial. JAMA Otolaryngol Head Neck Surg 139: 471–478.
28. Zhou H, Xu H, Zhang J, Wang W, Wang Y, et al. (2012) Combination of dexamethasone and tropisetron before thyroidectomy to alleviate postoperative nausea, vomiting, and pain: randomized controlled trial. World J Surg 36: 1217–1224.
29. Bononi M, Amore Bonapasta S, Vari A, Scarpini M, De Cesare A, et al. (2010) Incidence and circumstances of cervical hematoma complicating thyroidectomy and its relationship to postoperative vomiting. Head Neck 32: 1173–1177.
30. Fujii Y, Tanaka H, Kobayashi N (2000) Granisetron/dexamethasone combination for the prevention of postoperative nausea and vomiting after thyroidectomy. Anaesth Intensive Care 28: 266–269.
31. Hozo SP, Djulbegovic B, Hozo I (2005) Estimating the mean and variance from the median, range, and the size of a sample. BMC Med Res Methodol 5: 13.
32. Wang JJ, Ho ST, Tzeng JI, Tang CS (2000) The effect of timing of dexamethasone administration on its efficacy as a prophylactic antiemetic for postoperative nausea and vomiting. Anesth Analg 91(1): 136–9.
33. Watcha MF, White PF (1992) Postoperative nausea and vomiting: its etiology, treatment, and prevention. Anesthesiology 77: 162–84.
34. Kovac AL (2000) Prevention and treatment of postoperative nausea and vomiting. Drugs 59: 213–43.
35. White PF, Watcha MF (1993) Are new drugs cost-effective for patients undergoing ambulatory surgery? Anesthesiology 78(1): 2–5.

12

A Role of Supraspinal Galanin in Behavioural Hyperalgesia in the Rat

Diana Amorim[1,2], Ana David-Pereira[1,2], Patrícia Marques[1,2], Sónia Puga[1,2], Patrícia Rebelo[1,2], Patrício Costa[1,2], Antti Pertovaara[3], Armando Almeida[1,2], Filipa Pinto-Ribeiro[1,2]*

1 Life and Health Sciences Research Institute (ICVS), School of Health Sciences (ECS), University of Minho, Braga, Portugal, **2** ICVS/3B's - PT Government Associate Laboratory, Braga/Guimarães, Portugal, **3** Institute of Biomedicine/Physiology, University of Helsinki, Helsinki, Finland

Abstract

Introduction: In chronic pain disorders, galanin (GAL) is able to either facilitate or inhibit nociception in the spinal cord but the contribution of supraspinal galanin to pain signalling is mostly unknown. The dorsomedial nucleus of the hypothalamus (DMH) is rich in galanin receptors (GALR) and is involved in behavioural hyperalgesia. In this study, we evaluated the contribution of supraspinal GAL to behavioural hyperalgesia in experimental monoarthritis.

Methods: In Wistar-Han males with a four week kaolin/carrageenan-induced monoarthritis (ARTH), paw-withdrawal latency (PWL) was assessed before and after DMH administration of exogenous GAL, a non-specific GALR antagonist (M40), a specific GALR1 agonist (M617) and a specific GALR2 antagonist (M871). Additionally, the analysis of c-Fos expression after GAL injection in the DMH was used to investigate the potential involvement of brainstem pain control centres. Finally, electrophysiological recordings were performed to evaluate whether pronociceptive On- or antinociceptive Off-like cells in the rostral ventromedial medulla (RVM) relay the effect of GAL.

Results: Exogenous GAL in the DMH decreased PWL in ARTH and SHAM animals, an effect that was mimicked by a GALR1 agonist (M617). In SHAM animals, an unselective GALR antagonist (M40) increased PWL, while a GALR2 antagonist (M871) decreased PWL. M40 or M871 failed to influence PWL in ARTH animals. Exogenous GAL increased c-Fos expression in the RVM and dorsal raphe nucleus (DRN), with effects being more prominent in SHAM than ARTH animals. Exogenous GAL failed to influence activity of RVM On- or Off-like cells of SHAM and ARTH animals.

Conclusions: Overall, exogenous GAL in the DMH had a pronociceptive effect that is mediated by GALR1 in healthy and arthritic animals and is associated with alterations of c-Fos expression in RVM and DRN that are serotonergic brainstem nuclei known to be involved in the regulation of pain.

Editor: Yvette Tache, University of California, Los Angeles, United States of America

Funding: This study was supported by grants from the Portuguese Science Foundation (FCT) Project n° PTDC/SAU-NEU/108557/2008, FEDER-COMPETE, by the Academy of Finland and the Sigrid Jusélius Foundation, Helsinki, Finland. DA was supported by FCT grant SFRH/BD/71219/2010 and ADP was supported by FCT grant SFRH/BD/90374/2012. The funders had no role in study design, data collection and analysis, decision to publish, or preparation of the manuscript.

Competing Interests: The authors have declared that no competing interests exist.

* Email: filiparibeiro@ecsaude.uminho.pt

Introduction

Galanin (GAL) is an injury-responsive peptide that is dramatically upregulated in the dorsal root ganglia and spinal dorsal horn interneurones during inflammation [1] or after nerve injury [2]. In healthy animals, GAL's action on nociceptive processing in the spinal cord is bidirectional, with low concentrations eliciting pronociceptive actions [3] and high concentrations promoting antinociception [4]. Differences in spinal actions of GAL also vary with the differential availability/activation of GAL receptor (GALR) subtypes. GALR1 has an inhibitory action and is more abundant than GALR2 (excitatory) and GALR3 (inhibitory) in the superficial dorsal horn [5]. Despite the considerable number of works evaluating its action in the peripheral nervous system and at the spinal cord level, the role of GAL in pain modulation at the supraspinal level is mostly unknown.

In basal conditions several studies showed that, both in humans and rodents, GAL is expressed in the supraoptic nucleus, the paraventricular nucleus of the hypothalamus, the dorsomedial hypothalamic nucleus (DMH), the arcuate nuclei, the lateral hypothalamic area, the locus coeruleus (LC), the amygdala (AMY) and the median raphe nucleus [6], all areas involved in supraspinal pain modulation [7–11]. In relation to receptor expression, GALR1 is greatly expressed in the LC, dorsal raphe nucleus (DRN), the paraventricular nucleus of the hypothalamus, DMH, AMY, thalamus and medulla oblongata [12–15]. However, in the AMY, GALR2/R3 are also significantly expressed [12]. Similarly, all types of GAL receptors are expressed in the prefrontal cortex and the hippocampus but to a lesser extent [12,14,15]. GALR2 is highly expressed in the hypothalamus, dentate gyrus, piriform cortex and mammillary nuclei [14,15], while the expression of GALR3 has been reported mainly in the hypothalamus (preoptic, DMH, lateral and posterior hypothalamic, ventromedial and premammillary nuclei) [15], the bed nucleus of the stria terminalis, periaqueductal grey matter (PAG), lateral parabrachial nucleus and medial reticular formation [16]. Again, most brain areas mentioned above are involved in the codification and modulation of nociceptive inputs [7,10].

The administration of exogenous GAL to the arcuate [17], tuberomammillary [18], nucleus accumbens [19], central nucleus of the AMY [20,21] and PAG [22] decreases nociception in healthy rats, an effect that is mediated by GalR1 in rodents [23]. A similar effect is observed in some pathological conditions, such as acute inflammation or mononeuropathy [22], where the microinjection of supraspinal exogenous GAL also decreases nociception. Albeit the apparent antinociceptive role of supraspinal GAL in pain modulation, the intracerebroventricular administration of a GALR1 agonist in rats increased c-Fos expression in the DMH [24], an area that facilitates nociception by promoting behavioural hyperalgesia [9,25]. As hyperalgesia is one of the hallmarks of chronic pain, activation of the DMH promotes behavioural hyperalgesia and GAL receptors are strongly expressed in the DMH, here we evaluated the contribution of GAL receptors in the DMH to the descending control of inflammatory hyperalgesia in monoarthritis as well as nociception in healthy controls.

Methods

1. Animals, ethical issues and anaesthesia

The experiments were performed in adult male Wistar Han rats with 175–250 g (Charles Rivers, Barcelona, Spain). A total of 96 animals (SHAM, n = 48 and ARTH, n = 48) were used in the experiments herein, 40 animals (SHAM, n = 20 and ARTH, n = 20) were used in the behavioural assessment, 32 animals (SHAM, n = 16 and ARTH, n = 16) in the c-Fos protocol and 24 animals (SHAM, n = 12 and ARTH, n = 12) in the electrophysiological evaluation. Animals were randomly assigned two by two to boxes upon arrival; a blue line was painted in the tail of one rat and a red line in the tail of the other. Each box was numbered from 1 to 48, no indication concerning if the animals were assigned to the SHAM or ARTH group was displayed. The list discriminating the boxes corresponding to the SHAM or ARTH groups was kept by an independent party. Each animal was considered a single unit within its experimental group. Animals were housed two per cage, except for animals with chronic intracerebral cannulae implanted that were housed individually. Food and water were available *ad libitum* and animals were maintained in a climate-controlled room, under 22±2°C of temperature, 55±5% of humidity and under a 12 h light/dark cycle with lights on at 8:00am. The experimental protocol followed the European Community Council Directive 86/609/EEC and 2010/63/EU concerning the use of animals for scientific purposes and was approved by the Institutional Ethical Commission (Permit Number: 23248). All efforts were made to minimize animal suffering and to use only the number of animals necessary to produce reliable scientific data.

For cannula implantation the animals were anaesthetized i.p. with a mixture 1:1.5 of ketamine (Imalgene, Merial, Oeiras, Portugal) and medetomidine (Dorbene, Esteve, Carnaxide, Portugal). After the surgical procedure, the anaesthesia was reversed using atipamezole (Antisedan, Pfizer, Oeiras, Portugal, i.p.) and the animals were monitored until fully awake (grooming and eating).

Anaesthesia was induced by administering pentobarbitone (50 mg/kg, i.p., Eutasil, CEVA, Algés, Portugal) and maintained by infusing pentobarbitone (15–20 mg/kg/h, i.p.). The level of anaesthesia was frequently assessed by determining behavioural responses to noxious pinching. Body temperature was maintained within physiological range with the help of a warming blanket (DC Temperature Controller, FHC, Bowdoin, ME, USA). At the end of the experiment, animals received a lethal dose of pentobarbitone.

2. Induction of arthritis

The induction of monoarthritis (ARTH) was performed four weeks before the actual experiments, as described in detail elsewhere [9,26]. In order to maintain the researcher blind in relation to whether the animals from a specific box were assigned to the SHAM or ARTH groups, the animals were anaesthetized (section 2.1) by a third party in an adjacent room and then brought to the chirurgical table in groups of two for the injection of SAL or K/C in the right knee joint. Briefly, in anaesthetised animals a mixture of 3% kaolin and 3% carrageenan (K/C, Sigma-Aldrich, St. Louis, MO, USA) dissolved in saline was injected into the synovial cavity of the right knee joint at a volume of 0.1 mL. This model produces mechanical hyperalgesia, which begins a few hours after surgery and extends up to 8 weeks [27]. After the procedure, animals returned to the adjacent room, the anaesthesia was reversed and animals were monitored until fully recovered (eating and grooming). At the end of the induction session all boxes were returned to the animal house. In each animal, development of arthritis was verified again 1 h prior to each behavioural session. While confirming the arthritic status of the animals, through the flexion and extension of the right leg, the experimenter was handed the animals by a third party without any specific order and without prior knowledge of the box number. Only those rats that vocalized every time after five flexion–extension movements of the knee joint were considered to have arthritis, and they were included in the ARTH group. SHAM animals were injected with 0.1 mL saline in the synovial cavity of the right knee joint. SHAM animals did not vocalize to any of the five consecutive flexion–extension movements of the knee joint. After the test, the animals were returned to their home cages by a person other than the evaluator.

3. Behavioural assessment of nociception

All behavioural tests were performed during the day time, starting at 9:30am and ending at 1:30pm after which the animals were returned to the animal house.

3.1 Mechanical hyperalgesia. The application of noxious pressure to the primary site of injury is a classical approach to measure mechanical hyperalgesia [28], both in humans and animals [29]. Here, the pressure-application measurement (PAM; Ugo Basile, Comerio, Italy) method was used. It allows an accurate behavioural measurement of mechanical hypersensitivity in rodents with chronic inflammatory joint pain [30] by the application of a force range of 0–1500 g. To perform the test and with the animal securely held, the force transducer unit (fitted to the experimenter's thumb) is placed on one side of the animal's knee joint and the forefinger on the other and an increasingly force is applied across the joint until a behavioural response is observed (limb-withdrawal, freezing of whisker movement, wriggling or vocalization) with a cut-off of 5 s. The peak force applied immediately prior to the behavioural response is recorded as the response threshold (RT). RT was measured twice in the ipsilateral and contralateral limbs at 1 min intervals. The mean RTs were calculated per animal. At the end of the session animals were returned to their home cage.

3.2 Thermal hyperalgesia (heat). Heat hyperalgesia was evaluated using the Hargreaves test [31]. The rats were habituated to the experimental conditions by allowing them to spend 1–2 h daily in the experimental room for the three days preceding any behavioural tests [9]. For assessing heat hyperalgesia, a radiant heat source was placed under the hindpaws in awake animals and the time spent between the heat application and the withdrawal response (Plantar Test Instrument, Model 37370, Ugo Basile, Varese, Italy) was registered as the paw-withdrawal latency (PWL). In each session, the PWL was assessed prior to drug administration in the DMH and 20 min after. In each time point, the PWL was repeated twice at an interval of 1 min and the mean of these values was used in further calculations. Cut-off time was 15 s.

4. Procedures for intra-DMH microinjections

Before the placement of the guide cannulas the animals were anaesthetized (section 2.1) by a third party in an adjacent room and then brought to the chirurgical table one at the time. For intra-DMH drug administration, four weeks before the actual experiments (at the same time that arthritis was induced), animals were anaesthetised and placed in a stereotaxic frame, and one stainless steel guide cannula (26 gauge; PlasticsOne, Roanoke, VA, USA) was then implanted in the DMH according to the coordinates of the atlas by Paxinos and Watson [32]. The tip of the guide cannula was positioned 1 mm above the desired injection site in the DMH [AP, −3.24 mm from bregma; LM, 0.4 mm lateral from the midline (right side); DV, 7.5 mm below the surface of the skull]. The guide cannula was kept in place through the use of two dental screws and dental cement. A dummy cannula was inserted into the guide cannula to close the top. After the procedure, the anaesthesia was reversed and animals were monitored until being fully recovered (eating and grooming) in the adjacent room and returned to the animal house.

In order for the experimenter to remain blinded in relation to which animals were SHAMs or ARTHs, prior to the beginning of the behavioural session, the cards displaying the number of the box were substituted by cards displaying letters. Test drugs were administered in the DMH through a 33-gauge injection cannula (PlasticsOne) inserted into and protruding 1 mm beyond the tip of the guide cannula. The microinjection was made using a 10.0-μL-Hamilton syringe connected to the injection cannula by a polyethylene catheter (PE-10; Plastics One). The injection volume was 0.5 μL and therefore, the spread of the injected drugs within the brain was expected to be 1 mm [33]. The efficacy of injection was monitored by observing the movement of a small air bubble through the tubing. The injection lasted 20 s and the injection cannula was left in place for additional 30 s to minimize the return of drug solution back to the injection cannula. Brain injection sites were histologically verified from post-mortem sections and plotted on standardized sections from the stereotaxic atlas [32] (**Fig. 1**). After the completion of the tests and animals were returned to the animal house, the cards were switch again. The attribution of the letter cards was recorded in a lab book separate from the one used to register the results. The order of attribution of the letter cards was random and changed in each experimental session. The order of the administration of the drugs to each animal was defined at the beginning of the experiment to avoid potential confounding effects related to this parameter. The results of the tests were only associated with the respective animal after the end of the experiment.

5. Drugs

Solutions for drug administration in the DMH were prepared in sterilized saline 0.9% (Unither, Amiens, France; pH 7.2). All the experimental drugs used in this work were acquired from Tocris (Bristol, UK). Each injection had a volume of 0.5 μL and contained either GAL (1.0 nmol), a non-specific GAL receptor antagonist (M40, 1.0 nmol), a specific GALR1 agonist (M617, 1.0 nmol) or a specific GALR2 antagonist (M871, 1.0 nmol) [17,20,23]. Control injections were performed with SAL in order to avoid any confounding effect that might result from injecting the liquid itself.

6. Course of the pharmacological study

Four weeks following induction of arthritis and insertion of the guide cannula for DMH injections, the efficacy of DMH-induced phasic and tonic modulation of nociception was determined by assessing the effect of DMH injection of exogenous GAL, M40, M671 and M871 upon the PWL in awake SHAM and ARTH animals. SAL was used in control injections. The latency of the withdrawal response was assessed 20 min [18,34] following the intra-DMH injections. The interval between behavioural assessments of different drug treatment conditions in the same animal was at least two days. The order of testing different drugs varied between the animals.

7. Recording of neuronal activity in nociceptive RVM cells

For the electrophysiological study, animals were removed from the animal house in a random order, one per day, already anaesthetized, by a person other than the experimenter. Anaesthesia (section 2.1) was administered at 9:30am, the electrophysiological recordings started between 10am and 10:30 am and lasted for 3 h. The order of the administration of the drugs varied between the animals. The electrophysiological recordings of the activity of RVM neurones followed a protocol described in Pinto-Ribeiro and colleagues [9]. In anaesthetised animals, a recording electrode was placed in the RVM (AP: 5.88 mm rostral to the interaural line, ML: −0.6 to 0.6 mm lateral from the midline, and DV: 10.0 mm below the surface of the skull) [32]. Single neurone activity was recorded extracellularly with tungsten electrodes (tip impedance 3–10 MΩ at 1 kHz), the signal was amplified and filtered and data sampling was performed through a CED Micro 1401 interface and Spike 2 software (Cambridge Electronic Design, Cambridge, UK).

Recording of RVM neurones was started after the animal was under light anaesthesia; i.e., the animals gave a brief withdrawal response to noxious pinch, but the pinch did not produce any longer lasting motor activity, nor did the animals have spontaneous limb movements. RVM neurones were classified based on their response to noxious heating of the tail with a tail-flick device (Ugo Basile). Heat stimulation of the tail was applied during 10 s. Functional classification of RVM neurones followed the scheme developed earlier by Fields and colleagues [35] and by Fields and Heinricher [36]. The neurones whose firing activity increased during heat stimulation of the tail were considered On-cells, those decreasing its activity were classified as Off-cells and finally, cells displaying only a negligible (<10%) or no alteration in discharge rates during noxious stimulation were considered Neutral-cells and were not analysed in this study. However, a significant difference with the classification scheme of Fields [35] is that in the present study the noxious stimulus-induced withdrawal reflex was not taken into account in the classification. Therefore, as in previous studies, RVM cells are here called On-like and Off-like cells [9,37,38] rather than On- or Off-cells.

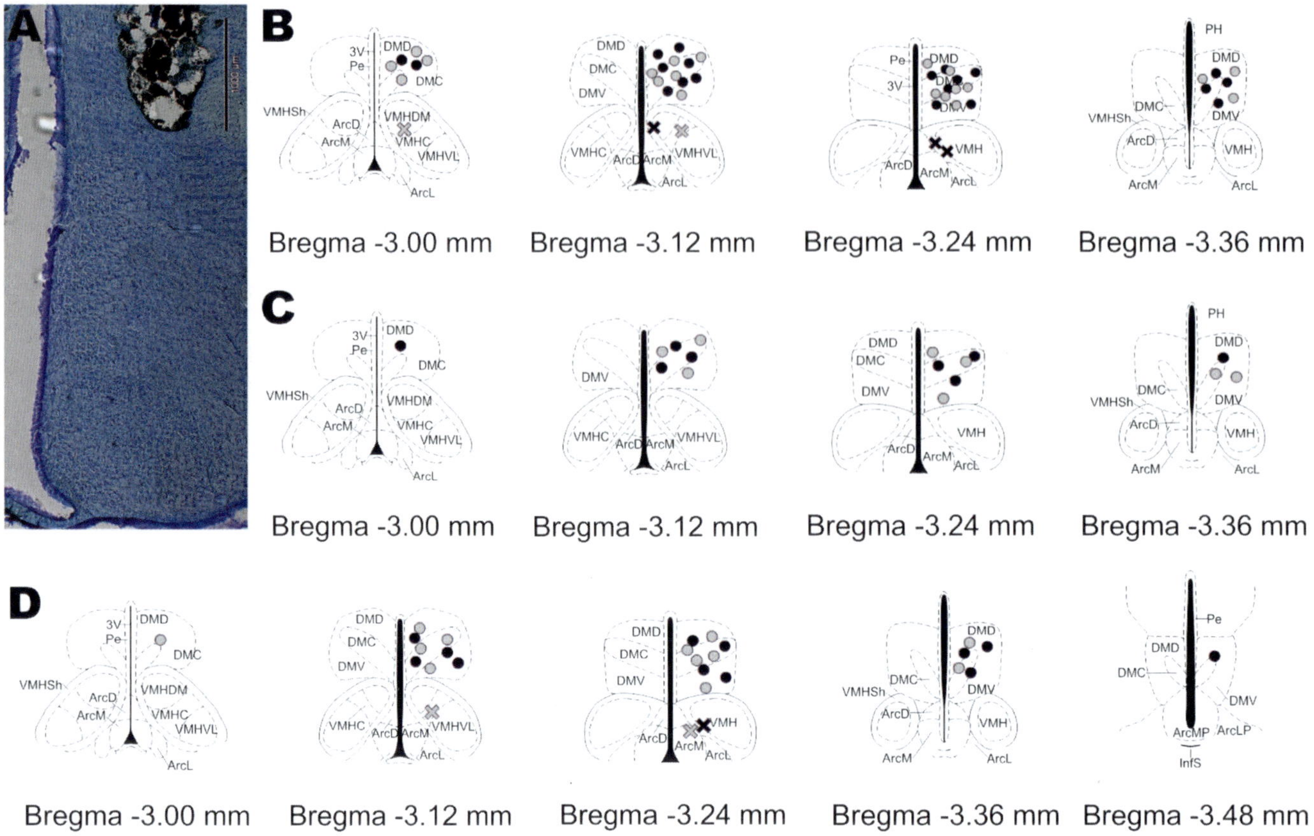

Figure 1. Anatomical confirmation of drug injection sites in the dorsomedial nucleus of the hypothalamus (DMH). (**A**) Photomicrograph of an example of the drug injection site in the right DMH of the rat brain (AP: −3.24 mm from bregma) superimposed with the appropriate plate of the Paxinos and Watson (2007) stereotaxic atlas. (**B**) Schematic representation of injection sites in the DMH during the behavioural study. The coordinates for the injection sites are as follow −3.00 mm, −3.12 mm, −3.24 mm and −3.36 mm from bregma. (**C**) Schematic representation of injection sites in the DMH during the protocol for the induction of c-Fos expression. The coordinates for the injection sites are as follow −3.00 mm, −3.12 mm, −3.24 mm and −3.36 mm from bregma. (**D**) Schematic representation of injection sites in the DMH during the electrophysiological study. The coordinates for the injection sites are as follow −3.00 mm, −3.12 mm, −3.24 mm, −3.36 mm and −3.48 mm from bregma. (Grey dots correspond to injection sites in the DMH of control (SHAM) animals and black dots show injection sites in the DMH of arthritic (ARTH) animals; grey and black crosses correspond to injection sites outside the DMH of SHAM and ARTH animals, respectively) ArcD- arcuate hypothalamic nucleus, dorsal; ArcL- arcuate hypothalamic nucleus, lateral; ArcM- arcuate hypothalamic nucleus, medial; DMC - dorsomedial hypothalamic nucleus, compact; DMD – dorsomedial hypothalamic nucleus, dorsal; DMV - dorsomedial hypothalamic nucleus, ventral; VMHDM - ventromedial hypothalamic nucleus, dorsomedial; VMHSh - ventromedial hypothalamic nucleus, shell; VMHVL - ventromedial hypothalamic nucleus, ventrolateral.

The characterization of the response properties of RVM cells consisted of the following assessments performed successively: (i) spontaneous activity; (ii) response to heating of the tail; (iii) recovery to the spontaneous activity level.

It should be noted that when analysing responses of RVM neurones to peripheral stimulation, the baseline discharge frequency (recorded just before the stimulation) was subtracted from the discharge frequency assessed during the stimulation using the following formula:

$$\begin{aligned}&\text{Evoked response}\\&=(\text{cell activity during acute noxious stimulation})\\&-(\text{basal cell activity prior to stimulus application})\end{aligned}$$

Thus, positive values represent an increase and negative ones represent a decrease in cell activity evoked by peripheral stimulation.

During the recordings, animals also had a guide cannula implanted for drug administration into the DMH. After determining the baseline spontaneous activity of RVM cells and their baseline noxious-evoked responses to peripheral stimulation, either exogenous GAL or a non-specific GALRs antagonist (M40) were microinjected in the DMH, in order to assess its phasic or tonic effect, respectively, upon the discharge rate of RVM neurones. All results from drug administrations were plotted for the variation in activity comparing baseline (before drug administration) and values obtained 20 min after the injection into the DMH. The results of the electrophysiological analysis were only associated with the respective animal after all recordings were performed.

8. Course of the electrophysiological study

Electrophysiological recordings of RVM neurones (SHAM: On-like cells, n = 58 and Off-like cells, n = 40; ARTH: On-like cells, n = 46 and Off-like cells, n = 47) were performed under pentobarbitone anaesthesia four weeks after the administration of K/C

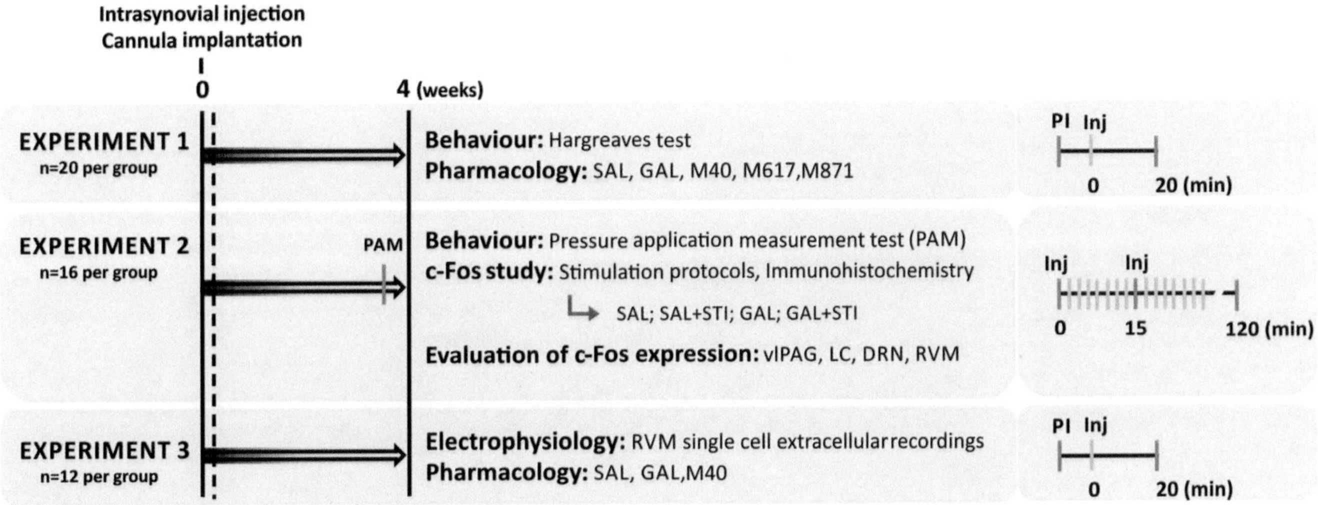

Figure 2. Schematic representation of the experimental design. In all experiments, animals were divided in two groups, control (SHAM) when injected with saline and arthritic (ARTH) when injected with a mixture of kaolin and carrageenan in the synovial capsule of the right knee joint. Three days after the intrasynovial injection, arthritis was confirmed by performing five consecutive movements of flexion/extension of the knee (dashed line). Animals in the ARTH group developed a clear swelling of the treated knee joint and all gave a vocalization response during a minor extension and flexion of the affected limb by the experimenter. SHAM animals displayed no obvious swelling of the knee joint and did not vocalize when the limb was flexed. Four weeks after the induction of monoarthritis animals were tested in three independent experiments. In experiment 1, the Hargreaves test was used to study the effect of exogenous galanin (GAL), a non-specific GAL receptor antagonist (M40), a specific GAL receptor-1 agonist (M617) and a specific GAL receptor-2 antagonist (M871) in the dorsomedial nucleus of the hypothalamus (DMH) upon paw-withdrawal latency (PWL) (n = 20 per experimental group). In each animal, the development of arthritis was confirmed again 1 h prior to each behavioural session by performing five consecutive movements of flexion/extension of the knee. During the experimental sessions, PWL was assessed before and 20 min after the administration of the drugs to the DMH. In experiment 2, two days prior the c-Fos study, the pressure application measurement (PAM) test was performed to confirm the arthritic state of the animals. c-Fos expression was evaluated in SHAM and ARTH animals after exogenous GAL or saline (SAL) administration in the DMH, peripheral noxious mechanical stimulation and the simultaneous application of noxious mechanical stimulation after the microinjection of exogenous GAL in the DMH (n = 16 per experimental group). Peripheral stimulation was applied each 2 minutes during 2 hours and two drug injections were made in the DMH, one at the beginning and another 15 minutes after the beginning of peripheral stimulation. Neurones expressing c-Fos were quantified bilaterally in the ventrolateral periaqueductal grey matter (vlPAG), locus coeruleus (LC), dorsal raphe nucleus (DRN) and rostral ventromedial medulla (RVM). In experiment 3, RVM neurones were recorded before and after the administration of exogenous GAL and M40 in the DMH. The assessment of neuronal activity includes a preliminary evaluation of spontaneous and noxious-evoked activity followed by the recording of these parameters 20 min after drug administration to the DMH (n = 12 animals per experimental group). PI – Pre-injection; Inj – Injection; SAL - saline microinjection in the dorsomedial nucleus of the hypothalamus; GAL - galanin microinjection in the dorsomedial nucleus of the hypothalamus; SAL+STI – saline microinjection in the dorsomedial nucleus of the hypothalamus and extension of right limb; GAL+STI – galanin microinjection in the dorsomedial nucleus of the hypothalamus and extension of right limb.

(ARTH) or SAL (SHAM) in the right knee of animals. In RVM recordings, the response properties of nociceptive neurones were assessed by determining their spontaneous activity and the response to noxious heating of the tail. Search for the next neurone to be studied started about 30 min after testing of the previous one was completed. At the end of the recording session, electrolytic lesions were made in the recording sites, the animals were given a lethal dose of pentobarbitone and the brains were removed for histological verification of the recording and injection sites.

9. c-Fos study

For the c-Fos induction protocol, animals were removed from the animal house in a random order, one per day, already anaesthetized, by a person other than the experimenter. Anaesthesia (section 2.1) was administered at 9:30 am; the protocol started between 10am and 10:30am and lasted for 2 h. To evaluate changes in brain activation after exogenous GAL administration in the DMH and/or peripheral noxious stimulation in SHAM and ARTH animals, c-Fos immunoreaction was performed following the protocol described elsewhere [39]. Animals were held in a stereotaxic frame. For drug administration, a guide cannula was placed in the DMH according to the coordinates of the atlas by Paxinos and Watson [32] and one of the following protocols was performed: (i) SAL microinjection in the DMH of SHAM animals; (ii) exogenous GAL microinjection in the DMH of SHAM animals; (iii) SAL microinjection in the DMH and extension of right limb of SHAM animals; (iv) exogenous GAL microinjection in the DMH and extension of right limb of SHAM animals; (v) SAL microinjection in the DMH of ARTH animals; (vi) exogenous GAL microinjection in the DMH of SHAM animals; (vii) extension of right limb of ARTH animals; (viii) exogenous GAL microinjection in the DMH and extension of right limb of ARTH animals. Two exogenous GAL (or SAL) doses were injected in the DMH with a 15 min interval (**Fig. 2**). Extension of the paw was performed 5 times every 2 minutes for 2 h. Two hours after the first injection and first knee extension (beginning of the protocol), the animals were transcardially perfused with 4% paraformaldehyde in 0.1 M phosphate buffer saline (PBS, pH = 7.4), brains were removed and then post-fixed overnight in the same fixative and kept in a solution of 8% sucrose in PBS. One in three coronal vibratome (Leica, Carnaxide, Portugal) sections (50 µm thick) were treated with a solution of 3.3% H_2O_2 in PBS (30 min) to inhibit endogenous peroxidase activity, and then sequentially washed thrice (10 min) in PBS and PBS-Triton (PBS-T; 0.3% triton X-100; Sigma-Aldrich, Sintra,

Portugal). Sections were then incubated in a blocking solution of 2.5% fetal bovine serum (FBS; Biochrom, Cambridge, United Kingdom) in PBS for 2 h, followed by the incubation overnight at 4°C in rabbit anti-Fos antibody (1:2000 in PBST and 2% FBS; Calbiochem, Merck, Algés, Portugal). The following day, after three washes (10 min) in PBST, sections were incubated in biotinylated polyclonal swine anti-rabbit antibody (1:200 in PBST; Dako, Denmark) for 1 h and again washed thrice (10 min) in PBS-T. Sections were then incubated in avidin–biotin complex (ABC; 1:200 in PBST; Vectastain, Vector Laboratories, Peterborough, USA) for 1 h followed by a series of washing steps with PBST (twice, 10 min), PBS (twice, 10 min) and Tris-HCl (0.05 M, pH 7.6) (twice, 10 min). Finally, sections were stained with diaminobenzidine (0.0125% in a solution of Tris-HCl with 0.02% H2O2; Sigma Aldrich) and washed twice (10 min) with Tris-HCl and PBS. After staining, the sections were mounted on SuperFrost slides (Braunschweig, Germany). c-Fos levels were determined by counting the number of Fos-immunoreactive neurones occurring bilaterally in the brainstem with the aid of a Stereo Investigator 10 Software (Microbrigthfield Bioscience, Madgedurg, Germany) using a video camera (Microbrigthfield Bioscience) attached to a microscope (BX51, Olympus Iberia, Lisboa, Portugal).

10. Statistics

For the effect of drugs upon PWL, the minimum number of animals needed was determine à priori using the G power software (version 3.1.9.2, University of Kiel, Germany) considering a ANOVA-2-way test, α err probability of 0.05, power of 0.95 and an effect size of 0.80 was n = 23. For the effect of drugs upon RVM neuronal activity, the minimum number of animals needed was determine à priori using the G power software considering a ANOVA-2-way test, α err probability of 0.05, power of 0.95 and an effect size of 0.80 was n = 28. For the effect of drugs upon c-Fos expression, the minimum number of animals needed was determine à priori using the G power software considering a ANOVA-2-way test, α err probability of 0.05, power of 0.95 and an effect size of 0.80 was n = 32. The results of the RT analysis correspond to the mean ± SD of raw data; no method of data normalization was used. To assess the effect of the drugs upon PWL for each behavioural session, the value of the basal withdrawal latency (withdrawal latency prior to drug administration) was subtracted from the value of the withdrawal latency at the peak effect of the drug, a negative value indicated the withdrawal latency decreased while a positive value corresponded to an increase in withdrawal latency after drug administration to the DMH. To perform this evaluation, raw data was used. To assess the effect of the drugs upon spontaneous neuronal activity, the value of the activity of RVM On- and Off-like cells without noxious peripheral stimulation prior to the administration of drugs in the DMH was subtracted from the activity of these cells without noxious peripheral stimulation at the peak effect of the drug. Similarly, to assess the effect of the drugs upon the noxious-evoked neuronal activity the value of the activity of RVM On- and Off-like cells during noxious peripheral stimulation prior to the administration of drugs in the DMH was subtracted from the activity of these cells during noxious peripheral stimulation at the peak effect of the drug. Only raw data was used in this analysis. To compare the level of c-fos in each area, the total number of cells stained was registered per area studied and only raw data was used in this analysis. The GraphPad Prism 6 software (GraphPad Software Inc, La Jolla, CA, USA) was used to perform the statistical analysis. The comparison of differences between RT in the PAM test and between the baseline of RVM neuronal spontaneous and heat-evoked activities of SHAM and ARTH animals were performed using a student's t-test for unpaired data. To compare differences in RT between the ipsilateral and the contralateral side in SHAM and ARTH animals a student's t-test for paired data was used. All other comparisons between groups were performed using a two-way ANOVA followed by a Bonferroni correction for multiple comparisons post-hoc test. Statistical significance was accepted for $P<0.05$.

Results

1. Monoarthritic animals developed ipsilateral mechanical allodynia

Three days after the intrasynovial injection, all animals in the ARTH group developed a clear swelling of the treated knee joint and all gave a vocalization response during a minor extension and flexion of the affected limb by the experimenter. SHAM animals displayed no obvious swelling of the knee joint and did not vocalize when the limb was flexed.

Mechanical hyperalgesia in the knee joint was assessed by determining RT to mechanical pressure over the knee joint. No differences were found between the RT of the ipsilateral and contralateral hindpaws in SHAM animals ($t_7 = 1.535$, $P = 0.169$) while in ARTH animals the ipsilateral RT was significantly lower than the contralateral ($t_7 = 3.377$, $P = 0.0118$). No differences were found between the contralateral RT of SHAM and ARTH animals ($t_{14} = 0.000$, $P > 0.999$). Four weeks after induction of monoarthritis, RT was significantly different between SHAM and ARTH animals ($t_{14} = 2.883$, $P = 0.012$). This result indicates that K/C induced a significant RT decrease, i.e., mechanical hyperalgesia (**Fig. 3**).

2. Exogenous GAL in the DMH decreases paw-withdrawal latency, an effect reversed by the administration of a GAL receptors antagonist

To investigate a possible role of supraspinal GAL in phasic and tonic pain facilitation in SHAM and ARTH animals, paw withdrawal latencies (PWL) were assessed after exogenous GAL or M40 microinjection, respectively, in the DMH. The PWL of SHAM and ARTH animals 20 min after exogenous GAL microinjection in the DMH was significantly decreased when compared with SAL injection (main effect of the drug: $F_{1,76} = 61.880$, $P<0.001$). The exogenous GAL-induced decrease in PWL was of the same magnitude in the SHAM and ARTH groups (main effect of the group: $F_{1,76} = 2.704$, $P = 0.104$). *Post hoc* tests confirmed that the PWL of SHAM and ARTH animals treated with exogenous GAL was significantly lower than the PWL of SHAM and ARTH animals treated with SAL (**Fig. 4A**).

Non-specific inhibition of GAL receptors induced by administration of M40 in the DMH significantly altered the PWL when compared with SAL injection (main effect of the drug: $F_{1,76} = 13.830$, $P<0.001$). The effect of M40 was significantly different between SHAM and ARTH animals (main effect of the group: $F_{1,76} = 10.070$, $P = 0.002$). The M40-induced effect on PWL varied with the experimental group (interaction between group and drug: $F_{1,76} = 8.048$, $P = 0.006$). *Post hoc* tests indicated that M40 significantly increased PWL in SHAM animals, but did not alter PWL in ARTH animals (**Fig. 4B**).

3. Nociceptive facilitation after exogenous GAL in the DMH is mediated by GAL receptors type-1

To determine which GAL receptor is involved in pain facilitation induced by exogenous GAL in the DMH, PWL was

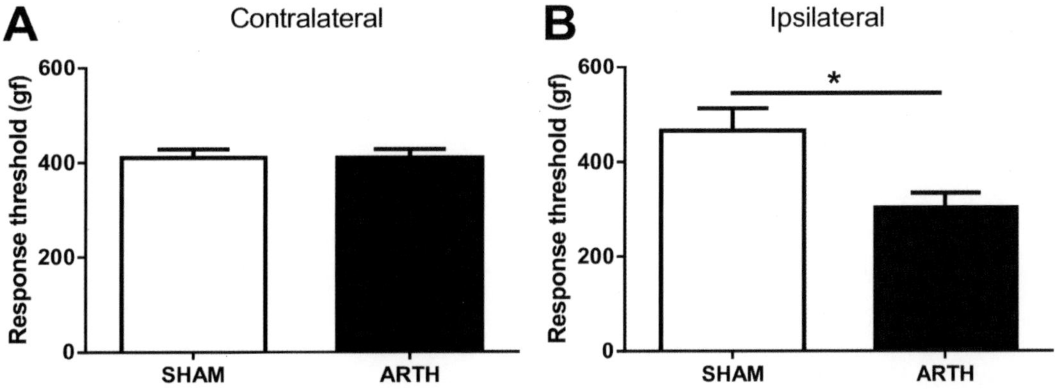

Figure 3. Response threshold. Four weeks after the induction of monoarthritis in the right hind limb, no differences were observed in the response threshold (RT) of the contralateral hindpaws between control (SHAM) and arthritic (ARTH) animals (**A**) in the pressure application measurement. In the ipsilateral side however ARTH animals displayed a decrease in RT during the pressure application measurement when compared to SHAM animals (**B**). Mean response threshold is presented as mean + SEM. (*$P<0.05$, t-test for unpaired data). gf – gram force.

assessed after the administration of M617 (a specific agonist of GAL receptor type-1 - GalR1) and M871 (a specific antagonist of GAL receptor type-2 - GalR2) into the DMH. Twenty minutes after microinjecting M617 in the DMH, PWL was significantly decreased when compared with SAL injection (main effect of the drug: $F_{1,76}=39.530$, $P<0.001$). The effect of M617 was not different between SHAM and ARTH groups (main effect of the group: $F_{1,76}=0.357$, $P=0.552$). *Post hoc* tests confirmed that PWL significantly decreased after M617 administration in the DMH both in SHAM and ARTH animals when compared to PWL after SAL administration (**Fig. 4C**).

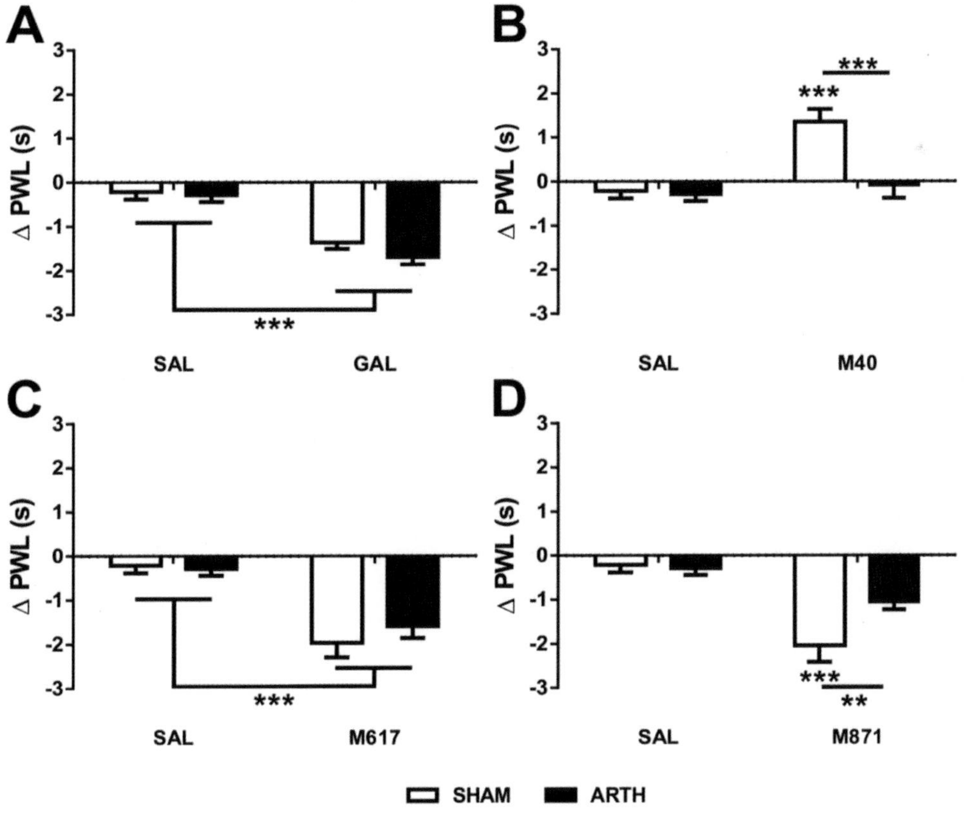

Figure 4. Paw-withdrawal latency after drug administration in the dorsomedial nucleus of the hypothalamus (DMH). In this experiment the analysis of the paw-withdrawal latencies in control (SHAM) and arthritic (ARTH) animals was performed 20 minutes after the intracerebral microinjection of either exogenous galanin (GAL) (**A**), a non-specific antagonist of GAL receptors (M40; **B**), a specific agonist of GAL receptor-1 (M617; **C**) or a specific antagonist of GAL receptor-2 (M871; **D**). Note that the pronociceptive action of exogenous GAL administration in the DMH in SHAM and ARTH animals (**A**) is only mimicked by the microinjection of M617 (**C**). Mean response latency is presented as mean + SEM. (*$P<0.05$, **$P<0.01$, ***$P<0.001$, t-test with a Bonferroni correction for multiple comparisons).

Administration of M871 in the DMH had a significant effect on PWL (main effect of the drug: $F_{1,76} = 29.820$, $P<0.001$), and the effect of M871 varied with the experimental group (interaction group x drug: $F_{1,76} = 5.089$, $P = 0.027$). *Post hoc* tests showed that M871 significantly decreased the PWL in SHAM animals but did not alter significantly the PWL of ARTH animals (**Fig. 4D**).

4. Expression of c-Fos in brainstem areas involved in pain control is altered by exogenous GAL in the DMH

Descending pain modulatory drive from the forebrain to the spinal cord may be relayed by multiple areas in the brainstem. To determine which brainstem areas mediate exogenous GAL-driven descending pain modulatory effects originating in the DMH, c-Fos expression was investigated in caudal brain areas that not only expressed GAL and/or its receptors but that are also involved in the descending modulation of nociception. Hence, we compared changes in c-Fos expression in the ventrolateral periaqueductal grey matter (VLPAG), the LC, the dorsal raphe nucleus (DRN) and the rostral ventromedial medulla (RVM) between SHAM and ARTH animals after (i) SAL microinjection in the DMH of SHAM animals; (ii) GAL microinjection in the DMH of SHAM animals; (iii) SAL microinjection in the DMH and extension of right limb of SHAM animals; (iv) GAL microinjection in the DMH and extension of right limb of SHAM animals; (v) SAL microinjection in the DMH of ARTH animals; (vi) GAL microinjection in the DMH of SHAM animals; (vii) extension of right limb of ARTH animals; (viii) GAL microinjection in the DMH and extension of right limb of ARTH animals.

Expression of c-Fos following injection of SAL in the DMH was considered to represent basal activation. The number of c-Fos positive neurones in the contralateral RVM varied with the stimulation protocol used (main effect of the protocol: $F_{3,24} = 22.570$, $P<0.001$) with different effects on SHAM and ARTH animals (interaction group x protocol: $F_{3,24} = 42.280$, $P<0.001$). *Post-hoc* testing showed that exogenous GAL in the DMH significantly increased c-Fos expression when compared to SAL-injected animals in both experimental groups, although a higher expression was observed in ARTH animals (**Fig. 5A**). The flexion-extension protocol (SAL+STI) increased c-Fos expression in SHAM animals when compared to SAL and GAL administration while it decreased its expression in ARTH animals when compared to GAL-Injected ARTH. The simultaneous infusion of GAL in the DMH and flexion-extension of the injected limb decreased c-Fos expression in SHAM when compared with its expression after the flexion-extension protocol and in ARTH when compared with GAL-injected ARTH (**Fig. 5A**). Similarly, in the ipsilateral RVM, the number of cells activated was significantly different depending on the protocols (main effect of the protocol: $F_{3,24} = 70.240$, $P<0.001$), an effect that varied with the experimental group (interaction group x protocol: $F_{3,24} = 20.240$, $P<0.001$). *Post-hoc* testing showed that GAL in the DMH increased the number of c-Fos expressing cells in both experimental groups when compared to SAL-injected animals, while its expression was different between SHAM and ARTH animals after repeated flexion-extension of the injected limb, with increased c-Fos expression in SHAM animals alone when compared with SAL and GAL-injected SHAM (**Fig. 5B**). The simultaneous injection of GAL in the DMH and flexion-extension of the injected limb significantly decreased the number of c-Fos positive cells in SHAM when compared to the flexion-extension protocol and in ARTH animals when compared with GAL administration and the flexion-extension protocols (**Fig. 5B**).

The number of c-Fos expressing neurones in the contralateral LC did not vary with the stimulation protocols (main effect of the protocol: $F_{3,24} = 0.413$, $P = 0.745$) although it was significantly different between experimental groups (main effect of the group: $F_{3,24} = 16.410$, $P<0.001$). *Post-hoc* testing did not show a specific alteration between each stimulation protocol (**Fig. 5C**). In the ipsilateral LC, the number of c-Fos positive cells varied with the stimulation protocol (main effect of the protocol: $F_{3,24} = 7.462$, $P = 0.001$), an effect that depended on the experimental group (interaction group x protocol: $F_{3,24} = 14.310$, $P<0.001$). *Post-hoc* testing showed an increase in the number of c-Fos expressing neurones after the simultaneous infusion of GAL in the DMH and flexion-extension of the injected limb in ARTH animals when compared with the same protocol in SHAM and with the SAL/GAL/flexion-extension protocols in ARTH (**Fig. 5D**).

In the contralateral vlPAG, the number of c-Fos expressing cells varied with the stimulation protocol (main effect of the protocol: $F_{3,24} = 19.200$, $P<0.001$), an effect that depended on the experimental group (interaction group x protocol: $F_{3,24} = 40.030$, $P<0.001$). *Post-hoc* testing showed a significant increase in the number of c-Fos positive cells in ARTH animals when compared to SHAM and after exogenous GAL in the DMH of SHAM animals when compared to SAL injected SHAM (**Fig. 5E**). In addition, in ARTH animals the number of c-fos expressing neurones was significantly lower in all protocols when compared to SAL injected ARTH animals (**Fig. 5E**). Similarly, the number of cells activated in the ipsilateral vlPAG was different after the stimulation protocols (main effect of the protocol: $F_{3,24} = 22.920$, $P<0.001$) and depended on the experimental group (interaction group x protocol: $F_{3,24} = 47.100$, $P<0.001$). *Post-hoc* testing (**Fig. 5F**) showed increased c-Fos expression in SAL-injected ARTH animals when compared with SAL-injected SHAM. GAL in the DMH significantly increased c-Fos expression in SHAM animals while it significantly decreased its expression in ARTH animals. c-Fos expression after the flexion-extension of the injected limb was not significantly different when compared to SAL-injected SHAM although it was significantly decreased when compared to GAL-injected SHAM (**Fig. 5F**). This protocol also significantly decreased c-Fos expression in ARTH animals when compared to SAL-injected ARTH although its expression was significantly higher when compared to GAL-injected ARTH. The simultaneous infusion of GAL in the DMH and flexion-extension of the injected limb did not significantly alter c-Fos expression when compared to SAL-injected SHAM but was significantly decreased when compared to its expression after GAL injection in the DMH. In ARTH animals, c-Fos expression was significantly decreased after the simultaneous infusion of GAL in the DMH and flexion-extension of the injected limb when compared to SAL-injected ARTH and the flexion-extension protocol (**Fig. 5F**).

Finally, In the DRN, the number of c-Fos positive cells varied with the stimulation protocol (main effect of the protocol: $F_{3,24} = 24.690$, $P<0.001$) and this effect was dependent of the experimental group (interaction group x protocol: $F_{3,24} = 14.140$, $P<0.001$). *Post-hoc* testing showed an increased DRN activation after GAL in the DMH in both experimental groups when compared to SAL-injected animals (**Fig. 5G**). The flexion-extension of the injured limb significantly increased c-Fos expression in SHAM animals when compared to ARTH animals and when compared with SAL- and GAL-injected SHAM. The simultaneous infusion of GAL in the DMH and flexion-extension of the injected limb increased c-Fos expression in SHAM animals when compared to ARTH and to its expression after SAL, but decreased when compared to the flexion-extension protocol. Additionally, it decreased c-Fos expression in ARTH animals when compared to GAL-injected ARTH (**Fig. 5G**).

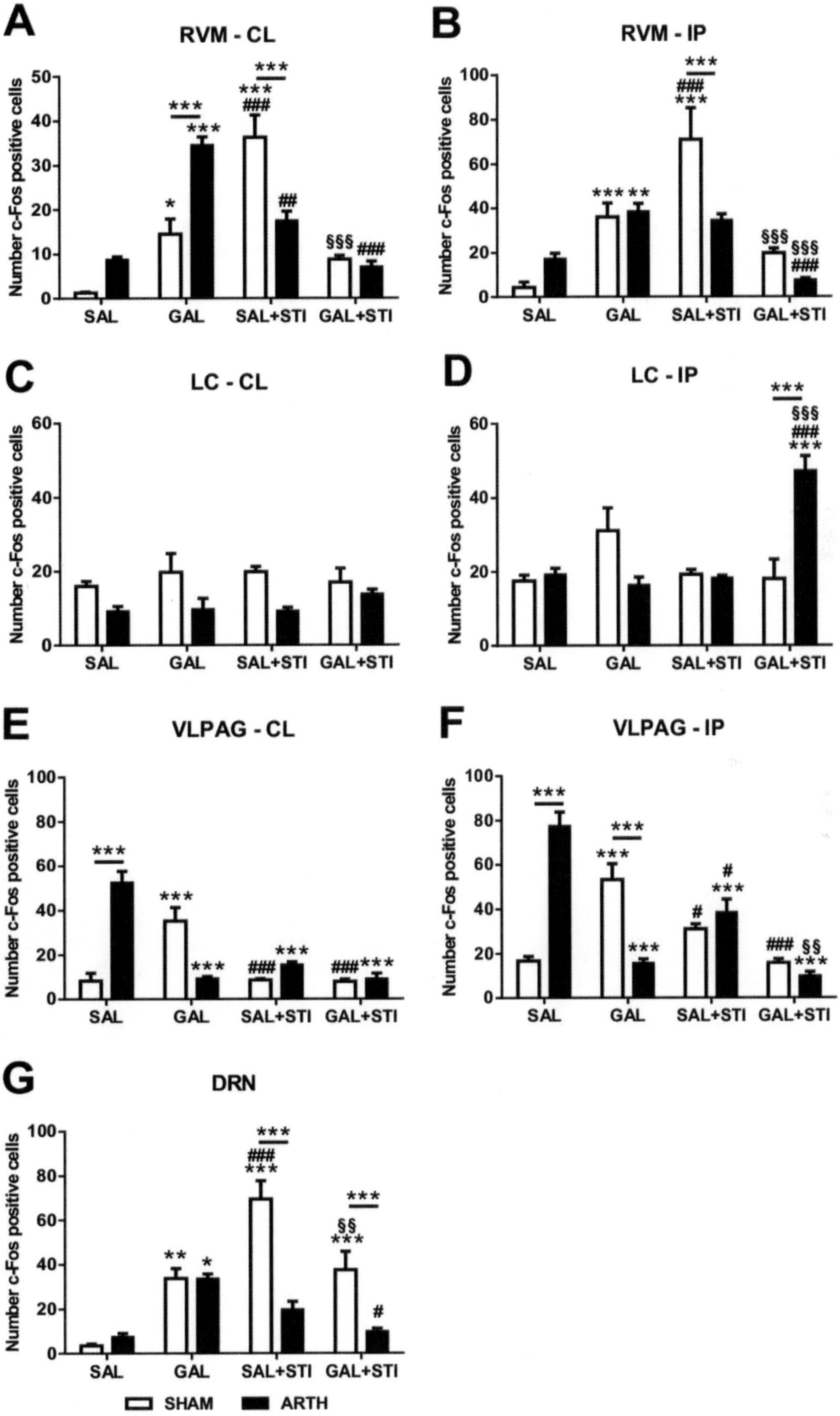
A
RVM - CL
B
RVM - IP
C
LC - CL
D
LC - IP
E
VLPAG - CL
F
VLPAG - IP
G
DRN
Number c-Fos positive cells
SAL
GAL
SAL+STI
GAL+STI
SHAM
ARTH

Figure 5. Brainstem c-Fos expression. Number of c-Fos positive cells in the contralateral (**A,C,E**) and ipsilateral (**B,D,F**) sides of the rostral ventromedial medulla (RVM; **A,B**), locus coeruleus (LC; **C,D**), ventrolateral periaqueductal matter (vlPAG; **E,F**) and dorsal raphe nucleus (DRN; **G**) after the administration of saline or exogenous galanin in the dorsomedial nucleus of the hypothalamus (DMH) with and without peripheral noxious stimulation. Data is presented as mean + SEM. SAL – Saline; GAL – Galanin; SAL+STI – SAL and peripheral noxious stimulation (limb flexion-extension); GAL+STI – GAL and peripheral noxious stimulation (limb flexion-extension). * indicates significant differences in c-Fos expression when compared to SAL injection in the DMH; * over line indicates differences in c-Fos expression between experimental groups; # indicates significant differences in c-Fos expression when compared to GAL injection in the DMH; § indicates significant differences in c-Fos expression when compared to the flexion-extension protocol (*, $^{\#}P<0.05$; **, $^{\#\#}$, $^{\S\S}P<0.01$; ***, $^{\#\#\#}$, $^{\S\S\S}P<0.001$).

5. The activity of pain modulatory On- or Off-like cells in the RVM is not altered by exogenous GAL in the DMH

To evaluate the effect of exogenous GAL administration in the DMH upon the activity of RVM neurones, the spontaneous and heat-evoked activities of presumably pronociceptive RVM On-like cells and antinociceptive RVM Off-like cells were recorded in SHAM and ARTH animals before and after the administration of exogenous GAL, M40 or SAL.

Before drug administration, the spontaneous activity of RVM On-like cells was significantly decreased in ARTH animals when compared to SHAM animals (**Table 1**). The magnitude of the response evoked by noxious heating of the tail in RVM On-like cells was not different between SHAM and ARTH animals. In RVM Off-like cells, the spontaneous activity before drug treatments was significantly decreased in ARTH animals when compared to SHAM animals. Similarly, the magnitude of the heat-evoked response in RVM Off-like cells of ARTH animals was significantly lower when compared to that in SHAM animals (**Table 1**).

Microinjection of drugs into the DMH did not alter the spontaneous activity of RVM On-like cells (main effect of the drug: $F_{2,98}=0.262$, $P=0.770$). Overall, after drug injection, On-like cell spontaneous activity was different between ARTH and SHAM animals (main effect of the group: $F_{1,98}=6.510$, $P=0.012$) (**Fig. 6A**), although *post-hoc* tests failed to show a significant difference between experimental groups at a specific time point. The administration of drugs to the DMH did not alter the spontaneous activity of RVM Off-like cells (main effect of the drug: $F_{2,81}=0.616$, $P=0.543$) and the spontaneous activity was not different between experimental groups (main effect of the group: $F_{1,81}=1.200$, $P=0.277$) (**Fig. 6B**) 20 min after drug administration.

Microinjection of drugs into the DMH altered the heat-evoked activity of RVM On-like cells (main effect of the drug: $F_{2,98}=5.010$, $P=0.009$) but this effect did not vary with the experimental group (interaction group x drug: $F_{2,98}=1.318$, $P=0.272$). *Post hoc* testing failed to find significant drug treatment-induced effects on the heat-evoked response of On-like cells (**Fig. 6C**). Similarly, drug administration in the DMH changed the heat-evoked activity of RVM Off-like cells (main effect of the drug: $F_{2,81}=4.967$, $P=0.009$) but these differences did not vary with the experimental group (interaction group x drug: $F_{2,81}=2.230$, $P=0.114$), 20 min after administration. Again, *post hoc* testing failed to find significant drug treatment-induced effects on the heat-evoked response of Off-like cells, except for the increase of response after exogenous GAL treatment in the SHAM group (**Fig. 6D**).

Discussion

This study demonstrates, for the first time, a pronociceptive role for supraspinal GAL, as the administration of this neuropeptide to the DMH significantly increased spinal nociception (as indicated by the decrease in PWL) in awake healthy and arthritic animals. Moreover, the microinjection of GAL receptor agonist/antagonist in the DMH showed that the exogenous GAL's pronociceptive effect was mediated by GALR1 but not GALR2. The analysis of c-Fos expression revealed the serotonergic RVM and DRN, particularly in SHAM animals, as caudal areas potentially involved in signalling this descending pronociceptive effect. The exogenous GAL-induced increase of c-Fos expression in the RVM may not be explained by action on RVM On-like or Off-like pain modulatory cells, as the discharge rates of these two non-serotonergic cell types remained unaltered during pharmacological manipulations in the present study.

1. Novel pronociceptive effect of supraspinal GAL

Administration of exogenous GAL into the DMH induced behavioural hyperalgesia (decreased PWL) in healthy and ARTH animals. This is a novel effect for GAL as previous studies had only reported an antinociceptive role of this neuropeptide after its administration in brain areas involved in pain modulation, such as the hypothalamic arcuate nucleus [40], central AMY [20] and the PAG [22]. Thus, and similarly to what is observed at the spinal cord level [41,42], GAL appears to have a bidirectional role in supraspinal descending pain modulation depending on the area where GALRs are activated. The demonstration of a tonic pronociceptive effect of GAL, by treatment of the DMH with a non-specific GALR antagonist, supports the proposal that the pronociceptive effect of GAL was mediated by GALRs.

Table 1. Spontaneous and heat-evoked baseline activities of rostral ventromedial medullary (RVM) On- and Off-like cells.

	Cell type	SHAM	ARTH	t	P
Spontaneous	**On-like**	**1.86±0.39 Hz**	**0.77±0.19 Hz**	$t_{102}=2.689$	$P=0.008$**
	Off-like	**4.77±0.46 Hz**	**3.37±0.26 Hz**	$t_{85}=2.833$	$P=0.006$**
Evoked	**On-like**	**2.51±0.31 Hz**	**2.82±0.37 Hz**	$t_{102}=0.601$	$P=0.549$
	Off-like	**-2.45±0.25 Hz**	**-1.72±0.26 Hz**	$t_{85}=2.782$	$P=0.007$**

Data presented as mean ± SEM.
**$P<0.01$.

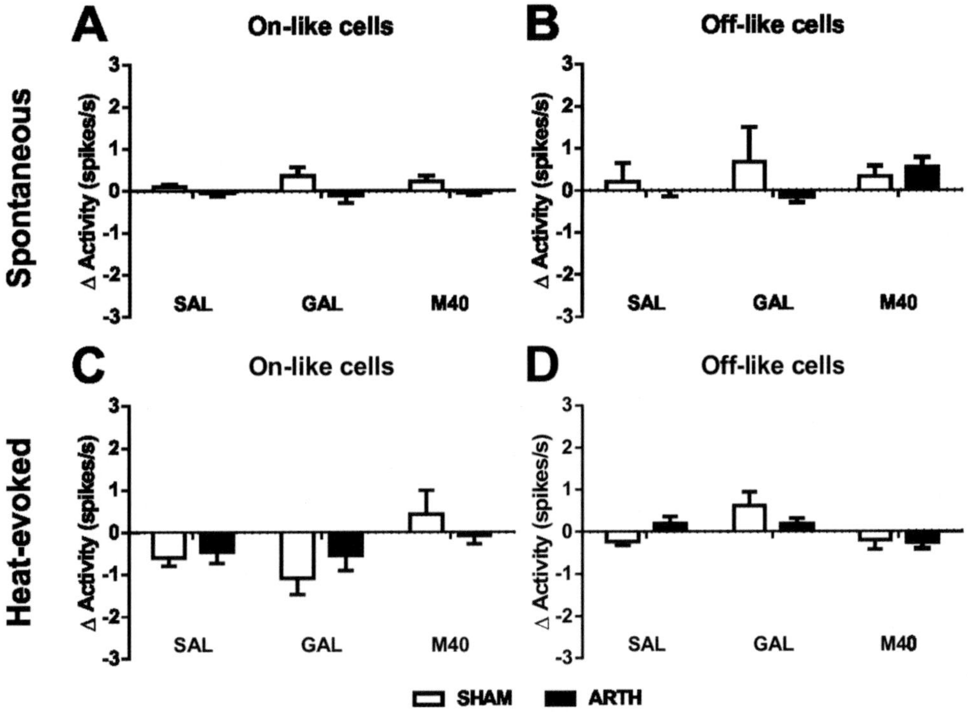

Figure 6. Spontaneous and noxious-evoked rostral ventromedial medulla (RVM) cell activity after the administration of exogenous galanin (GAL) or a non-selective GAL receptor antagonist (M40) in the dorsomedial nucleus of the hypothalamus (DMH). Overall, no changes were observed in the spontaneous (**A, B**) and noxious-evoked (**C, D**) activity of RVM pronociceptive On-like (**A, C**) and antinociceptive Off-like cells (B,D) before and 20 min after the intracerebral microinjection of exogenous GAL (**A–D**) and M40 (**A–D**). Data is presented as mean + SEM.

Administration of exogenous GAL in the DMH facilitated nociception in both ARTH and SHAM animals. This finding contrasts with the results of previous studies indicating that exogenous GAL is antinociceptive when administered in the hypothalamic arcuate nucleus of animals with inflammation [17], or in the PAG of animals with mononeuropathy [22]. Importantly, the present results show that the descending GAL-driven pathway originating in the DMH, unlike the glutamate-driven pathway [9], remains functional in animals with experimental monoarthritis. Administration of a non-specific GALR antagonist alone into the DMH of ARTH animals had no effect on nociception while it produced antinociception in SHAM controls. This finding suggests that the GAL-driven pathway descending from the DMH is not tonically active in ARTH as in SHAM animals, but its activation in ARTH animals depends on the activation of upstream pathways inducing the release of GAL in the DMH.

2. GAL-driven nociceptive facilitation is mediated by GALR1

Further analysis on the contributions of GALR1 and GALR2 to the pain modulatory role of GAL in the DMH demonstrated that the facilitatory effect of GAL is mediated by GALR1, a receptor that couples to the Gi/Go pathway to decrease adenylyl cyclase activity [43]. Once more, this result contrasts with the available literature, where the activation of this receptor at spinal and supraspinal levels is reported to elicit an antinociceptive effect [44–46]. In fact, in the spinal cord it was GALR2 that has been reported to have a pronociceptive effect [41]; however, the results on administration of a GALR2 antagonist in the present study indicated that endogenous GAL acting on GALR2 had a tonic antinociceptive action in SHAM animals, whereas blocking GALR2 did not alter nociception in ARTH animals. Another possibility would be that the differential distribution of GALR1 and GALR2 receptors in the DMH could contribute to enhance GALR1-dependent effects, however as demonstrated by Mitchell and collaborators [47], not only does mRNAs analysis confirm an overlapping of GAL-R1 and GAL-R2 in the DMH but both receptors are also highly expressed in this nucleus. On the other hand, the expression of both receptors in the DMH does not account *per se* for the GAL/DMH pronociceptive effect since these receptors are also highly expressed and overlapping in the arcuate nuclei, an area where the intracerebral administration of exogenous GAL promotes antinociception [17]. Overall, it is probable that the facilitation of nociceptive behaviour by GAL in the DMH of ARTH animals results (i) from disinhibition of pronociceptive pathways driven by GALR1 and/or (ii) from a decrease in the activity of antinociceptive GALR2-driven circuits.

It is also possible that behavioural hyperalgesia in ARTH animals is reinforced by their emotional-like status. A recent study from our group [48] showed that animals with experimental monoarthritis displayed depressive-like behaviour. Interestingly, Blackshear *et al.* [24] showed that the intracerebroventricular injection of GAL and M617 increased c-fos expression in the DMH and the AMY, a nuclei involved the modulation of the emotional component of pain. Another work [49] showed that acute activation of GALR1 promoted the expression of 'prodepressive-like' behaviours, while GALR2 mediated the 'antidepressant-like' effects of GAL. Hence, taking into account that depressive states heighten pain perception in humans [50] and rodents [51], the pronociceptive GALR1 and the antinociceptive GALR2 effects observed in this study may be related to comorbid mood alterations known to be associated with chronic pain [52,53].

3. Activation of serotonergic nuclei is influenced both by exogenous GAL in the DMH and noxious peripheral stimulation

The analysis of c-Fos expression was restricted to the VLPAG, DR, LC and RVM since these areas have been previously demonstrated to be strongly modulated by the DMH [54–56], while simultaneously implicated in nociceptive processing [57–59]. The limb extension-induced increase in c-Fos expression in the VLPAG and RVM of SHAM animals suggests that repetitive extension of a non-arthritic knee joint for a period of two hours can be considered a noxious stimulus [60]. In addition, the increased c-for expression in the VLPAG and RVM also suggests that repetitive knee joint extension activated the feedback loop of nociception involving the PAG-RVM-spinal dorsal horn circuitry, which may either inhibit or facilitate nociception [11,61,62].

Administration of exogenous GAL into the DMH increased the expression of c-Fos ipsilaterally in the VLPAG and bilaterally in the RVM, which suggests that DMH neurones expressing GALR are able to activate descending nociceptive controls. However, our electrophysiological data shows that exogenous GAL in the DMH did not alter the activity of RVM On- and Off-cells that are non-serotonergic pain control neurones. Therefore, we propose that the RVM cells expressing c-Fos following exogenous GAL treatment may have been RVM Neutral-cells, a subpopulation of which are serotonergic [63] and which were not studied in the present electrophysiological experiment. The fact that the DMH GAL-driven descending pronociceptive drive is independent of RVM On- and Off-like cell activity is very interesting in terms of pain management, since many centrally acting analgesic compounds (opioids, cannabinoids and non-steroidal anti-inflammatory drugs) reduce pain by increasing the discharge rate of antinociceptive RVM Off-cells and/or by inhibiting the discharge rate of pronociceptive RVM On-cells [61].

In SHAM animals, repetitive limb extension alone or exogenous GAL administration alone in the DMH activated the descending PAG-RVM-spinal cord pathway as revealed by c-Fos expression. However, application of exogenous GAL simultaneously with repetitive extension of the limb failed to increase c-Fos expression in the PAG-RVM circuitry of SHAM animals, suggesting that together the two stimulation procedures counteracted each other's effect, leading to a general inhibition of this circuitry. The increased c-Fos expression in the RVM by the pronociceptive exogenous GAL treatment alone might reflect activation of RVM serotonergic cells. While the serotonergic system has a complex role in pain control, there is evidence suggesting that the net effect induced by RVM serotonergic neurones is facilitation of nociception [64]. It should be noted here that serotonergic RVM neurones are not On- or Off- cells [63] that were studied in the present electrophysiological experiment using noxious heat and shown not to be influenced by exogenous GAL. We propose that the GAL-induced descending action may have induced activation of medullo-spinal serotonergic neurones shown as increased c-Fos expression in the RVM and resulting in the relay of pronociceptive action to the spinal cord.

The increased expression of c-Fos in the serotonergic DRN after limb extensions is in line with a role of this nucleus in ascending [65] and descending [66] pain modulatory pathways. Similarly, increased expression of c-Fos of DRN after exogenous GAL in the DMH is not unexpected as the DMH projects directly to the DRN [67] and the activity of DRN serotonergic neurones is influenced by GALR1 present on their soma and proximal dendrites [68]. It still remains to be studied through which mechanisms the DRN might be involved in the relay of the descending pronociceptive effect driven by exogenous GAL in the DMH.

4. Activation of the noradrenergic LC by exogenous GAL in the DMH and noxious peripheral stimulation varies between SHAM and ARTH animals

Previous studies have demonstrated that the LC responds to noxious stimulation, as revealed e.g. by c-Fos expression [69], while it is a major source of spinal noradrenaline and descending noradrenergic control of nociception [70,71]. In the present study, exogenous GAL treatment of DMH alone failed to influence c-Fos expression of LC in SHAM or ARTH animals. However, following repetitive limb extensions, c-Fos expression of LC was increased in SHAM but not ARTH animals. Interestingly, the peripheral stimulation-induced increase of c-Fos expression in the LC was predominantly ipsilateral, while ascending nociceptive signals activate the LC contra- or bilaterally [71]. A potential explanation for the ipsilaterally increased c-Fos expression after peripheral stimulation in the present study is that it reflected activation of descending pain modulation pathways descending predominantly ipsilaterally rather than processing of the ascending afferent volley that is expected to be contra- or bilateral. The DMH has a strong galaninergic output to various brain areas [72], including the LC [65], and GAL has been shown to decrease neuronal firing in LC [73]. While these findings suggest that the DMH may directly modulate activity of the LC, they still leave open what is the underlying mechanism and functional significance of the finding that exogenous GAL treatment of the DMH together with repetitive limb extensions increased c-Fos activity in the LC of ARTH but not SHAM animals.

5. Influence of arthritis and repetitive limb movement

The increase of c-Fos expression in the VLPAG and to a lesser extent in the RVM of SAL-treated ARTH animals indicates an overall increase in the tonic activity of the PAG-RVM-spinal cord pathways after the induction of experimental monoarthritis, which is in accordance with the enhancement of descending inhibitory circuits during chronic inflammation [74–77]. Interestingly, limb extension in the ARTH group decreased c-Fos expression in the VLPAG suggesting that acute noxious mechanical stimulation of the injured knee dampens tonic descending inhibition mediated by the VLPAG. On the other hand, the increase in c-Fos expression in the RVM, taking into account that the RVM can either facilitate or inhibit nociception [78], could indicate that this nucleus is engaged in descending facilitation during acute noxious stimulation of ARTH animals, as shown for other chronic pain disorders [79–81].

Our electrophysiological results showed that before any drug treatments both the baseline and the peripheral stimulus-evoked response in antinociceptive RVM Off-like cells were lower in ARTH than SHAM animals, while there was no difference in the pre-treatment heat-evoked activity of pronociceptive RVM On-like neurones of ARTH and SHAM animals. This finding suggests that a decreased activity of RVM Off-like cells contributes to hyperalgesia in ARTH animals. However, it does not exclude the possibility that among descending facilitatory mechanisms contributing to hyperalgesia in ARTH animals were other cell types of the RVM, in particular medullospinal serotonergic neurones, or other brainstem nuclei.

Concerning the DRN, the expression of c-Fos after repetitive limb extensions was increased, when compared with SAL-treated ARTH animals, but similar to the expression in c-Fos in SHAM after limb extensions, suggesting that the nociceptive processing through this pathway is not enhanced after the induction of experimental monoarthritis. By contrast, it is possible that the noxious stimulation-evoked activation of the LC is impaired in

ARTH animals, since c-Fos expression was decreased when compared to SHAM animals after limb extensions and unaltered when compared to SAL-treated ARTH animals.

Without noxious stimulation, exogenous GAL in the DMH of ARTH animals appeared to dampen tonic descending inhibition (as indicated by decreased c-Fos expression in the VLPAG) while it enhanced the tonic activity of pronociceptive serotonergic (indicated by increased c-Fos expression in the DRN and RVM), but not noradrenergic (unaltered c-Fos expression in the LC) circuits. However, when combined with limb extensions, both tonic descending inhibition (decreased c-Fos expression in the VLPAG) and the activity of pronociceptive serotonergic areas (decreased c-Fos expression in the RVM and DRN) were diminished. This finding indicates that in ARTH animals, exogenous GAL in the DMH exerts differential effects under basal and noxious stimulation-evoked conditions. A differential effect has also been reported while studying the role of GAL in the presence/absence of stress [49].

By contrast, only the combination of exogenous GAL injection in the DMH and limb stimulation was able to enhance the activity of the noradrenergic pain system as evidenced by the strong increase of c-Fos expression in the LC. Although noradrenergic pathways were up to recently considered to exert mostly inhibitory influences on spinal nociception, Hickey and collegues [59] recently demonstrated that a specific subpopulation of LC neurones enhances the processing of nociceptive information and could thus partly contribute to behavioural hyperalgesia in chronic inflammation. Further studies are needed to find out whether LC is involved in mediating the descending pronociceptive effect elicited by exogenous GAL in the DMH.

Conclusions

In the present study, we demonstrate a pronociceptive GALR1-mediated role for hypothalamic GAL in experimental monoarthritis. Exogenous GAL in the DMH appeared to exert differential effects upon the brainstem pain modulatory areas; the effect varied between the experimental group (healthy or arthritic animals), brainstem nucleus (PAG, RVM, DRN, or LC), and the presence or absence of concomitant noxious stimulation. Finally, the results suggest that further studies evaluating the potential applicability of GALR1 antagonists in the control of chronic inflammatory pain are needed.

Author Contributions

Conceived and designed the experiments: DA FPR. Performed the experiments: DA ADP PM SP PR. Analyzed the data: DA PC. Contributed reagents/materials/analysis tools: AA. Wrote the paper: DA FPR. Revised the manuscript: AP AA.

References

1. Jimenez-Andrade JM, Zhou S, Du J, Yamani A, Grady JJ, et al. (2004) Pronociceptive role of peripheral galanin in inflammatory pain. Pain 110: 10–21.
2. Liu HX, Hökfelt TG (2002) The participation of galanin in pain processing at the spinal level. Trends Pharmacol Sci 23: 468–474.
3. Reeve AJ, Walker K, Urban L, Fox A (2000) Excitatory effects of galanin in the spinal cord of intact, anaesthetized rats. Neurosci Lett 295: 25–28.
4. Yue H, Fujita T, Kumamoto E (2011) Biphasic modulation by galanin of excitatory synaptic transmission in substantia gelatinosa neurons of adult rat spinal cord slices. J Neurophysiol 105: 2337–2349.
5. Brumovsky P, Mennicken F, O'Donnell D, Hökfelt T (2006) Differential distribution and regulation of galanin receptors- 1 and -2 in the rat lumbar spinal cord. Brain Res 1085: 111–120.
6. Ch'ng JL, Christofides ND, Anand P, Gibson SJ, Allen YS, et al. (1985) Distribution of galanin immunoreactivity in the central nervous system and the responses of galanin-containing neuronal pathways to injury. Neuroscience 16: 343–354.
7. Millan MJ (2002) Descending control of pain. Prog Neurobiol 66: 355–474.
8. Pinto-Ribeiro F, Ansah OB, Almeida A, Pertovaara A (2008) Influence of arthritis on descending modulation of nociception from the paraventricular nucleus of the hypothalamus. Brain Res 1197: 63–75.
9. Pinto-Ribeiro F, Amorim D, David-Pereira A, Monteiro AM, Costa P, et al. (2013) Pronociception from the dorsomedial nucleus of the hypothalamus is mediated by the rostral ventromedial medulla in healthy controls but is absent in arthritic animals. Brain Res Bull 99: 100–108.
10. Pertovaara A, Almeida A (2006) Descending inhibitory systems. In: Cervero F, Jensen T, (eds) Handbook of Clinical Neurology, 3rd series, Elsevier, Amsterdam, pp 179–192.
11. Almeida A, Leite-Almeida H, Tavares I (2006) Medullary control of nociceptive transmission: reciprocal dual communication with the spinal cord. Drug Discov Today Dis Mech 3: 305–312.
12. Lu X, Lundström L, Langel Ü, Bartfai T (2005) Galanin receptor ligands. Neuropeptides 39: 143–146.
13. Mitchell V, Habert-Ortoli E, Epelbaum J, Aubert J, Beauvillain JC (1997) Semiquantitative distribution of galanin-receptor (GAL-R1) mRNA-containing cells in the male rat hypothalamus. Neuroendocrinology 66: 160–172.
14. Waters SM, Krause JE (2000) Distribution of galanin-1, -2 and -3 receptor messenger RNAs in central and peripheral rat tissues. Neuroscience 29: 265–271.
15. Webling KE, Runesson J, Bartfai T, Langel Ü (2012) Galanin receptors and ligands. Front Endocrinol 3: 146.
16. Mennicken F, Hoffert C, Pelletier M, Ahmad S, O'Donnell D (2002) Restricted distribution of galanin receptor 3 (GalR3) mRNA in the adult rat central nervous system. J Chem Neuroanat 24: 257–268.
17. Sun YG, Gu XL, Lundeberg T, Yu LC (2003) An antinociceptive role of galanin in the arcuate nucleus of hypothalamus in intact rats and rats with inflammation. Pain 106: 143–150.
18. Sun YG, Li J, Yang BN, Yu LC (2004) Antinociceptive effects of galanin in the rat tuberomammillary nucleus and the plasticity of galanin receptor 1 during hyperalgesia. J Neurosci Res 77: 718–722.
19. Xu SL, Li J, Zhang JJ, Yu LC (2012) Antinociceptive effects of galanin in the nucleus accumbens of rats. Neurosci Lett 520: 43–46.
20. Jin WY, Liu Z, Liu D, Yu LC (2010) Antinociceptive effects of galanin in the central nucleus of amygdala of rats, an involvement of opioid receptors. Brain Res 1320: 16–21.
21. Li J, Zhang JJ, Xu SL, Yu LC (2012) Antinociceptive effects induced by injection of the galanin receptor 1 agonist M617 into central nucleus of amygdala in rats. Neurosci Lett 526: 45–48.
22. Wang D, Lundeberg T, Yu LC (2000) Antinociceptive role of galanin in periaqueductal grey of rats with experimentally induced mononeuropathy. Neuroscience 96: 767–771.
23. Kong Q, Yu LC (2013) Antinociceptive effects induced by intra-periaqueductal grey injection of the galanin receptor 1 agonist M617 in rats with morphine tolerance. Neurosci Lett: 4–7.
24. Blackshear A, Yamamoto M, Anderson BJ, Holmes PV, Lundström L, et al. (2007) Intracerebroventricular administration of galanin or galanin receptor subtype 1 agonist M617 induces c-Fos activation in central amygdala and dorsomedial. hypothalamus. Peptides 28: 1120–1124.
25. Martenson ME, Cetas JS, Heinricher MM (2009) A possible neural basis for stress-induced hyperalgesia. Pain 142: 236–244.
26. Ansah OB, Pertovaara A (2007) Peripheral suppression of arthritic pain by intraarticular fadolmidine, an alpha 2-adrenoceptor agonist, in the rat. Anesth Analg 105: 245–250.
27. Radhakrishnan R, Moore SA, Sluka KA (2003) Unilateral carrageenan injection into muscle or joint induces chronic bilateral hyperalgesia in rats. Pain 104: 567–577.
28. Randall L, Selitto J (1957) A method for measurement of analgesic activity on inflamed tissue. Arch Int Pharmacodyn Thérapie 111: 409–419.
29. Rivat C, Richebé P, Laboureyras E, Laulin JP, Havouis R, et al. (2008) Polyamine deficient diet to relieve pain hypersensitivity. Pain 137: 125–137.
30. Barton NJ, Strickland IT, Bond SM, Brash HM, Bate ST, et al. (2007) Pressure application measurement (PAM): a novel behavioural technique for measuring hypersensitivity in a rat model of joint pain. J Neurosci Methods 163: 67–75.
31. Hargreaves K, Dubner R, Brown F, Flores C, Joris J (1988) A new and sensitive method for measuring thermal nociception in cutaneous hyperalgesia. Pain 32: 77–88.
32. Paxinos G, Watson C (2007) The rat brain in stereotaxic coordinates. 6th ed. Elsevier Inc.
33. Myers RD (1966) Injection of solutions into cerebral tissue: Relation between volume and diffusion. Physiol Behav 1: 171–174.
34. Sun YG, Gu XL, Yu LC (2007) The neural pathway of galanin in the hypothalamic arcuate nucleus of rats: Activation of beta-endorphinergic neurons projecting to periaqueductal gray matter. J Neurosci Res 85: 2400–2406.

35. Fields HL, Bry J, Hentall I, Zorman G (1983) The activity of neurons in the rostral medulla of the rat during withdrawal from noxious heat. J Neurosci 3: 2545–2552.
36. Fields H, Heinricher MM (1985) Anatomy and physiology of a nociceptive modulatory system. Philos Trans R Soc Lond B Biol Sci 308: 361–374.
37. Sanoja R, Tortorici V, Fernandez C, Price TJ, Cervero F (2010) Role of RVM neurons in capsaicin-evoked visceral nociception and referred hyperalgesia. Eur J Pain 14: 120.e1–9.
38. Song Z, Ansah OB, Meyerson BA, Pertovaara A, Linderoth B (2013) The rostroventromedial medulla is engaged in the effects of spinal cord stimulation in a rodent model of neuropathic pain. Neuroscience 247: 134–144.
39. Morgado C, Tavares I (2007) C-fos expression at the spinal dorsal horn of streptozotocin-induced diabetic rats. Diabetes Metab Res Rev 23: 644–652.
40. Gu XL, Sun YG, Yu LC (2007) Involvement of galanin in nociceptive regulation in the arcuate nucleus of hypothalamus in rats with mononeuropathy. Behav Brain Res 179: 331–335.
41. Liu H, Brumovsky P, Schmidt R, Brown W, Payza K, et al. (2001) Receptor subtype-specific pronociceptive and analgesic actions of galanin in the spinal cord: selective actions via GalR1 and GalR2 receptors. Proc Natl Acad Sci U S A 98: 9960–9964.
42. Hulse RP, Donaldson LF, Wynick D (2012) Differential roles of galanin on mechanical and cooling responses at the primary afferent nociceptor. Mol Pain 8: 41.
43. Wang S, Hashemi T, Fried S, Clemmons AL, Hawes BE (1998) Differential intracellular signaling of the GalR1 and GalR2 galanin receptor subtypes. Biochemistry 37: 6711–6717.
44. Blakeman KH, Hao JX, Xu XJ, Jacoby AS, Shine J, et al. (2003) Hyperalgesia and increased neuropathic pain-like response in mice lacking galanin receptor 1 receptors. Neuroscience 117: 221–227.
45. Hua XY, Hayes CS, Hofer A, Fitzsimmons B, Kilk K, et al. (2004) Galanin acts at GalR1 receptors in spinal antinociception: synergy with morphine and AP-5. J Pharmacol Exp Ther 308: 574–582.
46. Fu LB, Wanga XB, Jiao S, Wua X, Yua LC (2011) Antinociceptive effects of intracerebroventricular injection of the galanin receptor 1 agonist M 617 in rats. Neurosci Lett 491: 174–176.
47. Mitchell V, Bouret S, Howard AD, Beauvillain JC (1999) Expression of the galanin receptor subtype Gal-R2 mRNA in the rat hypothalamus. J Chem Neuroanat 16: 265–277.
48. Amorim D, David-Pereira A, Pertovaara A, Almeida A, Pinto-Ribeiro F (2014) Amitriptyline reverses hyperalgesia and improves associated mood-like disorders in a model of experimental monoarthritis. Behav Brain Res 265: 12–21.
49. Kuteeva E, Wardi T, Lundström L, Sollenberg U, Langel Ü, et al. (2008) Differential role of galanin receptors in the regulation of depression-like behavior and monoamine/stress-related genes at the cell body level. Neuropsychopharmacology 33: 2573–2585.
50. Murphy LB, Sacks JJ, Brady TJ, Hootman JM, Chapman DP (2012) Anxiety and depression among US adults with arthritis: prevalence and correlates. Arthritis Care Res (Hoboken) 64: 968–976.
51. Wang S, Tian Y, Song L, Lim G, Tan Y, et al. (2012) Exacerbated mechanical hyperalgesia in rats with genetically predisposed depressive behavior: role of melatonin and NMDA receptors. Pain 153: 2448–2457.
52. Verdu B, Decosterd I, Buclin T, Stiefel F, Berney A (2008) Antidepressants for the treatment of chronic pain. Drugs 68: 2611–2632.
53. Neugebauer V, Galhardo V, Maione S, Mackey SC (2009) Forebrain Pain Mechanisms. Brain Res Rev 60: 226–242.
54. Johnson P, Lowry C, Truitt W, Shekhar A (2008) Disruption of GABAergic tone in the dorsomedial hypothalamus attenuates responses in a subset of serotonergic neurons in the dorsal raphe nucleus following lactate-induced panic. J Psycopharmacology 22: 642–652.
55. Aston-Jones G, Chen S, Zhu Y, Oshinsky M (2001) A neural circuit for circadian regulation of arousal. Nat Neurosci 4: 732–738.
56. Wagner KM, Roeder Z, Desrochers K, Buhler AV, Heinricher MM, et al. (2013) The dorsomedial hypothalamus mediates stress-induced hyperalgesia and is the source of the pronociceptive peptide cholecystokinin in the rostral ventromedial medulla. Neuroscience 238: 29–38.
57. Wang QP, Nakai Y (1994) The dorsal raphe: an important nucleus in pain modulation. Brain Res Bull 34: 575–585.
58. De Luca MC, Brandão ML, Motta VA, Landeira-Fernandez J (2003) Antinociception induced by stimulation of ventrolateral periaqueductal gray at the freezing threshold is regulated by opioid and 5-HT2A receptors as assessed by the tail-flick and formalin tests. Pharmacol Biochem Behav 75: 459–466.
59. Hickey L, Li Y, Fyson SJ, Watson TC, Perrins R, et al. (2014) Optoactivation of locus ceruleus neurons evokes bidirectional changes in thermal nociception in rats. J Neurosci 34: 4148–4160.
60. Galbán CJ, Ling SM, Taub DD, Gurkan I, Fishbein KW, et al. (2007) Effects of knee injection on skeletal muscle metabolism and contractile force in rats. Osteoarthr Cartil 15: 550–558.
61. Ossipov MH, Dussor GO, Porreca F (2010) Central modulation of pain. J Clin Invest 120: 3779–3787.
62. Heinricher MM, Tavares I, Leith JL, Lumb BM (2009) Descending control of nociception: Specificity, recruitment and plasticity. Brain Res Rev 60: 214–225.
63. Potrebic SB, Fields HL, Mason P (1994) Serotonin immunoreactivity is contained in one physiological cell class in the rat rostral ventromedial medulla. J Neurosci 14: 1655–1665.
64. Wei F, Dubner R, Zou S, Ren K, Bai G, et al. (2010) Molecular depletion of descending serotonin unmasks its novel facilitatory role in the development of persistent pain. J Neurosci 30: 8624–8636.
65. Qiao JT, Dafny N (1988) Dorsal raphe stimulation modulates nociceptive responses in thalamic parafascicular neurons via an ascending pathway: further studies on ascending pain modulation pathways. Pain 34: 65–74.
66. Prado WA, Faganello FA (2000) The anterior pretectal nucleus participates as a relay station in the glutamate-, but not morphine-induced antinociception from the dorsal raphe nucleus in rats. Pain 88: 169–176.
67. ter Horst G, Luiten P (1986) The projections of the dorsomedial hypothalamic nucleus in the rat. Brain Res Bull 16: 231–248.
68. Larm JA, Shen PJ, Gundlach AL (2003) Differential galanin receptor-1 and galanin expression by 5-HT neurons in dorsal raphé nucleus of rat and mouse: evidence for species-dependent modulation of serotonin transmission. Eur - J Neurosci 17: 481–493.
69. Voisin DL, Guy N, Chalus M, Dallel R (2005) Nociceptive stimulation activates locus coeruleus neurones projecting to the somatosensory thalamus in the rat. J Physiol 566: 929–937.
70. Jones SL (1991) Descending noradrenergic influences on pain. Prog Brain Res 88: 381–394.
71. Pertovaara A (2006) Noradrenergic pain modulation. Prog Neurobiol 80: 53–83.
72. Jacobowitz DM, Kresse A, Skofitsch G (2004) Galanin in the brain: chemoarchitectonics and brain cartography - a historical review. Peptides 25: 433–464.
73. Sevcik J, Finta EP, Illes P (1993) Galanin receptors inhibit the spontaneous firing of locus coeruleus neurones and interact with mu-opioid receptors. Eur J Pharmacol 230: 223–230.
74. Ren K, Dubner R (2002) Descending modulation in persistent pain: an update. Pain 100: 1–6.
75. Cervero F, Schaible HG, Schmidt RF (1991) Tonic descending inhibition of spinal cord neurones driven by joint afferents in normal cats and in cats with an inflamed knee joint. Exp Brain Res 83: 675–678.
76. Ren K, Dubner R (1996) Enhanced descending modulation of nociception in rats with persistent hindpaw inflammation. J Neurophysiol 76: 3025–3037.
77. Terayama R, Guan Y, Dubner R, Ren K (2000) Activity-induced plasticity in brain stem pain modulatory circuitry after inflammation. Neuro Rep 26: 1915–1919.
78. Heinricher MM, Barbaro NM, Fields HL (1989) Putative nociceptive modulating neurons in the rostral ventromedial medulla of the rat: firing of on- and off-cells is related to nociceptive responsiveness. Somatosens Mot Res 6: 427–439.
79. Porreca F, Ossipov MH, Gebhart GF (2002) Chronic pain and medullary descending facilitation. Trends Neurosci 25: 319–325.
80. Herrero JF, Cervero F (1996) Supraspinal influences on the facilitation of rat nociceptive reflexes induced by carrageenan monoarthritis. Neurosci Lett 209: 21–24.
81. Kovelowski CJ, Ossipov MH, Sun H, Lai J, Malan TP, et al. (2000) Supraspinal cholecystokinin may drive tonic descending facilitation mechanisms to maintain neuropathic pain in the rat. Pain 87: 265–273.

13

Can Cognitive Activities during Breaks in Repetitive Manual Work Accelerate Recovery from Fatigue? A Controlled Experiment

Svend Erik Mathiassen[1]*, David M. Hallman[1], Eugene Lyskov[1], Staffan Hygge[2]

1 Centre for Musculoskeletal Research, Department of Occupational and Public Health Sciences, University of Gävle, Gävle, Sweden, 2 Department of Building, Energy and Environmental Engineering, University of Gävle, Gävle, Sweden

Abstract

Neurophysiologic theory and some empirical evidence suggest that fatigue caused by physical work may be more effectively recovered during "diverting" periods of cognitive activity than during passive rest; a phenomenon of great interest in working life. We investigated the extent to which development and recovery of fatigue during repeated bouts of an occupationally relevant reaching task was influenced by the difficulty of a cognitive activity between these bouts. Eighteen male volunteers performed three experimental sessions, consisting of six 7-min bouts of reaching alternating with 3 minutes of a memory test differing in difficulty between sessions. Throughout each session, recordings were made of upper trapezius muscle activity using electromyography (EMG), heart rate and heart rate variability (HRV) using electrocardiography, arterial blood pressure, and perceived fatigue (Borg CR10 scale and SOFI). A test battery before, immediately after and 1 hour after the work period included measurements of maximal shoulder elevation strength (MVC), pressure pain threshold (PPT) over the trapezius muscles, and a submaximal isometric contraction. As expected, perceived fatigue and EMG amplitude increased during the physical work bouts. Recovery did occur between the bouts, but fatigue accumulated throughout the work period. Neither EMG changes nor recovery of perceived fatigue during breaks were influenced by cognitive task difficulty, while heart rate and HRV recovered the *most* during breaks with the most difficult task. Recovery of perceived fatigue after the 1 hour work period was also most pronounced for the most difficult cognitive condition, while MVC and PPT showed ambiguous patterns, and EMG recovered similarly after all three cognitive protocols. Thus, we could confirm that cognitive tasks between bouts of fatiguing physical work can, indeed, accelerate recovery of some factors associated with fatigue, even if benefits may be moderate and some responses may be equivocal. Our results encourage further research into combinations of physical and mental tasks in an occupational context.

Editor: Naoyuki Hayashi, Tokyo Institute of Technology, Japan

Funding: The study was funded by internal grants at the University of Gävle. The funders had no role in study design, data collection and analysis, decision to publish, or preparation of the manuscript.

Competing Interests: The authors have declared that no competing interests exist.

* Email: SvendErik.Mathiassen@hig.se

Introduction

Introducing breaks is a key intervention to provide recovery after fatiguing physical work. Finding an optimal distribution across time of work periods and breaks has been a challenge in physiologic and ergonomics research for almost one century [1–6], and has also engaged management scientists [7,8]. Rest breaks have unambiguously been shown to alleviate fatigue in isometric, isotonic contractions, while the effect of added breaks in occupational work has been less obvious [9], even if recent theories explaining the origin and persistence of musculoskeletal disorders suggest that total rest will be a prerequisite for obtaining recovery of certain low-threshold "Cinderella" motor units that remain recruited as long as the muscle is active [10,11].

The basic rationale in ergonomics and management science for introducing breaks in occupational work is to maintain good productivity and a sustainable health and well-being of the individual worker by providing an opportunity to recover from tasks that might otherwise lead to a loss in performance [12]. In recent years, breaks have been explained and discussed as one option among others of how to obtain optimal variation in a job rather than as an initiative to specifically provide rest [9,13]. In line with this view, some occupational studies have investigated alternative non-rest "break" activities, including productive tasks. A majority of these studies have been devoted to physically "active" breaks, based on the notion that *more* activity will be a more effective source of variation than rest in occupations characterized by low-level, long-lasting muscle activity, such as office work or light industrial assembly [14–17].

Dating back more than 100 years and inspiring neurophysiological research since then, Sechenov (later cited in [18]) proposed that any type of "diverting" activity – physical as well as mental – would positively influence recovery from fatigue, the reason being that powerful processes leading to fatigue (in the sense of a decreased performance capacity) reside in the central nervous system and thus can be influenced by "diverting" central brain processes. As suggested in more recent studies, a mental activity may more effectively enhance recovery if it activates certain regions in the brain known to be involved in central fatigue processes, i.e. primarily the motor and prefrontal cortex [19]. Central fatigue processes add to and interact with peripheral physiologic responses locally in the exercising muscles, such as changes in the chemical environment [20,21], that may lead to a decreased force-generating capacity [22,23].

Following the ideas of Sechenov, "active" breaks with an organized mental activity between bouts of physical work might be more effective in alleviating fatigue than rest breaks without a focussed mental activation. This may appear a challenging and even awkward notion, considering that several studies have shown that mental tasks practiced "*on top*" of a physical work task may lead to increased muscle activity [24–29], and to more pronounced fatigue than the physical task alone [30,31], even if these results have been contested in other studies [32–34]. However, the effect of breaks with an organized mental activity between bouts of physical work has, to our knowledge, been empirically pursued only in very few studies. This is surprising, considering that alternating physical and mental work occurs in many occupations, and that organized breaks are probably often spent at activities that differ from rest and include cognitive engagement [35]. In one study of repeated elbow or finger flexor contractions, Asmussen and Mazin [36] found that the amount of work that could be performed until exhaustion was larger after a break containing mental arithmetic than after a passive rest break. As the authors did not observe any differences in muscle blood flow between active and passive breaks, they concluded that the mentally active breaks influenced recovery to a major extent via mechanisms in the central nervous system. In the 2002 Volvo Award in Biomechanics study, Davis and colleagues [37] showed that kinematics and muscle activation in the lower back during lifting was influenced by a preceding "complex" mental task (reading and interpreting an 8-digit number), particularly at a high lifting frequency. Thus, the biomechanical exposure was *larger* after the complex mental load than after a "simple" mental task involving an easy verbal command; the study did not explicitly evaluate recovery. Finally, in a recent study of repeated maximal isokinetic knee extensions, Stock and colleagues [38] found, in line with the results by Asmussen and Mazin, that a mental task (mathematical problem-solving) accelerated recovery between two exercise bouts as compared to quiet rest; a diverting physical task had the same positive effect. Thus, Stock and colleagues [38] agree with Asmussen and Mazin [39] in suggesting that the mental task most probably exerts its effect through processes in the central nervous system.

While a reasonable expectation would be that the possible ability of a mental activity to accelerate recovery depends on the specific combination of alternating physical and mental tasks, as well as the time pattern of alternation [31,34], the cited studies on serial combinations of physical and mental activity differ considerably in both physical and mental task protocols. Two of the studies used physical tasks requiring maximal effort, i.e. repeated maximal force exertions [38] or continuation of the task until exhaustion [39], which may be of limited validity as a model of occupational work. The study by Davis and colleagues did have an occupational basis, but investigated a lifting task. Thus, no evidence is available on effects of mental activity in combinations involving repetitive, sub-maximal work with the upper extremity, as in industrial assembly or cashier's work. Only the study by Davis and colleagues [37] addressed different levels of difficulty of the mental task, which can reasonably be expected to also influence its effect on recovery [28]. Furthermore, none of the three studies were devoted to multiple cycles of alternating physical and mental activity, and none of them followed physiologic responses using a comprehensive set-up of methods reflecting both central and peripheral factors of relevance to fatigue.

The present study therefore aimed at investigating the extent to which cognitive activities of different difficulty influence the development and recovery of fatigue resulting from repeated bouts of a repetitive, occupationally relevant reaching task in a population of young males.

Methods

Subjects

Eighteen healthy male volunteers aged 20–34 years (mean 24.2 (SD 4.3)), with BMI 18.6–29.0 kg·m^{-2} (mean 23.7 (SD 3.0)) participated in the study. Only males were recruited so as to avoid possible gender effects on the responses to the studied physical and mental task. The subjects answered to a public poster recruitment campaign at the University of Gävle, and entered into the study after providing their written consent, on the basis of information about the aim and experimental procedures of the study. The subjects had no self-reported history of major trauma to the back, arms, neck and shoulders, nor of diseases which could affect motor function or the autonomic nervous system; they did not use any medication regularly; and they reported to be free of upper extremity pain, fatigue and other signs of discomfort at the time of the study.

The study was approved by the Ethical Review Board in Uppsala, Sweden, and conducted in agreement with the Helsinki declaration.

Protocol

The study comprised three experimental sessions separated by at least one week. All three sessions were performed in a laboratory at a constant ambient temperature of 22°C. With very few exceptions, all sessions for any particular subject began at the same time of the day, selected according to the subject's preferences. On a separate day prior to the first session, subjects carried out a training and familiarisation trial. Training continued until the subject reached a stable work rhythm, or for a minimum of 3 minutes, corresponding to about 90 work cycles (see below).

Subjects were instructed to avoid smoking and caffeine intake thirty minutes before each experimental session, meals two hours before and intensive physical exercise two days before. During each session, subjects performed six bouts of a repetitive reaching task (see below) interrupted by rest breaks (Figure 1). During these breaks, subjects performed a mental task (a working memory test; see below) with three levels of cognitive difficulty, one in each experimental session. The order of sessions with different difficulties was balanced between subjects.

Physical task

The physical work task consisted of repeated movements of a 300 g manipulandum held in the right (dominant) hand, pushing two "near" and "far" buttons at 1 Hz (one complete cycle lasting 2 s) as guided by a metronome [40]. The distance between the two buttons were adjusted according to each subject's arm length so that the angle of the elbow was 90° and 160° when pressing the near and far buttons, respectively. The subject was seated comfortably at the work station in an adjustable chair with a knee angle of approximately 90°, the left arm resting on the table. A detailed description of the task is provided in a previous publication devoted specifically to fatigue effects on motor control

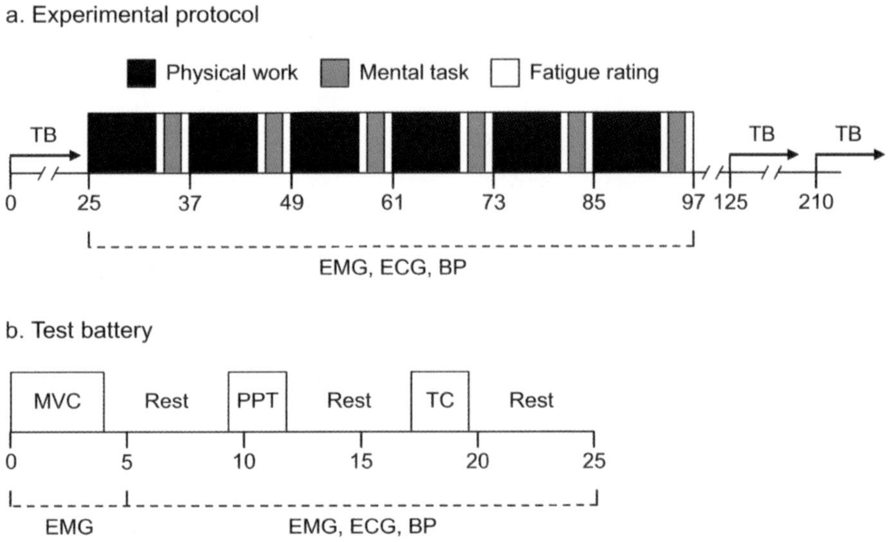

Figure 1. Experimental protocol and test battery. The protocol (Figure 1a) included six 7-minute bouts of a repetitive reaching task, interspersed by 5-minute breaks comprising two ratings of perceived fatigue and a 3-minute mental task. A test battery (TB, Figure 1b) was performed before, immediately after, and one hour after the work period. Both x-axes show time in minutes. EMG, electromyography; ECG, electrocardiography; BP, blood pressure; MVC, maximal voluntary contraction; PPT, pressure pain threshold; TC, test contraction.

during repetitive work, without any attention being paid to effects of mental tasks [41].

Mental task

During the breaks between physical work bouts, the subject performed a mental task (MT) often referred to as running memory span [42]. Eight series of 8–11 letters were presented on a computer screen in front of the subject. Letters were presented once per second with 0.8 s exposure time and 0.2 s of black screen. At the three levels of cognitive difficulty, the subject was asked to recall and orally report the last (MT1), two last (MT2) or three last (MT3) letters, respectively. MT1 was included to represent a condition in which the subject would have to focus his cognitive, visual, and motor attention on a similar activity as that eventually presented in the more difficult mental conditions MT2 and MT3, while at the same time being so easy that it could readily be accomplished by all subjects. Thus, MT1 represents a more consistent reference for evaluating the effects of MT2 and MT3 than the more common choice of passive rest as a control condition, during which the attention of subjects may differ widely in both focus and intensity. The subject's answer was scored by the examiner in terms of the number of correctly recalled letters in the correct order. The subject did not receive any feed-back on performance. Analyses after the full experiment confirmed that the three mental task conditions differed significantly in cognitive demands (ANOVA, $F = 88.17$; $p < 0{,}001$); MT3 was associated with a markedly reduced performance (83% correct answers) compared to MT2 (95%) and MT1 (99%).

Physiological and psychophysical measurements

Ratings of perceived fatigue. Before and after each of the six physical work bouts, the subject was asked to rate his perceived fatigue in the neck and shoulders on the 10-grade Borg CR10 scale [43], and to respond to items from the Swedish Occupational Fatigue Inventory (SOFI; [44]). SOFI measures, on a scale from 0 to 6, perceived fatigue in five dimensions, i.e. *lack of energy*, *physical exertion*, *physical discomfort*, *lack of motivation* and *sleepiness*. In the present study, a short version of SOFI was used, consisting of five items (*spent*, *breathing heavily*, *aching*, *uninterested* and *sleepy*), which have been shown to strongly represent each of the five fatigue dimensions [44].

Electromyography (EMG). EMG was recorded bilaterally from the upper trapezius muscles using pairs of self-adhesive surface electrodes with 20 mm inter-electrode distance, centres placed 2 cm lateral to the midpoint between vertebrae C7 and the acromion [45]. The trapezius muscle was selected as is standard in occupational studies [45–47], so as to represent a region often associated with work-related pain and discomfort [48]. The signal was amplified, band-pass filtered at 10–1000 Hz and sampled at 2000 Hz. Off-line, after cleaning the signal from obvious artefacts, it was root mean square (RMS) converted using consecutive 250 ms windows. The EMG RMS amplitude was then normalised to the mean amplitude during the test contraction in the baseline test battery (see below; [45]), and expressed in percent of reference voluntary exertion (%RVE). The normalized EMG amplitude and the raw EMG Mean Power Frequency (MPF) during the entire first and last minute of each physical work bout were retrieved for further analysis.

Electrocardiography (ECG). ECG was recorded from the thorax derivation (midaxillary sixth left rib – distal end of sternum) using a 0.5–200 Hz bandpass filter and a 2000 Hz sampling rate. R-R intervals were detected by a custom script (Spike 6.01, Cambridge Electronic Design. UK). After visual inspection of the signal and removal of artefacts, R-R intervalograms were further analysed in the time and frequency domains to provide measures of heart rate variability according to recommendations by the Task force of the European Society of Cardiology [49]; including inter-beat intervals (IBI), standard deviation of normal-to-normal inter-beat intervals (SDNN), the number of successive differences >50 ms between normal-to-normal intervals (NN50), spectral power in low frequency (LF 0,04–0,15 Hz) and high frequency (HF 0,15–0,4 Hz) bands, and the low-to-high frequency power ratio (LF/HF). These variables were retrieved for segments of 136 s during the physical work bouts (three segments in each bout) and while performing the mental task (one segment in each break).

After inspection of data, spectral power variables (but not their ratio) were log-transformed to ensure normal distribution.

Arterial Blood Pressure. Systolic and diastolic arterial blood pressure (BP) was measured using a non-invasive pressure sensor (NIBP100B-R; Biopac, CA, USA). The sensor was applied just above the radial artery on the left arm, and BP-values based on averaging approximately 15 pulse pressure waveforms were registered. BP was monitored during the entire experiment, and segments of 2 minutes were used for additional analyses; three segments for each physical work bout and one segment for each break.

Test battery

A test battery (TB, cf. [50]) was performed before, immediately after, and 1 hour after the work period, with 5 minutes of rest between different TB parts (Figure 1b). During the TB, subjects were instructed to sit quietly in their chair to avoid motion artefacts. Instructions for each TB part were orally presented by the examiner and also shown on a computer screen in front of the subject. ECG was monitored throughout the TB (cf. Figure 1b), which otherwise comprised the measurements described below.

Maximal voluntary contraction (MVC). MVC was obtained in bilateral isometric shoulder elevation, encouraging the subject to exert a maximal vertical shoulder "lift" while being fixed to straps connecting the shoulders and the floor. The developed force was read from a dynamometer placed in the right side strap (Somedic Production AB, Sollentuna, Sweden). The best of three attempts interspersed by one minute of rest was saved.

Pressure pain threshold (PPT). PPT was determined over both trapezius muscles using a pressure algometer (Somedic Production AB, Sollentuna, Sweden) applied halfway between C7 and acromion. Pressure was increased at a rate of approximately 50 $kPa{\cdot}s^{-1}$, and subjects pressed a button as soon as the sensation of pressure turned into pain. The corresponding pressure value was then noted by the examiner. Three measurements were collected from each of the left and right shoulders and averaged to give a PPT for each shoulder.

Isometric test contraction. The subject was instructed to raise his straight arms to 90° abduction in the frontal plane and keep them there for one minute. The EMG amplitude of the middle 10 s of this test contraction was retrieved for further analysis. The test contraction requires about 15 percent of the maximal voluntary capacity for an average male subject [50].

Further data analyses

Descriptive statistics for all variables were expressed as group means and SD between individuals, unless otherwise stated. For data averaged across the three experimental protocols, a pooled SD was calculated as the root of the average variance in the protocols.

In order to investigate the development of fatigue across repeated bouts of physical work, repeated-measure ANOVAs were constructed with work bout (WB, bout 1–6) and MT (MT1, MT2, MT3) as within-subject factors and the order of MT as a between-subjects factor. The effect of WB was modelled as a linear trend using polynomial contrasts. The ANOVA model included interactions between WB and MT. This ANOVA model was resolved for heart rate variability, arterial blood pressure, and amplitude and frequency of EMG (in all cases on results averaged across each WB), and perceived fatigue (using the ratings directly after each WB). If the main effect of MT and/or the interaction MT × WB was found to be significant, a series of post hoc tests were performed, in which the ANOVA model was run on data excluding either MT1, MT2 or MT3.

In order to analyse the immediate recovery effect of the break after each physical work bout, changes in EMG amplitude between the last part of one physical work bout and the initial part of the following bout were noted; i.e. five values in total for each work period. Recovery of cardiovascular variables was assessed by subtracting the value during each work bout from the value during the subsequent break; i.e. six change scores in total for each work period, including values immediately after the last bout. For perceived fatigue, recovery was measured by the difference between ratings early and late in each break; in total five change scores. Each set of change scores was analysed for effects of WB and MT using the ANOVA model described above, including the described post-hoc test procedure.

Recovery during prolonged rest after the entire work period was investigated by comparing the measurements of PPT, MVC, reference contraction EMG amplitude, perceived fatigue, and resting BP and heart rate variability obtained during the test battery before (pre-work), immediately after (post-work0h) and one hour after work (post-work1h). Measurement results were tested using ANOVAs with TB (three levels) and MT (three levels) as within-subject factors, followed by post hoc analyses of pre-work vs. post-work1h values (showing whether responses returned to baseline), post-work0h vs. post-work1h values (showing the extent of recovery during the first hour after work), and pre-work vs. post-work0h (giving a complementary measure of the overall development of fatigue during the work period).

All statistical analyses were performed using SPSS edition 18.0 or later (IBM Inc., Chicago, IL, USA).

Results

Complete data at the individual level are available on-line, as Dataset S1.

Exposure and response before and during the initial work bout

Before work, fatigue was, on average, rated 1.3 (SD 0.9) on the CR10 scale, and SOFI ratings were, "*spent*" 0.3, (SD 0.5), "*breathing heavily*" 0.1 (SD 0.3), "*aching*" 0.2 (SD 0.4), "*uninterested*" 1.2 (SD 1.2), and "*sleepy*" 1.7 (SD 1.3). None of these baseline ratings were influenced by the mental task condition in the following work period (all p-values ≥ 0.3, besides for "sleepy", $p = 0.06$). As expected, physiologic variables collected during the test battery preceding work (cf. Table 1) did not differ either between the three mental task conditions (MVC: $F = 0.20$, $p = 0.82$; ipsilateral PPT: $F = 0.81$, $p = 0.45$; contralateral PPT: $F = 0.56$, $p = 0.58$).

In the non-fatigued state, i.e. during the first minute of the initial work bout (WB1), the physical work task was performed with a mean ipsilateral trapezius EMG amplitude of 48 (SD 14) %RVE (mean across all subjects and conditions). The mean R-R interval was 794 (SD 92) ms during the first part of WB1 (rest: 856 (SD 93) ms), corresponding to a heart rate of 75.6 $beats{\cdot}min^{-1}$. Time domain HRV analyses showed a mean SDNN of 58 (SD 20) ms during WB1 (rest: 65 (SD 27) ms), and a NN50 of 17 (SD 14) counts/136s (rest: 28 (SD 20) counts/136s); both confirming the expected decrease in parasympathetic modulation of the heart during work compared to rest [51]. Arterial blood pressure increased as expected during WB1 (Systolic BP 150 (SD 16) mmHg; diastolic BP 85 (SD 10) mmHg) compared to resting values (Systolic BP 134 (SD 14) mmHg; diastolic BP 74 (SD 9) mmHg).

Table 1. Pre-work baseline values of maximal strength, pressure pain threshold and reference contraction EMG amplitude, and their recovery after work.

Measure	Mental task	Pre-work	Post-work0h	Post-work1h	Main effect TB, p-value	Interaction TB × MT, p-value
MVC (N)	MT1	662 (225)	596 (182)	625 (153)	**0.02**	**0.04**
	MT2	642 (132)	608 (153)	622 (127)		
	MT3	645 (170)	634 (208)	582 (161)		
PPT (kPa)						
Ipsilateral	MT1	448 (187)	427 (140)	434 (170)	**0.04**	>0.30
	MT2	443 (148)	425 (144)	415 (132)		
	MT3	467 (174)	444 (136)	432 (144)		
Contralateral	MT1	433 (174)	385 (106)	395 (123)	0.21	**0.03**
	MT2	408 (132)	382 (123)	385 (115)		
	MT3	416 (119)	428 (136)	422 (123)		
EMG amplitude, ipsilateral (%RVE[a])	MT1	100	113 (13)	106 (8)	**<0.003[b]**	>0.30[b]
	MT2	100	121 (34)	116 (30)		
	MT3	100	112 (17)	110 (21)		

[a]: EMG amplitude expressed in percent of the pre-work reference contraction value.
[b]: Main effect of TB tested using one sample t-tests for post-work0h and post-work1h values pooled across MT against the reference pre-work value (100); interaction effect (TB × MT) investigated by testing for the effect of MT in three separate ANOVAs on results from post-work0h, post-work1h, and the difference between post-work0h and post-work1h.
MVC, Maximum voluntary contraction; PPT, Pressure pain threshold; MT1, MT2, MT3, easy, medium and difficult mental task; TB, Test battery.
Table shows mean (SD between subjects) values of MVC, PPT and reference contraction EMG amplitude in the three test batteries (TB) preceding work, immediately after work and one hour into recovery after work including the three mental tasks (MT1, MT2, MT3). Right-most columns show results of the ANOVA tests (p-values less than 0.05 in bold) for a main effect of TB and an interaction TB × MT.

Fatigue during work bouts

Physical work led to a moderate perceived neck-shoulder fatigue already during the first WB according to ratings on the Borg CR10 scale (mean increase 3.7 (SD 1.3)), and perceived fatigue increased linearly across the whole work period as indicated by a significant WB effect (Table 2; $F = 38.4$, $p<0.001$). At the end of the experiment, Borg CR10 ratings had increased to, on the average, 5.8 (SD 1.9). For the SOFI ratings, significant increases across WB was found for *aching* ($F = 5.4$, $p = 0.04$), *spent* ($F = 44.3$, $p<0.001$), *heavy breathing* ($F = 9.1$, $p = 0.01$), and *uninterested* ($F = 5.8$, $p = 0.03$).

A significant linear increase across work bouts was found for the average ipsilateral trapezius EMG amplitude during bouts ($F = 32.1$, $p<0.001$), while MPF decreased ($F = 3.6$, $p = 0.08$). Trapezius EMG amplitude also increased at the contralateral side, but remained at considerably lower levels (Table 2, Figure 2).

Heart rate, calculated from IBI, decreased significantly with WB ($F = 7.7$, $p = 0.014$), while heart rate variability increased, as measured both by SDNN ($F = 4.4$, $p = 0.05$) and NN50 ($F = 8.2$, $p = 0.01$). Neither frequency-related variables of heart rate variability nor BP were significantly affected by WB.

Pre-post differences of test battery measurements confirmed that the work period led to fatigue (Table 1); the reference contraction EMG amplitude was, on average, 15 (SD 22) %RVE higher after work than before ($F = 11.2$, $p = 0.004$), and MVC had declined from 649 (SD 176) N to 610 (SD 185) N ($F = 6.0$, $p = 0.03$). The difficulty of the mental task did not have any significant main effect on perceived fatigue (Table 2). An interaction effect (WB × MT) was, however, found for the Borg CR10 ratings ($F = 4.4$, $p = 0.04$). Post-hoc tests showed that perceived muscle fatigue developed at a lower rate for the most difficult memory tasks than for the easy task (MT3 vs MT1: $F = 4.8$, $p = 0.04$.

The amplitude and frequency of EMG was not significantly influenced by MT (Table 2), and interactions between WB and MT were not found either. For heart rate variability and blood pressure during work, main effects of MT were observed in SDNN ($F = 8.6$, $p = 0.01$), NN50 ($F = 5.8$, $p = 0.03$), systolic BP ($F = 4.9$ $p = 0.05$) and diastolic BP ($F = 7.6$, $p = 0.02$). Post-hoc tests showed that MT1 was associated with lower heart rate variability than MT3, while blood pressure was elevated in the experiment with MT2 compared to MT3. No significant WB × MT interaction effects were found for these variables.

Recovery during breaks

Perceived neck-shoulder fatigue was significantly reduced during the breaks, indicating a rapid recovery after each WB, typically from "high" fatigue to "weak" fatigue at the Borg CR10 scale ($F = 69.8$, $p<0.001$). Recovery in CR10 ratings did not differ between the mental tasks ($F = 1.0$, $p = 0.40$). A tendency to higher alertness was, however, seen in breaks during the difficult mental task (MT3) condition, since the increase in SOFI rating of *sleepy* during those breaks was smaller than during breaks in the other two mental task conditions ($F = 7.9$, $p = 0.01$).

Trapezius EMG amplitude recovered between the last part of one WB and the first part of the next one (Figure 2). The extent of recovery in the ipsilateral EMG amplitude depended on WB ($F = 2.9$, $p = 0.04$); recovery diminishing slightly with time. The difficulty of the mental task had no significant effect on recovery of neither ipsilateral nor contralateral EMG (MT main effects: $F = 0.97$, $p = 0.39$ (ipsi) and $F = 2.34$, $p = 0.11$ (contra); interactions WB × MT: $F = 0.39$, $p = 0.93$ (ipsi) and $F = 1.0$, $p = 0.44$ (contra)).

Table 2. Development of perceived fatigue and muscle activity during work.

	MT1	MT2	MT3	WB Main effect p-value	MT Main effect p-value	Interaction WB × MT p-value
Borg CR10 (0–10)	2.6 (1.7)	2.2 (1.7)	1.6 (2.1)	**<0.001**	0.29	**0.04**
SOFI (0–6)						
Aching	0.8 (1.3)	0.8 (1.3)	0.4 (1.7)	**0.04**	0.14	>0.30
Spent	1.2 (0.8)	1.2 (0.8)	0.9 (1.3)	**<0.001**	>0.30	0.18
Sleepy	0.0 (1.3)	0.4 (1.3)	0.4 (1.3)	0.09	>0.30	>0.30
Heavy breathing	0.3 (0.4)	0.4 (0.4)	0.3 (0.8)	**0.01**	>0.30	>0.30
Uninterested	0.4 (0.8)	0.3 (1.3)	0.1 (0.8)	**0.03**	>0.30	>0.30
EMG amplitude (%RVE)						
Ipsilateral	7.6 (8.2)	5.7 (8.1)	9.5 (8.1)	**<0.001**	>0.30	>0.30
Contralateral	3.0 (8.5)	3.4 (7.2)	4.4 (5.1)	**<0.001**	>0.30	>0.30
EMG MPF (Hz)						
Ipsilateral	0.3 (3.0)	−1.2 (2.5)	−1.5 (3.0)	0.08	>0.30	>0.30
Contralateral	3.2 (8.9)	4.8 (8.9)	6.3 (8.1)	**0.003**	>0.30	0.26

MT1, MT2, MT3; easy, medium and difficult mental task.
The difference between work blocks 1 and 6 of perceived fatigue, and of ipsi- and contralateral trapezius EMG variables (means (SD between subjects)) is shown for each of the mental tasks (MT1, MT2, MT3); together with the corresponding results of the ANOVA tests, based on all six work blocks, for main effects and interaction of work bout (WB) and mental task (MT) condition (p-values less than 0.05 in bold).

Heart rate variability increased during breaks (Table 3). Enhanced recovery of heart rate and NN50 was found for the MT3 condition (Figure 3), as indicated by significant interactions between WB and MT ($F = 8.6$, $p = 0.009$; and $F = 6.8$, $p = 0.02$). Similarly, the LF/HF ratio during breaks was decreased for MT3 compared to MT1 (main effect of MT; $F = 6.7$, $p = 0.02$), mainly due to a larger HF content ($F = 10.3$; $p = 0.006$). Recovery of arterial blood pressure during the breaks did not show any dependence on MT.

Recovery after work

As expected, perceived fatigue diminished considerably during the first hour after the work period (Figure 4). Recovery of Borg CR10 ratings differed depending on the preceding mental task, and was most pronounced after the most difficult cognitive task, MT3 ($F = 7.8$, $p = 0.01$). SOFI ratings also recovered after work ($p < 0.05$), and trends suggesting an MT-by-time interaction were seen for *aching* ($F = 3.9$, $p = 0.07$) and *spent* ($F = 3.35$, $p = 0.05$), with recovery one hour after the work bout being most pronounced for the difficult mental condition MT3.

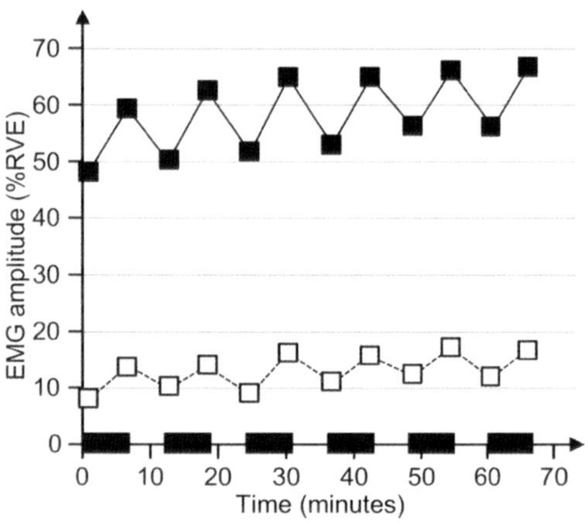

Figure 2. Trapezius EMG amplitude during the work period. EMG amplitude during the first and last minute of each of the six work bouts; mean across subjects and mental task conditions. X-axis shows time after commencing work; black zones mark physical work bouts. Filled and empty symbols with full-drawn and dashed line: ipsi- and contralateral trapezius EMG, respectively.

MVC was significantly reduced immediately after the experiments (Table 1; $F = 5.9$, $p = 0.03$) and did not recover fully during the hour after work ($F = 4.8$, $p = 0.04$). PPT on the ipsilateral side also decreased after the experiment ($F = 4.8$, $p = 0.04$). The extent of recovery after the experiment differed depending on the preceding mental task (MVC ($F = 5.3$, $p = 0.04$); contralateral PPT ($F = 5.4$, $p = 0.03$)). For PPT, recovery was slower (or even indiscernible) after MT3, while MVC was higher immediately after MT3 than after MT1 and MT2, but did then not recover during the following hour (Table 1). The reference contraction EMG amplitude had recovered significantly after one hour towards the value preceding work ($F = 5.1$, $p = 0.04$) (Table 1), and recovery did not differ depending on the mental condition. All cardiovascular indices were increased above baseline values immediately after work, and remained increased during the first hour of rest, yet to a similar extent irrespective of the preceding MT (values not shown).

Discussion

Motivated by our interest in fatigue and recovery in an occupational context, we selected a physical task for this experiment, which simulated repetitive manual handling of weights consistent with those occurring in many industrial settings, for instance in manufacturing [52–54] or slaughterhouses [55,56]. Fatigue and disorders in repetitive work is a major concern in occupational epidemiology, and the need to intervene has been emphasized in several reviews [57–60]. Our repetitive task did lead to pronounced, if not extreme, fatigue, as confirmed by subjective ratings (Table 2) and changes in the electromyographic

Table 3. Recovery of heart rate, heart rate variability, and blood pressure during the break after each bout of physical work (WB1-WB6), stratified by mental task (MT1, MT2, MT3); mean (SD between subjects)[a].

	Mental task	WB 1	WB 2	WB 3	WB 4	WB 5	WB 6
Heart Rate							
IBI (ms)	MT1	84 (59)	79 (42)	79 (47)	88 (49)	93 (57)	117 (58)
	MT2	96 (52)	107 (66)	99 (60)	98 (49)	103 (56)	103 (59)
	MT3	70 (58)	111 (65)	110 (63)	112 (74)	116 (60)	119 (58)
Heart Rate Variability							
NN50 (counts)	MT1	8 (18)	8 (14)	6 (11)	5 (15)	11 (13)	16 (15)
	MT2	12 (22)	11 (21)	12 (18)	8 (13)	15 (16)	15 (21)
	MT3	8 (17)	13 (19)	10 (18)	14 (18)	15 (12)	16 (15)
SDNN (ms)	MT1	11 (32)	16 (24)	10 (20)	13 (20)	21 (19)	28 (32)
	MT2	16 (25)	18 (21)	27 (34)	20 (22)	31 (40)	26 (33)
	MT3	7 (26)	19 (18)	14 (26)	27 (37)	21 (24)	26 (27)
ln LF (ms^{-2})	MT1	−0.4 (1.0)	0.5 (0.9)	0.3 (1.0)	0.3 (0.9)	0.5 (0.7)	0.6 (0.8)
	MT2	−0.3 (1.0)	0.2 (0.9)	0.4 (0.9)	0.5 (0.9)	0.8 (1.1)	0.6 (0.8)
	MT3	−0.3 (1.2)	0.6 (1.0)	0.1 (0.8)	0.4 (1.0)	0.4 (0.9)	0.4 (0.9)
ln HF (ms^{-2})	MT1	0.5 (1.1)	0.6 (0.9)	0.4 (1.0)	0.5 (1.0)	0.8 (0.6)	0.9 (1.0)
	MT2	0.6 (1.3)	0.7 (1.0)	0.8 (1.2)	0.8 (1.2)	0.9 (1.0)	0.8 (1.0)
	MT3	0.6 (1.0)	1.0 (0.9)	0.6 (0.8)	0.8 (1.0)	0.8 (0.6)	0.9 (1.1)
LF/HF ratio	MT1	−4.9 (6.6)	−1.9 (6.8)	−1.0 (5.1)	−2.7 (6.8)	−2.9 (8.4)	−2.6 (5.0)
	MT2	−5.0 (4.9)	−2.4 (4.5)	−2.0 (5.0)	−3.9 (9.9)	−2.2 (5.2)	−1.7 (4.8)
	MT3	−4.2 (4.1)	−2.1 (3.2)	−3.3 (5.2)	−3.0 (4.6)	−3.0 (6.6)	−2.5 (4.5)
Blood Pressure							
Systolic (mmHg)	MT1	−12.8 (9.6)	−15.2 (9.8)	−9.7 (9.1)	−13.4 (9.1)	−13.2 (10.0)	−13.3 (10.1)
	MT2	−14.3 (9.0)	−12.1 (14.2)	−11.8 (12.4)	−16.7 (9.0)	−14.8 (5.8)	−14.0 (7.1)
	MT3	−10.4 (7.9)	−11.1 (9.9)	−11.7 (12.3)	−12.9 (10.9)	−13.6 (9.5)	−9.8 (15.4)
Diastolic (mmHg)	MT1	−7.1 (5.8)	−11.0 (8.6)	−6.7 (8.1)	−7.8 (6.3)	−9.9 (7.4)	−9.7 (6.0)
	MT2	−10.5 (6.5)	−9.0 (7.0)	−6.5 (8.3)	−10.3 (6.8)	−9.4 (4.6)	−9.2 (5.4)
	MT3	−7.5 (6.2)	−8.2 (6.7)	−7.5 (7.4)	−7.3 (6.7)	−10.0 (7.5)	−8.1 (8.8)

[a]: scores were calculated by subtracting the value during work from the value during the subsequent break.
IBI, inter-beat interval. For Heart rate variability metrics, see methods section. MT1, MT2, MT3; easy, medium and difficult mental task.

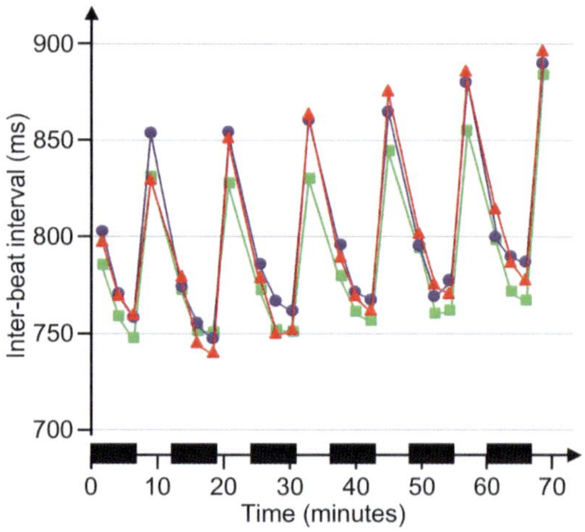

Figure 3. Heart rate during the work period. Heart rate (measured by inter-beat ECG intervals) during work and breaks in the easy (MT1, green squares), medium (MT2, blue circles), and difficult (MT3, red triangles) mental task protocols. X-axis shows time after commencing work; black zones mark physical work bouts.

(EMG) signal from the upper trapezius (Table 2) conventionally used as a sign of decreased force-generating capacity of the exercising muscles [47]. Also, subjects changed their motor strategy in the course of the work period, as shown in a previous publication of motor control in the physical task [41]. As expected from previous studies of intermittent work involving the arms [50,61], fatigue increased during each of the physical work bouts, and recovered partly, though not fully, in the subsequent break, such as illustrated by the EMG pattern in Figure 2. Also, signs of fatigue persisted one hour after work, as reflected in decreased maximal shoulder elevation strength (Table 1). This general pattern applied irrespective of the cognitive task performed during the breaks, even though maximal strength was reduced more one hour after the most difficult task, MT3, than after the two other conditions, MT1 and MT2.

We found indications that autonomic activity differed depending on the difficulty of the mental task; the most demanding task was associated with better recovery of heart rate and heart rate variability than the easy task, reflecting an accelerated return towards more parasympathetic cardiac activity (Table 3). Also, perceived fatigue developed slower during the protocol with the most demanding task (Table 2), and recovered faster after work (Figure 4), while muscle activity (as reflected by EMG) was not sensitive to the cognitive demands. One explanation that the most difficult mental task condition was associated with the largest parasympathetic involvement could be that the task was experienced to be so difficult that subjects gave in and lost motivation. However, this is not a likely explanation, considering that performance was consistently high (on average 83% correct answers) throughout the experimental session.

While these effects of a mental task on recovery after physical work were not very strong, and to some extent ambiguous, they do support the reports by Asmussen & Mazin [36] and Stock et al. [38] that a cognitive effort may enhance recovery compared to a passive break. This consistency is a remarkable result, considering that these two studies used physical task paradigms differing substantially from ours. In the Asmussen & Mazin study, subjects performed repeated submaximal force exertions using the flexors of the elbow or the middle finger till exhaustion, while Stock et al. had their subjects perform 50 fast and consecutive maximal isokinetic knee extensions. Thus, both studies used experimental tasks requiring a maximal effort, in terms of endurance and force, respectively, while our physical task required 5–10% of the maximal force-generating capacity, as judged from the average trapezius EMG amplitude in the first work bout, and was far from exhaustive. In keeping with their experimental tasks, both Asmussen & Mazin and Stock et al. measured fatigue using maximal performance metrics, while we applied a much wider selection of physiologic and psychophysical variables of relevance to central and peripheral fatigue.

Both Asmussen & Mazin and Stock et al. used a challenging, yet manageable mental arithmetic task during their "active" breaks, but did not explicitly assess neither intensity nor performance, beyond the instruction used by Stock et al. to "correctly answer as many problems as possible" in a 3-minute period. In our study, the mental task was strictly controlled in terms of speed and difficulty, and we kept track of the subjects' performance, i.e. the proportion of correct answers. As a "passive" reference condition, both Asmussen & Mazin and Stock et al. used quiet rest, while we used a standardized and very easy mental task, requiring subjects to devote their attention to the same cognitive activity which was then modified with respect to difficulty in the other experimental conditions. Any difference in physiologic response between the three mental conditions will therefore reflect a specific effect of changes in demands on the working memory, rather than an unspecific effect of mental attention, had the subjects been left in uncontrolled passive rest as the reference condition.

The studies by Asmussen & Mazin and Stock et al. presented evidence that a likely explanation why a mental task could influence recovery is that it changes the balance between inhibition and activation of brain centres involved in central fatigue [36,39]. The latter explanation is an extension of theories presented about a century ago by Sechenov (cited in [18]), who noted that both physical and mental "diverting activities" after a period of physical work seemed to improve performance in a subsequent work bout. Substantial research has confirmed that fatigue caused by muscle activity is, indeed, a complex result of both peripheral and central components [22,23], and that cognitive activity does change the activity in brain regions known to also be activated during a fatiguing physical task [62–64]. Our results corroborated that a possible recuperating effect of a demanding cognitive activity in short breaks between bouts of physical work, as well as during a longer rest period after work may, indeed, reside in the central nervous system, even though we did not explicitly measure brain activity using, e.g. electroencephalography or functional resonance imaging. The parasympathetic branch of the autonomic nervous system seemed to be involved in this modulation, as suggested even by studies showing that brain regions associated with parasympathetic activation are engaged during both mental and physical tasks [65,66]. The effect of a cognitive activity may thus be to change autonomic balance towards a larger parasympathetic involvement during recovery, rather than to promote an increased arousal as implied by Sechenov's theories. However, the modulating pathways remain to be verified by direct measurements of central nervous system activity.

While the available literature, including our study, suggests that the positive effect of a mental task on recovery may be found across a wide range of physical tasks, it appears reasonable to assume that the effect will be particularly pronounced in situations where, 1) fatigue caused by the physical task has a strong central component, 2) the physical work per se does not impose any strong cognitive demands, 3) the cognitive task is sufficiently demanding to activate the brain, but not so demanding that it leads to

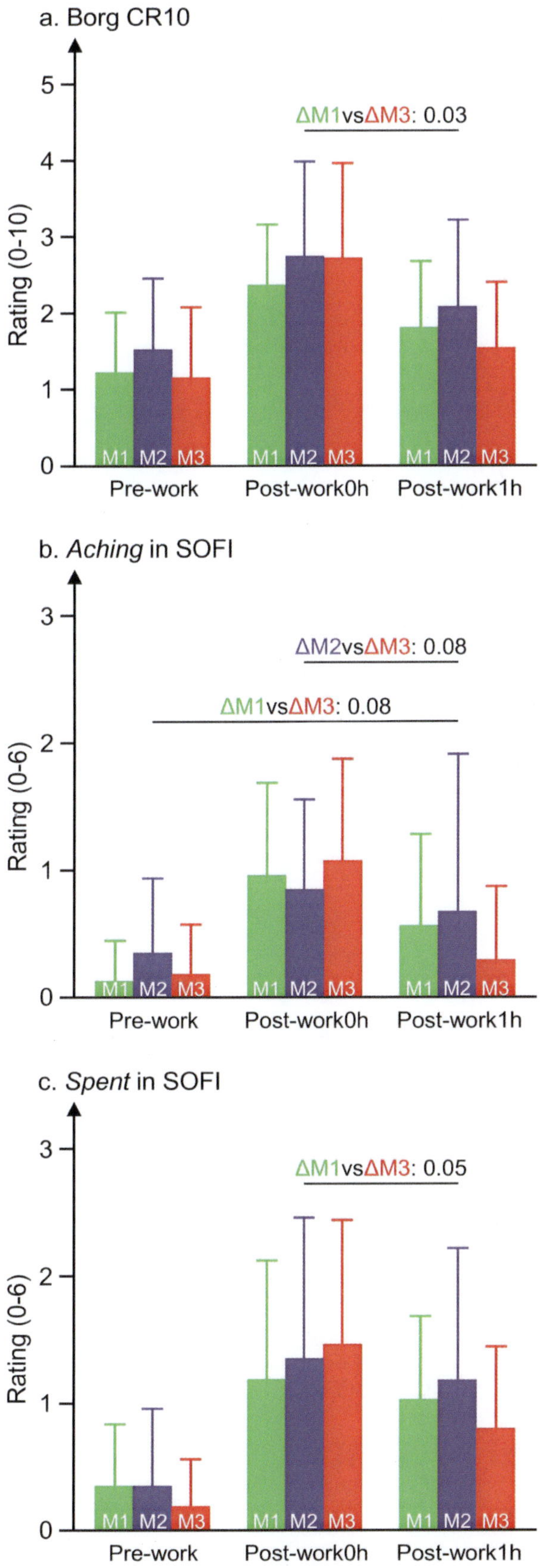

Figure 4. Ratings of perceived fatigue before, immediately after, and one hour after the work period. Perceived fatigue rated on, (a) the Borg CR10 scale, (b) *aching* in SOFI, and (c) *spent* in SOFI; before and after work in the easy (MT1, green), medium (MT2, blue) and difficult (MT3, red) mental task protocols. Mean values; bars illustrating SD between subjects. Text and numbers above columns mark differences in recovery between mental task conditions reaching a p-value less than 0.10. As an example, for *spent* the change from post-work0h to post-work1h differed between M1 and M3 at a p = 0.05 level of significance.

additional central fatigue or stress. Also, the specific effect of the mental task can be expected to differ between individuals according to their working memory and capacity for physical work. If this hypothesis is valid, the effect of a mental break should, for a particular individual, be most pronounced when performing a stereotyped physical task (i.e. a task with an automated motor control, [67] chapter 4) at a moderate intensity, and combining it with a mental task which is challenging but manageable, in a rotation scheme with reasonably frequent shifts (since frequent breaks lead to less fatigue than "rare" breaks [50]). Further research may examine this expectation, and the proposed occurrence of individual differences related to physical and mental capacity.

In an occupational interpretation, the idea that mental tasks in-between physical work bouts may be more beneficial to performance than passive breaks adds to a vivid discussion of the possible benefits of initiatives promoting variation, in particular in repetitive or constrained physical work. While passive rest breaks do, indeed, lead to a remarkable recovery of fatigue following from strictly controlled isometric and isotonic contractions [1–5], they show less encouraging effects when introduced in real occupational settings [9]. One reason may be that the proportion of a work day that can realistically be devoted to (non-productive) rest breaks is too small for the breaks to have any notable physiologic effect; intervention studies have, in general, implemented breaks corresponding to 5-10% of the total time at work [68,69]. This prompts the idea of identifying productive tasks that allow recovery from physical work, and that can feasibly be practiced for sufficient proportion of the work time to have a clear effect. In our study, about 30 percent of the "work cycle" was devoted to the mental task, and in many settings, even in industrial assembly, it may be feasible to introduce productive cognitive activities, such as administrative work [70]. Also, the suggested beneficial effect of mental activities may be realized by offering workers opportunities for cognitive stimulation during scheduled breaks off work.

In an even wider interpretation, alternating physical and mental tasks may be viewed as an idea for job rotation. The general aspiration in job rotation is to identify a combination of tasks that can be performed without loss in productivity or substantial fatigue (and, possibly, less risk of developing musculoskeletal disorders), compared to performing one of the component tasks alone [9,71,72]. While job rotation has generally been discussed in the context of mixing physical work tasks [17,73–78], and while effects of physical variation on fatigue and motor control are, indeed, promising [9,79,80], the present concept of alternating between physical and mental tasks widens job rotation to even include productive tasks that require cognitive efforts while posing very small biomechanical demands.

In conclusion, the results of the present study support a few previous investigations suggesting that mental tasks interspersed between bouts of fatiguing physical work may provide recovery more effectively than passive breaks, even if, in the present study, the benefits were moderate, mainly reflected in different cardio-vascular responses and perceived fatigue, and to some extent contested by the maximal strength response. Thus, our results encourage further research, both in a basic physiological context and motivated by questions of occupational relevance, such as which combinations of physical and mental tasks that may represent particularly attractive mutual effects; which time patterns of alternation that lead to the better results in terms of physiologic responses and acceptability; and which personal traits that may influence the outcome of alternating between physical and mental tasks.

Author Contributions

Conceived and designed the experiments: SEM EL SH. Performed the experiments: SEM DH. Analyzed the data: SEM DH. Contributed reagents/materials/analysis tools: SEM DH EL SH. Wrote the paper: SEM DH EL SH.

References

1. Monod H, Scherrer J (1957) Capacité de travail statique d'un groupe musculaire synergique chez l'homme. Soc Biol 151: 1358–1362.
2. Rohmert W (1960) Ermittlung von erholungspausen für statische arbeit des menschen. Int Z Angew Physiol Einschl Arbeitsphysiol 18: 123–164.
3. Mital A, Bishu RR, Manjunath SG (1991) Review and evaluation of techniques for determining fatigue allowances. Int J Ind Ergon 8: 165–178.
4. Price ADF (1990) Calculating relaxation allowances for construction operatives-part 2: local muscle fatigue. Appl Ergon 21: 318–324.
5. Konz S (1998) Work/rest: part II - The scientific basis (knowledge base) for the guide. Int J Ind Ergon 22: 73–99.
6. Vernon HM, Bedford T, Warner CG (1924) Two studies on rest pauses in industry; Council MR, editor. London: His Majesty's Stationery Office.
7. Bechtold SE, Janaro RE, DeWitt LS (1984) Maximization of labor productivity through optimal rest-break schedules. Mgmnt Sci 30: 1442–1458.
8. Janaro RE, Bechtold SE (1985) A study of fatigue impact on productivity through optimal rest break scheduling. Hum Factors 27: 459–466.
9. Mathiassen SE (2006) Diversity and variation in biomechanical exposure: what is it, and why would we like to know? Appl Ergon 37: 419–427.
10. Visser B, van Dieën JH (2006) Pathophysiology of upper extremity muscle disorders. J Electromyogr Kinesiol 16: 1–16.
11. Hägg GM (1991) Static work loads and occupational myalgia - a new explanation model. In: Anderson PA, Hobart DJ, Dainoff JV, editors.Elec-Electromyographical Kinesiology.Amsterdam: Elsevier. pp.141–144.
12. Wells RH, Mathiassen SE, Medbo L, Winkel J (2007) Time - a key issue for musculoskeletal health and manufacturing. Appl Ergon 38: 733–744.
13. Luger T, Bosch T, Veeger D, de Looze M (2014) The influence of task variation on manifestation of fatigue is ambiguous – a literature review. Ergonomics 57: 162–174.
14. Sundelin G, Hagberg M (1989) The effects of different pause types on neck and shoulder EMG activity during VDU work. Ergonomics 32: 527–537.
15. van den Heuvel SG, de Looze MP, Hildebrandt VH (2003) Effects of software programs stimulating regular breaks and exercises on work-related neck and upper-limb disorders. Scand J Work Environ Health 29: 106–116.
16. Henning RA, Jacques P, Kissel GV, Sullivan AB, Alteras-Webb SM (1997) Frequent short rest breaks from computer work: effects on productivity and well-being at two field sites. Ergonomics 40: 78–91.
17. Mathiassen SE, Winkel J (1996) Physiologic comparison of three interventions in light assembly work: reduced work pace, increased break allowance and shortened working days. Int Arch Occup Environ Health 68: 94–108.
18. Sechenov IM (1935) Zur Frage nach der Einwirking sensitiver Reize auf die Muskelarbeit des Menschen. Selected works. Moscow: State Publishing House for Biological and Medical Literature. pp. 246–260.
19. Gandevia SC, Macefield G (1989) Projection of low-threshold afferents from human intercostal muscles to the cerebral cortex. Respir Physiol 77: 203–214.
20. Sjøgaard G (1996) Potassium and fatigue: the pros and cons. Acta Physiol Scand 156: 257–264.
21. Flodgren G, Crenshaw A, Gref M, Fahlström M (2009) Changes in interstitial noradrenaline, trapezius muscle activity and oxygen saturation during low-load work and recovery. Eur J Appl Physiol 107: 31–42.
22. Enoka RM (2012) Muscle fatigue – from motor units to clinical symptoms. J Biomech 45: 427–433.
23. Gandevia SC (2001) Spinal and supraspinal factors in human muscle fatigue. Physiol Rev 81: 1725–1789.
24. Birch L, Juul-Kristensen B, Jensen C, Finsen L, Christensen H (2000) Acute response to precision, time pressure and mental demand during simulated computer work. Scand J Work Environ Health 26: 299–305.
25. Finsen L, Søgaard K, Christensen H (2001) Influence of memory demand and contra lateral activity on muscle activity. J Electromyogr Kinesiol 11: 373–380.
26. Lundberg U, Kadefors R, Melin B, Palmerud G, Hassmén P, et al. (1994) Psychophysiological stress and EMG activity of the trapezius muscle. Int J Behav Med 1: 354–370.
27. Au AK, Keir PJ (2007) Interfering effects of multitasking on muscle activity in the upper extremity. J Electromyogr Kinesiol 17: 578–586.
28. Leyman ELC, Mirka GA, Kaber DB, Sommerich CM (2004) Cervicobrachial muscle response to cognitive load in a dual-task scenario. Ergonomics 47: 625–645.
29. Wang Y, Szeto GP, Chan C-C (2011) Effects of physical and mental task demands on cervical and upper limb muscle activity and physiological responses during computer tasks and recovery periods. Eur J Appl Physiol 111: 2791–2803.
30. Mehta RK, Agnew MJ (2012) Influence of mental workload on muscle endurance, fatigue, and recovery during intermittent static work. Eur J Appl Physiol 112: 2891–2902.
31. Yoon T, Keller ML, Schlinder De-Lap B, Harkins A, Lepers R, et al. (2009) Sex differences in response to cognitive stress during a fatiguing contraction. J Appl Physiol 107: 1486–1496.
32. Blangsted AK, Søgaard K, Christensen H, Sjøgaard G (2004) The effect of physical and psychosocial loads on the trapezius muscle activity during computer keying tasks and rest periods. Eur J Appl Physiol 91: 253–258.
33. Mehta R, Agnew MJ (2011) Effects of concurrent physical and mental demands for a short duration static task. Int J Ind Ergon 41: 647–652.
34. Mehta R, Nussbaum MA, Agnew MJ (2012) Muscle- and task-dependent responses to concurrent physical and mental workload during intermittent static work. Ergonomics 55: 1166–1179.
35. Arvidsson I, Hansson G-Å, Mathiassen SE, Skerfving S (2006) Changes in physical workload with implementation of mouse-based information technology in air traffic control. Int J Ind Ergon 36: 613–622.
36. Asmussen E, Mazin B (1978) Recuperation after muscular fatigue by "diverting activities". Eur J Appl Physiol 38: 1–7.
37. Davis KG, Marras WS, Heaney CA, Watters TR, Gupta P (2002) The impact of mental processing and pacing on spine loading. Spine 27: 2645–2653.
38. Stock MS, Beck TW, DeFreitas JM (2011) The effects of diverting activities on recovery from fatiguing concentric isokinetic muscle actions. J Strength Cond Res 25: 1911–1917.
39. Asmussen E, Mazin B (1978) A central nervous component in local muscular fatigue. Eur J Appl Physiol 38: 9–15.
40. Björklund M, Crenshaw A, Djupsjöbacka M, Johansson H (2000) Position sense acuity is diminished following repetitive low-intensity work to fatigue in a simulated occupational setting. Eur J Appl Physiol 81: 361–367.
41. Bosch T, Hallman D, Mathiassen SE, De Looze M, Lyskov E, et al. (2012) Temporal strategy and performance during a fatiguing short-cycle repetitive task. Ergonomics 55: 863–873.
42. Bunting M, Cowan N, Scott Saults J (2006) How does running memory span work? Quart J Exp Psychol 59: 1691–1700.
43. Borg G (1998) Borg's perceived exertion and pain scales. Champaign, Illinois: Human Kinetics.
44. Åhsberg E (2000) Dimensions of fatigue in different working populations. Scand J Psychol 41: 231–241.
45. Mathiassen SE, Winkel J, Hägg G (1995) Normalization of surface EMG amplitude from the upper trapezius muscle in ergonomic studies - a review. J Electromyogr Kinesiol 5: 195–226.
46. Farina D, Madeleine P, Graven-Nielsen T, Merletti R, Arendt-Nielsen L (2002) Standardising surface electromyogram recordings for assessment of activity and fatigue in the human upper trapezius muscle. Eur J Appl Physiol 86: 469–478.
47. Hägg GM, Luttmann A, Jäger M (2000) Methodologies for evaluating electromyographic field data in ergonomics. J Electromyogr Kinesiol 10: 301–312.
48. Parent-Thirion A, Macías EF, Hurley J, Vermeylen G (2007) Fourth European Working Conditions Survey. Dublin: European Foundation for the Improvement of Living and Working Conditions.
49. Task force of the European Society of Cardiology, The North American Society of Pacing and Electrophysiology (1996) Heart Rate Variability: Standards of measurement, physiological interpretation, and clinical use. Eur Heart J 93: 1043–1065.
50. Mathiassen SE (1993) The influence of exercise/rest-schedule on the physiological and psychophysical response to isometric shoulder-neck exercise. Eur J Appl Physiol 67: 528–539.
51. Togo F, Takahashi M (2009) Heart Rate Variability in occupational health - A systematic review. Ind Health 47: 589–602.
52. Bao S, Mathiassen SE, Winkel J (1996) Ergonomic effects of a management-based rationalization in assembly work - a case study. Appl Ergon 27: 89–99.
53. Häkkänen M, Viikari-Juntura E, Takala E-P (1997) Effects of changes in work methods on musculoskeletal load. An intervention study in the trailer assembly. Appl Ergon 28: 99–108.

54. Punnett L, Fine LJ, Monroe Keyserling W, Herrin GD, Chaffin DB (2000) Shoulder disorders and postural stress in automobile assembly work. Scand J - Work Environ Health 26: 283–291.
55. Christensen H, Søgaard K, Pilegaard M, Olsen HM (2000) The importance of the work/rest pattern as a risk factor in repetitive monotonous work. Int J Ind Ergon 25: 367–373.
56. Arvidsson I, Balogh I, Hansson G-Å, Ohlsson K, Åkesson I, et al. (2012) Rationalization in meat cutting - Consequences on physical workload. Appl Ergon 43: 1026–1032.
57. van Rijn RM, Huisstede BM, Koes BW, Burdorf A (2010) Associations between workrelated factors and specific disorders of the shoulder – a systematic review of the literature. Scand J Work Environ Health 36: 189–201.
58. Côté P, van der Velde G, Cassidy JD, Carroll LJ, Hogg-Johnson S, et al. (2008) The burden and determinants of neck pain in workers: results of the Bone and Joint Decade 2000–2010 Task Force on Neck Pain and Its Associated Disorders. Spine 33 (4 suppl): S60–S74.
59. Palmer KT, Smedley J (2007) Work relatedness of chronic neck pain with physical findings – a systematic review. Scand J Work Environ Health 33: 165–191.
60. van der Windt DAWM, Thomas E, Pope DP, de Winter AF, Macfarlane GJ, et al. (2000) Occupational risk factors for shoulder pain: a systematic review. Occup Environ Med 57: 433–442.
61. Hermans V, Spaepen AJ (1997) Muscular activity of the shoulder and neck region during sustained and intermittent exercise. Clin Physiol 17: 95–104.
62. Zijdewind I, Van Duinen H, Zielman R, Lorist MM (2006) Interaction between force production and cognitive performance in humans. Clin Neurophysiol 117: 660–667.
63. Joyce J, Graydon J, McMorris T, Davranche K (2009) The time course effect of moderate intensity exercise on response execution and response inhibition. Brain and Cognition 71: 14–19.
64. Tomporowski P (2003) Effects of acute bouts of exercise on cognition. Acta Psychologica 112: 297–324.
65. Beissner F, Meissner K, Bär K-J, Napadow V (2013) The autonomic brain: An activation likelihood estimation meta-analysis for central processing of autonomic function. J Neurosci 33: 10503–10511.
66. Thayer JF, Åhs F, Fredrikson M, Sollers III JJ, Wager TD (2012) A meta-analysis of heart rate variability and neuroimaging studies: Implications for heart rate variability as a marker of stress and health. Neurosci Biobehav Rev 36: 747–756.
67. Schmidt RA, Lee T (2011) Motor Control and Learning: A Behavioral Emphasis. Champaign, IL, USA: Human Kinetics.
68. Dababneh AJ, Swanson N, Shell RL (2001) Impact of added rest breaks on the productivity and well being of workers. Ergonomics 44: 164–174.
69. Genaidy AM, Delgado E, Bustos T (1995) Active microbreak effects on musculoskeletal comfort ratings in meatpacking plants. Ergonomics 38: 326–336.
70. Christmansson M, Fridén J, Sollerman C (1999) Task design, psycho-social work climate and upper extremity pain disorders - effects of an organisational redesign on manual repetitive assembly jobs. Appl Ergon 30: 463–472.
71. Davis K, Jorgensen M (2005) Ergonomics. Pros and cons of job rotation as a means of reducing injury costs. J Occup Environ Hyg 2: D1–D3.
72. Diego-Mas JA, Asensio-Cuesta S, Sanchez-Romero MA, Artacho-Ramirez MA (2009) A multi-criteria genetic algorithm for the generation of job rotation schedules. Int J Ind Ergon 39: 23–33.
73. Kuijer PPFM, van der Beek AJ, van Dieën JH, Visser B, Frings-Dresen MHW (2005) Effect of job rotation on need for recovery, musculoskeletal complaints, and sick leave due to musculoskeletal complaints: a prospective study among refuse collectors. Am J Ind Med 47: 394–402.
74. Keir PJ, Sanei K, Holmes WR (2011) Task rotation effects on upper extremity and back muscle activity. Appl Ergon 42: 814–819.
75. Carnahan BJ, Redfern MS, Norman B (2000) Designing safe job rotation schedules using optimization and heuristic search. Ergonomics 43: 543–560.
76. Frazer MB, Norman RW, Wells RW, Neumann WP (2003) The effects of job rotation on the risk of reporting low back pain. Ergonomics 46: 904–919.
77. Vogel K, Karltun J, Eklund J, Engkvist I-L (2013) Improving meat cutters' work: Changes and effects following an intervention. Appl Ergon 44: 996–1003.
78. Horton LM, Nussbaum MA, Agnew MJ (2012) Effects of rotation frequency and task order on localised muscle fatigue and performance during repetitive static shoulder exertions. Ergonomics 55: 1205–1217.
79. Falla D, Farina D (2007) Periodic increases in force during sustained contraction reduce fatigue and facilitate spatial redistribution of trapezius muscle activity. Exp Brain Res 182: 99–107.
80. Srinivasan D, Mathiassen SE (2012) Motor variability in occupational health and performance. Clin Biomech 27: 979–993.

14

Nimesulide Improves the Symptomatic and Disease Modifying Effects of Leflunomide in Collagen Induced Arthritis

Ahmed M. Al-Abd[1]*, Fahad A. Al-Abbasi[2], Salwa M. Nofal[3], Amani E. Khalifa[4], Richard O. Williams[5], Wafaa I. El-Eraky[3], Ayman A. Nagy[6], Ashraf B. Abdel-Naim[4]

1 Department of Pharmacology and Toxicology, Faculty of Pharmacy, King Abdulaziz University, Jeddah, Saudi Arabia, **2** Department of Biochemistry, Faculty of Science, King Abdulaziz University, Jeddah, Saudi Arabia, **3** Department of Pharmacology, Medical Division, National Research Centre, Giza, Egypt, **4** Department of Pharmacology and Toxicology, Faculty of Pharmacy, Ain Shams University, Cairo, Egypt, **5** Kennedy Institute of Rheumatology, University of Oxford, Oxford, United Kingdom, **6** Department of Forensic Medicine and Clinical Toxicology, Faculty of Medicine, Tanta University, Egypt

Abstract

Nimesulide is a COX-2 inhibitor used for symptomatic relief of rheumatoid arthritis. Leflunomide is an anti-pyrimidine used to manage the progression of rheumatoid arthritis. Herein we studied the influence of nimesulide and leflunomide combination in terms of disease symptoms and progression using collagen-induced arthritis model in mice, as a model for rheumatoid arthritis. Collagen induced arthritis was induced by immunization with type II collagen. Assessment of joint stiffness and articular hyperalgesia were evaluated using a locomotor activity cage and the Hargreaves method, respectively. Disease progression was assessed via arthritic index scoring, X-ray imaging, myeloperoxidase enzyme activity and histopathologic examination. Nimesulide induced only transient symptomatic alleviation on the top of decreased leucocytic infiltration compared to arthritis group. However, nimesulide alone failed to induce any significant improvement in the radiological or pathological disease progression. Leflunomide alone moderately alleviates the symptoms of arthritis and moderately retarded the radiological and pathological disease progression. Combination of nimesulide and leflunomide significantly improved symptomatic (analgesia and joint stiffness) and arthritic disease progression (radiological, pathological and Myeloperoxidase enzyme activity) in collagen induced arthritis animal model.

Editor: David Douglass Brand, Veterans Affairs Medical Center, United States of America

Funding: This work was funded by the Deanship of Scientific Research (DSR), King Abdulaziz University, Jeddah, under grant No (9/166/1434). The authors, therefore, acknowledge with thanks, DSR for technical and financial support. The funders had no role in study design, data collection and analysis, decision to publish, or preparation of the manuscript.

Competing Interests: The co-author Ashraf B. Abdel-Naim is a PLOS ONE Editorial Board member. This does not alter the authors' adherence to PLOS ONE Editorial policies and criteria.

* Email: amalabd@kau.edu.sa

Introduction

Rheumatoid arthritis (RA) is a chronic progressive systemic inflammatory disorder characterized by synovial inflammation, cartilage damage, progressive bone erosion, and articular functional disability. The world wide incidence of RA ranges from 0.5% to 1.0% and it is more prevalent in women compared to men [1]. Historically, non-steroidal anti-inflammatory drugs "NSAIDs" have been considered to be the primary treatment option for RA. Yet, NSAID failed to exert any significant delay in RA disease progression. Accordingly, disease modifying anti-rheumatic drugs "DMARDs" have become the first treatment option [2]. NSAIDs can mediate short term symptomatic amelioration, but with very poor long term outcome [3]. On the other hand, DMARD based regimens mainly aim to intervene in disease progression, with limited or no short term symptomatic alleviation. Several novel treatments have been tested or suggested for managing rheumatoid arthritis symptoms and/or disease progression, such as lymphocyte co-stimulation-targeted therapy [4], TNFα blocking agents [5], B-cell targeted therapy [6] and novel anti-inflammatory drugs with antioxidant activity [7]. However, the economic burden and patient compliance to injectable drugs limited the widespread use of these agents [8,9].

Leflunomide (LEF) is a DMARD used for the treatment of several autoimmune disorders such as RA [10]. The active leflunomide metabolite, A771726LEF, is generated non-enzymatically or by hepatic microsomal enzymes (CYP 2C9) [11]. The active metabolite of leflunomide is considered to be dihydroorotate dehydrogenase (DHODH) enzyme inhibitor that decreases pyrimidine synthesis [12]. Yet, leflunomide is considered to be a selective anti- T cell agent for autoimmune disorders [13,14]. Leflunomide possesses other advantageous anti-inflammatory effects, such as COX-2 inhibition, matrix metalloproteinase inhibition and anti-chemotaxis, [15–18].

Nimesulide (NIM) is a selective potent cycloxygenase-2 (COX-2) inhibitor [19]. Besides its COX-2 inhibitory activity, nimesulide inhibits several superoxide anion generating enzymes such as myeloperoxidase (MPO) [20]. Other anti-inflammatory properties for nimesulide have been reported such as, suppression of the expression of platelet activation factor (PAF), tumor necrosis factor-α and inhibition of matrix metalloproteinase enzymes [21]. In view of these properties, nimesulide is a strong candidate for combination therapy with DMARDs for the treatment for RA.

Previously, we found that nimesulide improved the disease ameliorating effect of methotrexate in the CIA model [22]. Herein, we extended our finding by studying the influence of nimesulide and leflunomide combination in terms of clinical severity and disease progression in CIA in mice.

Results

Symptomatic assessment of arthritis

The Hargreaves's method for assessing articular hyperalgesia was used herein to monitor joint algesia and to check for the potential effect of combining nimesulide to leflunomide in mice with CIA. Before treatment, the CIA control group manifested pre-arthritic shortening in withdrawal latency (WDL) and algesic response prior to the appearance of clinical signs of arthritis. At the mid-arthritic phase, nimesulide and nimesulide+leflunomide significantly prolonged the WDL compared to CIA control group. On contrary, at the late arthritic phase, all single (LEF or NIM) and combination treatment regimens induced significant analgesic effects in terms of prolonged WDL. LEF and LEF+NIM groups induced equal prolongation in WDL with 55.3% compared to the CIA-group. Treatment with nimesulide alone resulted in weaker analgesia manifested as WDL prolongation of only 38.3% relative to CIA-group. Interestingly, WDL of animals treated with leflunomide or leflunomide/nimesulide combination was non-significantly different from normal non arthritic mice at the late arthritic phase Fig. 1-A.

Joint stiffness is one of the main symptoms of RA, leading to a reduction in mobility. As a measure of this, we recorded the number of movements each animal made within the open field instrument. Locomotor activity of CIA mice started to decline in the pre-arthritic phase with further deterioration up to the late-arthritic phase. In the mid-arthritic phase, nimesulide transiently improved joint stiffness with a significant increase in the total number of movements per minute. Nimesulide treatment did not induce any further improvement in joint stiffness at the late-arthritic phase. Leflunomide alone did not induce any significant improvement in joint stiffness at the mid-arthritic or late-arthritic phases. leflunomide+nimesulide combined treatment showed significant improvement in joint stiffness, which started from the mid-arthritic phase till the late-arthritic phase Fig. 1-B.

Assessment of disease progression

Arthritic index (AI) is a semi quantitative parameter that reflecting the severity of polyarthritis. Animals showed stable, low grade, and persistent polyarthritis after immunization with collagen. Animals treated with leflunomide+nemisulide showed the fastest onset of improvement in AI (31 days after the primary induction of arthritis). Animals treated with leflunomide or nimesulide alone started to show improvement in AI at day 35 after induction. After 40 days of induction, the reduction in AI scores was found to be 31.4%, 22.3%, and 43.8% in LEF-group, NIM-group, and (LEF+NIM)-group respectively compared to the CIA controlgroup Fig. 2-A.

After 40 days of primary immunization (arthritis induction), articular damage was assessed using diagnostic X-ray imaging. Significant periostitis, bone erosion, joint malalignment and cartilaginous deterioration was observed in CIA group indicative of severe articular damage. These radiological changes were also assessed in all other treatment groups Fig. 2-B. Nimesulide treatment alone did not show any radiological improvement. On the other hand, treatment with leflunomide improved the total radiological score by 16.5%, while treatment with leflunomide and nimesulide together provided 19.1% radiological protection Fig. 2-C.

In terms of detailed radiological assessment, leflunomide treatment significantly improved bone erosion, cartilage depth and joint alignment by 21.1%, 23.5% and 17.2%, respectively, compared to the CIA control group. However, combined leflunomide+nimesulide treatment significantly improved all radiological parameters compared to the CIA group. In addition, leflunomide+nimesulide treatment significantly improved bone erosion and periostitis compared to the LEF-group **Table 1**.

Histopathological assessment of articular damage

Articular damage was further confirmed pathologically in H&E stained sagittal sections in the joints of mice. CIA resulted in severe hyperplasia in the synovial membrane, irregularity and roughness of the articular surface, and narrowing of joint space as well as excessive leucocytic infiltration Fig. 3-A&B. Treatment with nimesulide alone resulted in decreased intra-articular leucocytic infiltration Fig. 3-D. Synovial membrane hyperplasia, articular surface roughness and narrowing of the joint space were decreased by leflunomide treatment Fig. 3-C. Of all the treatment groups, leflunomide+nimesulide showed the greatest histopathological improvement compared to the CIA group Fig. 3-E.

RA is characterized by leucocytic infiltration and the presence of neutrophils is often regarded as a marker of active disease. Herein, the activity of myeloperoxidase (MPO) was used as a marker for neutrophilic infiltration in the joints of mice with CIA. After 40 days of the primary induction of arthritis, the MPO level was elevated in the joints of mice with CIA-mice. However, all single and combination treatments significantly decreased the MPO activity compared to the CIA group (Fig. 4).

Discussion

Treatment options for RA warrants a lot of visionary decisions; it is not only confined to symptomatic alleviation [23]. NSAID's provide partial symptomatic alleviation in RA; however they do not generally induce long term joint protection. Nimesulide shows strong anti-inflammatory activity beyond COX-2 inhibition [24,25]. On the other hand DMARDS such as, leflunomide, can induce significant retardation in RA disease progression but they are relatively weak in improving key symptoms of RA such as joint stiffness and joint pain [3]. Hence, a DMARD/NSAID combination may provide long term prevention of disease progression on the top of short term symptomatic control [26]. In the current study, we have investigated the added value of combining nimesulide with leflunomide in controlling experimental arthritis.

Amelioration of the major symptoms of RA such as algesia and joint stiffness is necessary for patient compliance [27]. NSAID's are the major drug category used for this purpose [26]. Despite the huge number of existing NSAIDs, new agents with pharmacological properties and/or less toxic side effects are introduced to the field [7]. In our study, nimesulide alone alleviated joint pain at both the mid- and late arthritic phases (day 21 and day 40 after primary arthritis induction, respectively). However, nimesulide alone temporarily alleviated joint stiffness at mid-arthritic phase and failed at the late arthritic phase. Nimesulide is strong anti-inflammatory analgesic drug that possesses more than just COX-2 inhibition activity [24,25]. That might explain its ability for pain alleviation at all arthritic stages [28]; in addition, the transient improvement in joint stiffness might be partly attributed to the

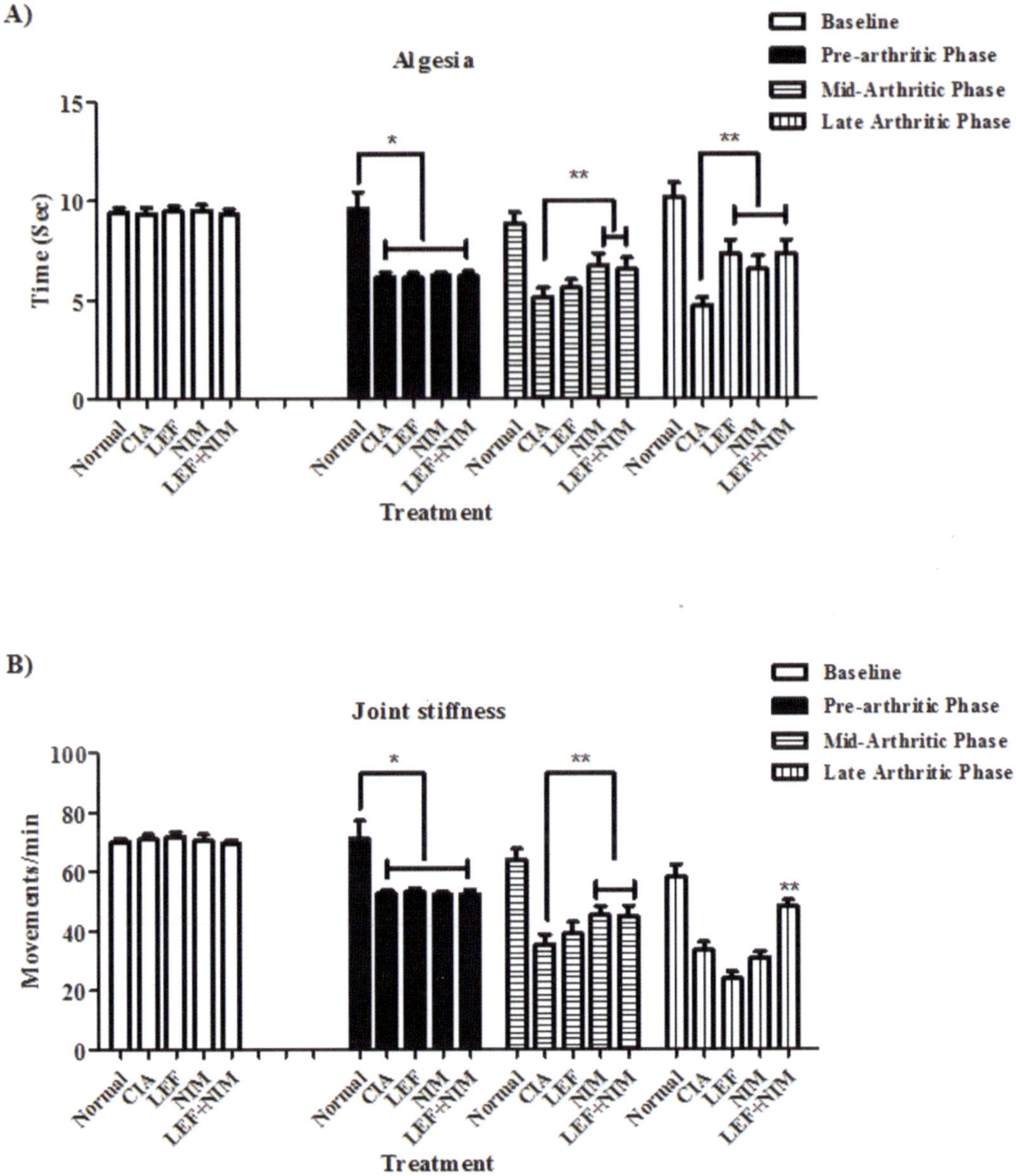

Figure 1. Symptomatic assessment of arthritis. Mice with CIA were treated with leflunomide (LEF), nimesulide (NIM), or leflunomide+ nimesulide (LEF+NIM) and compared to untreated arthritic and normal mice. Hyperalgesia (A) and joint stiffness (B) were recorded at pre-arthritic, mid-arthritic and late arthritic phases of arthritis and compared to base line readings. Data are presented as mean ± SD. * Significantly different from normal mice; ** significantly different from CIA-mice.

analgesic effect [22]. Leflunomide alone failed to induce any significant improvement in joint stiffness. This might be explained by the suboptimal dose level of leflunomide (3.75 mg/kg weekly) used in the current study compared to 10 mg/kg daily in other studies [29]. However, leflunomide at the current dose exerted some pain alleviation effect at the late arthritic phase which might be directly attributed to its moderate anti-inflammatory effects or secondary to its robust disease modifying anti-rheumatic activity [30]. The combination of nimesulide and suboptimal dose of leflunomide could be considered tentative evidence of a synergistic interaction which significantly improved both algesic and joint stiffness signs of CIA at the mid- and late arthritic stages. Symptomatic enhancement effect could be permeated partly to the shared COX-2 inhibition activity of both agents [16,19].

With respect to disease progression, leflunomide+nimesulide induced significant suppression of CIA progression in terms of time and magnitude. At day 33, the AI of LEF+NIM group was not significantly different from normal animals. In addition to the AI, the radiological evaluation showed significant protection for the leflunomide+nimesulide combination compared to either agent alone. Radiological progression is an important feature of RA, as well as CIA [31]. Despite the use of a sub-optimal dose of leflunomide in the current study, combination with nimesulide showed significant improvement in all aspects of the radiological evaluation of arthritis. Moreover, periostitis and bone erosion were significantly improved compared to the LEF-group. This strengthens the tentative synergistic interaction between leflunomide and nimesulide not only on the symptomatic level, but also on the disease modifying level [32].

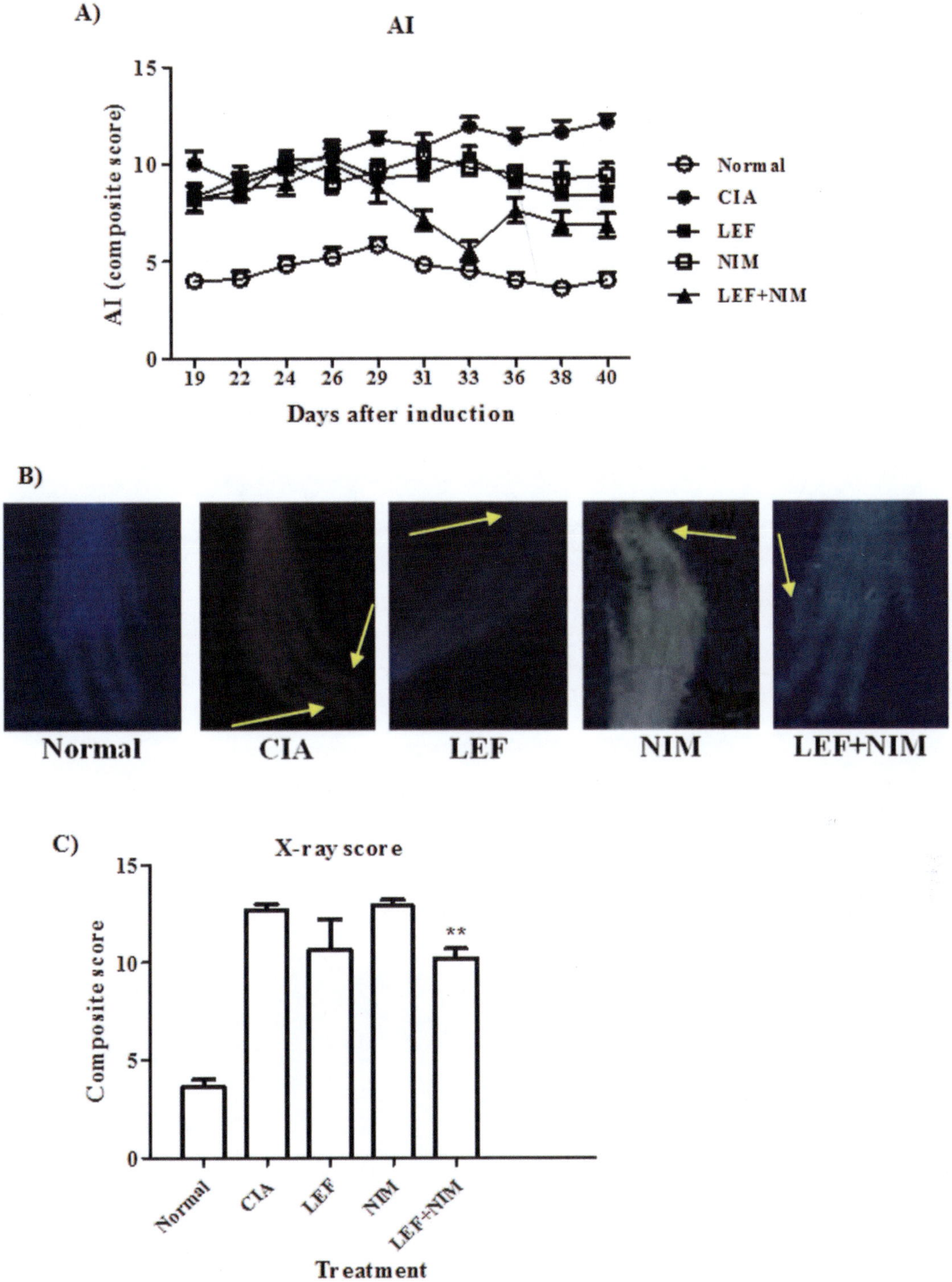

Figure 2. Assessment of disease progression. Mice with CIA were treated with leflunomide (LEF: ■), nimesulide (NIM: □), or leflunomide+ nimesulide (LEF+NIM: ▲) and compared to untreated arthritic (○) and normal mice (●). Arthritic index (AI) of mice was recorded over the duration of 40 days (A). Hind paws of mice were x-ray imaged at day 40 (B) and given a radiological score (C) as shown in the methods section. Data are presented as mean ± SD. ** Significantly different from CIA-mice.

The enhancement effect of nimesulide to leflunomide was further examined histopathologically. Nimesulide alone, significantly blunted the neutrophilic infiltration within joints of mice with CIA as shown by decreased MPO to almost normal levels. MPO is an enzyme known to be highly abundant to the azurophilic granules of neutrophils [33]. The role of neutrophil involvement in CIA and joint damage is well established. Yet, the anti-chemotaxis effect of nimesulide might partly explain the synergistic interaction with leflunomide in terms of disease progression [25,34].

Table 1. Detailed radiographic evaluation of articular damage.

Treatment group	CIA-group	LEF-group	NIM-group	LEF+NIM-group
Bone erosion	3.3 ± 0.1	$2.6^{a}\pm0.3$	3.6 ± 0.2	$2^{a,b}\pm0.2$
Cartilage distance	3.4 ± 0.1	$2.6^{a}\pm0.5$	3.1 ± 0.2	$2.9^{a}\pm0.2$
Periostitis	3.2 ± 0.2	3 ± 0.3	3.1 ± 0.2	$2.6^{a,b}\pm0.2$
Joint alignment	2.9 ± 0.1	$2.4^{a}\pm0.3$	3.1 ± 0.2	$2.9^{a}\pm0.3$

Data are presented as mean ± SEM.
n = 10.
a: significantly different from CIA-group at $p<0.05$.
b: significantly different from LEF-group at $p<0.05$.

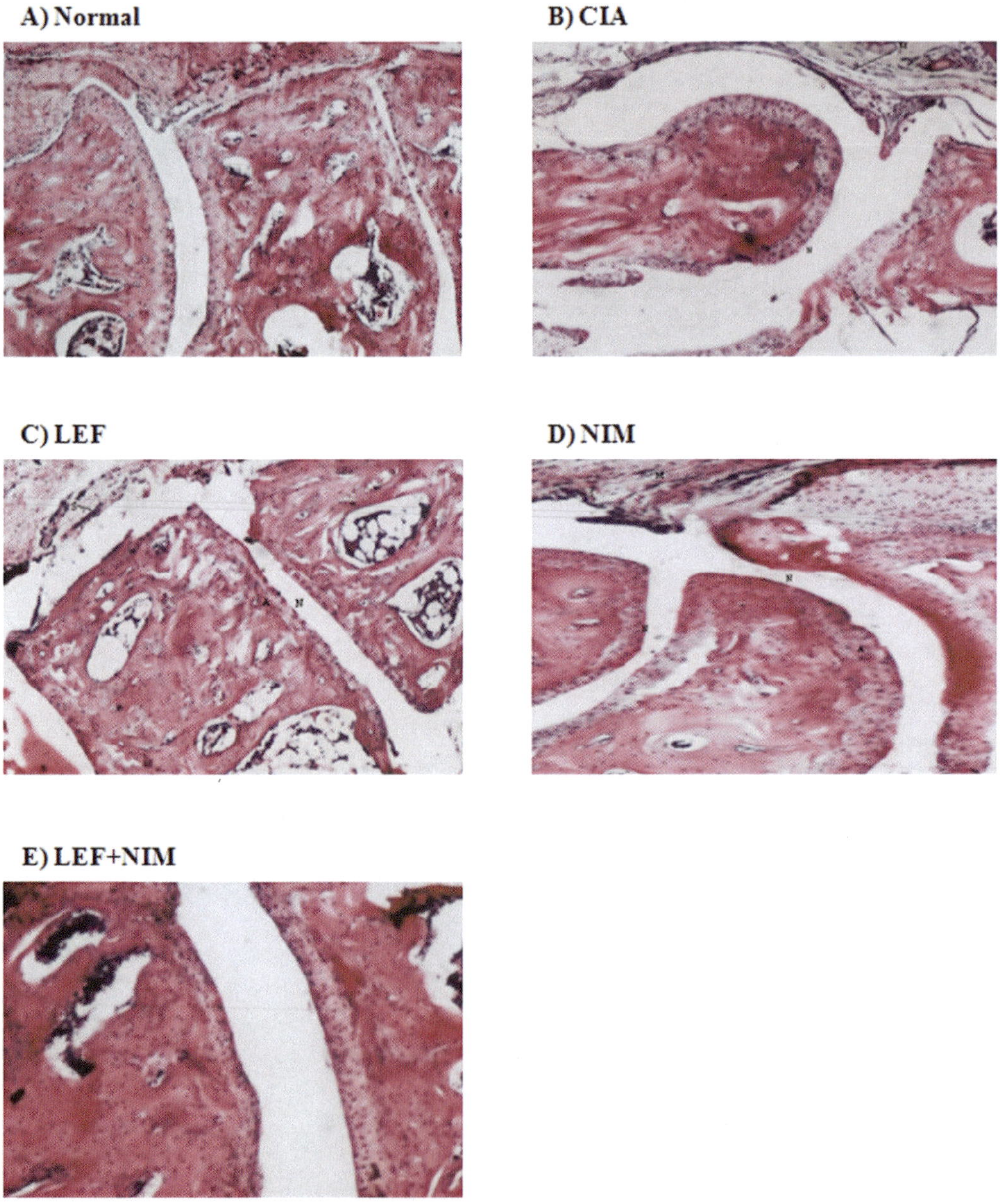

Figure 3. Histopathological assessment of articular damage. Mice with CIA were treated with leflunomide (LEF: Panel C), nimesulide (NIM: Panel D), or leflunomide+nimesulide (LEF+NIM: Panel E) for 40 days and the H&E stained joints were compared with untreated arthritic (CIA: Panel B) and normal mice (Panel A). Pathological findings were compared in terms of synovial hyperplasia (S), articular irregularity (A), narrowing of joint space (N), and lymphocytic infiltration (M).

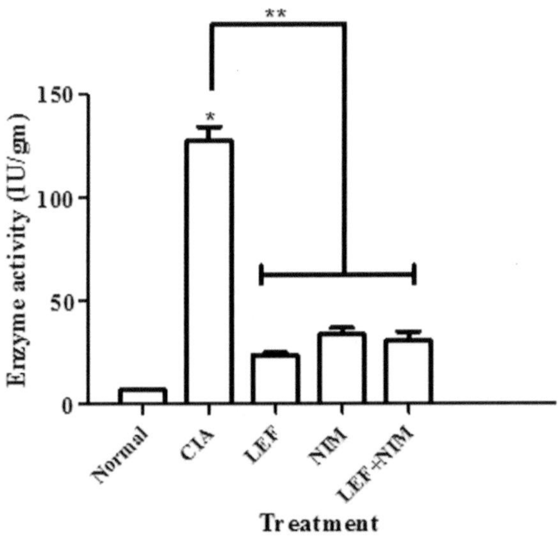

Figure 4. Intra-articular MPO activity. Mice with CIA were treated with leflunomide (LEF), nimesulide (NIM), or leflunomide+nimesulide (LEF+NIM) and compared to untreated arthritic and normal mice. Articular MPO activity was measured 40 days after treatment as a marker of leucocytic infiltration.

Conclusions

Nimesulide enhances the symptomatic, clinical and radiological anti rheumatic activity of Leflunomide in mice with CIA.

Materials and Methods

Chemicals and Drugs

Collagen Type II was prepared as previously described from bovine cartilage [35]. Complete Freund Adjuvant (CFA), leflunomide, hexadecyl trimethylammonium bromide (HTAB), and *o*-dianisidin were purchased from Sigma-Aldrich Chemical Company (St. Louis, MO, USA). Nimesulide was gifted from Alkan Pharmaceutical Co., (6th of October city, Egypt).

Arthritis induction

Male Swiss albino mice (7 weeks old, 30 g weight) were bred in the animal house of the National Research Center (Dokki, Giza, Egypt). Mice were left for one week to acclimatize in the local animal house facility of the Department of Pharmacology prior to experimentation. Animals were kept at controlled environmental conditions with 12 h day/night cycles (20±4°C and 65±10% relative humidity) during the whole experiment. Standardized food pellets and water were supplied *ad libitum*.

Collagen type II solution (4 mg/ml) was prepared by dissolution in 0.1 M acetic acid. Collagen solution was emulsified with an equal volume of CFA. A Volume of 100 µl of final emulsion was injected intradermally (day 0). Only animals with positive signs of arthritis after 2 weeks of induction (87% of animals developed arthritis) were assigned randomly into 5 treatment groups (n = 10 animals/group). After 7 days of the primary induction, another dose (100 µg collagen in CFA) was injected intradermally [36]. The LEF-group received leflunomide 3.75 mg/kg i.p every week; NIM-group received nimesulide 20 mg/kg i.p. every two day; and LEF+NIM-group received leflunomide (3.75 mg/kg i.p) every week and nimesulide (20 mg/kg i.p.) daily. All treatments started 7 days after induction. Treatment groups were compared to mice with CIA (CIA-group) that received no treatment and to a normal non-immunised group (Normal-group).

The Animal Care and Use Committee (IACUC) of the National Research Center (Animal Rights and ethics Committee) approved this complete study.

Assessment of arthritis severity

Arthritic index (AI) was recorded as previously described [37]. Briefly, mice paws were inspected every other day and AI was scored in each paw as follows: erythema and slight swelling in a single digit is given 0.5; erythema and slight swelling in two or more digits is given 1; erythend ma mild swelling in the whole limb is given 2; 3 = erythema and gross swelling in the whole limb is given 3; limb disability and massive limb deformity is given 4. Composite AI equals the sum of each animal's four paws. AI scores were assessed blindly by 2 independent observers starting 2 days before the primary induction of arthritis until the end of the experiment.

Assessment of articular hyperalgesia

Articular hyperalgesia was measured by Hargreaves method with minor in-house modifications [38]; briefly, mice were let to adapt in a designated chamber of planter test (Ugo Basile, Comerio, Italy) for 30 min. Inflamed joints were irradiated with an IR-beam from a movable bulb (Ugo Basile, Comerio, Italy) to induce algesia. The time taken for each animal to lick/withdraw IR-challenged limb was recorded and designated as withdrawal latency (WDL) [39]. The base-line for articular hyperalgesia was determined (2 days before the primary induction of arthritis) and compared to pre-arthritic phase (10 days after the primary induction of arthritis); mid-arthritic phase (25 days after the primary induction of arthritis); and late-arthritic phase (40 days after the primary induction of arthritis).

Assessment of joint stiffness

Joint stiffness was correlated to the locomotor activity of animlas and measured using open field activity cage method. As previously described [39], animals were left for five minutes in the grid floor activity cage (Ugo Basile, Comerio, Italy). The animals' movements with their paws were converted into electric signals and the number of movements per minute was recorded. The base-line for locomotor activity was recorded (2 days before the primary induction of arthritis) and compared to pre-arthritic phase (10 days after the primary induction of arthritis); mid-arthritic phase (25 days after induction); and late-arthritic phase (40 days after the primary induction of arthritis).

Determination of myeloperoxidase enzyme activity

MPO activity was determined in paws at the late-arthritic phase (40 days after the primary induction of arthritis) as previously described [40]. Briefly, mice were sacrificed; paws were immediately excised, weighed and rapidly homogenized for 15 minutes (0.5% hexadecyl trimethylammonuim bromide (HTAB) in 50 mM phosphate buffer, pH 6). Articular tissue homogenate (10% w/v) was centrifuged and 2.9 ml *o*-dianisidin (0.167 mg/ml) was added to 100 µL of the clear supernatant. Hydrogen peroxide (0.0005%) was finally added and absorbance was measured every 15 sec for 2 min (λ_{max} 460 nm). The rate of absorbance change was used to calculate the MPO activity per gram tissue (Molar absorbtivity of the color adduct is 1.13×10^4). [33].

X-rays analysis

Radiological assessment for joint damage was undertaken by X-ray imaging at the late-arthritic phase. Briefly, mice were sacrificed; anterior and hind limbs were excised and fixed in 10% buffered formalin solution. Paws were placed on an X-ray cassette (Medivance Instrument Limited, London, UK) and X-ray images were taken at 40 KV, 0.04 mA sec (Pioneer road-S-240 Salt Lake city, UT, USA). Radiological assessment for joint damage was performed as previously described [41]. Briefly, each limb's X-ray film was scored from 0–4 (4 is the worst) with respect to joint alignment, cartilage distance, bone erosion, and periostitis. The composite scores of each X-ray image represent the total radiological score. Each film was assessed blindly by 3 different observers [42].

Histopathological examination

Histological assessment for articular tissues was performed as follows. Paraformaldhyde fixed tissues were decalcified by EDTA and embedded in paraffin wax. Cross sagittal sections (5 μm) were obtained and after dewaxing and rehydration, sections were stained with H&E.

Statistical analysis

Data are presented as average ± SEM. Significance was tested using ANOVA) with LSD post hoc test was used for testing the significance of parametric data. Significance of non-parametric data was determined using the Mann-Whitney U test. All statistical calculations were carried out by SPSS software for windows, version 17.0.0.; $P<0.05$ was taken as the cut off value for significance.

Author Contributions

Conceived and designed the experiments: AMA WIE ROW ABA. Performed the experiments: AMA WIE ROW AAN. Analyzed the data: AMA FAA AEK AAN ABA. Contributed reagents/materials/analysis tools: FAA SMN AEK ROW. Wrote the paper: AMA AAN ABA. Fund raising: FAA.

References

1. Helmick CG, Felson DT, Lawrence RC, Gabriel S, Hirsch R, et al. (2008) Estimates of the prevalence of arthritis and other rheumatic conditions in the United States. Part I. Arthritis Rheum 58: 15–25.
2. Weinblatt ME (1996) Rheumatoid arthritis: treat now, not later! Ann Intern Med 124: 773–774.
3. Pincus T, O'Dell JR, Kremer JM (1999) Combination therapy with multiple disease-modifying antirheumatic drugs in rheumatoid arthritis: a preventive strategy. Ann Intern Med 131: 768–774.
4. Falgarone G, Semerano L, Rulle S, Boissier MC (2009) Targeting lymphocyte activation to treat rheumatoid arthritis. Joint Bone Spine 76: 327–332.
5. Wiens A, Correr CJ, Pontarolo R, Venson R, Quinalha JV, et al. (2009) A systematic review and meta-analysis of the efficacy and safety of etanercept for treating rheumatoid arthritis. Scand J Immunol 70: 337–344.
6. Bracewell C, Isaacs JD, Emery P, Ng WF (2009) Atacicept, a novel B cell-targeting biological therapy for the treatment of rheumatoid arthritis. Expert Opin Biol Ther 9: 909–919.
7. Khalil NA, Ahmed EM, El-Nassan HB, Ahmed OK, Al-Abd AM (2012) Synthesis and biological evaluation of novel pyrazoline derivatives as anti-inflammatory and antioxidant agents. Arch Pharm Res 35: 995–1002.
8. Schipper LG, Kievit W, den Broeder AA, van der Laar MA, Adang EM, et al. (2011) Treatment strategies aiming at remission in early rheumatoid arthritis patients: starting with methotrexate monotherapy is cost-effective. Rheumatology (Oxford) 50: 1320–1330.
9. Benucci M, Li Gobbi F, Sabadini L, Saviola G, Baiardi P, et al. (2009) The economic burden of biological therapy in rheumatoid arthritis in clinical practice: cost-effectiveness analysis of sub-cutaneous anti-TNFalpha treatment in Italian patients. Int J Immunopathol Pharmacol 22: 1147–1152.
10. Bartlett RR, Brendel S, Zielinski T, Schorlemmer HU (1996) Leflunomide, an immunorestoring drug for the therapy of autoimmune disorders, especially rheumatoid arthritis. Transplant Proc 28: 3074–3078.
11. Rozman B (2002) Clinical pharmacokinetics of leflunomide. Clin Pharmacokinet 41: 421–430.
12. Fox RI (1998) Mechanism of action of leflunomide in rheumatoid arthritis. J Rheumatol Suppl 53: 20–26.
13. Dimitrova P, Skapenko A, Herrmann ML, Schleyerbach R, Kalden JR, et al. (2002) Restriction of de novo pyrimidine biosynthesis inhibits Th1 cell activation and promotes Th2 cell differentiation. J Immunol 169: 3392–3399.
14. Fox RI, Herrmann ML, Frangou CG, Wahl GM, Morris RE, et al. (1999) Mechanism of action for leflunomide in rheumatoid arthritis. Clin Immunol 93: 198–208.
15. Kent EF Jr., Crawford J, Cohen HJ, Buckley RH (1990) Development of multiple monoclonal serum immunoglobulins (multiclonal gammopathy) following both HLA-identical unfractionated and T cell-depleted haploidentical bone marrow transplantation in severe combined immunodeficiency. J Clin Immunol 10: 106–114.
16. Hamilton LC, Vojnovic I, Warner TD (1999) A771726, the active metabolite of leflunomide, directly inhibits the activity of cyclo-oxygenase-2 in vitro and in vivo in a substrate-sensitive manner. Br J Pharmacol 127: 1589–1596.
17. Burger D, Begue-Pastor N, Benavent S, Gruaz L, Kaufmann MT, et al. (2003) The active metabolite of leflunomide, A77 1726, inhibits the production of prostaglandin E(2), matrix metalloproteinase 1 and interleukin 6 in human fibroblast-like synoviocytes. Rheumatology (Oxford) 42: 89–96.
18. Cao WW, Kao PN, Aoki Y, Xu JC, Shorthouse RA, et al. (1996) A novel mechanism of action of the immunomodulatory drug, leflunomide: augmentation of the immunosuppressive cytokine, TGF-beta 1, and suppression of the immunostimulatory cytokine, IL-2. Transplant Proc 28: 3079–3080.
19. Sengupta S (1998) Cyclooxygenase-2: a new therapeutic target. Indian J pharmacology 31: 322–332.
20. Bevilacqua M, Vago T, Baldi G, Renesto E, Dallegri F, et al. (1994) Nimesulide decreases superoxide production by inhibiting phosphodiesterase type IV. Eur J Pharmacol 268: 415–423.
21. Pelletier JP, Martel-Pelletier J (1993) Effects of nimesulide and naproxen on the degradation and metalloprotease synthesis of human osteoarthritic cartilage. Drugs 46 Suppl 1: 34–39.
22. Al-Abd AM, Inglis JJ, Nofal SM, Khalifa AE, Williams RO, et al. (2010) Nimesulide improves the disease modifying anti-rheumatic profile of methotrexate in mice with collagen-induced arthritis. Eur J Pharmacol 644: 245–250.
23. Walker-Bone K, Farrow S (2007) Rheumatoid arthritis. Clin Evid (Online) 2007.
24. Capecchi PL, Ceccatelli L, Beermann U, Laghi Pasini F, Di Perri T (1993) Inhibition of neutrophil function in vitro by nimesulide. Preliminary evidence of an adenosine-mediated mechanism. Arzneimittelforschung 43: 992–996.
25. Tool AT, Mul FP, Knol EF, Verhoeven AJ, Roos D (1996) The effect of salmeterol and nimesulide on chemotaxis and synthesis of PAF and LTC4 by human eosinophils. Eur Respir J Suppl 22: 141s–145s.
26. Ramiro S, Radner H, van der Heijde D, van Tubergen A, Buchbinder R, et al. (2011) Combination therapy for pain management in inflammatory arthritis (rheumatoid arthritis, ankylosing spondylitis, psoriatic arthritis, other spondyloarthritis). Cochrane Database Syst Rev: CD008886.
27. Inotai A, Meszaros A (2012) Determinants of NSAID choice in rheumatoid arthritis–a drug utilization study. Acta Pol Pharm 69: 773–777.
28. da Costa Araujo FA, de Santana Santos T, de Morais HH, Laureano Filho JR, de Oliveira ESED, et al. (2012) Comparative analysis of preemptive analgesic effect of tramadol chlorhydrate and nimesulide following third molar surgery. J Craniomaxillofac Surg 40: e346–349.
29. Coulthard LG, Costello J, Robinson B, Shiels IA, Taylor SM, et al. (2011) Comparative efficacy of a secretory phospholipase A2 inhibitor with conventional anti-inflammatory agents in a rat model of antigen-induced arthritis. Arthritis Res Ther 13: R42.
30. Curnock AP, Robson PA, Yea CM, Moss D, Gadher S, et al. (1997) Potencies of leflunomide and HR325 as inhibitors of prostaglandin endoperoxide H synthase-1 and -2: comparison with nonsteroidal anti-inflammatory drugs. J Pharmacol Exp Ther 282: 339–347.
31. Joosten LA, Helsen MM, Saxne T, van De Loo FA, Heinegard D, et al. (1999) IL-1 alpha beta blockade prevents cartilage and bone destruction in murine type II collagen-induced arthritis, whereas TNF-alpha blockade only ameliorates joint inflammation. J Immunol 163: 5049–5055.
32. Williams RO (1998) Combination therapy in mice: what can we learn that may be useful for understanding rheumatoid arthritis? Springer Semin Immunopathol 20: 165–180.
33. Bradley PP, Priebat DA, Christensen RD, Rothstein G (1982) Measurement of cutaneous inflammation: estimation of neutrophil content with an enzyme marker. J Invest Dermatol 78: 206–209.
34. de Mello SB, Laurindo IM, Cossermelli W (1994) Action of the 4-nitro-2-phenoximethanesulphonanilide (nimesulide) on neutrophil chemotaxis and superoxide production. Sao Paulo Med J 112: 489–494.
35. Miller EJ, Rhodes RK (1982) Preparation and characterization of the different types of collagen. Methods Enzymol 82 Pt A: 33–64.
36. Cook AD, Braine EL, Campbell IK, Rich MJ, Hamilton JA (2001) Blockade of collagen-induced arthritis post-onset by antibody to granulocyte-macrophage

colony-stimulating factor (GM-CSF): requirement for GM-CSF in the effector phase of disease. Arthritis Res 3: 293–298.

37. Urakawa K, Mihara M, Suzuki T, Kawamura A, Akamatsu K, et al. (2000) Polyglutamation of antifolates is not required for induction of extracellular release of adenosine or expression of their anti-inflammatory effects. Immunopharmacology 48: 137–144.

38. Hargreaves K, Dubner R, Brown F, Flores C, Joris J (1988) A new and sensitive method for measuring thermal nociception in cutaneous hyperalgesia. Pain 32: 77–88.

39. Chillingworth NL, Donaldson LF (2003) Characterisation of a Freund's complete adjuvant-induced model of chronic arthritis in mice. J Neurosci Methods 128: 45–52.

40. McVey DC, Vigna SR (2001) The capsaicin VR1 receptor mediates substance P release in toxin A-induced enteritis in rats. Peptides 22: 1439–1446.

41. Clark RL, Cuttino JT Jr., Anderle SK, Cromartie WJ, Schwab JH (1979) Radiologic analysis of arthritis in rats after systemic injection of streptococcal cell walls. Arthritis Rheum 22: 25–35.

42. Asanuma Y, Nagai K, Kato M, Sugiura H, Kawai S (2002) Weekly pulse therapy of methotrexate improves survival compared with its daily administration in MRL/lpr mice. Eur J Pharmacol 435: 253–258.

Methadone Induction in Primary Care for Opioid Dependence: A Pragmatic Randomized Trial (ANRS Methaville)

Patrizia Maria Carrieri[1,2,3]*, Laurent Michel[4,5,6], Caroline Lions[1,2,3], Julien Cohen[1,2,3], Muriel Vray[7,8], Marion Mora[1,2,3], Fabienne Marcellin[1,2,3], Bruno Spire[1,2,3], Alain Morel[9], Perrine Roux[1,2,3] and the Methaville Study Group[¶]

1 INSERM UMR912 (SESSTIM), Marseille, France, **2** Aix Marseille Université, UMR_S912, Marseille, France, **3** ORS PACA, Observatoire Régional de la Santé Provence Alpes Côte d'Azur, Marseille, France, **4** INSERM, Research Unit 669, Paris, France, **5** Univ Paris-Sud and Univ Paris Descartes, UMR-S0669, Paris, France, **6** Centre Pierre Nicole, Paris, France, **7** Unité de Recherche et d'Expertise en Epidémiologie des Maladies Emergentes, Institut Pasteur, Paris, France, **8** Institut National de la Santé et de la Recherche Médicale (INSERM), Paris, France, **9** Oppelia, Paris, France

Abstract

Objective: Methadone coverage is poor in many countries due in part to methadone induction being possible only in specialized care (SC). This multicenter pragmatic trial compared the effectiveness of methadone treatment between two induction models: primary care (PC) and SC.

Methods: In this study, registered at ClinicalTrials.Gov (NCT00657397), opioid-dependent individuals not on methadone treatment for at least one month or receiving buprenorphine but needing to switch were randomly assigned to start methadone in PC (N = 155) or in SC (N = 66) in 10 sites in France. Visits were scheduled at months M0, M3, M6 and M12. The primary outcome was self-reported abstinence from street-opioids at 12 months (M12) (with an underlying 15% non-inferiority hypothesis for PC). Secondary outcomes were abstinence during follow-up, engagement in treatment (i.e. completing the induction period), retention and satisfaction with the explanations provided by the physician. Primary analysis used intention to treat (ITT). Mixed models and the log-rank test were used to assess the arm effect (PC vs. SC) on the course of abstinence and retention, respectively.

Results: In the ITT analysis (n = 155 in PC, 66 in SC), which compared the proportions of street-opioid abstinent participants, 85/155 (55%) and 22/66 (33%) of the participants were classified as street-opioid abstinent at M12 in PC and SC, respectively. This ITT analysis showed the non-inferiority of PC (21.5 [7.7; 35.3]). Engagement in treatment and satisfaction with the explanations provided by the physician were significantly higher in PC than SC. Retention in methadone and abstinence during follow-up were comparable in both arms (p = 0.47, p = 0.39, respectively).

Conclusions: Under appropriate conditions, methadone induction in primary care is feasible and acceptable to both physicians and patients. It is as effective as induction in specialized care in reducing street-opioid use and ensuring engagement and retention in treatment for opioid dependence.

Trial registration: Number Eudract 2008-001338-28; ClinicalTrials.gov: NCT00657397; International Standard Randomized Controlled Trial Number Register ISRCTN31125511

Editor: John E. Mendelson, California Pacific Medical Center Research Institute, United States of America

Funding: The study received external funding by the French National Agency for Research on Aids and Viral Hepatitis (ANRS) and the French Ministry of Health. The funders had no role in study design, data collection and analysis, decision to publish, or preparation of the manuscript.

Competing Interests: The authors have declared that no competing interests exist.

* Email: pmcarrieri@aol.com

¶ Membership of the Methaville Study Group is provided in the Acknowledgments.

Introduction

Methadone is included in the WHO list of essential medicines thanks to its effectiveness in treating opioid dependence, preventing HIV [1] and improving adherence to antiretroviral treatment in HIV-infected individuals [2]. Despite this, access to methadone remains limited because of the risk of overdose during induction, especially in countries where the need for methadone is even greater.

While access to buprenorphine in primary care has been possible since 1996 thanks to its safety profile [3,4], methadone induction in France, as in most countries, is currently possible only in specialized centers caring for substance dependence (located in *ad hoc* sites or in hospitals) (hereafter specialized care or SC). In France these centers can refer patients to PC only after the end of methadone induction, i.e. when methadone doses are stabilized (after at least 14 days).

The specific model of care for regulating methadone induction can greatly influence its safety as the risk of overdose during the induction phase remains a major concern. Internationally, the regulations governing the extent to which methadone induction (i.e. until dosage stabilization) is authorized in primary care (PC) differ considerably. For example, methadone induction in PC is legal in the UK, in Switzerland and in Canada under different models of care. In contrast, France, the United States but also other countries have no such system currently in place.

This means that in the many geographic areas underserved by SC, opioid-dependent individuals seeking treatment have no access to methadone. To tackle this situation, one of the objectives of the French public health authorities' national strategic plan for prevention and care of Hepatitis was to consider using primary care as an entry point for methadone treatment, based on the results of a pragmatic trial. The trial, entitled Methaville, was designed both to evaluate the feasibility of methadone induction in PC and to compare outcomes in participants randomized into PC induction with those randomized into SC induction. Being a pragmatic trial, the objectives were to verify the feasibility and acceptability of the PC induction model to physicians and patients, and also to show that the main patient outcome (street-opioid abstinence after one year of treatment) and secondary outcomes (abstinence during follow-up, engagement in treatment, retention in treatment and satisfaction with the explanations provided by the physician) were all comparable between both induction arms.

Methods

The protocol for this trial and supporting CONSORT checklist are available as Checklist S1 and English protocol S1.

Ethics

The Methaville ANRS trial is registered with the French Agency of Pharmaceutical Products (AFSSAPS) under the number 2008-A0277-48, the European Union Drug Regulating Authorities Clinical Trials: Number Eudract 2008-001338-28, the ClinicalTrials.gov Identifier: NCT00657397 and the International Standard Randomized Controlled Trial Number Register ISRCTN31125511. The study protocol was approved by the Ethics Committee of Persons Protection in Paris, France. All individuals provided written, informed consent before participating in the study.

Physicians and Participants

In this multicenter, pragmatic, randomized trial, for each study site we selected an SC physician and nearby PC physicians who already had field experience in care for opioid dependence and/or training in care for drug dependence, and who were willing to participate. Only PC physicians with patients potentially eligible for enrollment in the study were selected because if methadone induction in PC is officially adopted in France in the future, only PC physicians meeting the above criteria will be targeted by authorities as methadone prescribers. Ten sites in four geographic areas (North, North-Eastern, South-Western and South-Eastern France) were included, with each site having at least one SC and one PC physician. These four geographical areas were chosen to better target the different types of populations who would benefit from access to methadone in primary care, as each geographical area is characterized by different drug markets and drug user practices/needs. Physicians (in PC and SC) enrolled opioid-dependent individuals who were randomized to start methadone either in PC or in SC.

Inclusion criteria were chosen to target a population representative of drug users needing/seeking methadone treatment in France as follows: aged over 18 years old, seeking care for opioid dependence and not prescribed methadone for at least one month or receiving buprenorphine but needing to switch to methadone for medical reasons (side effects, treatment misuse, etc.). Non-inclusion criteria were similar to those in other studies involving methadone prescription in PC [5,6] as follows: could not be reached by phone for an interview and screening positive for opioids/benzodiazepines/alcohol triple co-dependence, as assessed by the MINI [7] (as this condition exposed participants to a high risk of overdose [8,9]) and finally, for women, being pregnant.

Study design

The first visit took place when a patient seeking care for opioid dependence or needing to switch treatment from buprenorphine to methadone went to see a PC or SC physician participating in the trial. After providing consent to participate the patient was randomized into the PC or SC arm by this physician. To make patient randomization feasible, each site had one SC with at least one PC physician in the nearby vicinity. All PC and SC physicians involved underwent a one-day training course both to standardize methadone induction practices according to trial guidelines and to acquaint them with trial procedures [10]. Trial guidelines stipulated that the starting dose should be on average 30 mg and not exceed 40 mg, with 10 mg increases every 2–4 days thereafter until dose stabilization. This is comparable to methadone induction protocols used in other trials [5,11].

The "intervention" provided by trained physicians consisted in at least fourteen-day supervised methadone induction either in PC or in SC according to trial guidelines (Table 1). Thereafter, supervision was required only for patients who were deemed to be at risk of overdose. One main difference between both arms in the model of care was that delays in initiating treatment were more common in SC (see Table 1).

Participants were also followed up over one year through medical visits and phone interviews at months 0 (M0, enrolment), at 3, 6 and 12 months (M3, M6 and M12, respectively).

To emulate current care practices in France, patients could choose to change arm after the induction phase, i.e. SC physicians could refer their patient to a PC colleague who would prescribe methadone and vice versa. Accordingly, arm changes (PC to SC or SC to PC) were not considered as deviations from the protocol. Further details and the pre-trial phase of the protocol are described elsewhere [10].

Data sources and outcomes

The following 5 sources provided study data: a pre-enrollment medical questionnaire, a medical questionnaire at each scheduled visit (enrolment (M0), months 3, 6 and 12, respectively M3, M6 and M12), a short self-administered questionnaire (completed during scheduled visits), a Computer Assisted Telephone Interview (CATI) (conducted just after each scheduled visit) lasting no more than 30 minutes, and when available, urine rapid tests [10].

Abstinence from street-opioids at M12 was chosen as the primary outcome. Abstinence during the course of treatment, engagement in treatment, retention in methadone maintenance

Table 1. Features of the PC and SC model of care for methadone treatment (ANRS Methaville trial).

Methaville model for Primary Care (PC)	Current Methadone model for specialized care (SC)
• During induction, methadone intake is delivered and supervised daily at the pharmacy (with take home doses only for the weekend). Supervision is compulsory during induction.	• During induction, methadone is delivered daily at the center by the physician, the pharmacist or the nurse or is delivered at the pharmacy (with take home doses only for the weekend). Supervision is compulsory during induction.
• Psychosocial and health status assessment is not a necessary condition to start methadone – referral to specialized center if needed.	• It is recommended that Methadone induction is started after initial visits/interviews carried out by different members of health staff:
	a) A social counselor and/or a psychologist to obtain a psychosocial assessment of the patient;
	b) A physician or a nurse to obtain an assessment of the general health of the patient;
	c) An assessment of his/her social rights (health insurance, accommodation, resources, and previous access to care for drug dependence).
• Referral to psychosocial counseling in SC during methadone treatment if needed.	• Psychosocial counseling provided during methadone treatment.
• Methadone prescription possible the same day as the first medical visit.	• Time before methadone prescription may be delayed by some days after the first medical visit, depending on patient's conditions (withdrawal syndromes, pregnancy, etc.).
• Doses are prescribed according to Methaville guidelines.	• Doses are prescribed according to Methaville guidelines.
• Doses are reassessed at every medical visit (i.e. every 2–3 days) during induction.	• Doses are reassessed at every medical visit (i.e. every 2–3 days) during induction.
• Urine analyses at first dose prescription and monitoring once/twice a week during induction.	• Urine analyses at first dose prescription and monitoring once/twice a week during induction.

treatment and patient satisfaction with the explanations provided by the physician were secondary outcomes. The primary outcome, abstinence from street opioids during the previous month, was measured using a validated question [12], administered during phone interviews by trained non-judgmental staff. This question was also answered in the medical interviews at enrolment, M3, M6 and M12.

Methadone dose was defined as the number of mg/day of methadone prescribed by the physician for each patient at each medical visit.

Engagement in treatment was computed in those randomized to each specific arm as the proportion of patients who actually started methadone and remained in the trial until the stabilization of dosages (i.e. until the end of induction). Follow-up participation rates, i.e. participants who continued participating in study interviews until M12, were computed for each arm.

Retention in methadone maintenance treatment was defined, only for patients who actually started methadone treatment, as the time between the first day of methadone induction and the last known date that the patient was still receiving treatment. For individuals still on methadone at M12, retention was set at 12 months.

A 5-point Likert scale measured patient satisfaction with the explanations provided by his/her prescribing physician during CATI at M6 only. This outcome was then dichotomized (very satisfied vs. other).

There were three main reasons to justify the choice to use patient self-reported street-opioid use as the primary outcome. The first reason was to avoid introducing measures which would not reflect routine practices in the field of care for drug dependence in France (for example neither urine tests nor hair analysis are routinely performed). These alternative measures would have been negatively affected by several missing values. Furthermore, any cases with complete values would most likely have been biased, as urine testing is currently performed at the discretion of the physician if he/she is doubtful about patients' drug use. The second one was to place the patient at the center of the study and consider his/her self-reported experience with treatment (satisfaction with the explanations provided by the physician) as a major outcome. This choice reflects the work in other trials involving drug users and in other fields of medicine where patient's reported outcomes are considered as main outcome measures [13,14]. Third, patient self-reports are valid as PC physicians rely on them in clinical practice [15].

We chose the endpoint at M12 for the trial phase on the basis that any comparison between arms would not be significant enough immediately after the induction phase or indeed at M3, and that any possible benefit could be confirmed after one year of treatment.

The outcomes used in this pragmatic trial were those typically used in trials assessing the efficacy of a treatment for opioid dependence [5,6]. The only difference here is that they were used to assess methadone effectiveness (and not efficacy) by induction arm.

Safety issues

To ensure safety during induction, we implemented a wide range of strategies minimizing overdose risk in the trial's model of care, including a one-day training session for PC physicians, strict supervision of participants when they took their doses at the pharmacy during treatment initiation, and fostering strong collaboration between all the health professionals involved in the study, including pharmacists (shared-care model) [16]. The non-inclusion of patients with triple co-dependence (alcohol-opioid-benzodiazepine) [8,9] does not constitute a restrictive criterion and reflects standard practice for safety concerns. Methadone initiation in these patients is possible only after benzodiazepine detoxification.

Pharmacists and physicians involved in the trial had to signal overdoses, signs of intoxication and lost-to-follow-up patients to the center of methodology and management (CMM) (ORS PACA- INSERM-IRD UMR912). The latter was required to notify any severe adverse event, such as an overdose, to the French

National Agency for Research on Aids and Viral Hepatitis (ANRS) which in turn notified the French Agency of Pharmaceutical Products (ANSM).

A list of 50 health-related symptoms included in the questionnaire helped document self-reported symptoms during follow-up.

Statistical considerations

Sample size. Although retention in treatment is the most important outcome in patients receiving treatment for opioid dependence [17] and even more important in the context of decision-making by public health authorities, this trial was funded for HCV prevention purposes with opioid abstinence being considered the most pertinent primary outcome. It was therefore designed with an underlying hypothesis of non-inferiority in terms of the proportion of PC-inducted patients who were abstinent from street-opioids at 12 months (M12) of methadone treatment with respect to their SC counterparts.

The study hypothesis was that after one year of treatment, the proportion of patients abstinent from street-opioids would be 70% [18,19] for SC. Selecting an inferiority margin of 15 for patients starting methadone in PC entailed recruiting a minimum of 150 patients in order to show the non-inferiority, if any, of the PC arm for the primary outcome.

The choice of this margin reflected our willingness to accept decreased effectiveness in PC in return for increased attractiveness and engagement in PC treatment.

Randomization and masking. Randomization of patients was performed centrally by the study's methodology and data management center (ORS PACA- INSERM-IRD UMR912), via a secured intranet site, by simple random sampling with no block control on randomization rate. Information about patient randomization was confidentially stored and hidden from the study research team - except statisticians and the data manager - until the end of the last M12 interview, in December 2011. A randomization ratio 2:1 (PC: SC) was chosen to deliberately over-represent patients followed-up in PC to increase the probability of detecting possible intoxications in PC during induction.

Statistical analysis. Medians and interquartile ranges (IQR) and proportions were used to describe the distributions of continuous and categorical variables, respectively. Distributions of variables among the two groups were compared using Mann-Whitney U test for continuous variables, Chi-Squared or Fisher exact test for categorical variables.

The primary analysis used intention-to-treat (ITT) ($n = 221$) and the primary outcome was measured using a validated question [12] about opioid use during the previous month collected by CATI or medical interview (when CATI data was incomplete). The difference between both arms in the proportion of patients reporting abstinence from street-opioids during the previous month at M12 and the related 95% confidence interval (95% CI) were computed. In this ITT analysis all patients who discontinued follow-up before M12 for any reason (i.e. refused to start methadone after randomization or discontinued follow-up for any reason including treatment interruption, lost to follow-up, incarceration etc.) were classified as "failure" i.e. street-opioid users (see Fig. 1).

A "*per protocol*" analysis was also conducted only on individuals still followed-up at month 12 ($n = 162$).

Participants still followed up at M12 but with missing values for OTI (Opiate Treatment Index) at M12 were also classified as street-opioid users in both the ITT and *per protocol* analysis. The ITT classification for those who discontinued follow-up for any reason and for those with missing data is particularly pertinent in this population of opioid-dependent individuals because discontinuation is generally associated with relapse into street-opioid use.

Logistic mixed models assessed the effects of time on methadone and of each arm on the course of abstinence from street-opioids, and took into account whether patients were switching from buprenorphine to methadone at enrolment. Mixed models are currently considered the most appropriate methods to use in clinical trials with missing outcomes, as they meet intention-to-treat criteria [20]. A log-rank test was used to compare Kaplan–Meier curves for retention in treatment among patients who were engaged in treatment, i.e. completed the induction phase ($n = 188$). SAS (v.9.2) and STATA (v.12) statistical software packages were used for the statistical analyses.

Results

Sites and physicians included in the study

Of 12 sites contacted in France, two refused to participate for organizational reasons. The 10 participating sites each included a SC and between 1 to 3 PC physicians in the nearby vicinity. Among the 57 physicians (SC & PC) who agreed to participate, 32 (56%) enrolled at least one patient who met the inclusion criteria. These 32 physicians were significantly different from the other 25 in that they were significantly older ($p = 0.02$) and had more years of medical experience ($p = 0.002$).

Baseline data

The patients included were mainly men (84%), median [IQR] age was 32 [27–38] years and 51% were switching from buprenorphine. Table 2 reports the main patient characteristics for each induction arm.

Patient disposition

From January 2009 to December 2010, the 32 physicians in the 10 trial sites enrolled 221 eligible individuals who were to be followed up for 12 months. The flow of participants through each stage is reported in Figure 1. All participants approached agreed to participate in the trial before randomization. One pregnant woman was excluded.

Among the 221 eligible patients, 66 and 155 were randomly assigned to start methadone in SC and in PC, respectively. However, 18 (27%) and 8 (5%) subsequently refused to be inducted in SC and in PC ($p<0.001$), respectively. These 26 patients were classified as "failure" in the ITT analysis.

Of the 185 who started treatment, 5 SC and 2 PC patients dropped out (discontinued study visits) during induction ($p = 0.026$) (Figure 2) and were also classified as "failure" in the ITT analysis. Ten SC and 16 PC patients discontinued follow-up after induction ($p = 0.13$). They too were classified as "failure" in the ITT analysis.

Overall, 15 (31%) of the 48 SC-inducted patients and 18 (12%) of the 147 PC-inducted patients ($p = 0.0023$) discontinued follow-up. Reasons for discontinuation are reported in Figure 1.

Finally, 33 SC-inducted and 129 PC-inducted patients were present at M12 for the *per protocol* analysis. Data on the primary outcome was missing for four of these individuals (2 in SC and 2 in PC) who were therefore considered opioid users (i.e. "failure") in the ITT and *per protocol* analyses.

Participants who were switching from buprenorphine were older, more likely male, and, most importantly, had a higher abstinence rate from street-opioids (38% vs. 12.5%) and cocaine (78.5% vs. 68%) at baseline, than those who were out of opioid maintenance treatment. However, as these differences were similar

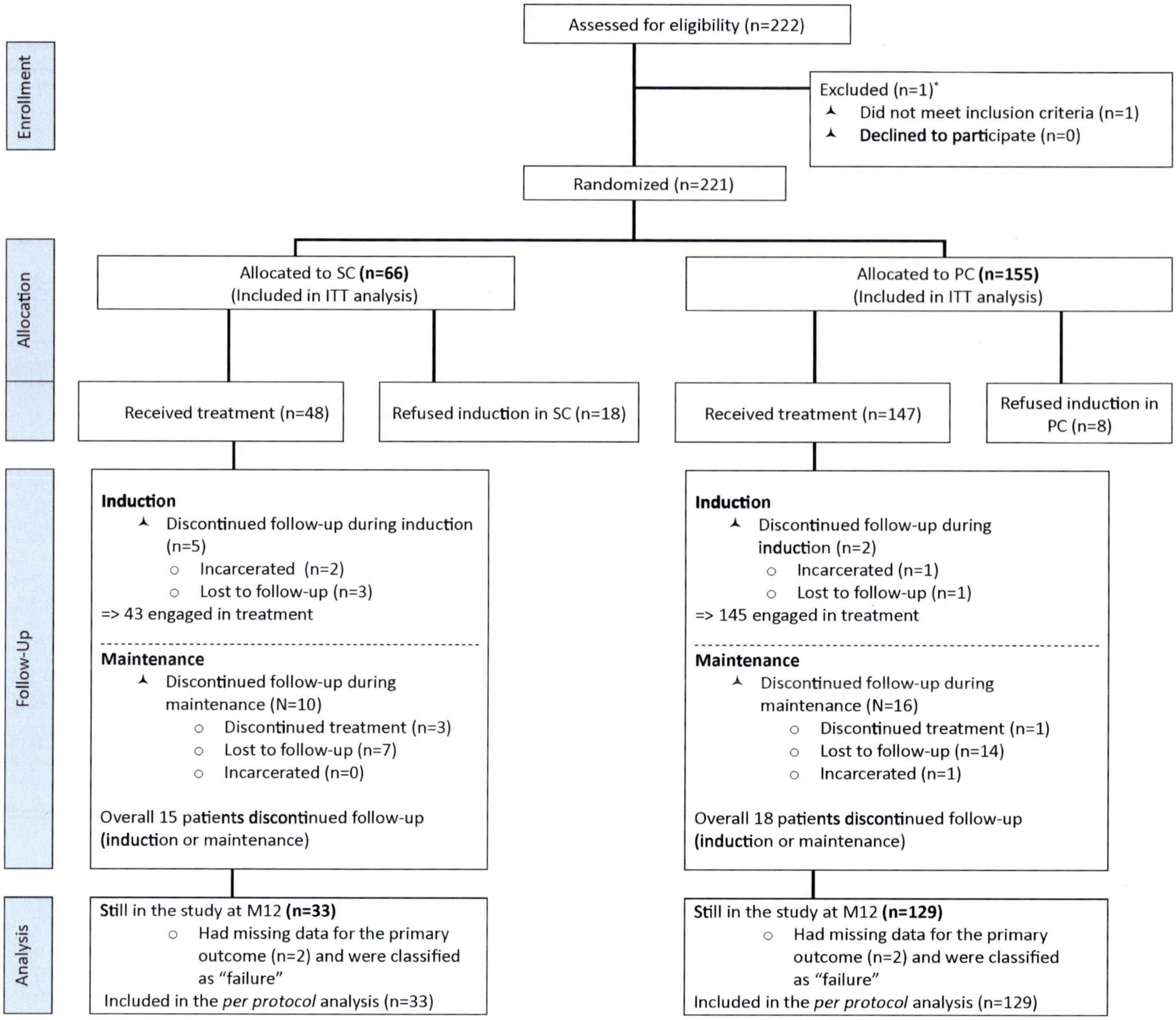

Figure 1. Flow chart of ANRS Methaville trial.

in both induction arms their compatibility in terms of the primary outcome remains unaffected.

Among the 48 SC patients, 18 (14 before M3 and 4 others before M6) changed to PC after induction, while one PC patient changed to SC. Nine patients were re-inducted during the study period after methadone interruption, two of these being re-inducted twice.

Sixty percent of the participants were prescribed methadone doses of between 60 and 80 mg between 11 and 17 days after initiation.

HIV and HCV self-reported prevalence rates were 2% and 19%, respectively.

The end of the study was set for the 1st January 2012 to allow one full year of follow-up for patients enrolled in December 2010.

Outcomes

Primary outcome was street opioid abstinence at 12 months and secondary outcomes: abstinence during follow-up, engagement in treatment, retention in treatment and satisfaction with the explanations provided by the physician.

The rates of participants included in the study and still in treatment at M12 were 129/155 = 83% for PC, 33/66 = 50% for SC and 162/221 = 73% for total sample.

The ITT and *per protocol* analyses reporting the difference in the proportions of street-opioid abstinent participants are described in Table 3. In the former (n = 155 in PC, 66 in SC), 85/155 (55%) and 22/66 (33%) were classified as street-opioid abstinent at M12 in PC and SC, respectively. The ITT analysis demonstrated the non-inferiority of the PC arm: the difference between the percentages of patients abstinent from street-opioids between both arms at M12 and the 95% CI was 21.5 [7.7; 35.3] in favor of PC. Although a *per protocol* analysis is not generally considered suitable in a pragmatic trial [15], it was computed for the sake of performing a comprehensive analysis. As expected, it provided inconclusive results, as the difference between the

Table 2. Patient characteristics by induction arm (SC and PC) at baseline (ANRS Methaville trial).

	SC (n = 48) % or median [IQR]	PC (n = 147) (%) or median [IQR]	Total % or median [IQR]
Gender	21	14	16
Male	79	86	84
Female	21	14	16
Age - *years*	30 [27–39]	32 [27–38]	32 [27–38]
Employment	44	53	51
High school certificate	43	32	35
Living in a couple	33	31	32
Children	33	39	38
Home owner or renter	56	64	62
Living area			
Urban	59	52	54
Suburban	13	26	23
Rural	28	22	23
Switching from buprenorphine	52	51	51
Age at first drug use - *years* (n = 176)	18 [17–21]	18 [17–22]	18 [17–21]
Age at first regular drug use - *years* (n = 160)	20 [18–24]	20 [18–25]	20 [18–24]
History of drug injection (n = 175)	55	47	49
Age at first drug injection (n = 86) – years	22 [20–25]	21 [19–26]	22 [19–26]
Drug injection (n = 162)*	21	14	15
Drug snorting (n = 162)*	74	61	64
Use of street opioids (n = 187)*	79	69	72
Cocaine use (n = 162)*	26	27	27
Use of psychotropic drugs (n = 162)*	13	23	20
Daily cannabis use (n = 176)*	20	17	18
Hazardous alcohol consumption (n = 172)**	33	32	33
Depressive symptoms (n = 170)***	32	41	39
History of suicide attempts (n = 157)	10	18	17
History of drug overdose (n = 188)	12	12	12
HIV+ (n = 152)****	3	2	2
HCV+ (n = 140) ****	18	19	19

*during the previous 4 weeks.
**AUDIT score ≥7 for males and ≥6 for females.
***CES-D score>17 for males and>23 for females.
****among those who had already done a test.

proportions and the non-inferiority margins was −0.8 [−18.8; 17.3], including the inferiority margin of −15.

Mixed models found no significant arm effect (p = 0.39) on abstinence during follow-up, even when adjusting for the switch from buprenorphine treatment. Abstinence from street-opioids significantly increased between enrolment and M3 and remained stable thereafter (Table 4). These results remained valid even after adjusting for a possible heterogeneity effect among sites (i.e. study sites with more than one PC physician versus sites with only one) which was tested as a random effect factor in the mixed models but which was not found to be statistically significant.

Engagement in treatment among those who were randomized only concerned patients who completed the methadone induction phase, i.e. 65% (43/66*100) for SC and 94% (145/155*100) for PC, p<0.001 (Fig. 1)).

When we computed "retention in treatment" we only focused on patients who had in fact started methadone treatment (i.e. 48 in SC and 147 in PC). At M12, thirty-three (33/48*100 = 69%) patients inducted in SC and 129 (129/147*100 = 88%) inducted in PC were still in treatment.

The Kaplan-Meier curves in Fig. 2 show that retention in methadone maintenance treatment was comparable between both induction arms.

Interestingly, PC-inducted patients reported high satisfaction with the explanations provided by their physician more often than their SC-inducted counterparts (p = 0.01).

Prescribed methadone dose during the study

Regarding the median dose of prescribed methadone, there were no significant differences between both arms. The median [IQR] dose of methadone at M12 was 60 [45–90] mg in primary care and 67.5 [50–82.5] mg in specialized care.

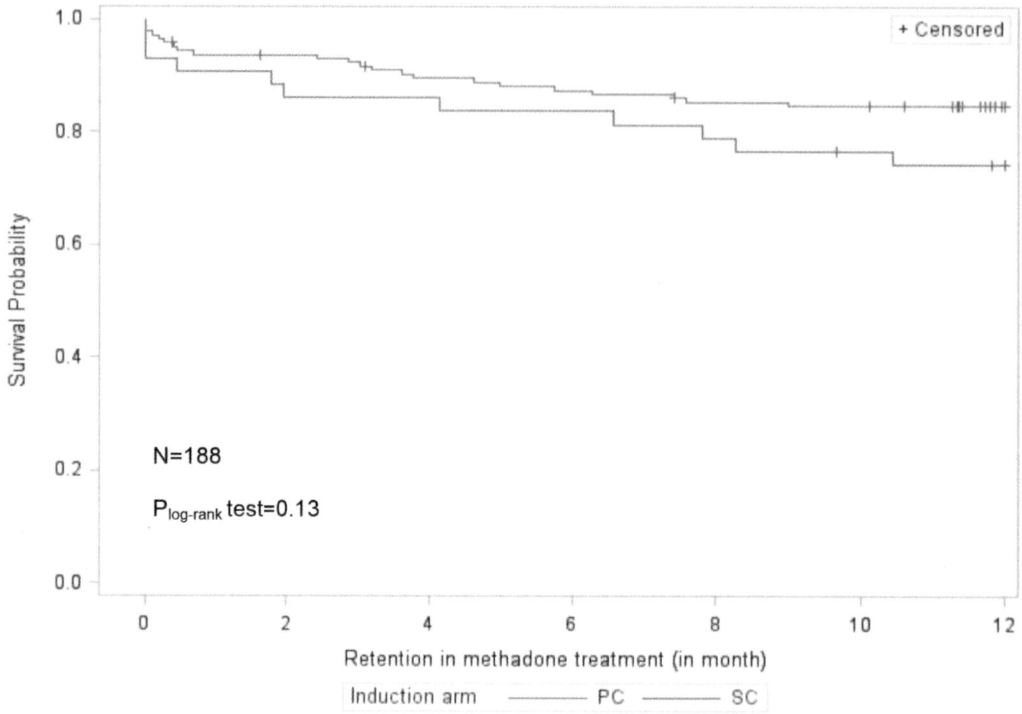

Figure 2. Retention in methadone maintenance treatment in patients (who completed the induction phase) in primary care (PC) versus those who started in specialized care (SC).

Adverse events and self-reported symptoms

No overdose was observed during the induction phase but one patient with a history of suicide attempts did intentionally overdose during methadone maintenance. Apart from this case, no other severe adverse events were reported during the trial.

The following symptoms were reported by more than 20% of patients at month 3: fatigue/energy loss (49%), difficulty sleeping (48%), constipation (40%), shortness of breath (33%), muscle pain (32%), tingling (32%), poor appetite (31%), wheezing (31%), loss of sexual desire (31%), stomach pain (28%), headaches (28%), joint pain (23%), weight loss (20%) and blackouts (20%).

Discussion

This study is the first to randomize methadone initiation in primary care. It was deliberately designed as a pragmatic trial [21,22], i.e. having a real-life context to ensure external validity and to provide information about methadone effectiveness, irrespective of the induction site. It was also designed to provide recommendations about the possible authorization of methadone induction in primary care in France.

The main result of the trial is that induction in primary care is feasible, as patients in primary care are not less likely to be abstinent from street opioids compared with those inducted in specialized care. Another interesting result is that PC appears to be more attractive for opioid-dependent individuals, first because patients randomized into primary care were more likely to accept

Table 3. ITT and *per protocol* analysis for the difference in the percentage of street-opioid abstinent patients by induction arm and its 95% confidence interval.

	Specialized care	Primary care	% [95% CI] of the difference
ITT analysis			
Number of street-opioid abstinent patients at M12	22	85	
Number of patients included	66	155	
Street-opioid abstinent patients	33%	54%	21.5 [7.7; 35.3]
***Per protocol* analysis**			
Number of street-opioid abstinent patients at M12	22	85	
Number of patients at M12	33	129	
Street-opioid abstinent patients at M12	67%	66%	−0.8 [−18.8; 17.3]

Table 4. Odds ratio from the adjusted mixed model for abstinence from opioids use during the treatment (n = 615 visits and 188 patients).

	OR (IC95%)
Time since methadone treatment initiation	
M3 vs. M0	19.62 (8.69–44.33)
M6 vs. M0	16.73 (7.73–36.19)
M12 vs. M0	19.42 (8.98–41.98)
Arm induction	
PC vs. SC	1.58 (0.57–4.37)
switching from buprenorphine	
Yes vs. No	1.99 (0.85–4.67)

treatment than those randomized in specialized centers. Secondly patients who were inducted (after randomization) in primary care were more likely to engage in treatment and report greater satisfaction with medical information provided by their physician. Furthermore, this study highlighted that once methadone treatment was started, retention in treatment was similar in both arms. These last two results reflect the two main criteria generally used for assessing the effectiveness of treatments for opioid dependence - namely retention and non-medical opioid use – and confirm the comparable effectiveness of PC and SC over one year.

Similar results were found in a previous pragmatic trial comparing maintenance in primary care and specialized care. That trial also showed comparable outcomes and better satisfaction with treatment in the primary care maintenance arm [5,19,23].

Engagement in treatment was significantly lower in specialized care than in primary care, with early discontinuation rates significantly higher in the former group. This may be directly attributable to the specific French context, where access to buprenorphine already exists in primary care [4]. Indeed, previous pragmatic trials for other treatments involving primary care [15] have highlighted that strong patient engagement is related to the high motivation of physicians enrolled in the trial. This was also the case for physicians who accepted to participate in the present trial. Indeed this is the population of physicians which will be targeted if methadone induction becomes authorized in France.

In addition, it is important to note that the results of this trial by and large are consistent with those found in previous literature [24]. This shows that patients receiving methadone in primary care have comparable treatment responses in terms of retention and opioid use.

Using primary care as an entry point for opioid dependence care (and also for associated comorbidities) has greatly contributed to the scaling-up of treatment for opioid dependence in countries such as the UK. Even more importantly it helps "normalize" care for drug users. The availability of buprenorphine in primary care has partially contributed to "normalize" care for drug users in France as it means they can initiate a treatment option for opioid dependence "free-of-charge" like any other patient, and do so in structures which also provide care for other medical conditions to the general population.

As the French public health authorities were particularly concerned by the overdose risk during induction, the design of the trial proposed a specific model of care for methadone induction in PC in order to maximize safety. Individuals inducted in PC were over-represented in order to better detect possible overdoses during induction in the PC arm. As it happened, no overdoses were observed during induction, confirming previous results about the importance of a shared-care model to minimize such a risk [16].

The strengths of this study lie in the following three key points: first the identification of physicians who will likely be authorized to induct methadone by public health authorities; second the choice of a population of patients which was highly representative of individuals seeking care for opioid dependence in France (non-inclusion criteria were based exclusively on clinical practice criteria to control the risk of overdose); third, the adoption of a flexible treatment protocol where patients could choose to change arm after induction reflecting current clinical practice in France.

One reason why equity of access to methadone and buprenorphine is important in France is because primary care physicians regularly have to manage persistent buprenorphine-injection practices and associated complications [25], which are often a consequence of inadequate dosage prescription [26] or patient dissatisfaction with treatment. For this reason it is important for France to also consider patients who need to switch from buprenorphine to methadone for medical reasons. Despite the wide availability of generic buprenorphine in France, switching from buprenorphine to methadone in primary care could result in reduced costs for care of opioid dependence. However, methadone is likely to present more drug-drug interactions than buprenorphine for those on HIV or HCV medication. Consequently, before starting methadone in patients already receiving such medication, physicians should know how to modify methadone doses accordingly. This is why primary care physicians involved in the present trial received training and appropriate guidelines for all possible drug-drug interactions with methadone treatment, together with guidance about the differences between starting methadone in buprenorphine patients compared with methadone induction in street-opioid users.

A substantial portion of the participants starting methadone in SC switched from buprenorphine to methadone. This is the usual treatment chain for opioid-dependent patients in France. This is not so frequent in other countries. However, switching in France is impossible in areas underserved by specialized centers for substance dependence (i.e. non-urban areas) where general methadone initiation is not available.

Although methadone induction is already possible in primary care in some countries including the UK and Switzerland, no previous trial has compared methadone outcomes over one year as a function of the site of induction. The randomization of a specific model of care for drug users has already been performed in other trials [5,27,28] which had similar public health objectives.

The population targeted in this trial is representative of those seeking care for opioid dependence in France [29] and in other countries where similar models of specialized care are available [30–33]. However it is difficult to say to what extent these results remain valid in countries where access to opioid maintenance treatment is not free for drug users. Nevertheless, the study was performed according to standard international guidelines [34,35] in order to make our results as relevant as possible for other contexts.

Among the limitations of the trial, the need for physical proximity between the primary care physician and specialized centers obliged us to target areas where patients' need for methadone was already being substantially met by the specialized centers rather than underserved areas. This resulted in slowed enrolment rates and the enforced extension of the duration of enrolment period. Certainly a larger sample size and longer follow-up would have provided long term comparisons and increased the study's power, but this was not feasible both because of the practical reasons outlined above and cost reasons. The possible effect of heterogeneity between sites (i.e. sites with more than one PC physician versus sites having only one) was tested as a random effect factor in mixed models but was not found to be significant. It is possible that a larger sample size could have altered these results. However, it was important to represent different site sizes (i.e. those with different numbers of participating PC physicians) in the trial for external validity reasons.

Today, many governments of countries with HCV and HIV epidemics driven by drug use are still reluctant to introduce or scale up methadone treatment using alternative models of care, even though such an approach would be cost-effective, especially for controlling HIV and HCV [36].

The model used for primary care in this study may be of interest in other settings where access to methadone is needed for HIV and HCV prevention purposes. However, it is important to remember that our results strongly depend on the specific context of France where primary care already plays an important role in engaging patients in treatment for opioid dependence.

In conclusion, methadone induction in primary care is feasible and acceptable for both physicians and patients. It is as effective as induction in specialized care in reducing street-opioid use and ensuring engagement and retention in treatment for opioid dependence.

Supporting Information

Checklist S1 CONSORT 2010 checklist for the ANRS-Methaville trial.

English protocol S1 Published protocol of ANRS-Methaville trial.

Acknowledgments

We thank all the members of the ANRS-Methaville Study Group. We especially thank all the physicians involved in the trial and all the patients who took part in this study. Finally, we thank Jude Sweeney for the English revision and editing of our manuscript.

The ANRS Methaville Study Group:

Scientific Committee: P.M. Carrieri (project director)[1,2,3], A. Morel (principal investigator)[4], L. Michel[5,6,7], M. Mora[1,2,3], P. Roux[1,2,3], JF. Aubertin[8], S. Robinet[8], JC. Desenclos[9], J. Cohen[1,2,3], A. Herszkowicz[10], C. Paul[11], I. Porteret[11], T. Sainte Marie[12].

Physicians who contributed to the study: Dr Achard (Private practice, Besançon); Dr Aubertin (Private practice, Thionville); Dr Balteau Bijeau (CSST Wads, Metz); Dr Bartolo (Protox, Marseille); Dr Bibette (Private practice; Biarritz); Dr Biderman (Private practice, Meudon); Dr. Bry (Private practice), Dr Cadart (Private practice, Avignon); Dr Dewost (CSST Le trait d'union; Boulogne); Dr. Daulouede (CSST Bizia, Bayonne); Dr Gassmann (Private practice, Strasbourg); Dr Guena (CSST La Boussole, Rouen); Dr Guillet (CSST Le trait d'union; Boulogne); Dr Gutekunst (Private practice, Buchviller); Dr Herouin (CSST La Boussole, Rouen); Dr Herran (CSST Bizia, Bayonne); Dr Jacob (CSST Centre Hospitalier du Jury, Metz); Dr Kerloc'h (CSST Bizia, Bayonne); Dr Khouri; Dr Lasalarié (Private practice, Marseille); Dr Lavignasse (CSST Bizia, Bayonne); Dr Magnin (Private practice, Besançon); Dr Marre (Private practice, Le Havre), Dr. Mauraycaplanne; Dr Michel (Private practice, Lillebonne); Dr. Alain Morel (CSST Le trait d'union; Boulogne); Dr Nemayechi (Private practice, Bordeaux); Dr Paillou (CSST CEID, Bordeaux); Dr Partouche (Private practice, Thionville); Dr Petit (CSST AVAPT, Avignon); Dr Pouclet (CSST Centre Hospitalier du Jury, Metz); Dr Raulin (Private practice, Maromme); Dr Regard (Private practice, Avignon); Dr Roch (Private practice, Besançon); Dr Rouille; Dr Truffy (Private practice, Metz); Dr Vergez (Private practice, Marseille); Dr Vincent (Private practice, Bayonne); Dr Wajsbrot (Private practice, Avignon).

[1] INSERM U912 (SESSTIM), Marseille, France

[2] Université Aix Marseille, IRD, UMR-S912, Marseille, France

[3] ORS PACA, Observatoire Régional de la Santé Provence Alpes Côte d'Azur, Marseille, France

[4] Oppelia, Paris, France

[5] INSERM, Research Unit 669, Paris, France.

[6] Univ Paris-Sud and Univ Paris Descartes, UMR-S0669, Paris, France.

[7] Centre Pierre Nicole, Paris, France.

[8] Private practice

[9] Institut de Veille Sanitaire, Saint Maurice, France.

[10] Ministry of Health, France.

[11] French National Agency of Research on AIDS and hepatitis (ANRS), France.

[12] Hôpital Bicêtre, AP-HP, Le Kremlin-Bicêtre, France.

Safety committee: J. Bachellier, P.Beauverie, M. Vray, B. Stambul, F. Questel.

International committee of experts: R. Baker, H. Catania, M. Gossop, R. Haemmig, M. Torrens, A. Wodak.

Center of Methodology and Management, INSERM U912:

Protocol, guidelines, training: P.M. Carrieri L. Michel, M. Mora, P. Roux.

Phone interviews, training, logistics: G. Maradan, J. Biemar, S. Huguet, C. Bravard

Data collection, management and statistical analyses: P. Kurkdji, C. Taieb, J. Cohen, C. Lions.

Administration: C. Giovannini, MP. Kissikian.

The French National Agency for Research on AIDS and Viral Hepatitis (ANRS): JC. Desenclos, N. Job-Spira, V. Dore, C. Paul, I. Porteret.

French agency for the safety of health products (AFSSPAS): N. Richard.

French Ministry of Health: A.Herszkowicz, N. Prisse.

ASUD association: F. Olivet; AIDES association

Center of evaluation and information on drug dependence (CEIP): J. Arditti

Author Contributions

Conceived and designed the experiments: PMC AM PR LM MV BS. Performed the experiments: AM PMC PR LM MM. Analyzed the data: JC CL FM PMC. Contributed reagents/materials/analysis tools: MM AM LM PR PMC. Wrote the manuscript: PMC. Contributed to the writing of the manuscript: PR.

References

1. Macarthur GJ, Minozzi S, Martin N, Vickerman P, Deren S, et al. (2012) Opiate substitution treatment and HIV transmission in people who inject drugs: systematic review and meta-analysis. Bmj 345: e5945.
2. Roux P, Carrieri MP, Villes V, Dellamonica P, Poizot-Martin I, et al. (2008) The impact of methadone or buprenorphine treatment and ongoing injection on highly active antiretroviral therapy (HAART) adherence: evidence from the MANIF2000 cohort study. Addiction 103: 1828–1836.
3. Carrieri MP, Amass L, Lucas GM, Vlahov D, Wodak A, et al. (2006) Buprenorphine use: the international experience. Clin Infect Dis 43 Suppl 4: S197–215.
4. Auriacombe M, Fatseas M, Dubernet J, Daulouede JP, Tignol J (2004) French field experience with buprenorphine. Am J Addict 13 Suppl 1: S17–28.
5. Fiellin DA, O'Connor PG, Chawarski M, Pakes JP, Pantalon MV, et al. (2001) Methadone maintenance in primary care: a randomized controlled trial. Jama 286: 1724–1731.
6. Strain EC, Bigelow GE, Liebson IA, Stitzer ML (1999) Moderate- vs high-dose methadone in the treatment of opioid dependence: a randomized trial. Jama 281: 1000–1005.
7. Sheehan DV, Lecrubier Y, Sheehan KH, Amorim P, Janavs J, et al. (1998) The Mini-International Neuropsychiatric Interview (M.I.N.I.): the development and validation of a structured diagnostic psychiatric interview for DSM-IV and ICD-10. J Clin Psychiatry 59 Suppl 20: 22–33; quiz 34–57.
8. Brands B, Blake J, Marsh DC, Sproule B, Jeyapalan R, et al. (2008) The impact of benzodiazepine use on methadone maintenance treatment outcomes. J Addict Dis 27: 37–48.
9. Kerr T, Fairbairn N, Tyndall M, Marsh D, Li K, et al. (2007) Predictors of non-fatal overdose among a cohort of polysubstance-using injection drug users. Drug Alcohol Depend 87: 39–45.
10. Roux PD, Michel LD, Cohen J, Mora M, Morel A, et al. (2012) Initiation of Methadone in primary care (ANRS-Methaville): a phase III randomized intervention trial. BMC Public Health 12: 488.
11. Schwartz RP, Jaffe JH, Highfield DA, Callaman JM, O'Grady KE (2007) A randomized controlled trial of interim methadone maintenance: 10-Month follow-up. Drug Alcohol Depend 86: 30–36.
12. Darke S, Hall W, Wodak A, Heather N, Ward J (1992) Development and validation of a multi-dimensional instrument for assessing outcome of treatment among opiate users: the Opiate Treatment Index. Br J Addict 87: 733–742.
13. Coons SJ, Kothari S, Monz BU, Burke LB (2011) The patient-reported outcome (PRO) consortium: filling measurement gaps for PRO end points to support labeling claims. Clin Pharmacol Ther 90: 743–748.
14. Snyder CF, Blackford AL, Aaronson NK, Detmar SB, Carducci MA, et al. (2011) Can patient-reported outcome measures identify cancer patients' most bothersome issues? J Clin Oncol 29: 1216–1220.
15. Fransen GA, van Marrewijk CJ, Mujakovic S, Muris JW, Laheij RJ, et al. (2007) Pragmatic trials in primary care. Methodological challenges and solutions demonstrated by the DIAMOND-study. BMC Med Res Methodol 7: 16.
16. Weinrich M, Stuart M (2000) Provision of methadone treatment in primary care medical practices: review of the Scottish experience and implications for US policy. Jama 283: 1343–1348.
17. Farre M, Mas A, Torrens M, Moreno V, Cami J (2002) Retention rate and illicit opioid use during methadone maintenance interventions: a meta-analysis. Drug Alcohol Depend 65: 283–290.
18. Teesson M, Ross J, Darke S, Lynskey M, Ali R, et al. (2006) One year outcomes for heroin dependence: findings from the Australian Treatment Outcome Study (ATOS). Drug Alcohol Depend 83: 174–180.
19. Wittchen HU, Apelt SM, Soyka M, Gastpar M, Backmund M, et al. (2008) Feasibility and outcome of substitution treatment of heroin-dependent patients in specialized substitution centers and primary care facilities in Germany: a naturalistic study in 2694 patients. Drug Alcohol Depend 95: 245–257.
20. Hamer RM, Simpson PM (2009) Last observation carried forward versus mixed models in the analysis of psychiatric clinical trials. Am J Psychiatry 166: 639–641.
21. Bouvenot G, Vray M (2006) Essais cliniques: théorie, pratique et critique; Medecine-Sciences, editor: Flammarion.
22. Vray M, Schwartz D (1996) Comments on a pragmatic trial. J Clin Epidemiol 49: 949–950.
23. Keen J, Oliver P, Rowse G, Mathers N (2003) Does methadone maintenance treatment based on the new national guidelines work in a primary care setting? Br J Gen Pract 53: 461–467.
24. MacGowan RJ, Swanson NM, Brackbill RM, Rugg DL, Barker T, et al. (1996) Retention in methadone maintenance treatment programs, Connecticut and Massachusetts, 1990–1993. J Psychoactive Drugs 28: 259–265.
25. Del Giudice P (2004) Cutaneous complications of intravenous drug abuse. Br J Dermatol 150: 1–10.
26. Roux P, Villes V, Blanche J, Bry D, Spire B, et al. (2008) Buprenorphine in primary care: Risk factors for treatment injection and implications for clinical management. Drug Alcohol Depend 97: 105–113.
27. O'Connor PG, Oliveto AH, Shi JM, Triffleman EG, Carroll KM, et al. (1998) A randomized trial of buprenorphine maintenance for heroin dependence in a primary care clinic for substance users versus a methadone clinic. Am J Med 105: 100–105.
28. Gibson AE, Doran CM, Bell JR, Ryan A, Lintzeris N (2003) A comparison of buprenorphine treatment in clinic and primary care settings: a randomised trial. Med J Aust 179: 38–42.
29. Cadet-Taïrou A, Cholley D (2004) Rapport 2004 - Approche régionale de la substitution aux opiacés, 1999–2002. OFDT. 28–36 p.
30. McCowan C, Kidd B, Fahey T (2009) Factors associated with mortality in Scottish patients receiving methadone in primary care: retrospective cohort study. Bmj 338: b2225.
31. Nosyk B, Sun H, Evans E, Marsh DC, Anglin MD, et al. (2012) Defining dosing pattern characteristics of successful tapers following methadone maintenance treatment: results from a population-based retrospective cohort study. Addiction 107: 1621–1629.
32. Hser YI, Saxon AJ, Huang D, Hasson A, Thomas C, et al. (2014) Treatment retention among patients randomized to buprenorphine/naloxone compared to methadone in a multi-site trial. Addiction 109: 79–87.
33. Schwartz RP, Kelly SM, O'Grady KE, Gandhi D, Jaffe JH (2012) Randomized trial of standard methadone treatment compared to initiating methadone without counseling: 12-month findings. Addiction 107: 943–952.
34. Fareed A, Casarella J, Amar R, Vayalapalli S, Drexler K (2010) Methadone maintenance dosing guideline for opioid dependence, a literature review. J Addict Dis 29: 1–14.
35. Soyka M, Kranzler HR, van den Brink W, Krystal J, Moller HJ, et al. (2011) The World Federation of Societies of Biological Psychiatry (WFSBP) guidelines for the biological treatment of substance use and related disorders. Part 2: Opioid dependence. World J Biol Psychiatry 12: 160–187.
36. Wolfe D, Carrieri MP, Shepard D (2010) Treatment and care for injecting drug users with HIV infection: a review of barriers and ways forward. Lancet 376: 355–366.

Knowledge, Practices, and Perceived Barriers Regarding Cancer Pain Management among Physicians and Nurses in Korea: A Nationwide Multicenter Survey

Hyun Jung Jho[1], Yeol Kim[2*], Kyung Ae Kong[3], Dae Hyun Kim[4], Jin Young Choi[1], Eun Jeong Nam[5], Jin Young Choi[5], Sujin Koh[6], Kwan Ok Hwang[7], Sun Kyung Baek[8], Eun Jung Park[1]

1 Hospice & Palliative Care Branch, National Cancer Control Institute, National Cancer Center, Goyang, Republic of Korea, **2** Division of Cancer Management & Policy, National Cancer Control Institute, National Cancer Center, Goyang, Republic of Korea, **3** Clinical Trial Center, Ewha Womans University Medical Center, Seoul, Republic of Korea, **4** Department of Pain and Anesthesiology, Hospital, National Cancer Center, Goyang, Republic of Korea, **5** Department of Nursing, Hospital, National Cancer Center, Goyang, Republic of Korea, **6** Department of Hematology and Oncology, Ulsan University Hospital, Ulsan, Republic of Korea, **7** Korean Hospice & Palliative Nurse Association, Daejeon, Republic of Korea, **8** Department of Medical Oncology and Hematology, Kyung Hee University Medical Center, Seoul, Republic of Korea

Abstract

Purpose: Medical professionals' practices and knowledge regarding cancer pain management have often been cited as inadequate. This study aimed to evaluate knowledge, practices and perceived barriers regarding cancer pain management among physicians and nurses in Korea.

Methods: A nationwide questionnaire survey was administered to physicians and nurses involved in the care of cancer patients. Questionnaire items covered pain assessment and documentation practices, knowledge regarding cancer pain management, the perceived barriers to cancer pain control, and processes perceived as the major causes of delay in opioid administration.

Results: A total of 333 questionnaires (149 physicians and 284 nurses) were analyzed. Nurses performed pain assessment and documentation more regularly than physicians did. Although physicians had better knowledge of pain management than did nurses, both groups lacked knowledge regarding the side effects and pharmacology of opioids. Physicians working in the palliative care ward and nurses who had received pain management education obtained higher scores on knowledge. Physicians perceived patients' reluctance to take opioids as a barrier to pain control, more so than did nurses, while nurses perceived patients' tendency to under-report of pain as a barrier, more so than did physicians. Physicians and nurses held different perceptions regarding major cause of delay during opioid administration.

Conclusions: There were differences between physicians and nurses in knowledge and practices for cancer pain management. An effective educational strategy for cancer pain management is needed in order to improve medical professionals' knowledge and clinical practices.

Editor: Richard E. Burney, University of Michigan, United States of America

Funding: This research was funded by National Cancer Center grant number 1032040-1. URL of funder http://ncc.re.kr/english/index.jsp. YK received the funding. The funders had no role in study design, data collection and analysis, decision to publish, or preparation of the manuscript.

Competing Interests: The authors have declared that no competing interests exist.

* Email: drheat@ncc.re.kr

Introduction

Pain management is an important aspect in the care of cancer patients. Although cancer pain can be controlled up to 90% of the cases through the use of appropriate methods [1,2], its prevalence has been reported to be as high as 64% among patients with advanced cancer [3] and pain control was found to be inadequate for more than 40% of patients [4]. Factors relating to the medical professional, patient, and the healthcare system have been identified as causes of this apparent under-treatment of cancer pain among patients [4]. Specifically, medical professionals' inadequacy in pain assessment and management has been pointed out as an important barrier to cancer pain control [5–9].

Studies have noted knowledge deficits in cancer pain management among medical professionals [10,11]. For example, physicians, especially oncologists, generally have general knowledge of cancer pain management, while seemingly lacking knowledge regarding opioid administration or alternate therapies for pain control [8]. This knowledge deficit typically emerged when physicians calculated opioid dosages for the management of breakthrough pain [12] and when attempting to select the correct response to challenging clinical vignettes [5]. Nurses' knowledge of opioids as a pain control measure was found to be as inadequate as that of the physicians referred to above [8], demonstrated by their exaggerated fear of the addictive nature of opioids or their potential to culminate in respiratory suppression [6]. In Korea, studies also have reported inadequate knowledge and incorrect attitudes among doctors and nurses [13–16]. Kim et al. surveyed 1,204 young doctors from all specialties and determined that the majority of doctors were not knowledgeable about equianalgesic opioid dosages, adjuvant analgesics, the numeric rating scale, and the fact that opioids have no ceiling effect [13].

In Korea, approximately 200,000 people are diagnosed with cancer annually, while more than 70,000 die from the condition [17]. According to another Korean study, 70% of patients with advanced cancer experienced pain, and pain management was inadequate in half of the patients [18].

Cancer pain control forms part of Korea's national healthcare policy. In order to improve knowledge and practices regarding cancer pain management among medical professionals, Korea's Ministry of Health and Welfare and the National Cancer Center have been publishing and distributing a national guideline known as the "Cancer Pain Management Guideline" across Korea since 2004. In the current study, we investigated and compared knowledge, practices and perceived barriers regarding cancer pain management among physicians and nurses to identify the need for improvement in clinical practice, education and policy.

Method

Study design, participants, and procedures

This survey took place from September 2010 until June 2011 at 11 hospitals (6 public and 5 private hospitals) across Korea. Doctors and nurses involved in the care of cancer patients were eligible for participation. The research coordinator contacted eligible participants at participating hospitals and subsequently delivered the questionnaires. All participants provided written consent to participate in the study. Upon completion of the questionnaire, participants received a voucher worth 10,000 KRW (approximately US $10) as a reward for their participation. This study was approved by the Institutional Review Board at 11 participating hospitals (National Cancer Center, Chonbuk National University Hospital, Chonnam National University Hospital, Chungbuk National University Hospital, Chungnam National University Hospital, Pusan National University Hospital, Good Samaritan Hospital, Korea Cancer Center Hospital, Korea University Kuro hospital, KyungHee University Medical Center, The Catholic University of Korea Seoul St. Mary's Hospital).

Questionnaire development

The questionnaire was developed by the researchers for the purposes of the current study and pilot-tested and revised by a panel of experts consist of 7 physicians (from specialty of pain, medical oncology, family medicine and preventive medicine) and 8 nurses working in oncology ward or palliative care unit. Questionnaire items relating to knowledge and practices regarding cancer pain management were generated on the basis of the contents of the Cancer Pain Management Guideline published by the Ministry of Health and Welfare and the National Cancer Center. The Guideline encompasses pain assessment, pharmacologic and non-pharmacologic pain management, radiation therapy for pain control, interventional pain management such as nerve block, and approaches towards refractory cancer pain.

Items relating to practices assessed the frequency of pain assessment for admitted patients, specific details of pain assessment, and documentation following assessment. Knowledge of cancer pain management was evaluated through 14 items (11 "true" or "false" questions and 3 multiple choice questions), tapping into the principles of cancer pain management, specific properties of analgesics, interventional pain management, opioid dose calculation, and the duration of re-assessment after opioid administration.

Questions on perceived barriers were extracted from the literature [19–23], and comprised 3 categories related to patients, medical staff, and the health care system. The following is an example of an item relating to perceived barriers: "how often does a particular barrier interfere with pain control?" Responses were organized on a 4-point scale, where a scale of 1 indicated "never," 2 = "sometimes," 3 = "often," and 4 = "always." For each item, frequency of scale 1 and 2 was combined as negative response, and frequency of scale 3 and 4 was combined as positive response for a statistical analysis.

Data analysis

Descriptive analysis was used to summarize the characteristics of participants and responses to items relating practice, knowledge, and perceived barriers. A chi-squared test was carried out to compare differences between physicians and nurses in terms of practices, knowledge, and perceived barriers to cancer pain control. We used multiple linear regression analysis to determine the relationship between participants' characteristics and the number of correct responses for knowledge of cancer pain management. β value is a regression coefficient which is interpreted as the difference in the number of correct answers according to the differences in age, sex, whether the participant is working in palliative care unit, and whether the participant had attended any type of cancer pain education. The statistical significance level was set at $p<0.05$. Statistical analyses were performed using the STATA SE version 12.0 software package (StataCorp, College Station, TX, USA).

Results

Sample Characteristics

A summary of the study participants' characteristics is presented in Table 1. A total of 335 questionnaires were collected from 11 hospitals. After excluding 2 incomplete questionnaires, 333 (149 physicians and 284 nurses) questionnaires were included in the final analysis. The participants' mean age was 33.2 and 29.0 (in years) for physicians and nurses, respectively. 70.8% of participating physicians specialized in internal medicine. 13.3% of physicians and 19.0% of nurses were working in the palliative care ward. More than 70% of physicians and nurses had received cancer pain education.

Pain assessment practices and documentation

Table 2 presents practices relating to pain assessment and documentation among physicians and nurses. Results showed that about three times more nurses indicated that they assessed patients' pain levels on every round than physicians did ($p<0.001$). In addition, nurses checked all items relating to pain assessment more frequently than physicians did. Further, a higher proportion of nurses, in comparison to physicians, reported that they documented pain assessment ($p<0.001$). In additional analysis, there was no significant difference in general characteristics among nurses according to the pain assessment and documentation practices. For physicians, having received cancer pain education and working in the palliative ward were positively associated with doing pain documentation ($p = 0.001$).

Table 1. Characteristics of participants.

Characteristics	Physician, N = 149 n (%)	Nurse, N = 284 n (%)
Gender		
Male	91 (61.5)	0 (0)
Female	57 (38.5)	283 (100)
Age (years) Mean (SD)	33.2 (6.9)	29.0 (5.8)
<40	119 (85.6)	251 (92.9)
≥40	20 (14.4)	19 (7.0)
Working experience in years, Mean (SD)	7.3 (6.5)	6.6 (5.8)
<10	111 (75.5)	207 (76.7)
≥10	36 (24.5)	63 (23.3)
Clinical specialty		
Internal medicine	104 (70.8)	
Surgery	24 (16.3)	
Family medicine	9 (6.1)	
Other*	10 (6.8)	
Working in palliative care unit	20 (13.3)	54 (19.0)
Having attended any type of cancer pain education	106 (72.1)	232 (78.8)

*Other includes gynecology, radiation oncology, and odontology.

Knowledge of cancer pain management

The rate of correct responses to each of the questions on knowledge for cancer pain management is shown in Table 3. The mean number of correct responses provided by physicians was higher than that of nurses, at 10.8 and 9.0, respectively. For both physicians and nurses, knowledge deficit was prominent in questions on tolerance for opioid-induced sedation (Question 8: the rate of correct responses was 48.0% and 35.0% for physicians and nurses, respectively) and the duration of re-assessment after intravenous morphine administration (Question 13: 51.0% and 48.4% for physicians and nurses, respectively). The rate of correct responses was higher among physicians for questions on NSAIDs (Question 3), specific properties of opioids and opioid dose calculation (Questions 7, 10, and 12), as well as the utilization of radiotherapy or interventional pain management as measures of pain control (Questions 9 and 11).

Table 2. Pain assessment and documentation practices.

	Physician %	Nurse %	P value
Occasion of pain assessment			
Every round*	24.8	75.2	<0.001
On selected occasions*†	67.1	23.2	<0.001
Seldom*	4.0	0.4	0.015
Items checked during pain assessment			
Location*	83.8	95.8	<0.001
Quality*	66.9	89.8	<0.001
Related factor*	55.4	68.8	0.006
Severity*	84.4	97.2	<0.001
Timing*	69.4	78.8	0.031
Documentation of pain assessment*	60.8	98.9	<0.001

*$P<0.05$.
†New admission, when patient complains of pain, or when patient seems to be in pain.

Table 3. Rate of correct responses regarding knowledge of cancer pain management.

Question	Physician %	Nurse %	P value
1. You should not trust patient's subjective reports of pain (F)	86.5	91.3	0.118
2. You should differentiable certain cause of pain which needs specific treatment (i.e. cord compression) (T)	96.6	96.7	0.943
3. Prescribing a few different types of NSAIDs will increase the analgesic efficacy and decreased adverse effect* (F)	77.7	52.7	<0.001
4. Pethidine can be prescribed for chronic cancer pain safely. (F)	81.8	81.2	0.880
5. Opioid analgesics have a high risk of addiction. (F)	91.9	86.3	0.087
6. The effect of immediate release oral opioid can be assessed at 1 hour after administration (T)	77.0	76.8	0.960
7. Opioid analgesics do not have a ceiling effect (T)*	78.4	55.2	<0.001
8. Tolerance for opioid-induced sedation develops within a few days* (T)	48.0	35.0	0.008
9. For painful bone metastasis, radiotherapy can alleviate the pain or help to reduce the amount of analgesics* (T)	82.3	53.1	<0.001
10. Opioid-induced respiratory suppression is common* (F)	82.4	54.9	<0.001
11. Celiac plexus block is effective for treating cancer pain at upper abdomen.* (T)	68.5	45.3	<0.001
12. Calculation of opioid rescue dose*	73.1	52.4	<0.001
13. Duration of evaluation following intravenous morphine administration	51.0	48.4	0.607
14. Knowledge regarding refractory cancer pain	96.0	93.6	0.314
Mean number of correct responses*, Mean (SD)	10.8 (2.4)	9.0 (2.5)	<0.001

*$P<0.05$.

A relationship between the number of correct responses given on knowledge of cancer pain management and the sample characteristics is shown in Table 4. Working in palliative care unit was associated with a higher number of correct responses for physicians. For nurses, being older and having received cancer pain education were related to a higher rate of correct responses.

Table 4. Relationship between knowledge and characteristics of participants.

	Physician β (95% CI)	Nurse β (95% CI)
Age	NS	0.07 (0.02, 0.12)
Sex*	NS	-
Working in palliative care unit†	1.25 (0.05, 2.44)	NS
Having attended any type of cancer pain education‡	NS	1.75 (0.95, 2.56)

Multiple linear regression analysis for the number of correct answers for knowledge with general characteristics of participants as independent variables.
β regression coefficient; NS not significant.
Reference values: *Male; †Not working in the palliative care ward; ‡Not having attended any type of cancer pain education.

Perceived barriers for cancer pain management

Perceived barriers for cancer pain control were compared; results are described in Table 5. Time constraints and insufficient knowledge of pain control were cited by both nurses and physicians as barriers to cancer pain management that were experienced more frequently than other barriers. Physicians perceived barriers such as the "patient's reluctance to take opioids" ($p = 0.011$) and "not prioritizing pain control" ($p = 0.003$) to a higher extent than nurses. In contrast, nurses perceived "insufficient communication with patients" ($p = 0.001$) and "patients' reluctance to report pain" ($p = 0.030$) as barriers to a higher extent than physicians.

Perceptions regarding processes delaying opioid administration

Figure 1 depicts differences in perceptions regarding processes considered to be major sources of delay in the administration of opioids between physicians and nurses. In this regard, "obtaining opioids from pharmacy" was cited by 57.1% of physicians, while 53.4% of nurses cited "contacting physician for prescription of opioid" ($p < 0.001$).

Discussion

This is the first nationwide study to evaluate knowledge and practices relating to cancer pain management among doctors and nurses in Korea, on the basis of the national Cancer Pain Management Guideline. Overall, results showed that doctors have better knowledge of cancer pain management than nurses, while the latter tended to conduct regular pain assessment and documentation practice more frequently. In addition, doctors and nurses held different perceptions regarding barriers to cancer pain management and the opioid administration process.

The differences found between nurses and doctors in knowledge and practices reflect areas requiring improvement in cancer pain management within these professions. Similarly to results from previous studies [10,24,25], our findings showed that doctors scored higher on knowledge than nurses. In our study, both doctors and nurses displayed substantial knowledge deficits regarding tolerance for opioid-induced sedation, the duration of evaluation after opioid administration, calculation of rescue opioid dosages, and utilization of other modalities, such as celiac plexus block. This result is also consistent with findings from previous studies [5,8,12]. The low rate of correct responses obtained for knowledge regarding celiac plexus block indicates limited understanding of specialist areas within the medical field, which could lead to less referrals to other specialists. It was reported in a previous study that less than 20% of oncologists referred their

Table 5. Perceived barriers to cancer pain control.

	Physician	Nurse	P value
	%	%	
Related to medical staff			
Inadequate pain assessment	37.6	36.8	0.864
Inadequate experience on pain control	42.3	35.7	0.180
Insufficient knowledge of pain control	45.0	40.8	0.403
Time constraints*	75.8	66.1	0.036
Reluctance to prescribe opioid	23.5	25.8	0.599
Insufficient communication with patient*	30.2	47.0	0.001
Patient-related			
Reluctance to report pain*	36.1	47.0	0.030
Reluctance to take opioid*	54.1	41.1	0.011
Insufficient communication with medical staff	44.6	49.1	0.373
Financial constraints	12.8	13.3	0.891
Insufficient knowledge of pain control	60.5	57.7	0.572
Related to the health care system			
Strict regulation of opioids	29.1	36.5	0.120
Inadequate staffing	41.9	39.7	0.662
Limited stock of different types of opioids	29.1	27.1	0.675
Cancer pain management is not considered as important*	43.5	29.3	0.003
Medication and intervention costs*	32.7	23.6	0.044

*$P < 0.05$.

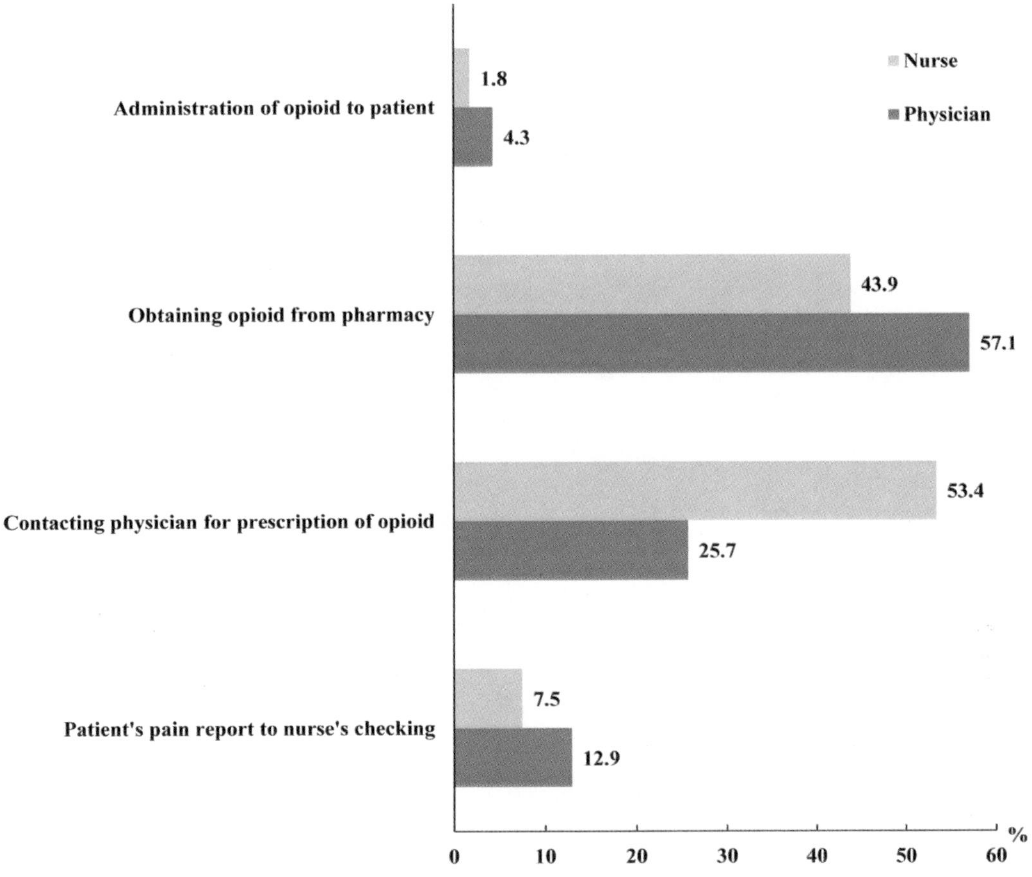

Figure 1. The most delayed process during opioid administration perceived by physicians and nurses.

patients to palliative or pain specialists [5]. Moreover, medical staff with insufficient knowledge of pain control may delay the administration of opioids to patients [15].

It is generally agreed that the education of medical professionals is necessary to improve cancer pain management. Findings from our study showed that having received cancer pain education was significantly associated with better knowledge among nurses, which was compatible with findings from other study [26]. However, this benefit of education is unclear among physicians. In our finding, knowledge regarding cancer pain management was not significantly different between physicians who received cancer pain education and who didn't. This echoes with previous study [5] which showed increased continued medical education for pain management could not satisfy the clinical need in pain management. In comparison, projects based approaches which utilized developing action plan [27] or continued quality improvement [28] for pain management reported improved practice and knowledge among medical professionals. This suggests that delivering knowledge alone is not enough to promote cancer pain management, and additional educational strategy such as combining different education methods is needed [29]. For example, the didactic lecture is used for delivering general principles, while small group discussions are more suitable for discussions of clinical cases [29]. This issue relating to educational methods seems to be applicable to the Korean context, where didactic lectures are most widely used for medical education.

In the current study, nurses practiced pain assessment and documentation more regularly than physicians. This is compatible with findings from a previous study which reported that nurses were more skilled at pain assessment, as compared to doctors or pharmacists [8]. This difference could be explained by the roll allocation between nurses and physicians, since nurses are usually required to monitor and report patient's symptom to physicians. Another consideration which could have influenced nurses' pain assessment and documentation practice in our survey is the institutional accreditation standard. In this regard, all but one participating hospitals in the current study were accredited by Korea Institute for Healthcare Accreditation (KOIHA), which recommends to assess pain using assessment tool for inpatients.

Time constraints and insufficient knowledge regarding pain management of medical professional were the most commonly encountered barriers to effective pain management for both physicians and nurses. Interestingly, physicians and nurses held different perceptions regarding patient-related barriers. Physicians perceived the "patient's reluctance to take opioid" as a barrier more often, while nurses perceived the "patient underreporting pain" more often. This is comparable to findings from a previous study, wherein doctors tended to believe that patients over-reported their pain, more so than nurses [8].

There were differences between the nurses and the physicians in perceptions regarding factors that contributed the most towards the delay in the opioid administration process. This discordance of perception between physicians and nurses seems to reflect insufficient coordination of the opioid administration process. For example, in many hospital wards in Korea, nurses are often required to confirm the administration of opioids with physicians, even when there is an "as needed" opioid prescription for breakthrough pain. Moreover, opioids are usually kept in hospital pharmacies, rather than wards, due to the strict regulation policy. In such instances, traveling between the pharmacy and the ward to obtain opioids is time-consuming. In order to reduce the duration of this process, there is a need for institutional policy change, which could advocate the storage of opioids in hospital wards as well as clear team communication about executing standing order for breakthrough pain.

This study has a few limitations. First, although we performed a multicenter study, the results may not represent practices and knowledge of all medical professionals in Korea. Second, in order to accurately measure actual pain assessment and documentation practices, additional monitoring, such as auditing charts, is needed. Third, in this study, we simply asked whether participants had attended pain education before, so as to determine exposure to the educational experience, without considering the level of such exposure. However, the content and methods used in cancer pain management education could be diverse; this, however, was not considered in the current study. Finally, the actual duration of the each process for the administration of opioid was not measured. Therefore we couldn't verify the medical professional's perception for the delayed process.

In conclusion, physicians showed better knowledge of cancer pain management, while nurses performed better in pain assessment and documentation practices. Although time constraints were perceived more frequently as a barrier to cancer pain management, physicians perceived patients' reluctance to take opioids as a barrier, more so than nurses, while nurses deemed patients' underreporting of pain as a barrier to pain control, more so than physicians. The findings in this study indicate that changes in the educational strategy are required to enhance clinical practice among healthcare professionals in relation to cancer pain management.

Acknowledgments

The authors are grateful for the participation of the 11 institutions below.

National Cancer Center, Chonbuk National University Hospital, Chonnam National University Hospital, Chungbuk National University Hospital, Chungnam National University Hospital, Pusan National University Hospital, Good Samaritan Hospital, Korea Cancer Center Hospital, Korea University Kuro hospital, KyungHee University Medical Center, The Catholic University of Korea Seoul St. Mary's Hospital.

Author Contributions

Conceived and designed the experiments: HJJ YK KAK DHK JYC EJN JYC SK KOH EJP. Performed the experiments: SK SKB. Analyzed the data: HJJ YK KAK. Contributed to the writing of the manuscript: HJJ YK KAK DHK JYC EJN JYC SK KOH SKB EJP.

References

1. Cancer pain relief: with a guide to opioid availability - second edition. (1996) World Health Organization.
2. Meuser T, Pietruck C, Radbruch L, Stute P, Lehmann KA, et al. (2001) Symptoms during cancer pain treatment following WHO-guidelines: a longitudinal follow-up study of symptom prevalence, severity and etiology. Pain 93: 247–257.
3. Van den Beuken-van Everdingen M, De Rijke J, Kessels A, Schouten H, Van Kleef M, et al. (2007) Prevalence of pain in patients with cancer: a systematic review of the past 40 years. Annals of oncology 18: 1437–1449.
4. Deandrea S, Montanari M, Moja L, Apolone G (2008) Prevalence of undertreatment in cancer pain. A review of published literature. Annals of oncology 19: 1985–1991.
5. Breuer B, Fleishman SB, Cruciani RA, Portenoy RK (2011) Medical oncologists' attitudes and practice in cancer pain management: A national survey. Journal of Clinical Oncology 29: 4769–4775.
6. Bernardi M, Catania G, Lambert A, Tridello G, Luzzani M (2007) Knowledge and attitudes about cancer pain management: a national survey of Italian oncology nurses. Eur J Oncol Nurs 11: 272–279.
7. Sapir R, Catane R, Strauss-Liviatan N, Cherny NI (1999) Cancer pain: knowledge and attitudes of physicians in Israel. Journal of pain and symptom management 17: 266–276.
8. Xue Y, Schulman-Green D, Czaplinski C, Harris D, McCorkle R (2007) Pain attitudes and knowledge among RNs, pharmacists, and physicians on an inpatient oncology service. Clinical journal of oncology nursing 11: 687–695.
9. Pargeon KL, Hailey BJ (1999) Barriers to effective cancer pain management: a review of the literature. Journal of pain and symptom management 18: 358–368.
10. Lebovits AH, Florence I, Bathina R, Hunko V, Fox MT, et al. (1997) Pain knowledge and attitudes of healthcare providers: practice characteristic differences. The Clinical journal of pain 13: 237–243.
11. Yanjun S, Changli W, Ling W, Woo JC, Ai L, et al. (2010) A survey on physician knowledge and attitudes towards clinical use of morphine for cancer pain treatment in China. Supportive Care in Cancer 18: 1455–1460.
12. Gallagher R, Hawley P, Yeomans W (2004) A survey of cancer pain management knowledge and attitudes of British Columbian physicians. Pain research & management: the journal of the Canadian Pain Society = journal de la societe canadienne pour le traitement de la douleur 9: 188.
13. Kim M-H, Park H, Park EC, Park K (2011) Attitude and knowledge of physicians about cancer pain management: young doctors of South Korea in their early career. Japanese journal of clinical oncology 41: 783–791.
14. Kim HJ, Park IS, Kang KJ (2012) Knowledge and Awareness of Nurses and Doctors Regarding Cancer Pain Management in a Tertiary Hospital. Asian Oncol Nurs 12: 147–155.
15. Jun M-H, Park K-S, Gong S-H, Lee S-H, Kim Y-H, et al. (2006) Knowledge and Attitude toward Cancer Pain Management: Clinical Nurses Versus Doctors. Korean Acad Soc Nurs Edu 12: 115–123.
16. Park H, Koh MJ, Lee HS, Kim YM, Kim MS (2003) Nurses' knowledge about and attitude toward cancer pain management: a survey from korean cancer pain management project. Journal of Korean Academy of Adult Nursing 15: 205–214.
17. Jung K-W, Won Y-J, Kong H-J, Oh C-M, Seo HG, et al. (2013) Cancer Statistics in Korea: Incidence, Mortality, Survival and Prevalence in 2010. Cancer Res Treat 45: 1–14.
18. Yun YH, Heo DS, Lee IG, Jeong HS, Kim HJ, et al. (2003) Multicenter Study of Pain and Its Management in Patients with Advanced Cancer in Korea. Journal of Pain and Symptom Management 25: 430–437.
19. Gunnarsdottir S, Donovan HS, Serlin RC, Voge C, Ward S (2002) Patient-related barriers to pain management: the Barriers Questionnaire II (BQ-II). Pain 99: 385–396.
20. Jeon YS, Kim HK, Cleeland CS, Wang XS (2007) Clinicians' practice and attitudes toward cancer pain management in Korea. Support Care Cancer 15: 463–469.
21. Ger L-P, Ho S-T, Wang J-J (2000) Physicians' knowledge and attitudes toward the use of analgesics for cancer pain management: a survey of two medical centers in Taiwan. Journal of Pain and Symptom management 20: 335–344.
22. Sun VC, Borneman T, Ferrell B, Piper B, Koczywas M, et al. (2007) Overcoming barriers to cancer pain management: an institutional change model. J Pain Symptom Manage 34: 359–369.
23. International Associations for the Study of Pain. (2008) Barriers to Cancer Pain Treatment; Cancer Pain Fact Sheet.
24. Furstenberg CT, Ahles TA, Whedon MB, Pierce KL, Dolan M, et al. (1998) Knowledge and attitudes of health-care providers toward cancer pain management: a comparison of physicians, nurses, and pharmacists in the state of New Hampshire. Journal of pain and symptom management 15: 335.
25. Visentin M, Trentin L, de Marco R, Zanolin E (2001) Knowledge and attitudes of Italian medical staff towards the approach and treatment of patients in pain. Journal of pain and symptom management 22: 925–930.
26. Lui LYY, So WKW, Fong DYT (2008) Knowledge and attitudes regarding pain management among nurses in Hong Kong medical units. Journal of Clinical Nursing 17: 2014–2021.
27. Weissman DE, Dahl JL (1995) Update on the cancer pain role model education program. Journal of pain and symptom management 10: 292–297.
28. Bookbinder M, Coyle N, Kiss M, Goldstein ML, Holritz K, et al. (1996) Implementing national standards for cancer pain management: program model and evaluation. Journal of pain and symptom management 12: 334–347.
29. Weissman DE (1996) Cancer pain education for physicians in practice: Establishing a new paradigm. Journal of pain and symptom management 12: 364–371.

A Capsaicin (8%) Patch in the Treatment of Severe Persistent Inguinal Postherniorrhaphy Pain: A Randomized, Double-Blind, Placebo-Controlled Trial

Joakim M. Bischoff[1]*, Thomas K. Ringsted[1], Marian Petersen[1], Claudia Sommer[2], Nurcan Üçeyler[2], Mads U. Werner[1]

1 Multidisciplinary Pain Center 7612, Neuroscience Center, Rigshospitalet, Copenhagen University, Copenhagen, Denmark, **2** Department of Neurology, University Hospital of Würzburg, Würzburg, Germany

Abstract

Background: Persistent pain after inguinal herniorrhaphy is a disabling condition with a lack of evidence-based pharmacological treatment options. This randomized placebo-controlled trial investigated the efficacy of a capsaicin 8% cutaneous patch in the treatment of severe persistent inguinal postherniorrhaphy pain.

Methods: Forty-six patients with persistent inguinal postherniorrhaphy pain were randomized to receive either a capsaicin 8% patch or a placebo patch. Pain intensity (Numerical Rating Scale [NRS 0–10]) was evaluated under standardized conditions (at rest, during movement, and during pressure) at baseline and at 1, 2 and 3 months after patch application. Skin punch biopsies for intraepidermal nerve fiber density (IENFD) measurements were taken at baseline and 1 month after patch application. Quantitative sensory testing was performed at baseline and at 1, 2, and 3 months after patch application. The primary outcome was comparisons of summed pain intensity differences (SPIDs) between capsaicin and placebo treatments at 1, 2 and 3 months after patch application (significance level $P<0.01$).

Results: The maximum difference in SPID, between capsaicin and placebo treatments, was observed at 1 month after patch application, but the pain reduction was not significant (NRS, mean difference [95% CI]: 5.0 [0.09 to 9.9]; $P=0.046$). No differences in SPID between treatments were observed at 2 and 3 months after patch application. Changes in IENFD on the pain side, from baseline to 1 month after patch application, did not differ between capsaicin and placebo treatment: 1.9 [−0.1 to 3.9] and 0.6 [−1.2 to 2.5] fibers/mm, respectively ($P=0.32$). No significant changes in sensory function, sleep quality or psychological factors were associated with capsaicin patch treatment.

Conclusions: The study did not demonstrate significant differences in pain relief between capsaicin and placebo treatment, although a trend toward pain improvement in capsaicin treated patients was observed 1 month after patch application.

Trial Registration: Clinicaltrialsregister.eu 2012-001540-22 ClinicalTrials.gov NCT01699854

Editor: T. Mark Doherty, Glaxo Smith Kline, Denmark

Funding: The study was supported by an unrestricted research grant from Astellas Pharma a/s, Kastrup, Denmark (http://www.astellas.dk/). The funders had no role in study design, data collection and analysis, decision to publish, or preparation of the manuscript.

Competing Interests: The authors have read the journal's policy and have the following conflicts: JMB and MW have received an unrestricted research grant from Grünenthal GmbH, Aachen, Germany. CS and NÜ have been speakers for Astellas GmbH, Germany and NÜ has received travel grants from Astellas GmbH, Germany. CS and NÜ are PLOS ONE Editorial Board members. The study was supported by an unrestricted research grant from Astellas Pharma a/s, Kastrup, Denmark. This does not alter the authors' adherence to PLOS ONE policies on sharing data and materials.

* Email: jomutahi@hotmail.com

Introduction

Inguinal herniorrhaphy is a common surgical procedure with more than 800.000 repairs annually in the United States [1]. Persistent severe pain affecting daily activities is present in 5% of patients [2,3] and in spite of exploratory surgery including selective neurectomy [4,5], that has been associated with a satisfactory outcome, the invasive nature of the procedure requires availability of medical treatment options for patients reluctant to undergo repeat surgery or not fit for a surgical procedure. The evidence-base for pharmacological treatment of persistent pain following inguinal hernia repair is nearly non-existent and therefore it is of considerable clinical relevance to identify the efficaciousness of drug therapy.

The capsaicin 8% cutaneous patch is used in the treatment of peripheral neuropathic pain and significant pain-relief for up to 12 weeks has been observed in randomized, controlled trials in post-herpetic neuralgia and HIV-related distal neuropathy [6–10]. Capsaicin is a selective agonist for the transient receptor potential vanilloid (TRPV1) receptor residing on nociceptive peripheral nerve fibers and keratinocytes [11]. The effect of capsaicin is assumed to be mediated by a reversible defunctionalization of cutaneous nociceptors thereby inhibiting transmission of nociceptive signals [12,13]. The long lasting pain relieving effect, up to three months after a single capsaicin 8% patch application, is of particular clinical interest. From a pharmacodynamic view, the localized action of the capsaicin patch confers a reduced risk of systemic side effects and a lessened potential for drug interactions. In an un-controlled prospective study (n = 1,044) the capsaicin 8% patch relieved pain and improved sleep quality in patients with various peripheral neuropathic pain states [14]. Interestingly, in this cohort 23% of the patients experienced persistent postsurgical pain of differing etiologies. However, the efficacy of capsaicin 8% patch treatment has never been evaluated in a randomized controlled trial in persistent postsurgical pain. Purified capsaicin has been shown to reduce acute postoperative pain following inguinal hernia repair. In a randomized placebo-controlled trial intraoperative wound instillation of purified capsaicin significantly reduced pain scores in the capsaicin group during the first 4 days after inguinal hernia repair [15].

In the present study we tested the hypothesis that capsaicin 8% patch treatment would be associated with a higher analgesic efficacy compared to placebo in patients suffering from severe persistent inguinal postherniorrhaphy pain.

Since changes in intraepidermal nerve fiber density (IENFD) have been observed following capsaicin 8% patch application in healthy volunteers [16,17], we investigated the effect of capsaicin on IENFD and sensory function, assessed by thermal and mechanical thresholds, as secondary outcomes. Additional secondary outcomes were changes in ratings of sleep quality, catastrophizing behaviour, anxiety and depression, associated with capsaicin 8% patch treatment.

Materials and Methods

A randomized, double-blind, placebo-controlled, parallel-group study was conducted at the Multidisciplinary Pain Center, Rigshospitalet, Copenhagen with patients recruitment from August 2012 to May 2013 and follow-up from September 2012 to September 2013. Study approval was obtained from the Committee on Health Research Ethics of the Capital Region of Denmark (H-4-2012-055), the Danish Data Protection Agency, the Danish Medicines Agency (EudraCT-Nr. 2012-001540-22) and the study was registered at ClinicalTrials.gov (NCT01699854). The study was conducted in accordance with Good Clinical Practice (GCP) Guidelines and was monitored by the Copenhagen University Hospital GCP Unit. The protocol for this trial and supporting CONSORT checklist are available as supporting information; see Checklist S1 and Protocol S1.

Patients eligible in the study were referred to the Multidisciplinary Pain Center by a surgeon or a general practitioner and written informed consent was obtained from all patients. Patients were ≥18 years with severe unilateral persistent inguinal postherniorrhaphy pain (numerical rating scale [NRS, 0–10] ≥ 5) for more than 6 months. Concomitant analgesic medication was allowed if patients had maintained a stable regimen for at least 4 weeks prior to study entry and stayed on stable doses throughout the study period. Exclusion criteria were allergy to capsaicin or vehicle-ingredients in the patch, skin lesions or inflamed skin at the application site, bilateral groin pain, severe cardiac impairment, known diseases impairing nervous system function, alcohol or drug abuse, inability to understand Danish, and in female patients lactation or pregnancy (negative pregnancy test required for females of fertile age).

Randomization

Randomization was done by Herning Hospital Pharmacy according to a computer-generated randomization list (http://randomization.com/) and a block-size of four was used.

Pain assessment

Patients evaluated pain intensities (NRS) every morning and evening, at rest in the supine position, during transition from supine to standing position, and during the patient's palpation of the point of maximum pain in the groin. Assessments were made in the 3 days preceding the patch treatment (baseline) and in the 3 days preceding the clinical visits at 1, 2 and 3 months after patch application.

Questionnaires

Questionnaires were completed at baseline and at 1, 2 and 3 months after patch application. Anxiety and depression were evaluated with the Hospital Anxiety and Depression Scale (HADS) [18] and the level of catastrophizing behaviour with the Pain

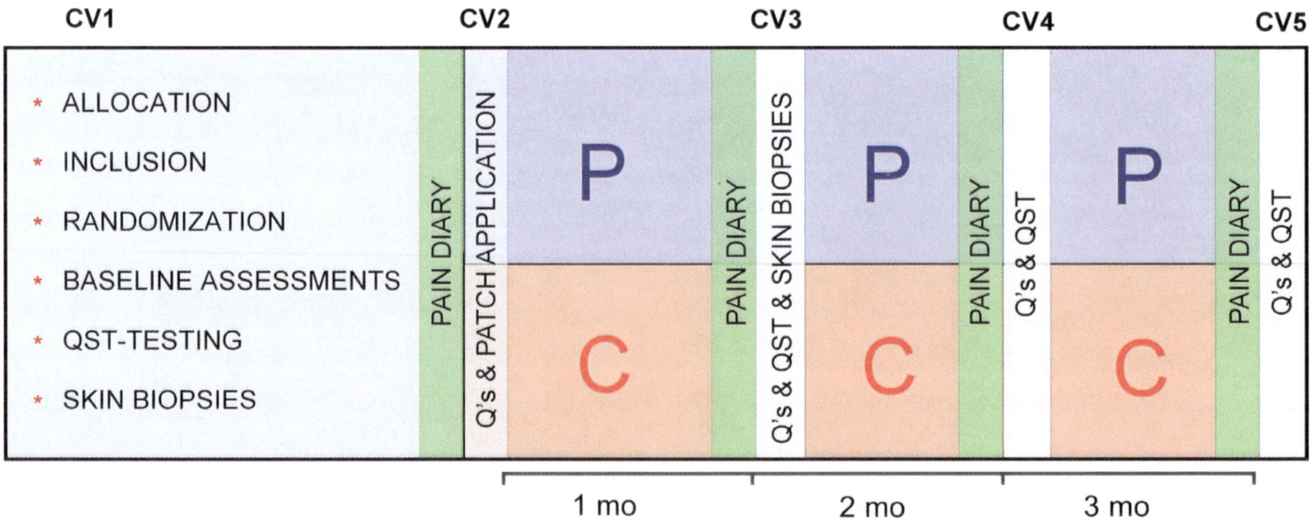

Figure 1. Study algorithm, CV = Clinical visit, Q's = Questionnaires.

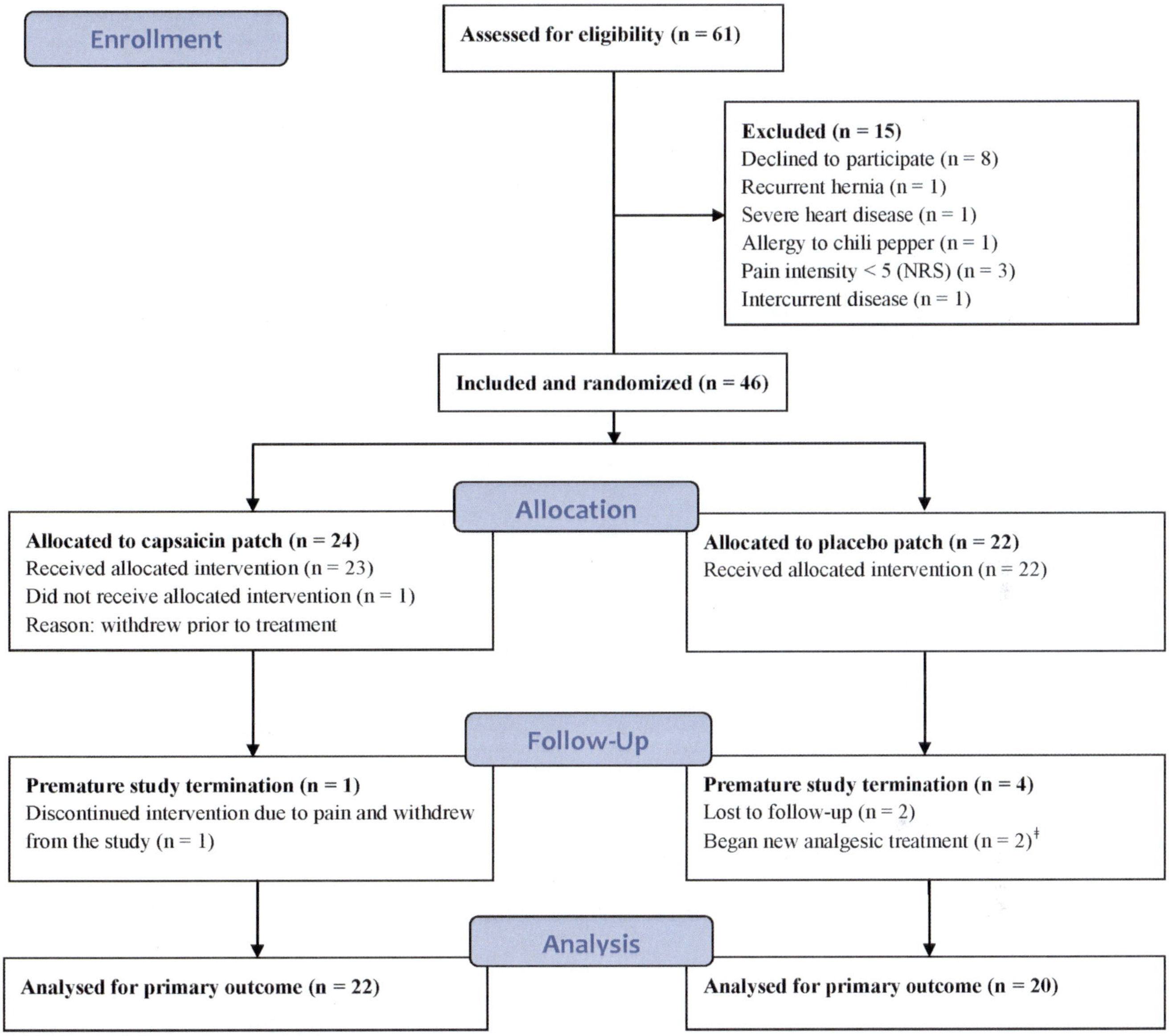

Figure 2. Flow diagram of patients in the study. ‡ Data from these two patients were included in the analyses up to the time of the medication violation. NRS = Numerical Rating Scale.

Catastrophizing Scale (PCS) [19]. Pain-related sleep interference was evaluated with the Daily Sleep Interference Scale (DSIS [0–10, 0 = pain did not interfere with sleep, 10 = pain completely interfered with sleep]) [20]. The self-report version of the Leeds Assessment of Neuropathic Symptoms and Signs pain scale (S-LANSS) was used for assessment of neuropathic pain components [21].

Quantitative sensory testing (QST)

Prior to the QST, hair growth in the inguinal and suprapubic areas was carefully trimmed using a surgical clipper (3M-9671, St. Paul, MN). The QST assessments were performed in accordance with previous studies in persistent inguinal postherniorrhaphy pain [22,23]. The sensory testing area on the pain side included the point of maximum pain and in addition the contralateral inguinal region was used as a control area. The warmth and cool detection thresholds (WDT, CDT) and the heat pain threshold (HPT) were determined using a computer controlled thermode (Somedic AB, Hörby, Sweden; contact area 2.5×5.0 cm^2). The baseline temperature was 32°C and thermal stimuli were delivered with a ramp rate of ±1°C/s with cut-off values of 50°C for heat, and 5°C for cold stimuli. The pressure pain threshold (PPT) was assessed at the point of maximum pain using a handheld pressure algometer (Somedic AB, Hörby, Sweden; 1 cm^2 felt-tipped probe) applied perpendicularly to the skin, until the pressure was perceived as painful or exceeded the cut-off value of 350 kPa. A heat stimulus (5 s at 47°C, ramp rate 1°C/s) was delivered at the point of maximum pain to evaluate the suprathreshold heat pain perception (STH) rated by the patient (NRS). All QST parameters were assessed three times and the median values were used. The QST was performed at baseline and at the clinical visits: at 1 month (day 30–36), 2 months (day 60–66), and 3 months (day 90–96) after patch application (fig. 1).

Table 1. Baseline patient characteristics.

	Capsaicin (n = 24)	Placebo (n = 22)
Age (yrs)†	52 (17)	55 (14)
Sex (male/female)	20/4	22/0
BMI (kg/m²) ‡	25 (23–30)	26 (23–28)
Duration of pain (mo)‡	37 (22–58)	39 (18–63)
Primary/recurrent operation§, *n*	20/4	20/2
Open mesh/laparoscopic§, *n*	21/3	17/5
Unilaterally/bilaterally operated, *n*	23/1	17/5
Exploratory surgery for pain, yes/no, *n*	10/14	7/15
Concomitant pain medication, yes/no, *n*	11/13	13/9
- Acetaminophen, *n*	7	7
- NSAIDs, *n*	3	7
- Gabapentin, *n*	2	4
- Tricyclic antidepressants, *n*	1	2
- Opioids, *n*	2	2
Baseline pain ratings¶		
- Pain at rest (NRS)	4 (3–7)	4 (3–6)
- Pain during movement (NRS)	5 (4–7)	6 (3–7)
- Pain during palpation (NRS)	7 (5–9)	7 (5–8)

†Mean (standard deviation).
‡Median (25–75% interquartile range).
§Pain-generating inguinal hernia operation.
¶Pain ratings at baseline assessed at rest in the supine position, during transition from supine to standing position, and during the patient's palpation of the point of maximum pain in the groin. Values are medians (25–75% interquartile range). Two patients who withdrew early from the study and one patient who was lost to follow-up did not report baseline pain ratings and were not included in the analyses of pain ratings.
BMI = Body Mass Index, NRS = Numerical Rating Scale (0–10), NSAIDs = Non-steroidal Anti-inflammatory Drugs.

Skin biopsies

At baseline and at the clinical visit at 1 month after patch application two 3-mm skin punch biopsies (disposable biopsy punch, Miltex, York, PA) were performed, using a sterile technique, at the point of maximum pain in the groin and on the contralateral control side. Prior to biopsies, the skin areas were anesthetized with 1–2 ml of mepivacaine (10 mg/ml, AstraZeneca AB, Södertälje, Sweden). The IENFD was estimated in agreement with previously described methods [23,24]. After fixation with 4% paraformaldehyde, the biopsies were washed in phosphate buffer and then stored in 10% sucrose with 0.1 M phosphate buffer at 4°C, until analysis. Sections of 50-μm thickness were immunostained with the pan-neuronal marker PGP-9.5 (1:800, Ultraclone, Wellow, UK) and visualized with Cy3-coupled anti-rabbit antibodies (1:100, Amersham Biosciences, Piscataway, NJ). Intraepidermal nerve fiber counting was performed with a light-microscope (Zeiss Axiophot 2, Wetzlar, Germany) and Spot advanced software (Windows Version 4.5, Sterling Heights, MI). The skin biopsies were analyzed blinded in regard to side.

Treatment procedure and blinding method

The research nurse and the physician responsible for the intervention did only meet the patient on the day of treatment and were not further involved in the study. The research nurse delineated the patch area corresponding to the inguinal pain distribution including the point of maximum pain. Patients were pre-treated with a topical local anesthetic cream (EMLA, lidocaine/prilocaine 25 mg/25 g, AstraZeneca AB, Södertälje, Sweden) 60 min before patch application. The patch application, patch removal, and skin cleansing were done by a physician. During this procedure the research nurse was not allowed presence in the treatment room since minute quantities of aerosolized capsaicin-particles during patch handling could have led to accidental un-blinding of the research nurse.

The capsaicin patches (capsaicin 640 μg/cm², 8% w/w; Astellas Pharma Europe B.V., Leiderdorp, The Netherlands) and the inactive placebo patches were identical in appearance and composition (in regard to vehicle substances). An inactive placebo patch was used since an active placebo patch was not obtainable from the manufacturer of the capsaicin patch. The patients were informed that they might experience pain during and after the patch application. The patches were applied in the groin area for 60 min. After patch removal a cleansing gel (Astellas Pharma Europe B.V., Leiderdorp, The Netherlands) was applied in order to remove capsaicin residues. In order to decrease local irritation of the skin cool packs (assistCo AS, Rjukan, Norway) were administered for 45–60 minutes after patch removal. Patients were told to use oral acetaminophen 1 g every 6 h and ibuprofen 400 mg every 6 h for up to 3 days as needed after patch application. The patients and investigators were blinded to the treatment allocation throughout the study. At the clinical visit 1 month after patch application patients were asked to report if they had experienced application site skin reactions (erythema, pain, burning sensation) or any other adverse events. To evaluate patient blinding we asked patients at the clinical visit 1 month after patch application to verbally report which treatment they had received.

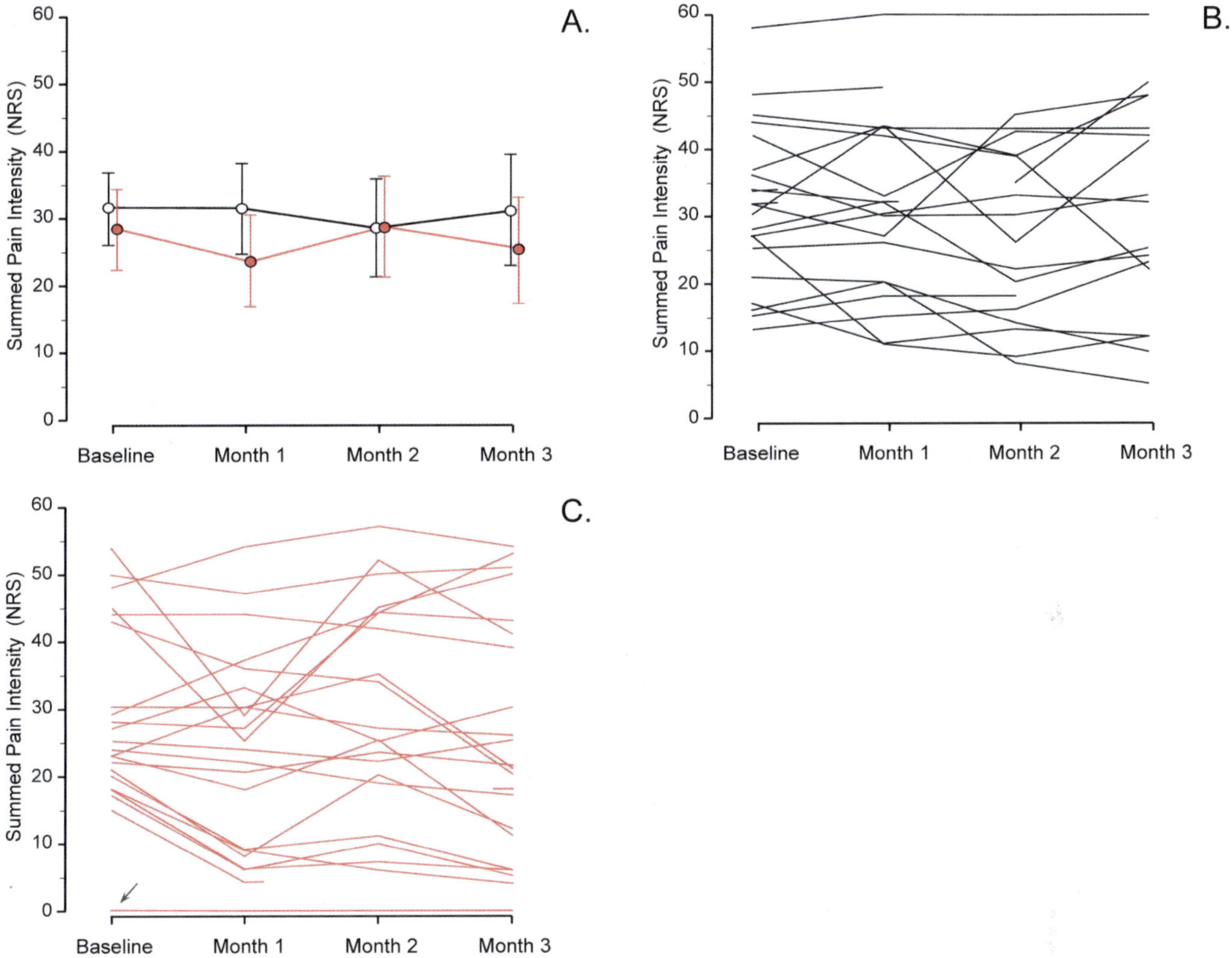

Figure 3. Panel A. Summed pain intensity (SPI) values assessed on a Numerical Rating Scale (NRS) at baseline and at 1, 2 and 3 months after patch application. Each SPI-value contains six median values (pain assessments twice daily for three days) and the maximum SPI-value is 60 NRS units. Values are mean (95% confidence interval). Black line (○) placebo treated patients. Red line (●) capsaicin treated patients. Individual time profiles are displayed for placebo treated patients (panel B, black lines) and capsaicin treated patients (panel C, red lines). The arrow (panel C) indicates patient #10 with baseline median NRS-value of 0 (see text for explanation).

Statistical analyses

The pain intensities during the 3 standardized conditions (at rest, during movement and pressure evoked), were evaluated twice daily in the 3 days preceding patch treatment (baseline) and in the 3 days preceding the clinical visit at 1, 2 and 3 months after patch application. The median value of the 3 standardized pain assessments was used to calculate the summed pain intensity (SPI) values (containing 6 median values [pain assessments twice daily for 3 days]) in accordance with a previously described method [23]. The summed pain intensity differences (SPID) were

Table 2. Changes in pain intensity between baseline and 1 month after patch application presented as SPID for capsaicin and placebo patch treatments, and the mean difference.

	Capsaicin (n = 22)	Placebo (n = 20)	Difference	*P*-value
SPID (NRS)	4.8 (1.4 to 8.2)	−0.2 (−3.8 to 3.4)	5.0 (0.09 to 9.9)	0.046
SPID %	19.8 (7.5 to 32.1)	−1.0 (−14.1 to 12.1)	20.9 (2.9 to 38.9)	0.024

The SPID was calculated as the difference between the baseline SPI-value and the SPI-value at 1 month after patch application. Each SPI- value contains six median values (pain assessments twice daily for three days). Values are mean (95% CI). Positive values of SPID indicate pain reduction after treatment. *P*-values indicate comparisons of SPID (capsaicin *vs.* placebo).
NRS = Numerical Rating Scale (0–10), SPID = Summed pain intensity difference, SPI = summed pain intensity.

Table 3. Differences in quantitative sensory assessments on the pain side from baseline to 1 month after patch application.

Δ-value	Capsaicin (n = 21)	Placebo (n = 19)	*P*-value
ΔWDT§ (°C)	0.2 (−0.9 to 1.2)	0.6 (−0.1 to 1.3)	0.52‡
ΔCDT (°C)	0.0 (−0.8 to 0.7)	−0.1 (−0.7 to 0.8)	0.96
ΔHPT (°C)	0.3 (−0.4 to 1.5)	0.3 (−0.2 to 1.2)	0.91
ΔPPT§ (kPa)	1.5 (−24.8 to 27.8)	−0.4 (−23.2 to 22.4)	0.91‡
ΔSTH (NRS)	0.0 (−1.0 to 0.0)	0.0 (−1.0 to 1.0)	0.56

Values are mean (95% CI)§ or median (95% CI). Δ value = post-treatment minus baseline value. *P*-values indicate comparisons of Δ-values (capsaicin *vs.* placebo [unpaired t-test‡ or the Mann-Whitney test). Positive Δ-values for WDT, HPT, PPT and CDT indicate increased thresholds after treatment.
WDT = warmth detection threshold, CDT = cool detection threshold, HPT = heat pain threshold, PPT = pressure pain threshold, STH = suprathreshold heat pain perception, NRS = Numerical Rating Scale (0–10).

calculated for 1, 2 and 3 months after patch application, as the difference between the baseline SPI-value and the post-treatment SPI-value. The primary outcome was comparisons of SPIDs between capsaicin and placebo treatments at 1, 2 and 3 months after patch application. No data from previous studies were available and the *a priori* sample size calculation was therefore based on the best estimates for the study cohort. Based on a significance level of 0.01 (α), a power of 0.9 (β = 0.1), an estimated standard deviation for the SPI assessments of 3.1 (NRS), and a minimal relevant difference for the six SPI assessments of 4.5 (NRS), the estimated number of patients needed in each group were 24 (48 in total). In order to compensate for dropouts the number of patients was set to 50. Due to uncertainties in the power calculation an interim analysis by an independent statistician was planned *a priori* following completion of the first 32 patients.

Linear regression analyses for repeated measures (a mixed model method) were used to evaluate the treatment effects over time. The summed pain intensity difference (SPID) was the outcome variable and treatment group (capsaicin or placebo) and time (1, 2 and 3 months after patch application) were explanatory variables. While measurements taken at different time points were expected to correlate, we also assumed that measurements taken at adjacent time points were more correlated than measurements further apart, and therefore we used an unstructured covariance structure (all covariance parameters are freely estimated). We used the PROC MIXED procedure and the repeated statement in SAS software (9.3, SAS Institute Inc., Cary, NC) to estimate the model. We included the interaction because we were interested in testing whether potential group differences changed over time. The mixed model is dealing with missing longitudinal measures and the analysis included all patients with at least one SPID-value. For secondary outcomes, including QST variables and questionnaire scores (DSIS, HADS, PCS, S-LANNS), differences (Δ) between post-treatment follow-up and baseline values were used to compare capsaicin and placebo patch treatments. The numbers of patients included in the data analyses vary for different outcome measures and are indicated in the tables for each analysis.

The normality of data was assessed with the Kolmogorov-Smirnov test and visual estimation of relevant residual distribution plots. Comparisons between treatment groups were performed with unpaired t-tests (normally distributed data) and the Mann-Whitney tests (non-normally distributed data). Fischer's exact test was used to compare proportions. Statistical analyses were conducted using SPSS software (SPSS 20.0, Chicago, IL) and MedCalc Software (12.3.0.0, Mariakerke, Belgium). The linear regression analyses for repeated measures were performed with SAS software. Due to the three statistical tests performed (comparisons 1, 2 and 3 months after patch application) and the planned interim analysis, thus increasing the probability of a type I error, all results were considered significant at $P<0.01$ (two-tailed).

Results

A total of 46 patients were randomized (fig. 2). Baseline patient characteristics and pain ratings are shown in table 1. In one patient (#46) severe pain at the application site necessitated premature patch removal leading to study withdrawal. In two patients (#16, #34) add-on treatment with other analgesics was initiated during the study. Data from these two patients were included in the analyses only up to the time of the violation of the medication criterion. One patient (#10) reported severe pain (NRS ≥5) at the first clinical visit and was thus included in the study in accordance with the protocol. However, in the pain diary evaluations preceding the patch application the patient only reported pain during palpation (NRS = 5), and, no pain (NRS = 0) at rest and during movement Therefore, the median NRS-value of the three standardized pain assessments at baseline was 0 for this patient (indicated in Fig. 3C). Five patients had one or more missing SPID values. Three patients (#4, #15, #49) had one

Table 4. Assessments of intraepidermal nerve fiber density (IENFD) on the pain side at baseline and at 1 month after patch application.

	Baseline (IENFD/mm)	1 month (IENFD/mm)	Δ value	*P*-value
Capsaicin (n = 18)	4.8 (2.5 to 7.2)	2.9 (1.2 to 4.7)	1.9 (−0.1 to 3.9)	0.32
Placebo (n = 20)	5.8 (3.2 to 8.3)	5.2 (2.2 to 8.1)	0.6 (−1.2 to 2.5)	

Values are mean (95% CI). The *P*-value indicates comparison of Δ values (capsaicin *vs.* placebo unpaired t-test). Δ value = baseline −1 month value. Δ values are normally distributed while baseline and 1 month IENFD values are non-normally distributed.

Table 5. Skin reactions at application site.

	Capsaicin (n = 23)	Placebo (n = 20)
Any application site reaction, *n* (%)	17 (74)	6 (30)
- Erythema, *n*	9	3
- Pain, *n*	12	6
- Burning sensation, *n*	12	1

missing SPID value and two patients (#2, #34) had two missing SPID values.

As previously mentioned, an interim analysis was planned for the first 32 patients, but due to a lower patient-recruitment rate than anticipated and a premature expiry date of the placebo patches (May 2013) an interim analysis could not be performed. The interim analysis would have impeded study progression and prolonged the study for an estimated period of at least three months (time from patch application to study completion; fig. 1). Therefore, it was decided to continue the study without an interim analysis and to recruit patients until the expiration date of the placebo patch: the actual number of randomized patients (n = 46) in the study were thus lower than the originally estimated sample size of 50 patients.

Pain

The summed pain intensity (SPI) values (NRS) at baseline and at 1, 2 and 3 months after patch application are presented in (fig. 3). A linear regression analysis for repeated measures with SPID as outcome variable and treatment group (capsaicin [n = 22] or placebo [n = 20]) and time (1, 2 and 3 months after patch application) as explanatory variables revealed a significant interaction for group * time ($F_{2,37.4} = 5.53$, $P = 0.008$). The analysis showed that the maximum difference in SPID between capsaicin and placebo treated patients was observed at 1 month after patch application, although statistical significance at the 0.01 level was not achieved. The mean difference [95% CI] in SPID at 1 month after patch application was (5.0 [0.09 to 9.9] NRS-units; $P = 0.046$, table 2), corresponding to a mean difference [95% CI] in SPID percentage of (20.9% [2.9 to 38.9%]; $P = 0.024$). Similarly, there were no significant differences in SPID between capsaicin and placebo patch treatments at 2 months after patch application (mean difference [95% CI]: −1.7 [−6.4 to 3.1] NRS-units; $P = 0.48$) or at 3 months after patch application (mean difference [95% CI]: 3.6 [−3.1 to 10.2] NRS-units; $P = 0.29$).

Sensory Function

Analyses of changes in QST assessments from baseline to 1 month after treatment are presented in table 3. No significant differences between capsaicin and placebo patch treated patients for thermal thresholds, suprathreshold heat pain perception, and pressure pain thresholds were observed.

Skin innervation

The median (95% CI) IENFD at baseline was significantly lower on the pain side, i.e. 4.3 (1.5 to 6.8) fibers/mm compared with the non-pain side 8.6 (7.4 to 11.0) fibers/mm, ($P < 0.0001$, Wilcoxon signed rank test). Changes in IENFD, from baseline to 1 month after patch application on the pain side, did not differ between capsaicin and placebo treated patients ($P = 0.32$, table 4).

S-LANSS, Sleep Quality and Psychological Factors

At baseline the median (95% CI) S-LANSS score was 15 (10 to 17) and 26 of 42 patients (62%) reported a S-LANSS score of ≥12 indicating pain components of predominantly neuropathic origin [21]. Changes from baseline to 1 month after patch application with regard to sleep quality, PCS, S-LANSS, and HADS scores did not differ between capsaicin and placebo treated patients.

Adverse Events

Seventeen of 23 (74%) capsaicin treated patients and 6 of 20 (30%) placebo treated patients reported one or more skin reactions on the application site ($P = 0.006$, Fischer's exact test, table 5). No other adverse events or complications were observed in the study.

Patient Blinding

Sixteen of 23 patients (70%) treated with the capsaicin patch and 17 of 21 patients (81%) treated with the placebo patch correctly identified their treatment allocation ($P = 0.49$, Fischer's exact test).

Discussion

The present study in patients with severe persistent inguinal postherniorrhaphy pain, comparing the pain relief of a capsaicin 8% patch with an inactive placebo patch, was not able to demonstrate significant differences in pain reduction during standardized testing conditions. In addition, we did not observe any changes in secondary outcome variables including sensory function, IENFD, sleep quality, catastrophizing behaviour (PCS), or anxiety and depression (HADS) scores associated with capsaicin patch treatment.

Statistical Issues

Interpretation of the study's main finding should consider the *a priori* assigned significance level of 0.01. The authors regarded this conservative statistical measure a precaution against the introduction of type I errors due to the use of multiple comparisons and interim analysis. However, the statistical comparisons of SPID-scores, one month after patch application, yielding *P*-values of 0.024 and 0.046, indicated a trend of an improved pain relief in capsaicin treated patients. A potential contributing factor to the non-significant findings is obviously the premature discontinuation of the study after 46 randomized patients compared to the *a priori* estimated sample size of 50 patients. This circumstance may have introduced a type II error. A post hoc power calculation could be considered but is generally not recommended [25].

Skin innervation

The study corroborates our previous findings of a reduced IENFD on the pain side compared to the contralateral side in persistent inguinal postherniorrhaphy pain patients, most likely caused by surgical nerve injury [23,26]. Several studies in healthy volunteers have demonstrated a 60–80% reduction in IENFD one week after capsaicin 8% patch treatment [16,17,27]. The current study, the first to evaluate changes in IENFD following capsaicin patch treatment in patients, failed to show a significant difference in IENFD between treatment groups. A plausible explanation is the low baseline IENFD on the pain side in postherniorrhaphy pain patients compared to healthy volunteers, making it difficult to demonstrate a further reduction in IENFD following capsaicin treatment. The small group size may be another reason why the observed reduction of IENFD in the capsaicin group did not reach significance. However, it should be emphasized that none of the studies investigating IENFD after application of an 8% capsaicin patch in healthy volunteers provide data at 4 weeks after application [16,17,27], and it cannot be excluded that partial regeneration of nerve fibers already may have taken place [28].

Sensory Assessments

The QST assessment did not demonstrate any differences in cutaneous (thermal) or deep tissue (mechanical) sensory function between capsaicin and placebo treatment. A possible explanation is the previously mentioned lack of a significant reduction in IENFD after capsaicin treatment. In addition, sensory nerve endings not expressing TRPV1 receptors, i.e. Aβ-fibers, the majority of Aδ-fibers, and a subgroup of C-fibers, remain intact after capsaicin treatment and are thus still capable of transmitting sensory stimuli [12]. Accordingly, previous studies in neuropathic pain patients have failed to demonstrate sensory impairment after capsaicin patch treatment. In painful HIV-related neuropathy no differences in thermal and vibration detection thresholds were observed between capsaicin treated patients and controls at 4 and 12 weeks after patch application [9]. Furthermore, no differences between treatment groups were found in two studies investigating detection thresholds for brush, punctate stimulation, vibration and warmth in patients with post-herpetic neuralgia at 4 and 12 weeks after patch application [8,29].

Limitations

A confounding factor for the study is the patient-blinding. The higher incidence of local side effects experienced by patients in the capsaicin group (74%) compared to the placebo group (30%), and the correspondingly high proportion of patients who correctly identified their treatment allocation, indicate an insufficient blinding-technique. Therefore, it cannot be excluded that the potential analgesic effect experienced by the capsaicin treatment may in fact represent a placebo effect. The short duration of the potential analgesic effect (i.e. one month) also may connote to a placebo effect. The study thus supports the use of an active placebo (e.g. low-dose of capsaicin) in order to ensure adequate blinding in future studies assessing the effects of topical capsaicin.

Pathophysiological Mechanism

Pain relief up to 12 weeks after capsaicin patch application has been observed in previous randomized, controlled trials in post-herpetic neuralgia and HIV-related distal neuropathy [6–10]. The lack of a significant analgesic effect in the present study may be explained by a different pain mechanism in persistent inguinal postherniorrhaphy pain. The S-LANNS findings in the present study and the QST results in previous studies [30,31] point towards neuropathic pain components in this patient cohort, which is also underscored by the reduced IENFD on the painful side, specifying a small-fiber neuropathy. However, a number of postherniorrhaphy pain patients demonstrate decreased pain thresholds to pressure algometry indicating increased deep tissue sensitivity and suggesting deep pain components that may be caused by an untoward inflammatory reaction to the implanted mesh [31]. The negative findings in our study suggest that interruption of cutaneous nerve transmission alone may be insufficient to relieve pain substantially in these patients and seem to indicate that nerve injury, as well as deep tissue inflammation, may contribute to the development and maintenance of persistent postherniorrhaphy pain. Further studies are needed to elucidate the pathophysiological contributors in persistent postherniorrhaphy pain in order to guide future treatment strategies.

In conclusion capsaicin patch 8% did not significantly reduce combined static and dynamic pain components compared to placebo in persistent inguinal postherniorrhaphy pain, albeit a trend towards pain relief was observed 1 month after capsaicin patch application.

Acknowledgments

The authors would like to thank Morten Aagaard Petersen, M.Sc., Department of Palliative Medicine, Bispebjerg Hospital, Copenhagen University Hospitals, DENMARK for statistical assistance, Manuel Pedro Pereira M.D., Department of Anaesthesia, Center of Head and Orthopaedics, Rigshospitalet, Copenhagen University Hospitals, DENMARK for assistance during patch application and Kathleen Stahl, Department of Neurology, University Hospital of Würzburg, GERMANY, for technical help during skin biopsy staining.

Author Contributions

Wrote the paper: JMB MW. Critically revising the manuscript: TR MP CS NÜ. Conceived and designed the experiments: JMB MW CS NÜ. Performed the experiments: JMB TR MP. Analyzed the data: JMB MW. Contributed reagents/materials/analysis tools: MW CS NÜ.

References

1. Rutkow IM (2003) Demographic and socioeconomic aspects of hernia repair in the United States in 2003. Surg Clin North Am 83: 1045-10vi. S0039-6109(03)00132-4 [pii]; 10.1016/S0039-6109(03)00132-4 [doi].
2. Franneby U, Sandblom G, Nordin P, Nyren O, Gunnarsson U (2006) Risk factors for long-term pain after hernia surgery. Ann Surg 244: 212–219.
3. Kalliomaki ML, Meyerson J, Gunnarsson U, Gordh T, Sandblom G (2008) Long-term pain after inguinal hernia repair in a population-based cohort; risk factors and interference with daily activities. Eur J Pain 12: 214–225.
4. Chen DC, Hiatt JR, Amid PK (2013) Operative management of refractory neuropathic inguinodynia by a laparoscopic retroperitoneal approach. JAMA Surg 148: 962–967. 1722800 [pii]; 10.1001/jamasurg.2013.3189 [doi].
5. Bischoff JM, Enghuus C, Werner MU, Kehlet H (2013) Long-term follow-up after mesh removal and selective neurectomy for persistent inguinal postherniorrhaphy pain. Hernia 17: 339–345. 10.1007/s10029-013-1073-z [doi].
6. Derry S, Sven-Rice A, Cole P, Tan T, Moore RA (2013) Topical capsaicin (high concentration) for chronic neuropathic pain in adults. Cochrane Database Syst Rev 2: CD007393. 10.1002/14651858.CD007393.pub3 [doi].
7. Backonja M, Wallace MS, Blonsky ER, Cutler BJ, Malan P Jr, et al. (2008) NGX-4010, a high-concentration capsaicin patch, for the treatment of postherpetic neuralgia: a randomised, double-blind study. Lancet Neurol 7: 1106–1112. S1474-4422(08)70228-X [pii]; 10.1016/S1474-4422(08)70228-X [doi].
8. Irving GA, Backonja MM, Dunteman E, Blonsky ER, Vanhove GF, et al.(2011) A multicenter, randomized, double-blind, controlled study of NGX-4010, a

high-concentration capsaicin patch, for the treatment of postherpetic neuralgia. Pain Med 12: 99-109. 10.1111/j.1526-4637.2010.01004.x [doi].

9. Simpson DM, Brown S, Tobias J (2008) Controlled trial of high-concentration capsaicin patch for treatment of painful HIV neuropathy. Neurology 70: 2305–2313. 70/24/2305 [pii]; 10.1212/01.wnl.0000314647.35825.9c [doi].
10. Webster LR, Malan TP, Tuchman MM, Mollen MD, Tobias JK, et al. (2010) A multicenter, randomized, double-blind, controlled dose finding study of NGX-4010, a high-concentration capsaicin patch, for the treatment of postherpetic neuralgia. J Pain 11: 972–982. S1526-5900(10)00296-8 [pii]; 10.1016/j.jpain.2010.01.270 [doi].
11. Ringkamp M, Raja SN, Campbell JN, Meyer RA (2013) Peripheral mechanisms of cutaneous nociception. In: McMahon SB, Koltzenburg M, Tracey I, Turk DC, editors. Wall and Melzack's textbook of pain. Elsevier Saunders. pp. 1–30.
12. Anand P, Bley K (2011) Topical capsaicin for pain management: therapeutic potential and mechanisms of action of the new high-concentration capsaicin 8% patch. Br J Anaesth 107: 490–502. aer260 [pii]; 10.1093/bja/aer260 [doi].
13. Treede RD, Wagner T, Kern KU, Husstedt IW, Arendt G, et al. (2013) Mechanism- and experience-based strategies to optimize treatment response to the capsaicin 8% cutaneous patch in patients with localized neuropathic pain. Curr Med Res Opin 29: 527–538. 10.1185/03007995.2013.781019 [doi].
14. Maihofner C, Heskamp ML (2013) Prospective, non-interventional study on the tolerability and analgesic effectiveness over 12 weeks after a single application of capsaicin 8% cutaneous patch in 1044 patients with peripheral neuropathic pain: first results of the QUEPP study. Curr Med Res Opin 29: 673–683. 10.1185/03007995.2013.792246 [doi].
15. Aasvang EK, Hansen JB, Malmstrom J, Asmussen T, Gennevois D, et al. (2008) The effect of wound instillation of a novel purified capsaicin formulation on postherniotomy pain: a double-blind, randomized, placebo-controlled study. Anesth Analg 107: 282–291.
16. Malmberg AB, Mizisin AP, Calcutt NA, von ST, Robbins WR, et al. (2004) Reduced heat sensitivity and epidermal nerve fiber immunostaining following single applications of a high-concentration capsaicin patch. Pain 111: 360–367. 10.1016/j.pain.2004.07.017 [doi];S0304-3959(04)00344-6 [pii].
17. Kennedy WR, Vanhove GF, Lu SP, Tobias J, Bley KR, et al. (2010) A randomized, controlled, open-label study of the long-term effects of NGX-4010, a high-concentration capsaicin patch, on epidermal nerve fiber density and sensory function in healthy volunteers. J Pain 11: 579–587.
18. Zigmond AS, Snaith RP (1983) The hospital anxiety and depression scale. Acta Psychiatr Scand 67: 361–370.
19. Sullivan MJL, Bishop SR, Kivik J (1995) The pain catastrophizing scale: development and validation. Psych Assess 7: 524–532.
20. Vernon MK, Brandenburg NA, Alvir JM, Griesing T, Revicki DA (2008) Reliability, validity, and responsiveness of the daily sleep interference scale among diabetic peripheral neuropathy and postherpetic neuralgia patients. J Pain Symptom Manage 36: 54–68.
21. Bennett MI, Smith BH, Torrance N, Potter J (2005) The S-LANSS score for identifying pain of predominantly neuropathic origin: validation for use in clinical and postal research. J Pain 6: 149–158.
22. Bischoff JM, Koscielniak-Nielsen ZJ, Kehlet H, Werner MU (2012) Ultrasound-guided ilioinguinal/iliohypogastric nerve blocks for persistent inguinal post-herniorrhaphy pain: a randomized, double-blind, placebo-controlled, crossover trial. Anesth Analg 114: 1323–1329. ANE.0b013e31824d6168 [pii]; 10.1213/ANE.0b013e31824d6168 [doi].
23. Bischoff JM, Petersen M, Uceyler N, Sommer C, Kehlet H, et al. (2013) Lidocaine Patch (5%) in Treatment of Persistent Inguinal Postherniorrhaphy Pain: A Randomized, Double-blind, Placebo-controlled, Crossover Trial. Anesthesiology 119: 1444–1452. 10.1097/ALN.0b013e3182a2a243 [doi].
24. Torvin MA, Winther BF, Feldt-Rasmussen U, Rasmussen A, Hasholt L, et al. (2009) Functional and structural nerve fiber findings in heterozygote patients with Fabry disease. Pain 145: 237–245.
25. Moher D, Hopewell S, Schulz KF, Montori V, Gotzsche PC, et al. (2010) CONSORT 2010 explanation and elaboration: updated guidelines for reporting parallel group randomised trials. BMJ 340: c869.
26. Kehlet H, Jensen TS, Woolf CJ (2006) Persistent postsurgical pain: risk factors and prevention. Lancet 367: 1618–1625.
27. Knolle E, Zadrazil M, Kovacs GG, Medwed S, Scharbert G, et al. (2013) Comparison of cooling and EMLA to reduce the burning pain during capsaicin 8% patch application: a randomized, double-blind, placebo-controlled study. Pain 154: 2729–2736. S0304-3959(13)00437-5 [pii]; 10.1016/j.pain.2013.08.001 [doi].
28. Rage M, Van AN, Facer P, Shenoy R, Knaapen MW, et al. (2010) The time course of CO2 laser-evoked responses and of skin nerve fibre markers after topical capsaicin in human volunteers. Clin Neurophysiol 121: 1256–1266. S1388-2457(10)00263-4 [pii]; 10.1016/j.clinph.2010.02.159 [doi].
29. Webster LR, Tark M, Rauck R, Tobias JK, Vanhove GF (2010) Effect of duration of postherpetic neuralgia on efficacy analyses in a multicenter, randomized, controlled study of NGX-4010, an 8% capsaicin patch evaluated for the treatment of postherpetic neuralgia. BMC Neurol 10: 92. 1471-2377-10-92 [pii]; 10.1186/1471-2377-10-92 [doi].
30. Mikkelsen T, Werner MU, Lassen B, Kehlet H (2004) Pain and sensory dysfunction 6 to 12 months after inguinal herniotomy. Anesth Analg 99: 146–151.
31. Aasvang EK, Brandsborg B, Jensen TS, Kehlet H (2010) Heterogeneous sensory processing in persistent postherniotomy pain. Pain 150: 237–242.

Asymptomatic Bacteriuria *Escherichia coli* Are Live Biotherapeutics for UTI

Charles N. Rudick[1]⁹, Aisha K. Taylor[1]⁹¤, Ryan E. Yaggie[1], Anthony J. Schaeffer[1], David J. Klumpp[1,2]*

1 Department of Urology, Feinberg School of Medicine, Northwestern University, Chicago, Illinois, United States of America, **2** Microbiology-Immunology, Feinberg School of Medicine, Northwestern University, Chicago, Illinois, United States of America

Abstract

Urinary tract infections (UTI) account for approximately 8 million clinic visits annually with symptoms that include acute pelvic pain, dysuria, and irritative voiding. Empiric UTI management with antimicrobials is complicated by increasing antimicrobial resistance among uropathogens, but live biotherapeutics products (LBPs), such as asymptomatic bacteriuria (ASB) strains of *E. coli*, offer the potential to circumvent antimicrobial resistance. Here we evaluated ASB *E. coli* as LBPs, relative to ciprofloxacin, for efficacy against infection and visceral pain in a murine UTI model. Visceral pain was quantified as tactile allodynia of the pelvic region in response to mechanical stimulation with von Frey filaments. Whereas ciprofloxacin promoted clearance of uropathogenic *E. coli* (UPEC), it did not reduce pelvic tactile allodynia, a measure of visceral pain. In contrast, ASB *E. coli* administered intravesically or intravaginally provided comparable reduction of allodynia similar to intravesical lidocaine. Moreover, ASB *E. coli* were similarly effective against UTI allodynia induced by *Proteus mirabilis, Enterococccus faecalis* and *Klebsiella pneumoniae*. Therefore, ASB *E. coli* have anti-infective activity comparable to the current standard of care yet also provide superior analgesia. These studies suggest that ASB *E. coli* represent novel LBPs for UTI symptoms.

Editor: Neil A. Bhowmick, Cedars Sinai Medical Center, United States of America

Funding: These studies were funded by the National Institute of Diabetes and Digestive and Kidney Diseases (http://www.niddk.nih.gov/Pages/default.aspx). Funding was through awards R01 DK042648 and U01 DK8234201 to D.J.K. and A.J.S. Award U01 DK8234201 is within the Multi-Disciplinary Approaches to Chronic Pelvic Pain Research Network (MAPP, www.mappnetwork.org). This work was approved for publication by the MAPP Publications Committee. The funders had no role in study design, data collection and analysis, decision to publish, or preparation of the manuscript.

Competing Interests: The authors have the following interests: Northwestern University holds a patent for skewing immune responses by strains with altered LPS structures (Billips et al., Live-attenuated compositions for bacterial infections, US 8,709,444 B2, issued 29 April, 2014) and a pending application for pain therapies based on analgesic bacteria (Rudick et al., Compositions and methods for treatment of pain, provisional 61.450,937, filed 09 March, 2011). D.J.K. and A.J.S. are incorporated in the State of Illinois as ProbioTx, Inc. and pursue commercial development of strains described here, with the support of Northwestern University and the Chicago Innovation Mentors program. D.J.K. and A.J.S. are also officers in Gold Coast Therapeutics, Inc., a company targeting mast cells in urologic disease. This does not alter the authors' adherence to all the PLOS ONE policies on sharing data and materials. All proprietary bacterial strains from Northwestern University described in provisional patent 61.450,937 and this article will be shared upon request through Northwestern's INVO under a Material Transfer Agreement authorizing non-commercial use.

* Email: d-klumpp@northwestern.edu

¤ Current address: Department of Urology, Case Western Reserve, Cleveland, OH, United States of America

⁹ These authors contributed equally to this work.

Introduction

Urinary tract infection (UTI) is the second-most common infectious disease, resulting in millions of cases in the U.S. annually and costing billions of dollars for associated treatment [1,2]. The standard of care for UTI is antimicrobial therapy, where such therapy effectively sterilizes the urine of susceptible bacteria [3]. Unfortunately, uropathogenic bacteria are increasingly resistant to frontline antimicrobials, and multi-drug resistant strains are emerging rapidly [4,5]. In addition to waning efficacy due to resistance, it is unclear that acute antimicrobial therapy is sufficient to prevent recurrent UTI. Data from murine models and clinical studies demonstrate that UPEC and other uropathogens establish quiescent reservoirs within bladder urothelium that can trigger subsequent acute infection [6]. These quiescent reservoirs are resistant to antimicrobial therapy, indicating a need for alternative approaches. While antimicrobial therapies are effective at sterilizing urine of susceptible bacteria, it is unclear that antimicrobial activity is the basis for symptomatic relief of UTI [4]. Indeed, recent studies in murine UTI suggest that symptom kinetics are mediated by initial receptor-mediated responses to bacterial surface molecules, not bacterial loads [7].

Given the rapid rise in antimicrobial resistance and the potential for collateral damage caused by conventional therapies [8–11], alternative approaches are needed, and live biotherapeutic products (LBPs) such as vaccines and probiotics offer the potential to treat UTIs without concerns about antimicrobial resistance. Lactobacilli are normally a major component of the vaginal microflora of fertile women that act as a natural barrier against ascending infection by uropathogens [12]. Clinical trials have demonstrated that vaginal application of *L. crispatus* reduces UTI occurrence, presumably by restoring or augmenting the natural

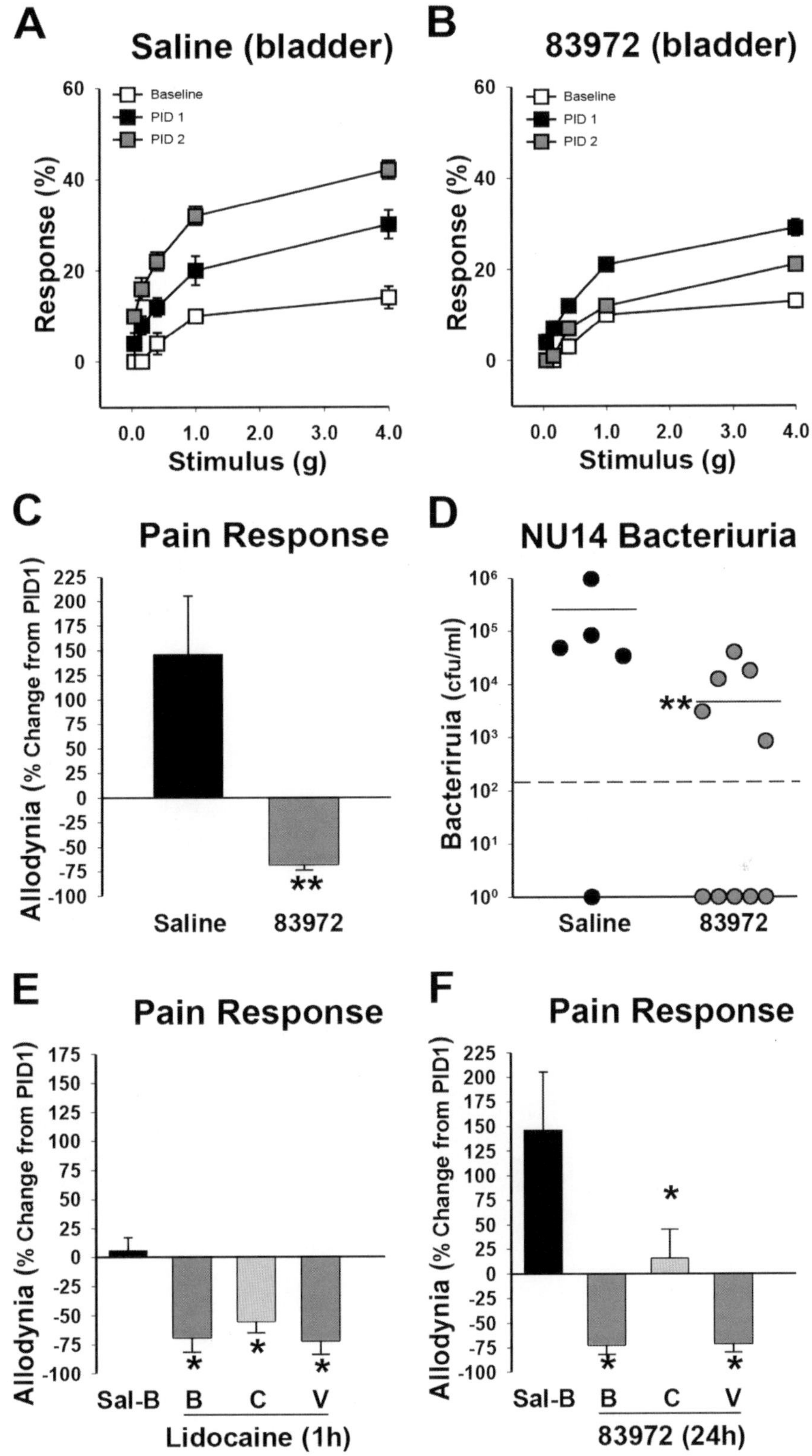

Figure 1. ***E. coli*** **83972 attenuates NU14-induced bacteriuria and pelvic pain.** A) Referred visceral hyperalgesia was measured as responses to mechanical stimulation of the pelvic region with von Frey filaments of 5 intensities. Responses were quantified at baseline, PID1 following NU14 infection, and 24 hours following of saline (n = 5) or 83972 (n = 10) instillation (PID2). B) NU14-infected mice exhibited a significant decrease in allodynia 24 hours following 83972 instillation. C) Percent increase in allodynia from PID1 was 146.2% in saline-treated mice, but decreased by over 68.9% in 83972-treated mice ($P<0.01$). D) Mice treated with 83972 exhibited a significantly less NU14 bacteriuria compared to saline-treated mice ($P<0.01$). Dashed line represents limit of detection. E) At PID1, NU14-infected mice were instilled with saline into the bladder or 2% lidocaine in the

bladder, vaginal introitus or colon. Allodynia was significantly reduced at 1 h after lidocaine into any compartment, relative to bladder saline (*P< 0.05; n = 9 saline, n = 10 bladder lidocaine, n = 11 colon lidocaine, n = 12 vaginal lidocaine). F) NU14-infected mice exhibited increased allodynia 24 hours after bladder instillation of saline, relative to PID1 (n = 10). Allodynia was significantly decreased at 24 hours following 83972 instillation into the bladder, colon or vaginal introitus (*P<0.05, n = 10 all groups). Data are reported as the mean ± SEM (A–C, E & F).

protective barrier against ascending infection [13–15]. Alternatively, asymptomatic bacteriuria (ASB) *E. coli* have been harnessed to prevent UTI. Since the American Urologic Association Guidelines are to not treat ASB, ASB *E. coli* have been instilled into patients to occupy this biological niche and thereby prevent infection by "bacterial interference" [16]. Clinical inoculation of the prototypic ASB *E. coli* strain 83972 was shown to significantly reduce UTI among spinal cord injury patients with chronic indwelling or intermittent catheterization while protecting patients with incomplete bladder emptying from recurrent UTI [17]. Similarly, clinical trials with HU2117, a P fimbriae-deficient mutant of 83972, demonstrated significantly increased time between symptomatic UTI in neurogenic bladder patients [18]. These studies with 83972 suggest that ASB *E. coli* strains possess biologic activities that thwart uropathogens and/or alter UTI symptoms. These clinical studies were not designed to test the bacterial interference hypothesis directly so mechanism of ASB *E. coli* impact UTI pathogenesis is unknown.

We recently characterized pelvic pain responses in a murine model of UTI. Using tactile allodynia as a behavioral correlate to pelvic pain, we quantified pelvic allodynia in response to UPEC strain NU14 or ASB strain 83972. NU14 induced pelvic allodynia that was not observed in response to 83972, yet similar inflammatory responses were induced by either bacterial infection or by lipopolysaccharide (LPS) purified from either strain [7,19]. Although neither instillation of 83972 nor its purified LPS induced pelvic allodynia, we found that 83972 LPS significantly reduced allodynia associated with NU14 infection, suggesting that ASB *E. coli* possess analgesic activity [19]. Here, we evaluated ASB *E. coli* strains for efficacy treating colonization of the urinary tract by uropathogens and for efficacy treating pain associated with UTI. We found that ASB *E. coli* exhibit anti-infective and analgesic activities in murine UTI, suggesting a potential use of ASB *E. coli*-based LBPs for treating UTI and other symptom-based disorders.

Methods

Animals

Adult female mice C57BL/6J 10–14 weeks of age were purchased from Jackson Laboratory. All experiments were performed using protocols approved by Northwestern University Animal Care and Use Committee as previously described [7,19].

Bacterial strains

NU14 is a clinical isolate of *E. coli* originally obtained from the urine of a cystitis patient and is considered archetypal for UPEC [20]. ASB strain 83972 was isolated from a young Swedish girl who was infected for at least 3 years without symptoms [21,22] and is one of the most extensively characterized ABS strains [23,24]. ASB *E. coli* strains were previously collected as a panel of consecutive clinical isolates [25] or isolates from the Northwestern Urology Clinic for the purposes of this study. *Proteus mirabilis*, *Enterococcus faecalis* and *Klebsiella pneumoniae* were isolated from discarded urine of uncomplicated cystitis patients. All clinical isolates obtained for this study were identified by standard microbiologic testing, including Gram staining and Microscan (Siemens Healthcare). Bacteria were cultured by serial passage in Luria broth at 37° in static broth [26,27]. *E. coli* strains were differentiated by plating onto selective agar: NU14 is resistant to streptomycin, 2–12 is resistant to streptomycin/ampicillin, and 83972 is resistant to chloramphenicol.

Infection and behavioral testing

Female mice were anesthetized with isoflurane and instilled via transurethral catheter with a volume of 10 μl containing 1×10^8 CFU bacteria in saline [28]. Following termination of the experiment the bladders were harvested, homogenized and plated on agar with or without antibiotic selection for colonization. Mice were tested prior to bacterial infection (baseline) and up to PID 20. Referred hyperalgesia and tactile allodynia was tested, as previously described [29,30], using von Frey filaments applied to the abdomen [29,30].

Treatments

Lidocaine was administered as a 2% lidocaine solution in water that was instilled via a Hamilton syringe and polyethylene catheter as previously described [30]. Ciprofloxacin (10 mg/kg/0.15 ml) drug therapy was administered daily as a 3-day course via I.P. via injection.

Statistical analyses

Colonization, inflammation and behavioral data were analyzed with the student t-test or a Kruskal-Wallis test followed by Dunn's post test or repeated ANOVA followed by a Dunnett's post test using Prism software from GraphPad Inc. as appropriate. A value of $P<0.05$ was considered statistically significant.

Ethics statement

These studies were conducted under Northwestern University IACUC protocols 2010–1788 and 2009–1677.

Results

ASB isolate 83972 attenuates UTI allodynia and bacteriuria

Since 83972 LPS attenuated UTI-associated allodynia [19], we hypothesized that intact 83972 bacteria would exhibit similar analgesic activity. To test this, female B6 mice were instilled with the UPEC strain NU14 via transurethral catheter to initiate UTI; after 24 h, mice were instilled with saline or 83972. Allodynia was quantified at baseline and daily throughout the experiment by assessing responsiveness to stimulation of the pelvic region with a graded series of von Frey filaments [30]. Saline-treated mice exhibited significant pelvic allodynia (Figs. 1A and C) relative to 83972-treated mice that showed a significantly reduced allodynia (Figs. 1B and C, P<0.01). Since 83972 is thought to prevent UTI by bacterial interference, we also quantified bacteriuria. 83972 significantly reduced urinary NU14, relative to saline instillation (Fig. 1D, P<0.01).

ASB isolate 83972 mediates analgesia via crosstalk

We have shown previously that colonic lidocaine attenuates pelvic pain in a neurogenic cystitis model as effectively as intravesical lidocaine, demonstrating organ crosstalk in pelvic pain relief [30]. We used a similar strategy to evaluate whether

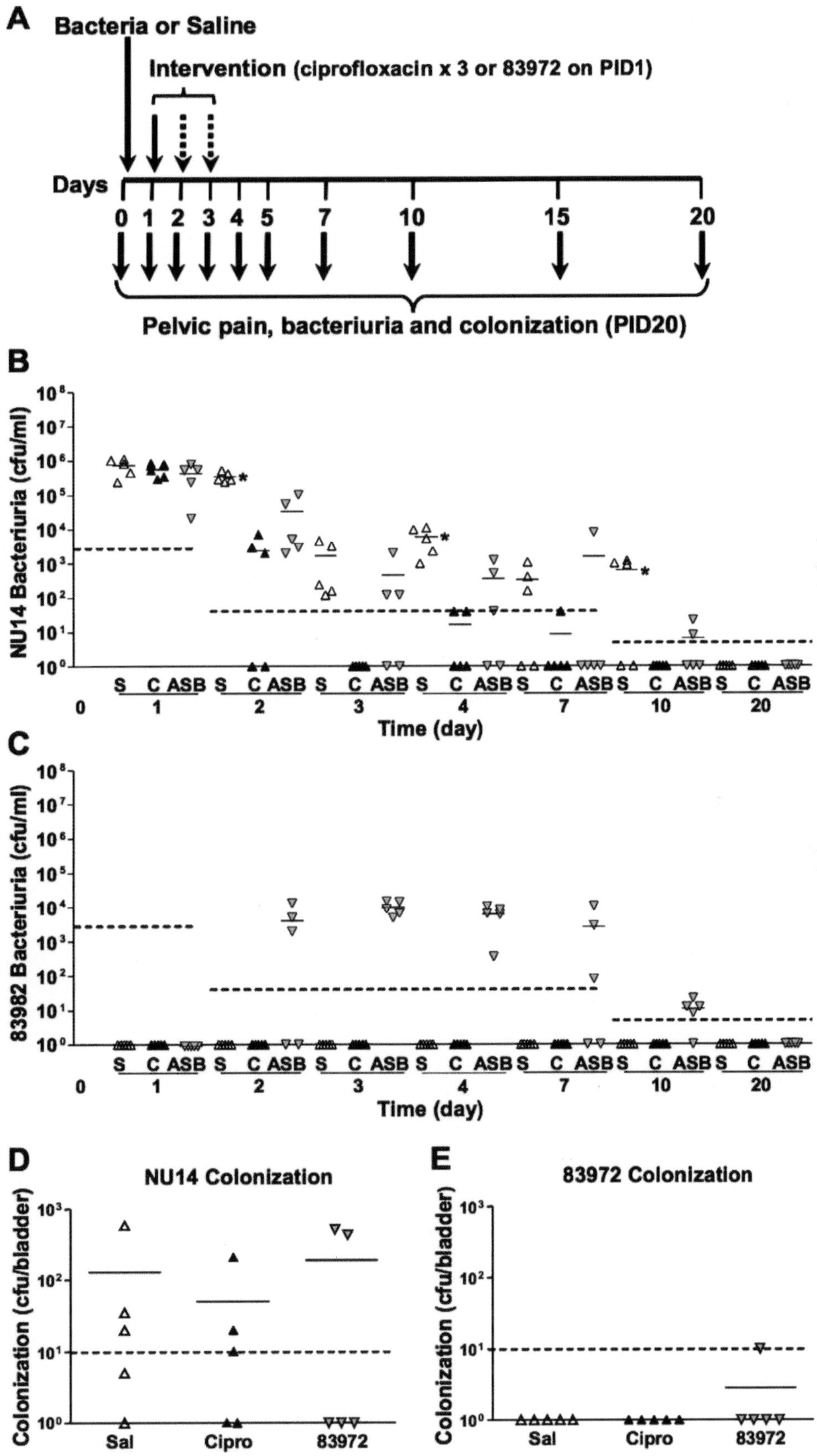

Figure 2. ***E. coli*** **83972 attenuates NU14 bacteriuria.** A) Experimental scheme for assessing efficacy of a single administration of ASB therapy relative to 3-day course of ciprofloxacin (n = 5 for all groups). B) Mice infected with NU14 exhibited a significant decrease in NU14 bacteriuria 24 hours

after initiation of ciprofloxacin (group C, back triangles, PID2, 4, 10), relative to saline-treated mice (group S, white triangles, *$P<0.05$). A single instillation of 83972 (group ASB, grey inverted triangles) also resulted in a significant decrease in NU14 bacteriuria after 24 hours (PID2, 4, 10, *$P<0.05$). C) Urinary 83972 for all three groups during the experiment. D and E) Bladder colonization on PID20 was not significantly different between the groups tested. Dashed lines represent limits of detection.

analgesic activity of ASB *E. coli* was capable of crosstalk during UTI. Allodynia was quantified 1 hour after lidocaine administration to mice that were infected with NU14 24 h prior (Fig. 1E); as a result, allodynia was not increased in the saline group (compare saline group in Fig. 1F). Relative to bladder instillation of saline, 2% lidocaine significantly and similarly attenuated UTI allodynia whether administered into the bladder, colon, or vagina (Fig. 1E, $P<0.05$). Analgesic activity of 83972 was evaluated at 24 h, and colonic 83972 significantly reduced saline-treated UTI allodynia (Fig. 1F, $P<0.05$), consistent with our previous findings for colonic modulation of cystitis pain [30]. 83972 significantly and similarly attenuated NU14-induced allodynia when administered intravesically or intravaginally ($P<0.05$). Remarkably, 83972 analgesic activity was comparable to lidocaine, whether acting directly or via crosstalk from the vagina (compare Figs. 1E and F).

ASB isolate 83972 attenuates bacteriuria comparable to ciprofloxacin

Since 83972 significantly reduced NU14 bacteriuria (Fig. 1D), we evaluated the anti-infective activity of intravesical 83972 relative to a three-day course of ciprofloxacin, a standard clinical regimen for uncomplicated UTI. All three groups exhibited similar levels of bacteriuria at post-infection day 1 (PID1) and had sterile urine by PID20 (Fig. 2B). Mice receiving ciprofloxacin or 83972 exhibited significantly reduced NU14 bacteriuria from PID2, 4 and 10, compared to the saline group (Fig. 2B, $P<0.05$). 83972 also became transiently established in the urinary tract, as indicated by 83972 bacteriuria from PID2 to PID10 (Fig. 2C). At PID20, most mice exhibited low levels of residual bladder colonization consistent with previous reports [31], no differences in NU14 colonization were observed between bladders of treated and untreated mice, and 83972 was largely cleared (Figs. 2D and E). While not significantly different here, we cannot exclude the possibility that ciprofloxacin therapy would exhibit increased antimicrobial activity relative to 83972 with larger samples. Nonetheless, these data suggest that the antimicrobial activity of ciprofloxacin and the anti-infective activity of 83972 are comparable and are manifested at the level of bacteriuria without fully sterilizing the bladder of bacterial reservoirs.

ASB *E. coli* differentially attenuate UTI allodynia

To determine whether analgesic activity was a unique property of 83972, we screened a panel of ASB *E. coli* strains including 3 strains collected from the Northwestern Urology Clinic for this study and 12 ASB strains from a panel of 54 consecutive clinical isolates [25]. As in Figure 1, mice were instilled with NU14 and then instilled with saline or an ASB panel strain 24 hours later and evaluated for pelvic responsiveness prior to instillation, 24 hours after NU14 instillation, and daily after saline or ASB treatment; strains were then grouped arbitrarily by relative analgesic activity (panels of Fig. 3A). All ASB isolates attenuated NU14-induced pelvic allodynia when compared to saline-instilled controls, but the magnitude of attenuation varied (Figs. 3A & B). While some mice exhibited an increase in pelvic pain 24 hours after infection with an ASB isolate (Fig. 3A, left panel), indicating only modest analgesic activity, they were significantly decreased compared to the saline-instilled control (Fig. 3B, black bars, $P<0.05$). Eight strains exhibited an intermediate analgesic phenotype, ranging from no increase in allodynia from PID1 to 70% reduction in allodynia (Fig. 3A, middle panel, and Fig. 3B, white bars). A third group was comprised of 6 ASB isolates that displayed a high analgesic phenotype, relative to PID1, attenuating cystitis allodynia from 75% to 85% (Fig. 3A, right panel, and Fig. 3B, grey bars). Since we recently showed that serial infections with could reveal a pain phenotype in an *E. coli* strain otherwise exhibiting no pain phenotype [7], three serial infections were performed with strains from the ASB panel (Fig. 3C). None of the ASB isolates tested induced pain following serial infections, consistent with our recent report that serial infection with 83972 did not induce pain [7]. These data demonstrate that ASB *E. coli* exhibit a range of analgesic phenotypes, and that the prototypic ASB strain, 83972, possesses a highly analgesic phenotype. However, since strain 2–12 had the greatest analgesic activity against cystitis pain, 85%, we focused on 2–12 for further study.

ASB isolate 2–12 is superior to ciprofloxacin for analgesia

We evaluated the effect of 2–12 on NU14-induced cystitis pain, relative to sham treatment or a 3-day course of ciprofloxacin using the schemed depicted in Figure 2A. Since we observed that 83972 could exert analgesic activity via crosstalk (Fig. 1F), we also evaluated 2–12 administered intravesically and intravaginally. Control groups instilled with saline then treated with 3 injections of saline or ciprofloxacin did not develop detectable allodynia (Fig. 4A). Consistent with previous observations [19], mice instilled with NU14 developed allodynia that decayed over two or three weeks, but ciprofloxacin therapy did not reduce allodynia better than saline during the course of the experiment (Fig. 4A). In contrast, mice receiving a single therapeutic dose of ASB isolate 2–12 exhibited a rapid and significant decrease in allodynia, whether that dose was administered to the bladder or vaginal introitus (Fig. 4A, $P<0.05$).

ASB isolate 2–12 is a superior analgesic against diverse uropathogens

Since ASB *E. coli* strains possess anti-infective and analgesic activity against UPEC, we examined effects against non-*E. coli* uropathogens. Allodynia was quantified in murine models of UTI Gram-positive bacteria, and responses to 2–12 therapy were compared with saline and ciprofloxacin. A single clinical isolate of *Proteus mirabilis* (PM1, Gram negative), *Enteroccus faecalis* (EF1, Gram positive) and *Klebsiella pneumoniae* (KP1, Gram negative) was obtained from urines of the Northwestern Urology Clinic and typed using standard microbiologic procedures. PM1-induced acute pelvic allodynia that was unaltered by a 3-day course of ciprofloxacin (Fig. 4B). However, PM1-induced allodynia was significantly attenuated in mice instilled with 2–12 on PID3 and PID4 ($P<0.05$). Similarly, 2–12 significantly reduced allodynia associated with EF1 or KP1 infection (Figs. 4C and D, respectively, $P<0.05$). Thus, 2–12 exhibits superior analgesic activity to current antimicrobial therapy in multiple urine UTI models.

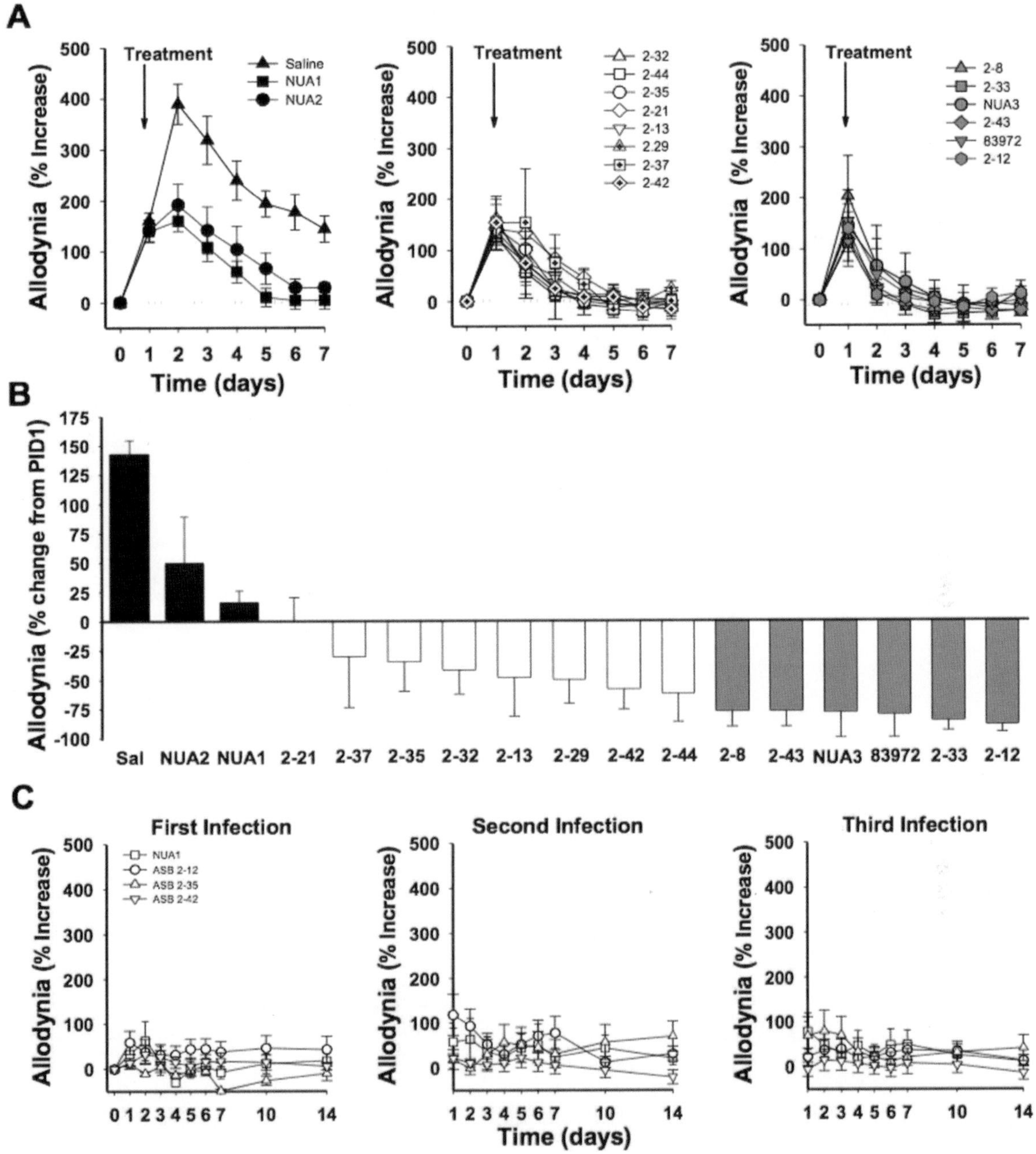

Figure 3. ASB strains differentially attenuate UTI visceral pain. Modulation of UTI visceral pain by a panel of 16 ASB *E. coli* strains. A) Mice were infected with NU14 and then instilled with saline or ASB *E. coli* at PID1, and allodynia was quantified through PID7 (n = 6 for all groups). For clarity, timecourses of allodynia for all 17 conditions were divided among 3 panels. All 16 ASB strains attenuated NU14-induced pelvic pain compared to the saline treated group. B) The relative analgesic activity of ASB strains was arbitrary grouped according to the magnitude of analgesia: strains with analgesic relative to saline but increased allodynia from PID1 (black bars), those that exhibited no increase in allodynia from PID1 to less than 75% reduction in visceral pain from PID1 (white bars), and those that exhibited greater than 75% reduction (gray bars). C) Representative ASB strains from each group in (B) were used in serial infections at two-week intervals. Serial infection did not induce allodynia. Data are reported as the mean ± SEM.

Discussion

Our findings demonstrate that ASB *E. coli* 83972 exhibit anti-infective activities comparable to ciprofloxacin in a murine UTI model. While ciprofloxacin promoted clearance of uropathogenic *E. coli* (UPEC), it did not reduce pelvic tactile allodynia, a measure of visceral pain. In contrast, ASB *E. coli* administered intravesically or intravaginally provided comparable reduction of allodynia similar to intravesical lidocaine. Moreover, ASB *E. coli* were similarly effective against UTI allodynia induced by *Proteus mirabilis*, *Enterococccus faecalis* and *Klebsiella pneumoniae*. Therefore, ASB *E. coli* have anti-infective activity comparable to the current standard of care yet also provide superior analgesia suggesting that ASB *E. coli* represent novel LBPs for UTI..

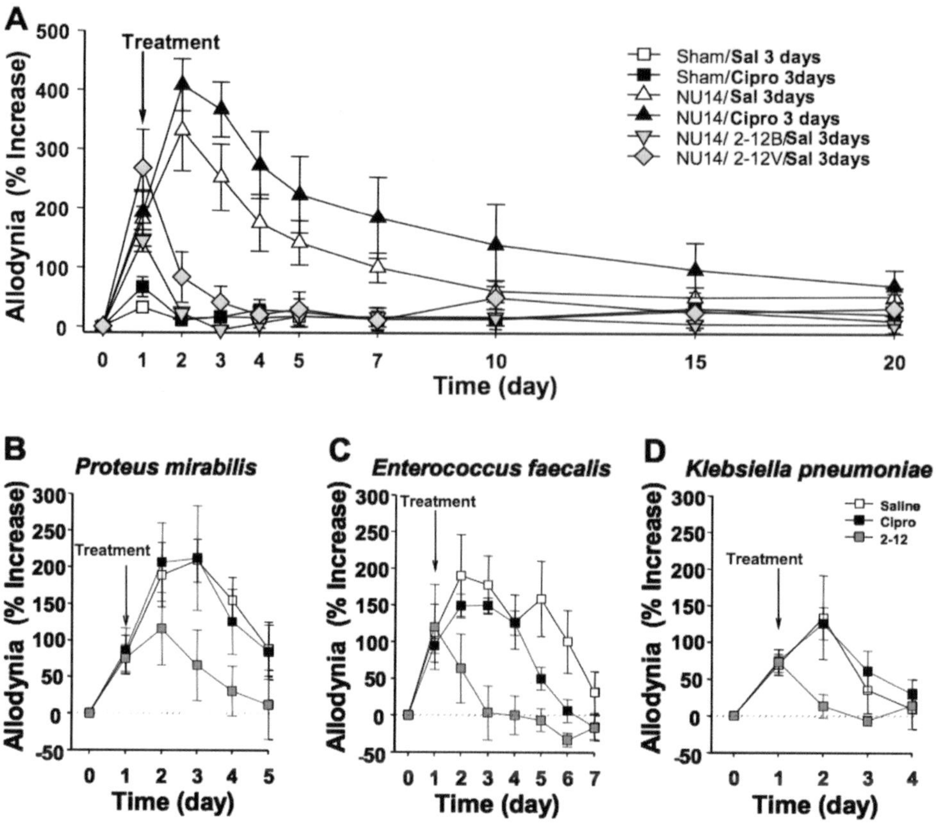

Figure 4. ASB *E. coli* isolate 2–12 rapidly attenuates UTI visceral pain of diverse uropathogens. A) Allodynia was quantified daily in groups of sham– or NU14-infected mice that were then treated at PID1 with saline, a three-day course of ciprofloxacin, or a single dose of intravesical or intravaginal 2–12 as described in Figure 2A (n = 8 in all groups except the 2–12 intravaginal group where n = 6). NU14-infected mice exhibited a significant decrease in pelvic pain 24 hours following treatment with 2–12 via the bladder or vaginal introitus ($P<0.05$). Allodynia was quantified in mice infected via transureathral catheter with *Proteus mirabilis* (PM1), *Enterocccus faecalis* (EF1) and *Klebsiella pneumoniae* (KP1) and then treated with a three-day course of ciprofloxacin initiated at PID1 or a single intravesical dose of 2–12 (n = 5). B) PM1 induced pelvic allodynia that was significantly attenuated on PID3 and PID4 by 2–12 treatment, relative to the ciprofloxacin or saline groups ($P<0.05$). C) EF1 induced allodynia that was significantly attenuated on PID2-PID4 by 2–12 treatment, relative to ciprofloxacin or saline groups ($P<0.05$). Allodynia was also significantly reduced on PID5–6 compared to the saline group ($P<0.05$). D) KP1 induced allodynia that was significantly attenuated on PID2 by 2–12 treatment, relative to ciprofloxacin or saline groups ($P<0.05$).

UTI is associated with a leukocytic influx dominated by neutrophils to drive clearance of UPEC [32,33]. Quantifying urinary myeloperoxidase (MPO) as a marker of bladder neutrophil influx, we previously found that 83972 and UPEC strain NU14 similarly induce MPO and inflammation [7,19]. We also observed that purified LPS preparations from 83972 and NU14 resulted in similar levels of neutrophil recruitment when instilled into the bladder and similarly activated splenic macrophages in culture [19], so it is unlikely that 83972 markedly enhances neutrophil influx. Another potential mechanism is the rapid urothelial apoptotic host defense response that is induced by the interaction of the UPEC type 1 pilus adhesin (FimH) with uroplakins [20,34–36], however 83972 do not express type 1 pili. We speculate that one anti-infective effect of ASB *E. coli* is to function as an adjuvant that enhances immune responses to uropathogens.

Ciprofloxacin and other antimicrobials sterilize the urine of susceptible bacteria, but the relationship between antimicrobial activity and symptomatic relief is increasingly unclear. A recent study revealed that ibuprofen was as effective as ciprofloxacin at ameliorating symptoms of dysuria and frequency during acute, uncomplicated UTI [37]. This is consistent with previous observations that UTI symptoms resolve spontaneously in the majority of patients and do not correlate with urinary bacterial loads [38,39]. We observed that ciprofloxacin did not alter pelvic allodynia in murine UTI (Fig. 4A), reinforcing clinical findings and consistent with our recent report that pelvic allodynia can persist long after bacterial clearance [7]. In contrast, we find ASB *E. coli* significantly reduce UPEC-induced allodynia, suggesting analgesic activity that is not unique to a single ASB strain but rather but varies across a spectrum. We find several aspects of this analgesic effect remarkable. First, ASB *E. coli* can exhibit analgesic activity comparable to intravesical lidocaine (Figs. 1E and F), suggesting clinical utility. Second, the significant reduction in allodynia when 83972 was administered in the vagina or colon indicates that the analgesic activity against UPEC can be mediated via organ crosstalk, similar to lidocaine (Fig. 1E and F; [30]). The physiologic basis for organ crosstalk is visceral convergence of sensory pathways among pelvic organs such as the bladder and bowel [40–42] and this observation of organ crosstalk in ASB *E. coli* analgesia is evidence that ASB *E. coli* may mediate effects independent of bacterial interference. Since prior clinical studies of 83972 and HU2117 demonstrated significant reduction in symptomatic events in patients prone to recurrent UTI [17,18,43], an alternative explanation for those findings is that

83972 analgesic activity masked symptoms that would have been scored as a symptomatic recurrence. Third, 2–12 reduced allodynia induced by infection with non-UPEC uropathogens, demonstrating that ASB *E. coli* exhibit analgesic activity against diverse insults. Since we reported that LPS purified from 83972 reduced allodynia in NU14 infection [19], it is likely that the analgesic activity of other ASB *E. coli* strains is generally mediated by LPS through the cognate receptor TLR4 [7,19].

The anti-infective and analgesic properties of ASB *E. coli* described here suggest several clinical applications, in addition to the use as a prophylactic for catheterized patients as reported previously [16,43]. The anti-infective activity of 83972 was comparable to ciprofloxacin in promoting clearance for acute UTI, suggesting that ASB *E. coli* could be administered as a therapy of uncomplicated UTI. In both acute and recurrent UTI, the analgesic effect would be an advantage of ASB *E. coli* therapy over conventional antimicrobials. Finally, we observe that ASB *E. coli* reduced allodynia associated with diverse acute insults, suggesting general analgesic effects could be exploited to treat non-infectious pain conditions. Patients suffering chronic pelvic pain of interstitial cystitis/bladder pain syndrome (IC) can gain temporary relief from intravesical lidocaine [44]. Since ASB strains exert analgesic activity comparable to lidocaine and mediate these effects via organ crosstalk, ASB *E. coli* therapy could be used for chronic pelvic pain conditions such as IC, vulvodynia, or endometriosis.

The U.S. FDA classifies whole, live microorganisms that exhibit drug activities as LBPs. LBPs are subject to FDA oversight using the same Investigational New Drug regulatory pathway as small molecule drugs [45]. Given that ASB *E. coli* are considered harmless and clinical guidelines are to not treat ASB, therapeutic use of ASB *E. coli* would be safe. We find that ASB *E. coli* is cleared from the urinary tracts of healthy mice within days and consistent with clinical studies revealing the prevalence of ASB among healthy young women is approximately 5% [46]. Thus, the urinary tract appears similarly resistant to stable colonization by ASB *E. coli* in both healthy young women and mice, suggesting that ASB *E. coli* would be safe for clinical use as an LBP. ASB *E. coli* therapy also would not contribute to resistance against conventional antimicrobials. Finally, ASB *E. coli* address unmet needs for effective therapies against recurrent UTI and chronic pelvic pain, representing novel LBP candidates for urologic disease.

Acknowledgments

We thank Dr. Catharina Svanborg for generously providing the asymptomatic bacteriuria strain 83972. We thank Joseph Done for assistance quantifying allodynia and Eduardo and Faye Sarmiento for identifying uropathogens. These studies were as part of the NIH/NIDDK Multi-Disciplinary Approaches to Chronic Pelvic Pain (MAPP) Research Network (www.mappnetwork.org).

Author Contributions

Conceived and designed the experiments: CNR AKT REY AJS DJK. Performed the experiments: CNR AKT REY. Analyzed the data: CNR AKT REY AJS DJK. Contributed reagents/materials/analysis tools: AJS. Wrote the paper: CNR AKT REY AJS DJK.

References

1. Foxman B, Barlow R, D'Arcy H, Gillespie B, Sobel JD (2000) Urinary tract infection: self-reported incidence and associated costs. Ann Epidemiol 10: 509–515.
2. Schappert SM (1999) Ambulatory care visits to physician offices, hospital outpatient departments, and emergency departments: United States, 1997. PG - i–iv. Vital Health Stat 13.
3. Schaeffer AJ, Schaeffer EM (2012) Infections of the urinary tract. In: Wein A, Kavoussi L, Novick A, Partin A, Peters C, editors. Campbell-Walsh Urology. 8th ed. Philadelphia: Elsevier. pp. 223–303.
4. Foxman B (2010) The epidemiology of urinary tract infection. Nat Rev Urol 7: 653–660.
5. Karlowsky JA, Kelly LJ, Thornsberry C, Jones ME, Sahm DF (2002) Trends in antimicrobial resistance among urinary tract infection isolates of Escherichia coli from female outpatients in the United States. Antimicrob Agents Chemother 46: 2540–2545.
6. Hunstad DA, Justice SS (2010) Intracellular lifestyles and immune evasion strategies of uropathogenic Escherichia coli. Annu Rev Microbiol 64: 203–221.
7. Rudick CN, Jiang M, Yaggie RE, Pavlov VI, Done J, et al. (2012) O-antigen modulates infection-induced pain States. PLoS ONE 7: e41273.
8. Stewardson AJ, Huttner B, Harbarth S (2011) At least it won't hurt: the personal risks of antibiotic exposure. Curr Opin Pharmacol 11: 446–452.
9. Naber KG, Wullt B, Wagenlehner FM (2011) Antibiotic treatment of uncomplicated urinary tract infection in premenopausal women. Int J Antimicrob Agents 38 Suppl: 21–35.
10. Wise BL, Peloquin C, Choi H, Lane NE, Zhang Y (2012) Impact of age, sex, obesity, and steroid use on quinolone-associated tendon disorders. Am J Med 125: 1228 e1223–1228 e1228.
11. Looft T, Allen HK (2012) Collateral effects of antibiotics on mammalian gut microbiomes. Gut Microbes 3: 463–467.
12. Gupta K, Stapleton AE, Hooton TM, Roberts PL, Fennell CL, et al. (1998) Inverse association of H2O2-producing lactobacilli and vaginal Escherichia coli colonization in women with recurrent urinary tract infections. J Infect Dis 178: 446–450.
13. Czaja CA, Stapleton AE, Yarova-Yarovaya Y, Stamm WE (2007) Phase I trial of a Lactobacillus crispatus vaginal suppository for prevention of recurrent urinary tract infection in women. Infect Dis Obstet Gynecol 2007: 35387.
14. Stapleton A (2003) Novel approaches to prevention of urinary tract infections. Infect Dis Clin North Am 17: 457–471.
15. Reid G, Bruce AW (2006) Probiotics to prevent urinary tract infections: the rationale and evidence. World J Urol 24: 28–32.
16. Hull R, Rudy D, Donovan W, Svanborg C, Wieser I, et al. (2000) Urinary tract infection prophylaxis using Escherichia coli 83972 in spinal cord injured patients. J Urol 163: 872–877.
17. Sunden F, Hakansson L, Ljunggren E, Wullt B (2010) Escherichia coli 83972 bacteriuria protects against recurrent lower urinary tract infections in patients with incomplete bladder emptying. J Urol 184: 179–185.
18. Darouiche RO, Green BG, Donovan WH, Chen D, Schwartz M, et al. (2011) Multicenter Randomized Controlled Trial of Bacterial Interference for Prevention of Urinary Tract Infection in Patients With Neurogenic Bladder. Urology 78: 341–346.
19. Rudick CN, Billips BK, Pavlov VI, Yaggie RE, Schaeffer AJ, et al. (2010) Host-pathogen interactions mediating pain of urinary tract infection. J Infect Dis 201: 1240–1249.
20. Klumpp DJ, Weiser AC, Sengupta S, Forrestal SG, Batler RA, et al. (2001) Uropathogenic Escherichia coli potentiates type 1 pilus-induced apoptosis by suppressing NF-kappaB. Infect Immun 69: 6689–6695.
21. Lindberg U (1975) Asymptomatic bacteriuria in school girls. V. The clinical course and response to treatment. Acta Paediatr Scand 64: 718–724.
22. Andersson P, Engberg I, Lidin-Janson G, Lincoln K, Hull R, et al. (1991) Persistence of Escherichia coli bacteriuria is not determined by bacterial adherence. Infect Immun 59: 2915–2921.
23. Klemm P, Hancock V, Schembri MA (2007) Mellowing out: adaptation to commensalism by Escherichia coli asymptomatic bacteriuria strain 83972. Infect Immun 75: 3688–3695.
24. Bergsten G, Wullt B, Schembri MA, Leijonhufvud I, Svanborg C (2007) Do type 1 fimbriae promote inflammation in the human urinary tract? Cell Microbiol 9: 1766–1781.
25. Hultgren SJ, Schwan WR, Schaeffer AJ, Duncan JL (1986) Regulation of production of type 1 pili among urinary tract isolates of Escherichia coli. Infect Immun 54: 613–620.
26. Old DC, Duguid JP (1970) Selective outgrowth of fimbriate bacteria in static liquid medium. J Bacteriol 103: 447–456.
27. Billips BK, Schaeffer AJ, Klumpp DJ (2008) Molecular basis of uropathogenic Escherichia coli evasion of the innate immune response in the bladder. Infect Immun 76: 3891–3900.
28. Hopkins WJ, Hall JA, Conway BP, Uehling DT (1995) Induction of urinary tract infection by intraurethral inoculation with Escherichia coli: refining the murine model. J Infect Dis 171: 462–465.
29. Rudick CN, Bryce PJ, Guichelaar LA, Berry RE, Klumpp DJ (2008) Mast cell-derived histamine mediates cystitis pain. PLoS ONE 3: e2096.

30. Rudick CN, Chen MC, Mongiu AK, Klumpp DJ (2007) Organ Crosstalk Modulates Pelvic Pain. Am J Physiol Regul Integr Comp Physiol 293: R1191–1198.
31. Mulvey MA, Schilling JD, Hultgren SJ (2001) Establishment of a persistent Escherichia coli reservoir during the acute phase of a bladder infection. Infect Immun 69: 4572–4579.
32. Hang L, Frendeus B, Godaly G, Svanborg C (2000) Interleukin-8 receptor knockout mice have subepithelial neutrophil entrapment and renal scarring following acute pyelonephritis. J Infect Dis 182: 1738–1748.
33. Mulvey MA, Schilling JD, Martinez JJ, Hultgren SJ (2000) From the cover: bad bugs and beleaguered bladders: interplay between uropathogenic Escherichia coli and innate host defenses. Proc Natl Acad Sci U S A 97: 8829–8835.
34. Klumpp DJ, Rycyk MT, Chen MC, Thumbikat P, Sengupta S, et al. (2006) Uropathogenic Escherichia coli induces extrinsic and intrinsic cascades to initiate urothelial apoptosis. Infect Immun 74: 5106–5113.
35. Mulvey MA, Lopez-Boado YS, Wilson CL, Roth R, Parks WC, et al. (1998) Induction and evasion of host defenses by type 1-piliated uropathogenic Escherichia coli. Science 282: 1494–1497.
36. Thumbikat P, Berry RE, Zhou G, Billips BK, Yaggie RE, et al. (2009) Bacteria-induced uroplakin signaling mediates bladder response to infection. PLoS Pathog 5: e1000415.
37. Bleidorn J, Gagyor I, Kochen MM, Wegscheider K, Hummers-Pradier E (2010) Symptomatic treatment (ibuprofen) or antibiotics (ciprofloxacin) for uncomplicated urinary tract infection?—results of a randomized controlled pilot trial. BMC Med 8: 30.
38. Christiaens TC, De Meyere M, Verschraegen G, Peersman W, Heytens S, et al. (2002) Randomised controlled trial of nitrofurantoin versus placebo in the treatment of uncomplicated urinary tract infection in adult women. Br J Gen Pract 52: 729–734.
39. Ferry SA, Holm SE, Stenlund H, Lundholm R, Monsen TJ (2004) The natural course of uncomplicated lower urinary tract infection in women illustrated by a randomized placebo controlled study. Scand J Infect Dis 36: 296–301.
40. Malykhina AP, Wyndaele JJ, Andersson KE, De Wachter S, Dmochowski RR (2012) Do the urinary bladder and large bowel interact, in sickness or in health? ICI-RS 2011. Neurourol Urodyn 31: 352–358.
41. McMahon SB, Morrison JF (1978) Convergence of visceral and somatic axons on neurones which ascend in the lateral funiculus of the cat [proceedings]. J Physiol 275: 56P.
42. Pezzone MA, Liang R, Fraser MO (2005) A model of neural cross-talk and irritation in the pelvis: implications for the overlap of chronic pelvic pain disorders. Gastroenterology 128: 1953–1964.
43. Darouiche RO, Thornby JI, Cerra-Stewart C, Donovan WH, Hull RA (2005) Bacterial interference for prevention of urinary tract infection: a prospective, randomized, placebo-controlled, double-blind pilot trial. Clin Infect Dis 41: 1531–1534.
44. Parsons CL (2006) Advances in the treatment of interstitial cystitis. Expert Opin Pharmacother 7: 411–419.
45. Fiore C (2010) Regulatory considerations for the safety assessment of live biotherapeutic products in clinical trials. New York Academy of Sciences: U.S. Food and Drug Administration.
46. Hooton TM, Scholes D, Stapleton AE, Roberts PL, Winter C, et al. (2000) A prospective study of asymptomatic bacteriuria in sexually active young women. N Engl J Med 343: 992–997.

Opioid-Induced Mitogen-Activated Protein Kinase Signaling in Rat Enteric Neurons following Chronic Morphine Treatment

Celine Durafourd[1,2], Erica Kumala[1,2], Laura Anselmi[1], Nicholas C. Brecha[1,2,3], Catia Sternini[1,2,3]*

1 CURE Digestive Diseases Research Center, Division of Digestive Diseases and Department of Medicine, David Geffen School of Medicine, University of California Los Angeles, Los Angeles, California, United States of America, **2** CURE Digestive Diseases Research Center, Division of Digestive Diseases and Department of Neurobiology, David Geffen School of Medicine, University of California Los Angeles, Los Angeles, California, United States of America, **3** Veteran Administration Greater Los Angeles Healthcare System, Los Angeles, California, United States of America

Abstract

Opioids, acting at μ opioid receptors, are commonly used for pain management. Chronic opioid treatment induces cellular adaptations, which trigger long-term side effects, including constipation mediated by enteric neurons. We tested the hypothesis that chronic opioid treatment induces alterations of μ opioid receptor signaling in enteric neurons, which are likely to serve as mechanisms underlying opioid-induced constipation. In cultured rat enteric neurons, either untreated (naïve) or exposed to morphine for 4 days (chronic), we compared the effect of morphine and DAMGO (D-Ala2,MePhe4,Gly-ol5 enkephalin) on μ opioid receptor internalization and downstream signaling by examining the activation of the mitogen-activated protein kinase/extracellular signal-regulated kinases 1 and 2 (MAPK/ERK) pathway, cAMP accumulation and transcription factor cAMP Response Element-Binding protein (CREB) expression. μ opioid receptor internalization and MAPK/ERK phosphorylation were induced by DAMGO, but not morphine in naïve neurons, and by both opioids in chronic neurons. MAPK/ERK activation was prevented by the receptor antagonist naloxone, by blocking receptor trafficking with hypertonic sucrose, dynamin inhibitor, or neuronal transfection with mutated dynamin, and by MAPK inhibitor. Morphine and DAMGO inhibited cAMP in naïve and chronic enteric neurons, and induced desensitization of cAMP signaling. Chronic morphine treatment suppressed desensitization of cAMP and MAPK signaling, increased CREB phosphorylation through a MAPK/ERK pathway and induced delays of gastrointestinal transit, which was prevented by MAPK/ERK blockade. This study showed that opioids induce endocytosis- and dynamin-dependent MAPK/ERK activation in enteric neurons and that chronic morphine treatment triggers changes at the receptor level and downstream signaling resulting in MAPK/ERK-dependent CREB activation. Blockade of this signaling pathway prevents the development of gastrointestinal motility impairment induced by chronic morphine treatment. These findings suggest that alterations in μ opioid receptor downstream signaling including MAPK/ERK pathway in enteric neurons chronically treated with morphine contribute to the development of opioid-induced constipation.

Editor: Wenhui Hu, Temple University School of Medicine, United States of America

Funding: This work was supported by National Institutes of Health (NIH) grants R01-DK054155 and P30-DK041301, and UCLA Academic Senate. The funders had no role in study design, data collection and analysis, decision to publish, or preparation of the manuscript.

Competing Interests: The authors have declared that no competing interests exist.

* Email: csternin@ucla.edu

Introduction

The long-term use of opioids for the treatment of moderate to severe pain is a common clinical practice and has increased exponentially during the past decade in the United States [1]. Opioid drugs exert their pharmacological effects by interacting with the opioid receptors (ORs), mostly targeting the μORs. Binding of opioids with μORs in neurons of the central nervous system (CNS) induces analgesia, whereas activation of μORs in neurons of the enteric nervous system (ENS) inhibits gastrointestinal (GI) motility and secretion [2–5]. Unfortunately, the beneficial, analgesic effect of opioids decreases with time due to tolerance [6,7], thus requiring increasing concentrations of opioids for pain control [1]. This intensifies the inhibitory effects of opioids in the GI tract, resulting in the development of opioid bowel dysfunction, a serious condition characterized by abdominal pain and constipation [1,8], which significantly hampers opioid treatment. Opioid-induced constipation is the most common adverse GI effect resulting from chronic opioid exposure, with a prevalence of 41% in non-cancer patients up to 95% in cancer-patients [9,10]. Unlike analgesia, the constipating effect of chronic opioid treatment does not subside with time and it is likely that the different outcome of prolonged stimulation in CNS and ENS neurons is due to different signaling of μORs in distinct neuronal populations.

Activated μORs undergo desensitization due to β-arrestin interaction and G proteins uncoupling, dynamin-dependent internalization and resensitization [7]. μORs signal by coupling to inhibitory Gi/Go proteins and activating several effectors, including inhibition of cAMP, modulation of cation channels and activation of mitogen-activated protein kinase (MAPK) pathway to induce a functional response, which results in inhibition of cellular activity by reducing transmitter release [4,7]. Opioids can be distinguished by their internalization profiles and downstream effectors, which reflect functional selectivity at μOR or ligand-directed signaling [6,7]. Indeed, many opioid drugs (e.g. fentanyl, etorphine) and endogenous opioids are efficient in internalizing and desensitizing μORs in multiple cell types, whereas morphine does not [6,11–13]. However, morphine can induce desensitization in the absence of internalization [14] and trigger μOR internalization in certain opioid-responsive CNS neurons [15]. Interestingly, in enteric neurons, chronic *in vivo* treatment with morphine enhances the ability of acute morphine to internalize μORs through a dynamin-mediated pathway [16]. Internalization and desensitization are critical events regulating downstream signaling and receptor function, and alteration of these regulatory processes induced by long-term opioid treatment results in intracellular adaptations underlying the development of opioid-induced side effects [6]. In addition, differences in μOR downstream signaling with chronic opioid treatment have been described. Indeed, chronic opioid stimulation results in up-regulation of the cAMP pathway through activation of Gβγ proteins, whereas acute μOR activation inhibits cAMP through activation of Gα protein. cAMP superactivation together with persistent activation of the MAPK cascade that has also been reported in chronically treated neurons represent intracellular adaptations underlying the development of long-term treatment side effects [7]. Opioid-induced constipation results from disruption of GI motility mediated by μORs in enteric neurons [4,5,17], thus an elucidation of μOR signaling in these neurons is essential to understand the mechanisms underlying the development of GI side effects such as motility impairment following chronic opioid treatment. μOR signaling is regulated by multiple factors including the type of opioid agonist, and magnitude and length of stimulation, which induce compensatory changes in signal transduction [6]. However, little is known about μOR signaling in enteric neurons. In this study, we tested the hypothesis that μOR agonists differing in their efficiency to induce receptor internalization in enteric neurons [12,13], differentially regulate MAPK in enteric neurons untreated (naive) or chronically treated with morphine (chronic), and that chronic morphine modulates downstream events mediating alterations of GI motility. We focused on extracellular signal-regulated kinase 1 and 2 (ERK1/2) members of the MAPK family, which are upregulated in different neuronal populations by chronic morphine and produce long-lasting changes [7,18,19]. We found that DAMGO, an internalizing opioid, but not morphine, a poor internalizing agonist, induces MAPK/ERK phosphorylation in naïve enteric neurons, whereas both DAMGO and morphine activate MAPK/ERK pathway in chronic enteric neurons. By contrast, opioids inhibit cAMP signaling in acute and chronic neurons irrespective of their internalization efficiency. Chronic morphine triggers activation of the transcription factor, cAMP Response Element-Binding protein (CREB) via a MAPK-dependent pathway and suppresses opioid-induced μOR desensitization. Finally, blockade of MAPK/ERK pathway reversed the delay of GI transit induced by chronic morphine. These findings support the concept that changes in μOR downstream signaling in enteric neurons induced by chronic morphine treatment are important factors underlying the development of long-term GI opioid effects.

Materials and Methods

Five to 10 day-old (Harlan Labs, San Diego, CA) and adult (200–225 g from Charles River Laboratory International, Inc., Hollister, CA) Sprague Dawley rats were used for this study. Pups and adult rats were housed in rooms with controlled temperature and light-dark cycles. Adult rats had unrestricted access to standard rat chow and tap water and acclimated for 1 week before experimentation.

Ethics Statement

Animal care and procedures were in accordance with the National Institutes of Health recommendations for the humane use of animals. Experimental procedures were reviewed and approved by the Animal Research Committee of the University of California, Los Angeles (ARC protocol # 2002-012). All efforts were made to minimize the number of animals used and their suffering.

Preparation of primary cultures of enteric neurons

Primary cultures of myenteric neurons were prepared as described [20]. Pups were euthanized by isoflurane (5%; Phoenix Pharmaceuticals Inc, Burlingame, CA) followed by decapitation. The small intestine was removed, and the longitudinal muscle with attached the myenteric plexus was separated from the whole thickness of the specimen and processed for enzymatic and mechanical dissociation. Neurons were plated at 2.5×10^5 cells/mL on cover slips coated with poly-L-Lysine (Sigma-Aldrich, St Louis, MO) in DMEM supplemented with 100 U/mL penicillin, 100 U/mL streptomycin (Invitrogen, Carlsbad, CA) and 10% fetal bovine serum (FBS, Life Technologies, Grand Island, NY) at 37°C for 4 hours. Cover slips were placed cell side facing down, which reduces oxygen tension environment and proliferation of non-neuronal cells, in new wells containing Neurobasal-A medium (Invitrogen) with 1% FBS, penicillin, streptomycin and B27-supplement (Invitrogen).

Effects of μOR-agonists on ERK pathway and μOR internalization

We used the endogenous opioid analogue, DAMGO (D-Ala2,MePhe4,Gly-ol5 enkephalin; Sigma-Aldrich), which is a potent internalizing agonist, and morphine (Sigma-Aldrich), which is a poor internalizing opioid in enteric neurons [13,16]. Cultured enteric neurons were exposed to medium (naïve neurons) or medium with 10 μM morphine for 4 days (chronic neurons) following plating. Medium was changed every 2 days. On day 5, cover slips were rotated so that cells were facing up and incubated at 37°C for 1 hour in agonist- and serum-free Neurobasal-A medium, then treated with DAMGO (1 μM), morphine (10 μM) or medium alone for 5, 10, 20, and 30 minutes at 37°C. Initial dose-response study tested DAMGO 10 nM–10 μM and morphine 100 nM–100 μM and showed that 1 and 10 μM, respectively were the lowest doses with the highest effect on ERK1/2, thus were selected for subsequent experiments.

To confirm that ERK1/2 activation is receptor mediated and is not due to endogenous opioid release, cells were incubated with the opioid receptor antagonist, naloxone (Sigma-Aldrich, St Louis, MO; 10 μM) for 1 hour or a blocker of endogenous neurotransmitter release, tetrodotoxin (TTX, Sigma-Aldrich; 10 μM) for 1.5 hours prior to opioid stimulation. Enteric neurons were pre-incubated with MEK inhibitor, U0126 (1,4-diamino-2,3-dicyano-1, 4-bis[2-aminophenylthio]butadiene; Cell Signaling, Danvers, MA; 10 μM), which blocks the MAPK cascade leading to ERK, for 1.5 hours [21]. To establish whether opioids induce desensitization, we treated enteric neurons for 2 hours with 1 μM DAMGO or 10 μM morphine, washed and then exposed them to a second stimulation with the same dose of agonist for 5 minutes.

To determine whether DAMGO and morphine induced μOR internalization in cultured enteric neurons, we exposed either naïve or chronic enteric neurons to DAMGO (1 μM), morphine (10 μM) or medium alone for 1 hour at 4°C to allow ligand-receptor binding, then transferred to ligand-free medium at 37°C for 30 minutes to allow receptor internalization and processed for immunohistochemistry [13,16]. Briefly, cultured neurons were fixed in 4% paraformaldehyde in 0.1 M phosphate buffer (PB), pH 7.4 for 2 hours, washed and incubated in rabbit polyclonal, affinity-purified μOR antibody (Incstar Science, Technology and Research, Stillwater, MN; 1:3,000) directed to the C-terminus region of rat μ-OR (384–398) in 0.1 M PB/0.5% Triton X-100 (Sigma-Aldrich), and 10% goat serum (Invitrogen, Carlsbad, CA) (overnight at 4°C) followed by Alexa Fluor 488 affinity-purified donkey anti-rabbit (1:1000; Invitrogen Molecular Probes, Eugene, OR) (1 hour at room temperature). The μOR antibody has been previously characterized [13,16,17]. μOR immunoreactivity was visualized using a Zeiss 510 META laser scanning upright compound confocal microscope (Axioplan 2) using the 488 nm line of the argon laser. All images were acquired with a PlanApo 63×1.4 NA objective. Images were processed and labeled using Adobe Photoshop 7.0 (Adobe Systems, Mountain View, CA).

To determine the involvement of μOR internalization in opioid-induced ERK1/2 phosphorylation, enteric neurons were pre-incubated with an hypertonic sucrose solution (Sigma-Aldrich) for 1 hour to block clathrin-coated pits formation. Since upregulation of dynamin facilitates the endocytosis of morphine-activated μORs in chronic enteric neurons [16], we tested whether dynamin plays a role in opioid-induced ERK1/2 activation. We treated enteric neurons for 15 minutes with dynasore (Calbiochem, San Diego, CA; 10 μM), a cell-permeable inhibitor of dynamin [22], prior to opioid stimulation. We also transfected enteric neurons with a mutated dynamin (K44E-dynamin, mutation leading to lack of GTP activity [23,24], provided by Dr. Bunnett, Monash University, Australia) or wild type (WT) dynamin using the lentiviral transfection method.

Lentivirus WT or mutated K44E-dynamin constructs and transfection of enteric neurons

WT and mutated rat dynamin sequences were amplified from rat dynamin-HA WT pIRES2 GFP or rat dynamin-HA K44E pIRES2 GFP plasmids by PCR. PCR products were cloned into plasmid pRRL-sin-cPPT-CMV-MCS-IRES-GFP encoding a HIV-derived lentiviral vector with a cytomegalovirus (CMV) promoter to drive high gene expression. Lentivirus-based vectors encoding different isoforms of dynamin were generated by transient co-transfection of 293T cells with a three-plasmid combination [25]. Briefly, 100 mm dishes of nonconfluent 293T cells were co-transfected with 6.5 μg of packaging construct pMDLg/pRRE, 3.5 μg of pMDG (construct encoding the VSV-G envelope), 2.5 μg of pRSV–REV and 10 μg of pRRL-sin-cPPT-CMV-dynamin-IRES-GFP, by CaPi-DNA co-precipitation method. The following day, cells were incubated for 8 hours in 10 mM sodium butyrate to obtain high-titer virus production [25]. Conditioned medium was harvested 16 hours later and passed through 0.45 μm filters. Viral titer was determined by assessing viral p24 antigen concentration by ELISA (Alliance HIV-I p24 ELISA Kit, Perkin Elmer). Transfections were carried out in 1 mL of DMEM, including serial dilutions of lentiviral vector supernatant and 1 mg/mL of protamine sulfate. One day post-transfection, cells were incubated in Neurobasal-A medium complemented with 1% FBS, 100 U/mL penicillin, 100 U/mL streptomycin and B27-supplement for 3 days, then treated with either 1 μM DAMGO, 10 μM morphine, or medium for 5 minutes. Dynamin expression was measured by Western blot (see below) using anti-dynamin 1 antibody (C-16, sc-6402, Santa Cruz), which recognizes the C-terminal part of the protein. This antibody detects both the WT and mutated form of dynamin, since the mutation appears in the 44th amino acid corresponding at the GTPase activity domain, present in the N-terminal part of the protein [23,24].

Dynamin, ERK and CREB Western blot assays

Cells were extracted using Laemmli buffer, separated by SDS-polyacrylamide gel electrophoresis and transferred onto PVDF membranes. Membranes were blocked 1 hour at room temperature in LI-COR Blocking buffer (LI-COR Biosciences, Lincoln, NE) and incubated at 4°C overnight with rabbit anti-dynamin 1 antiserum (1:200), mouse monoclonal antibody to phospho-p44/42 (Thr202/Tyr204) ERK1/2 (pERK1/2) (1:1000; Cell Signaling, Danvers, MA) or anti phosphorylated-CREB 1 (pCREB) antibody (Ser 133; 1:1000; Cell Signaling). Total ERK (tERK) or CREB (tCREB) were determined after stripping and reprobing the membranes previously incubated with pERK1/2 or pCREB with rabbit polyclonal anti tERK1/2 (C14) (1:500; Santa Cruz Biotechnology, CA) or anti tCREB (1:1000; Cell Signaling), respectively. Antibodies recognizing total proteins (ERK and CREB) were used to verify that the cell treatments did not affect the total level of these proteins and to confirm equal gel loading [26]. To verify equal loading of the gels for dynamin Western blot, a mouse antibody against the housekeeping protein, glyceraldehyde-3-phosphate dehydrogenase (GAPDH), was used (1:000; Cell Signaling). Immunoreactive bands were visualized by using infrared fluorescent secondary antibodies IRDye 800 Goat anti Mouse (1:10000) for pERK and GAPDH, and IRDye 680 Goat anti Rabbit (1:10000) for tERK quantification; and IRDye 800 Goat anti Rabbit (1:10000) for tCREB, pCREB and dynamin. Images were collected using the LI-COR Odyssey infrared imaging system and staining intensities were quantified with Odyssey Application Software Version 3.0. Values were expressed as a ratio of control at 0 minute.

cAMP assay

A cAMP assay was used to determine whether morphine induces desensitization in naïve neurons and whether chronic morphine induces cAMP superactivation, a hallmark of chronic opioids treatment [7]. Briefly, naïve or chronically treated enteric neurons were exposed to forskolin (10 μM) and IBMX 0.5 mM for 15 min at 37°C, before addition of opioids, or control solution for 15 min and intracellular cAMP was measured using the Amersham cAMP Biotrak Enzyme Immunoassay System [27].

Chronic treatment with morphine and assessment of gastrointestinal transit

To determine whether disruption of μOR signaling affects GI transit delay in animal chronically treated with morphine, we used a MEK1/2 inhibitor *in vivo* and measured total GI transit following chronic morphine treatment with or without MEK1/2 inhibitor. Rats received one of the following treatment: saline, MEK1/2 inhibitor (40 mg/kg) [28], morphine (day 1–2, 10 mg/kg; day 3–4, 20 mg/kg; days 5–6, 40 mg/kg) or morphine and MEK1/2 inhibitor twice a day subcutaneously for 6 days ($n = 5$ per group). GI transit was measured as previously described by evaluating the distribution of non-absorbable fluorescent 70,000 MW dextran (150 μL, 5 mg/mL) administered intragastrically by gavage [29]. Animals received their last injection of saline or drugs 30 minutes after gavage, then they were euthanized by an overdose of isoflurane (5%) followed by thoracotomy. The entire GI tract was excised and divided into 15 segments: stomach, small intestine (10 segments of equal length), cecum and colon (3 segments of equal length). The luminal content of each segment was collected, suspended in 1 mL of distilled water, clarified by centrifugation (15 min at 14,000 rpm at 4°C). The supernatants of individual samples were collected and the fluorescence signal was determined in triplicates by using a fluorescence plate reader (excitation wavelength 485 nm and emission wavelength 528 nm, FLX800 Microplate Fluorescence Reader, Bio-Tek instruments Inc., Winooski, VT). The averaged fluorescent intensity of each segment in triplicate and the sum of all fluorescent averages were measured. The GI transit was expressed as the geometric center (GC) of the distribution of labeled fluorescent dextran along the entire GI tract using the following equation: GC = sum of the products of the fraction of the marker in each segment times the segment number [30].

Statistical analysis

Data are expressed as mean ± SEM. Statistical differences were analyzed by a one-way ANOVA with Bonferroni post-tests. A $p < 0.05$ was considered significant. Statistical analyses were performed using Prism 5.0 software (GraphPad Software, San Diego, CA).

Results

Ligand-directed μOR internalization in cultured enteric neurons

DAMGO, but not morphine induced rapid μOR internalization in cultured naïve enteric neurons, whereas both DAMGO and morphine induced comparable μOR translocation in chronically treated neurons (Figure 1). These results are comparable to published data *in vivo* and *in vitro* [12,13,16].

Effects of DAMGO and morphine on ERK activation in enteric neurons

In naïve neurons, DAMGO induced a marked and significant increase of ERK1/2 phosphorylation with peaks at 5 and 10 minutes ($p<0.01$ vs. controls) and returned to baseline at 20 minutes (Figure 2). By contrast, ERK1/2 phosphorylation levels in naïve neurons exposed to morphine were similar to controls (Figure 2), suggesting ligand selectivity of ERK1/2 activation. However, in neurons treated chronically with morphine, both DAMGO and morphine induced significant ERK phosphorylation at 5 and 10 minutes ($p<0.01$).

Naloxone prevented opioid-induced ERK1/2 phosphorylation in naïve and chronic enteric neurons (Figure 3 A, B). Regardless of opioid stimulation, ERK activation in acute and chronic enteric neurons was unaffected by the sodium channel blocker TTX, indicating it was not due to endogenous opioid release (data not shown).

ERKs are the direct downstream proteins activated by MEK via phosphorylation [7]. To characterize the pathway of opioid-induced ERK1/2 activation, we pretreated naïve and chronic enteric neurons with a MEK1/2 inhibitor (U0126) prior to opioid stimulation. There was no ERK1/2 activation in DAMGO- and morphine-stimulated enteric neurons pretreated with U0126, supporting that opioid-induced ERK1/2 activation is MEK1/2 dependent (Figure 3 C, D).

Opioid-induced ERK1/2 activation in enteric neurons was blocked by pretreatment with hypertonic sucrose solution (Figure 3 E, F) and with the dynamin inhibitor, dynasore (Figure 4 A and D). Furthermore, ERK1/2 phosphorylation was observed in opioid-stimulated enteric neurons transfected with WT dynamin, but not in those expressing the mutated dynamin (Figure 4 B, E). Western blot analysis showed a significant increase ($p<0.01$) in the expression of dynamin in enteric neurons transfected with either WT or mutated dynamin compared to non transfected neurons, showing that transfection was effective (Figure 4 C). These findings confirmed that opioid-induced ERK1/2 activation in enteric neurons is endocytosis- and dynamin-dependent.

Desensitization of opioid-induced ERK activation

In naïve enteric neurons exposed to DAMGO (1 μM) for 2 hours, a second exposure to the same concentration of DAMGO did not induce ERK1/2 phosphorylation suggesting desensitization of MAPK signaling (Figure 5 A). By contrast, in chronic enteric neurons stimulated with DAMGO (1 μM) or morphine (10 μM) for 2 hours, a second exposure to either DAMGO or

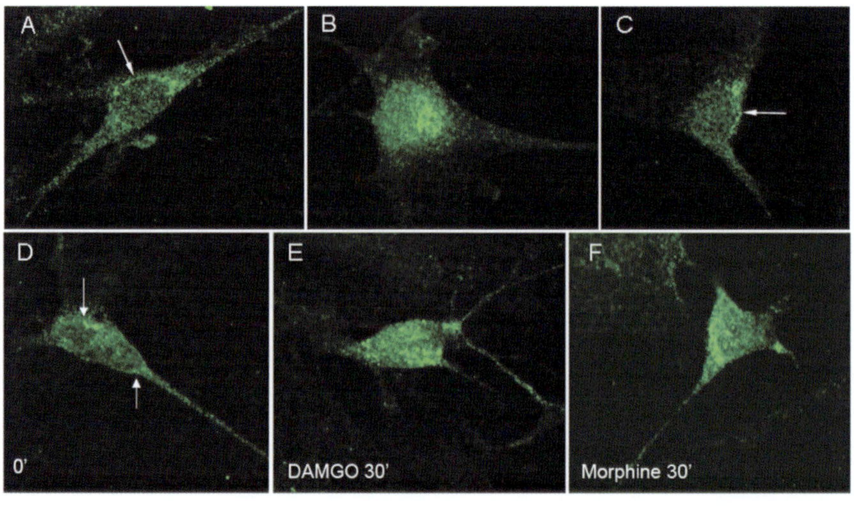

Figure 1. μOR immunoreactivity in naïve enteric neurons (A–C) and in neurons chronically treated with morphine (D–F). μOR immunoreactivity is at the cell surface in unstimulated and morphine-stimulated neurons (A, C arrows), and it is in the cytosol following stimulation with DAMGO (B) in naïve enteric neurons. μOR immunoreactivity is at the cell surface in unstimulated neurons (D, arrows), but in the cytosol following DAMGO or morphine stimulation (E, F) in chronic enteric neurons.

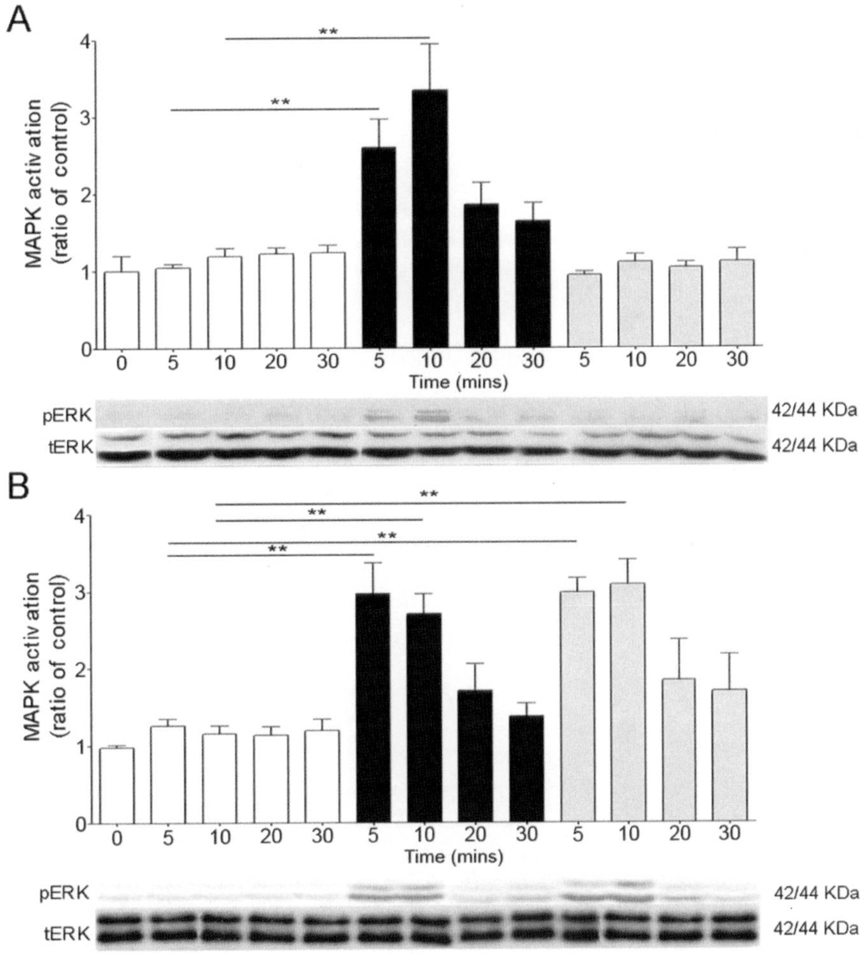

Figure 2. Opioid-induced MAPK activation in naïve (A) and chronically treated (B) enteric neurons. DAMGO (1 μM, black bars) induced a transient MAPK/ERK1/2 activation in naïve (A) and chronic (B) neurons at 5 and 10 minutes, whereas morphine (grey bars) induced MAPK/ERK1/2 activation only in chronic (B) neurons. $^{**}p<0.01$ compared to controls (white bars). N = 4–7 experiments in triplicate. Representative gels of pERK1/2 and tERK are shown at the bottom of each graph. tERK was used to verify that the treatment did not affect the total level of this protein and to confirm equal gel loading.

morphine (at the same concentration) induced significant ERK1/2 phosphorylation, indicating suppression of desensitization of MAPK signaling (Figure 5 B). This prolonged signaling could be the initiating factor leading to cellular adaptations induced by prolonged opioid stimulation.

cAMP signaling in enteric neurons and desensitization of cAMP inhibition

In naïve neurons, both DAMGO and morphine inhibit forskolin-stimulated cAMP. When naïve neurons were exposed for 2 hours to either DAMGO (1 μM) or morphine (10 μM), then stimulated again with the same opioid at the same concentration, there was no inhibition of cAMP indicating desensitization (Figure 5 C). In chronically treated enteric neurons, there was cAMP superactivation, which was inhibited by either DAMGO or morphine. Opioid-inhibition of forskolin-stimulated cAMP persisted in neurons exposed to a second dose of DAMGO or morphine following a previous incubation with the same agonist for 2 hours indicating loss of desensitization in chronic enteric neurons (Figure 5 D).

ERK activation mediated CREB phosphorylation in enteric neurons chronically treated with morphine

DAMGO and morphine induced significant CREB phosphorylation at 5 and 10 minutes in enteric neurons chronically treated with morphine compared to controls, but not in naïve neurons (Figure 6). Opioid-induced CREB phosphorylation was abolished by MEK1/2 inhibitor treatment (Figure 6), indicating that CREB activation is MAPK/ERK pathway-dependent.

Effect of MAPK pathway disruption on chronic morphine-induced GI transit delay

We tested whether there was a correlation between MAPK signaling and functional response of GI transit to chronic morphine treatment. The pronounced delay of GI transit observed in rats chronically treated with morphine, was reversed to normal in rats chronically treated with morphine and MEK1/2 inhibitor (Figure 7). These data suggest that MAPK/ERK pathway plays a role in the opioid-induced impairment of GI motility, which is likely to involve CREB phosphorylation.

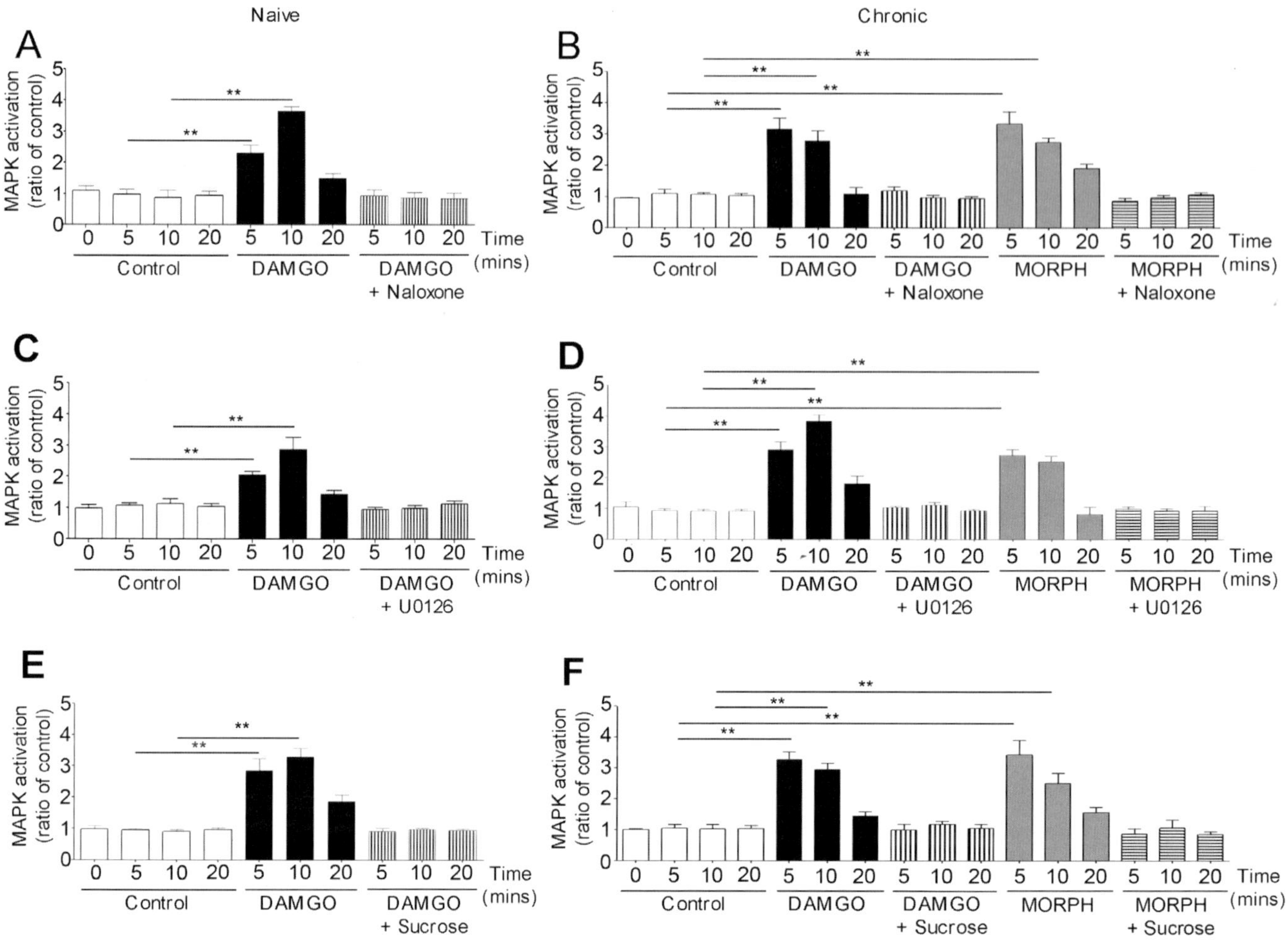

Figure 3. Characterization of opioid-induced MAPK pathway in enteric neurons. DAMGO-induced MAPK activation in naive (A, C, E) and DAMGO- and morphine-activation of MAPK in chronic (B, D, F) enteric neurons. Naloxone (A, B), MEK1/2 inhibitor, U0126 (C, D) and hypertonic sucrose (E, F) prevented opioid induced MAPK activation in naïve (A, C, E) and chronic (B, D, F) neurons. **$p<0.01$ significantly different from control. N = 4–7 experiments in triplicate per group.

Discussion

This study showed that opioids induce activation of MAPK/ERK1/2 in enteric neurons of the small intestine through a pathway requiring μOR internalization, whereas opioid inhibition of cAMP signaling is independent of ligand internalization efficiency. Chronic morphine treatment suppressed opioid-induced desensitization of cAMP and MAPK signaling and induced activation of the transcription factor, CREB through a MAPK/ERK pathway, since it was prevented by a selective MEK inhibitor, an upstream protein of ERK. Finally, MAPK/ERK blockade reversed total GI transit delay induced by chronic morphine treatment. These findings provide novel information on μOR signaling in rat enteric neurons, which mediate opioid-induced GI effects [4,5], and suggest that prolonged μOR signaling and MAPK/ERK activation induced by long-term opioid treatment contribute to the development of opioid-induced constipation and are likely to involve CREB phosphorylation.

Several lines of evidence support the internalization-dependency of opioid-mediated MAPK/ERK activation in enteric neurons of the small intestine. Significant ERK1/2 phosphorylation was observed only in conditions in which opioids triggered endocytosis and was blocked by hypertonic sucrose, or dynasore, a dynamin inhibitor, and in enteric neurons transfected with a dominant negative K44E mutant dynamin, which prevent clathrin-dependent, dynamin-mediated endocytosis [13,22–24,31]. Our data in enteric neurons are consistent with previous reports of endocytosis as a prerequisite for opioid-induced MAPK activation in cell lines [27,32], but in contrast with other studies indicating internalization-independence [33,34], but dynamin-dependence [33], of opioid-stimulated MAPK pathway in heterologous cells and neuronal cell lines expressing endogenous μORs. Furthermore, the failure of morphine to activate ERK1/2 in naïve enteric neurons is consonant with findings in cultured striatal neurons [19], whereas in naïve neurons of the midbrain (Duraffourd and Sternini, unpublished) and in cell lines, morphine was effective in activating MAPK/ERK1/2 [27,32–34]. Similarly, opioid internalization efficiency varies in different cell populations. Indeed, morphine fails to internalize μORs in enteric neurons of the small intestine, dorsal root ganglion cells, and subpopulations of CNS neurons, whereas it elicits internalization in other neuronal populations [11–13,15,16,35]. Furthermore, chronic treatment with morphine reverses the resistance of morphine-activated μORs to internalize in enteric neurons of the small intestine *in vivo* [16] and *in vitro* (this study). Moreover, prolonged (2–

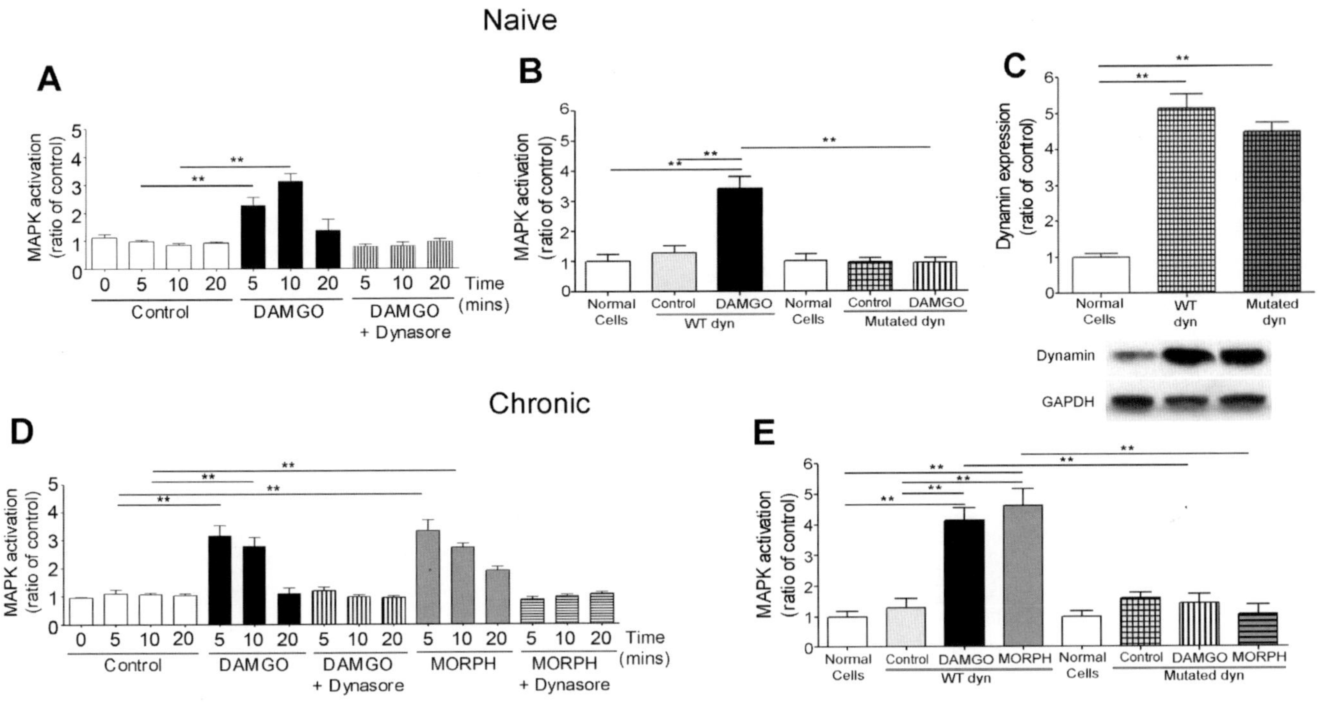

Figure 4. Role of dynamin on MAPK activation in enteric neurons. DAMGO-induced MAPK in naïve neurons is inhibited by dynasore, a dynamin inhibitor (A) and it is not observed in neurons transfected with mutated K44E dynamin (B). Both DAMGO- and morphine-induced MAPK activation in chronic neurons is blocked by dynasore (D) and is not detected in neurons transfected with mutated dynamin (E). C shows the increased expression of dynamin (dyn) immunoreactivity in enteric neurons transfected with wild type (WT) or mutated dynamin, confirming effectiveness of neuronal transfection. $^{**}p<0.01$ compared to controls; $n=5–7$ performed in triplicate per group. Representative immunoblots of dynamin immunoreactivities are shown at the bottom of histogram in C. GAPDH served as housekeeping protein to verify that the same amount of proteins was loaded on each gel.

24 hours) morphine stimulation results in μOR internalization in cultured dorsal root ganglion cells [35], but not in heterologous cell lines [36]. Taken together, these findings support the notion of cell specific μOR trafficking and signaling.

To determine μOR desensitization in naïve enteric neurons, we used the cAMP assay, since cAMP signaling is internalization-independent [37]. These studies showed that morphine induces the same level of desensitization of cAMP inhibition in enteric neurons as DAMGO, extending previous observations of morphine-induced desensitization in absence of internalization in different cell types [38,39], indicating dissociation between internalization and desensitization [33,38]. Furthermore, chronic morphine treatment suppresses μOR desensitization in enteric neurons as shown by the inability of opioids to activate MAPK/ERK and to inhibit cAMP, whereas it does not affect the magnitude of ligand-induced μOR internalization. This further supports the dissociation between these two regulatory processes, unlike previous findings in cell lines reporting that chronic morphine inhibits both opioid receptor desensitization and internalization [40]. Chronic morphine treatment does not affect opioid-evoked functional response in enteric neurons, as indicated by the same magnitude of opioid-induced μOR internalization and the same degree of MAPK/ERK activation and cAMP inhibition by opioids in naïve and chronic enteric neurons.

Together, these findings challenge the concept that morphine's inefficiency to internalize and desensitize μORs serves as the initial step to promote intracellular mechanisms, at least in enteric neurons of the small intestine, leading to long-term opioid side effects [6,41], whereas receptor endocytosis would prevent compensatory downstream changes by limiting signaling [33]. Other mechanisms are likely to be involved in the development of long-term opioid side effects, including changes of G protein levels, trafficking of proteins and kinases, which would alter downstream signaling and resensitization [42]. We investigated whether in enteric neurons, opioids activate the transcription factor CREB, which has been shown to be involved with opioid-induced effects [7,18,19]. Significant increase in CREB phosphorylation was observed in chronically treated neurons in response to either DAMGO or morphine compared to naïve neurons and was prevented by MEK inhibitor. The activation of the transcription factor CREB in enteric neurons chronically stimulated with opioids is in agreement with previous studies in different types of neurons [7,18,19] and is likely to represent one of the intracellular adaptations induced by prolonged activation of μORs, though the exact mechanism behind this change remains to be fully elucidated. Activated ERK1/2 has different intracellular localization, which might vary according to the activation pathway and downstream cascade [43]. Studies in different types of cells including primary CNS neurons have shown that morphine activates ERK via protein kinase C (PKC) pathway and morphine-induced ERK phosphorylation remains in the cytosol inducing CREB, whereas internalizing opioids such as etorphine and fentanyl activate ERK in a ß arrestin-dependent pathway resulting in ERK nuclear translocation and activation of G protein kinase2 and ß arrestin2 transcription [43]. In our study, both morphine and the internalizing opioid, DAMGO induce internalization- and dynamin-dependent ERK phosphorylation and CREB phosphorylation in chronic neurons. However, ERK compartmentalization as well as the relative role of PKC or ß-arrestin in ERK activation were not investigated and further studies are required to determine

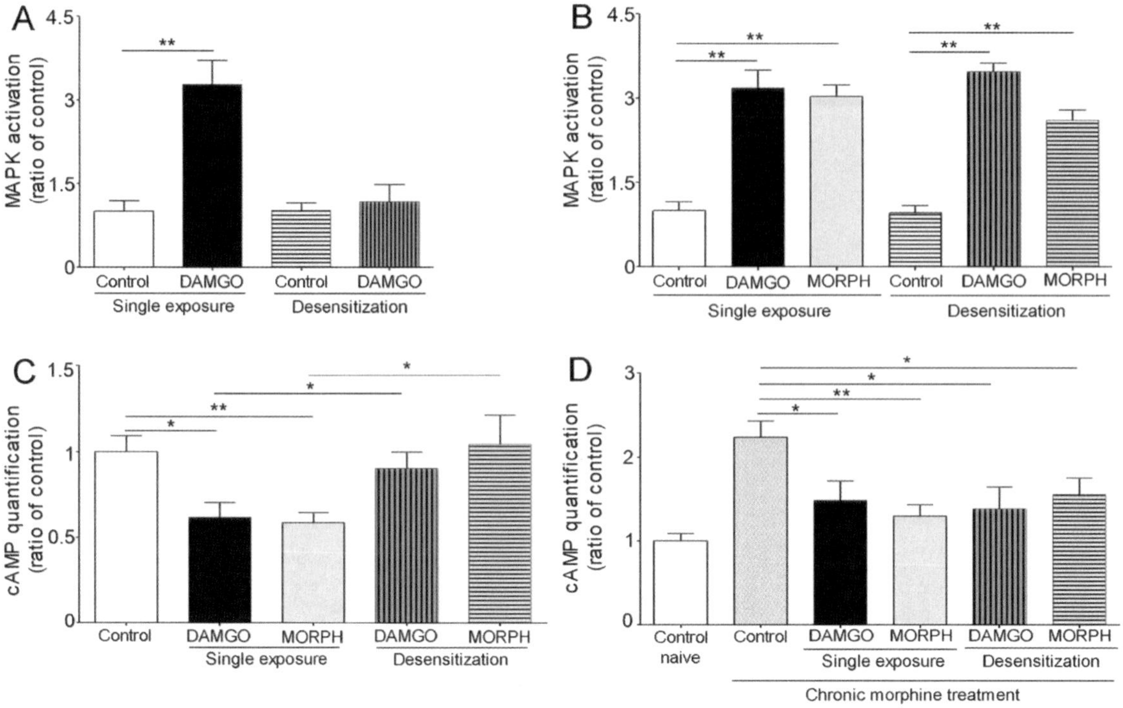

Figure 5. Desensitization of μOR signaling in enteric neurons. A: Single exposure to DAMGO (1 μM, 5 min) induced significant MAPK activation in naïve enteric neurons, whereas a second exposure to the same DAMGO dose following 2 hours DAMGO pretreatment abolished DAMGO-mediated MAPK response, indicating desensitization. B: Single exposure to DAMGO (1 μM) or morphine (10 μM) activated MAPK in chronic neurons. A second exposure to the same dose of DAMGO or morphine following 2 hours DAMGO or morphine pretreatment induced the same effect in chronic neurons as single exposures, indicating suppression of desensitization. (** $p<0.01$ vs. control in A and B). C and D: DAMGO and morphine inhibit forskolin-stimulated cAMP in naïve (C) and chronic (D) enteric neurons. This effect was not observed in naïve enteric neurons (C) with a second opioid stimulation following a prior 2 hour exposure, indicative of desensitization. D: Note the over 2 fold increase in cAMP in unstimulated chronic neurons (cAMP superactivation or "overshooting") vs. naïve control; DAMGO and morphine inhibition of cAMP was not prevented by 2 hours DAMGO or morphine pretreatment in chronic neurons, indicating suppression of desensitization. **$p<0.01$ vs. controls. N = 5–7 experiments performed in duplicate per group.

the mechanism underlying CREB phosphorylation induced by chronic opioid treatment.

μOR enteric neurons are a heterogeneous population comprising ascending and descending neurons, interneurons and motor neurons [17]. μORs are Gi/Go coupled and when activated inhibit neurotransmitter release by modulating neuronal excitability [4,5] in different neuronal pathways thus impairing motility and transit. Prolonged opioid exposure induces inhibition of neurotransmitter release thus impairing intestinal peristalsis and propulsion and inhibition of intestinal secretion further exacerbating GI transit delay [4,5,44,45]. Our study shows that blocking the MAPK/ERK1/2 pathway and CREB activation with a selective MEK1/2 inhibitor reversed the GI transit delay induced by chronic morphine, suggesting that MAPK/ERK pathway plays a role in motility impairment resulting in constipation, which is likely to involve CREB. Since upregulation of CREB phosphorylation has been shown to affect neuronal excitability in CNS and ENS neurons [46,47], it is tempting to speculate that activation of CREB contributes to GI transit delay by altering the neuronal circuits mediating GI motility. However, this remains to be elucidated. Finally, further studies are required to determine whether μOR signaling differs in enteric neurons of the colon compared to the ileum. This is likely based on previous findings of different functional responses of the ileum and colon following chronic morphine as indicated by the reduction of the neurogenic response of neuromuscular preparations of the ileum but not colon, which involves ß arrestin [48,49].

In summary, this study shows that opioid activation of MAPK/ERK signaling pathway in enteric neurons is endocytosis- and dynamin-dependent, whereas cAMP signaling is inhibited by opioids irrespective of their internalization efficiency. Chronic morphine treatment suppressed μOR desensitization thus resulting in prolonged signaling, and induced MAPK/ERK-dependent activation of the transcription factor, CREB. Opioid-induced CREB upregulation is likely due, at least in part, to cytosolic ERK since it was observed only in neurons chronically treated with morphine and morphine-activated ERK has been reported to be retained in the cytosol [43], though the contribution of nuclear ERK cannot be discounted at this point. Finally, the prevention of morphine-induced delay of GI transit by blockade of MAPK/ERK/CREB cascade in enteric neurons strongly supports the involvement of this downstream signaling pathway in the development of opioid-induced constipation in chronic conditions, a major limiting factor in the use of opioids in pain management. Intervention at the level of the μOR-mediated activation of the MAPK/ERK signaling pathway in enteric neurons might provide a novel, potential therapeutic target for opioid-induced GI dysfunction following chronic opioid exposure.

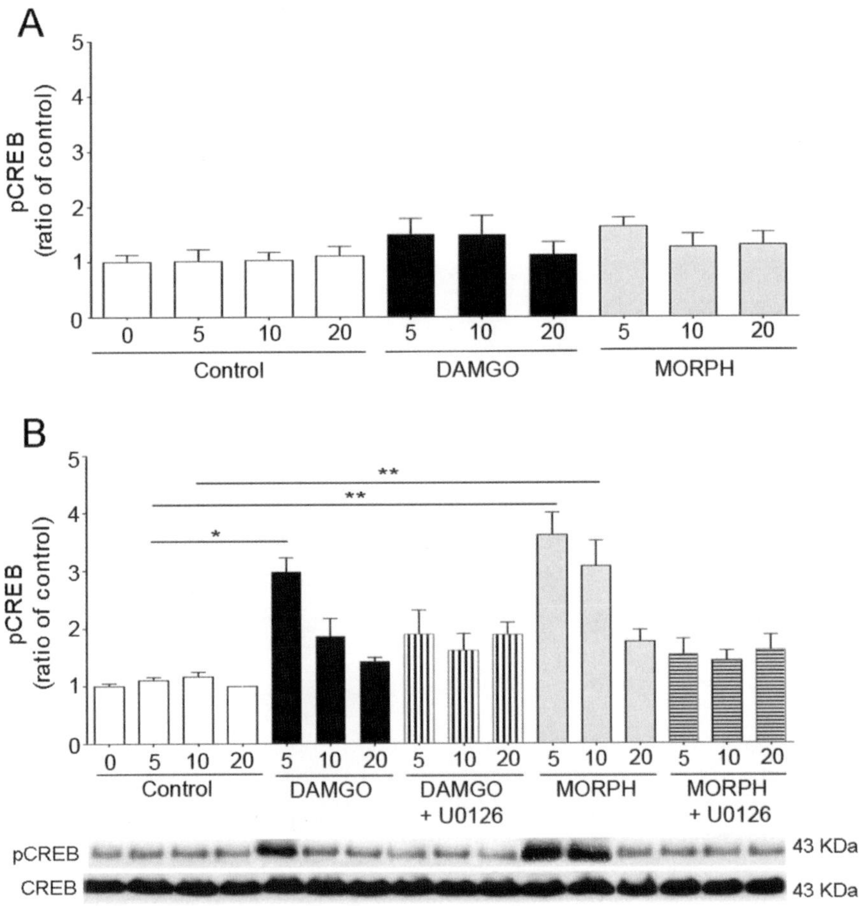

Figure 6. Effect of opioids on CREB phosphorylation in enteric neurons. Naïve (A) and chronic (B) neurons were stimulated with 1 μM DAMGO, 10 μM morphine or medium (control) for 0–20 minutes. DAMGO and morphine induced a significant, transient CREB activation in chronic, but not naïve enteric neurons. CREB phosphorylation in chronic neurons was blocked by the MEK1/2 inhibitor (U0126) treatment. *$p<0.05$ and **$p<0.01$ vs. control; $n=4$–7 experiments in triplicate per group. Representative gels of pCREB and CREB are shown at the bottom of the figure. Total CREB was used to verify that the treatment did not affect the total level of this protein and to confirm equal gel loading.

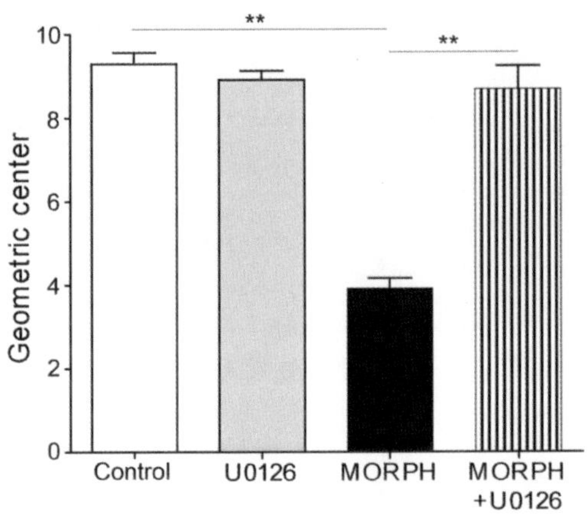

Figure 7. Effect of MEK1/2 inhibitor (U0126) on GI transit delay induced by chronic morphine in rats. Chronic morphine (MORPH) significantly delayed GI transit (reduction of geometric center) (**$p<0.01$ vs. control). MEK1/2 inhibitor alone (U0126) did not affect transit. Administration of MEK1/2 inhibitor together with morphine (MORPH+U0126) reversed the delay in GI transit (**$p<0.01$ vs. MORPH). $N=5$ per group.

Acknowledgments

The authors would like to thank Dr. Nigel Bunnett, Monash University, Melbourne, Australia, for providing the WT and K44E-dynamin dominant negative plasmids, Dr. Emmanuelle Faure of the CURE Integrated Molecular Technologies Core for the preparation of Lentivirus WT and K44E-dynamin constructs, and Jennifer Huynh and Dr. Steve Young of the CURE Morphology and Cell Imaging Core for their assistance with the use of the confocal microscope.

Author Contributions

Conceived and designed the experiments: CD CS. Performed the experiments: CD EK LA. Analyzed the data: CD EK LA CS. Contributed reagents/materials/analysis tools: NCB CS. Wrote the paper: CD LA NCB CS. Obtained the funds to support the study: CS NCB.

References

1. Camilleri M (2011) Opioid-induced constipation: challenges and therapeutic opportunities. Am J Gastroenterol 106: 835–842; quiz 843.
2. Matthes HW, Maldonado R, Simonin F, Valverde O, Slowe S, et al. (1996) Loss of morphine-induced analgesia, reward effect and withdrawal symptoms in mice lacking the μ-opioid receptor gene. Nature 383: 819–823.
3. Roy S, Liu H-C, Loh HH (1998) μ-opioid receptor-knockout mice: the role of μ-opioid receptor in gastrointestinal transit. Mol Brain Res 56: 281–283.
4. Wood JD, Galligan JJ (2004) Function of opioids in the enteric nervous system. Neurogastroenterol Motil 16 Suppl 2: 17–28.

5. Holzer P (2009) Opioid receptors in the gastrointestinal tract. Regul Pept 155: 11–17.
6. Martini L, Whistler JL (2007) The role of mu opioid receptor desensitization and endocytosis in morphine tolerance and dependence. Curr Opin Neurobiol 17: 556–564.
7. Williams JT, Ingram SL, Henderson G, Chavkin C, von Zastrow M, et al. (2013) Regulation of mu-opioid receptors: desensitization, phosphorylation, internalization, and tolerance. Pharmacol Rev 65: 223–254.
8. Kurz A, Sessler DI (2003) Opioid-induced bowel dysfunction: pathophysiology and potential new therapies. Drugs 63: 649–671.
9. Kalso E, Edwards JE, Moore RA, McQuay HJ (2004) Opioids in chronic non-cancer pain: systematic review of efficacy and safety. Pain 112: 372–380.
10. Robinson CB, Fritch M, Hullett L, Petersen MA, Sikkema S, et al. (2000) Development of a protocol to prevent opioid-induced constipation in patients with cancer: a research utilization project. Clin J Oncol Nurs 4: 79–84.
11. Keith DE, Anton B, Murray SR, Zaki PA, Chu PC, et al. (1998) μ-opioid receptor internalization: opiate drugs have differential effects on a conserved endocytic mechanism in vitro and in mammalian brain. Mol Pharmacol 53: 377–384.
12. Sternini C, Spann M, Anton B, Keith DE Jr, Bunnett NW, et al. (1996) Agonist-selective endocytosis of μ opioid receptor by neurons *in vivo*. Proc Natl Acad Sci USA 93: 9241–9246.
13. Minnis J, Patierno S, Kohlmeier SE, Brecha N, Tonini M, et al. (2003) Ligand-induced μ opioid receptor endocytosis and recycling in enteric neurons. Neuroscience 119: 33–42.
14. Arttamangkul S, Quillinan N, Low MJ, von Zastrow M, Pintar J, et al. (2008) Differential activation and trafficking of micro-opioid receptors in brain slices. Mol Pharmacol 74: 972–979.
15. Haberstock-Debic H, Kim KA, Yu YJ, von Zastrow M (2005) Morphine promotes rapid, arrestin-dependent endocytosis of mu-opioid receptors in striatal neurons. J Neurosci 25: 7847–7857.
16. Patierno S, Anselmi L, Jaramillo I, Scott D, Garcia R, et al. (2011) Morphine induces μ opioid receptor endocytosis in guinea pig enteric neurons following prolonged receptor activation. Gastroenterology 140: 618–626.
17. Ho A, Lievore A, Patierno S, Kohlmeier SE, Tonini M, et al. (2003) Neurochemically distinct classes of myenteric neurons express the μ-opioid receptor in the guinea pig ileum. J Comp Neurol 458: 404–411.
18. Ma W, Zheng WH, Powell K, Jhamandas K, Quirion R (2001) Chronic morphine exposure increases the phosphorylation of MAP kinases and the transcription factor CREB in dorsal root ganglion neurons: an in vitro and in vivo study. Eur J Neurosci 14: 1091–1104.
19. Macey TA, Lowe JD, Chavkin C (2006) μ opioid receptor activation of ERK1/2 is GRK3 and arrestin dependent in striatal neurons. J Biol Chem 281: 34515–34524.
20. Anselmi L, Stella SL Jr, Brecha NC, Sternini C (2009) Galanin inhibition of voltage-dependent Ca(2+) influx in rat cultured myenteric neurons is mediated by galanin receptor 1. J Neurosci Res 87: 1107–1114.
21. Duncia JV, Santella JB 3rd, Higley CA, Pitts WJ, Wityak J, et al. (1998) MEK inhibitors: the chemistry and biological activity of U0126, its analogs, and cyclization products. Bioorg Med Chem Lett 8: 2839–2844.
22. Macia E, Ehrlich M, Massol R, Boucrot E, Brunner C, et al. (2006) Dynasore, a cell-permeable inhibitor of dynamin. Dev Cell 10: 839–850.
23. Schmidlin F, Dery O, DeFea KO, Slice L, Patierno S, et al. (2001) Dynamin and rab5a dependent trafficking and signaling of the neurokinin 1 receptor. J Biol Chem 276: 25427–25437.
24. Herskovits JS, Burgess CC, Obar RA, Vallee RB (1993) Effects of mutant rat dynamin on endocytosis. J Cell Biol 122: 565–578.
25. Sakoda T, Kasahara N, Hamamori Y, Kedes L (1999) A high-titer lentiviral production system mediates efficient transduction of differentiated cells including beating cardiac myocytes. J Mol Cell Cardiol 31: 2037–2047.
26. Soares HP, Ni Y, Kisfalvi K, Sinnett-Smith J, Rozengurt E (2013) Different patterns of Akt and ERK feedback activation in response to rapamycin, active-site mTOR inhibitors and metformin in pancreatic cancer cells. PLoS One 8: e57289.
27. Polakiewicz RD, Schieferl SM, Dorner LF, Kansra V, Comb MJ (1998) A mitogen-activated protein kinase pathway is required for mu-opioid receptor desensitization. J Biol Chem 273: 12402–12406.
28. Karim F, Hu HJ, Adwanikar H, Kaplan D, Gereau RWt (2006) Impaired inflammatory pain and thermal hyperalgesia in mice expressing neuron-specific dominant negative mitogen activated protein kinase kinase (MEK). Mol Pain 2: 2.
29. Saccani F, Anselmi L, Jaramillo I, Bertoni S, Barocelli E, et al. (2012) Protective role of μ opioid receptor activation in intestinal inflammation induced by mesenteric ischemia/reperfusion in mice. J Neurosci Res 90: 2146–2153.
30. Miller MS, Galligan JJ, Burks TF (1981) Accurate measurement of intestinal transit in the rat. J Pharmacol Methods 6: 211–217.
31. Heuser JE, Anderson RG (1989) Hypertonic media inhibit receptor-mediated endocytosis by blocking clathrin-coated pit formation. J Cell Biol 108: 389–400.
32. Ignatova EG, Belcheva MM, Bohn LM, Neuman MC, Coscia CJ (1999) Requirement of receptor internalization for opioid stimulation of mitogen-activated protein kinase: biochemical and immunofluorescence confocal microscopic evidence. J Neurosci 19: 56–63.
33. Whistler JL, Chuang H-H, Chu P, Jan LY, von Zastrow M (1999) Functional dissociation of μ opioid receptor signaling and endocytosis: implications for the biology of opiate tolerance and addiction. Neuron 23: 737–746.
34. Trapaidze N, Gomes I, Cvejic S, Bansinath M, Devi LA (2000) Opioid receptor endocytosis and activation of MAP kinase pathway. Brain Res Mol Brain Res 76: 220–228.
35. Walwyn WM, Wei W, Xie CW, Chiu K, Kieffer BL, et al. (2006) μ opioid receptor-effector coupling and trafficking in dorsal root ganglia neurons. Neuroscience 142: 493–503.
36. Arden JR, Segredo V, Wang Z, Lameh J, Sadee W (1995) Phosphorylation and agonist-specific intracellular trafficking of an epitope-tagged μ-opioid receptor expressed in HEK293 cells. J Neurochem 65: 1636–1645.
37. Zhao H, Loh HH, Law PY (2006) Adenylyl cyclase superactivation induced by long-term treatment with opioid agonist is dependent on receptor localized within lipid rafts and is independent of receptor internalization. Mol Pharmacol 69: 1421–1432.
38. Arttamangkul S, Torrecilla M, Kobayashi K, Okano H, Williams JT (2006) Separation of μ-opioid receptor desensitization and internalization: endogenous receptors in primary neuronal cultures. J Neurosci 26: 4118–4125.
39. Borgland SL, Connor M, Osborne PB, Furness JB, Christie MJ (2003) Opioid agonists have different efficacy profiles for G protein activation, rapid desensitization, and endocytosis of mu-opioid receptors. J Biol Chem 278: 18776–18784.
40. Eisinger DA, Ammer H, Schulz R (2002) Chronic morphine treatment inhibits opioid receptor desensitization and internalization. J Neurosci 22: 10192–10200.
41. Whistler JL, von Zastrow M (1998) Morphine-activated opioid receptors elude desensitization by ß-arrestin. Proc Natl Acad Sci USA 95: 9914–9919.
42. Dang VC, Christie MJ (2012) Mechanisms of rapid opioid receptor desensitization, resensitization and tolerance in brain neurons. Br J Pharmacol 165: 1704–1716.
43. Zheng H, Loh HH, Law PY (2008) ß-arrestin-dependent μ-opioid receptor-activated extracellular signal-regulated kinases (ERKs) translocate to nucleus in contrast to G protein-dependent ERK activation. Mol Pharmacol 73: 178–190.
44. Kromer W (1990) Endogenous opioids, the enteric nervous system and gut motility. Dig Dis 8: 361–373.
45. Kromer W (1990) Regulation of intestinal motility by peripheral opioids: facts and hypotheses. In: Almeida OFX, Shippenberg TS, editors. Opioid peptides and receptors. Berlin: Springer.
46. Chen Z, Suntres Z, Palmer J, Guzman J, Javed A, et al. (2007) Cyclic AMP signaling contributes to neural plasticity and hyperexcitability in AH sensory neurons following intestinal Trichinella spiralis-induced inflammation. Int J Parasitol 37: 743–761.
47. Lopez de Armentia M, Jancic D, Olivares R, Alarcon JM, Kandel ER, et al. (2007) cAMP response element-binding protein-mediated gene expression increases the intrinsic excitability of CA1 pyramidal neurons. J Neurosci 27: 13909–13918.
48. Kang M, Maguma HT, Smith TH, Ross GR, Dewey WL, et al. (2011) The role of ß-arrestin2 in the mechanism of morphine tolerance in the mouse and guinea pig gastrointestinal tract. J Pharmacol Exp Ther 340: 567–576.
49. Ross GR, Gabra BH, Dewey WL, Akbarali HI (2008) Morphine tolerance in the mouse ileum and colon. J Pharmacol Exp Ther 327: 561–572.

20

Butanol Isomers Exert Distinct Effects on Voltage-Gated Calcium Channel Currents and Thus Catecholamine Secretion in Adrenal Chromaffin Cells

Sarah McDavid[1]⁹, Mary Beth Bauer[1]⁹, Rebecca L. Brindley[1], Mark L. Jewell[2], Kevin P. M. Currie[3]*

1 Department of Anesthesiology, Vanderbilt University School of Medicine, Nashville, Tennessee, United States of America, 2 Department of Pharmacology, Vanderbilt University School of Medicine, Nashville, Tennessee, United States of America, 3 Department of Anesthesiology, Department of Pharmacology, and Vanderbilt Brain Institute, Vanderbilt University School of Medicine, Nashville, Tennessee, United States of America

Abstract

Butanol ($C_4H_{10}OH$) has been used both to dissect the molecular targets of alcohols/general anesthetics and to implicate phospholipase D (PLD) signaling in a variety of cellular functions including neurotransmitter and hormone exocytosis. Like other primary alcohols, 1-butanol is a substrate for PLD and thereby disrupts formation of the intracellular signaling lipid phosphatidic acid. Because secondary and tertiary butanols do not undergo this transphosphatidylation, they have been used as controls for 1-butanol to implicate PLD signaling. Recently, selective pharmacological inhibitors of PLD have been developed and, in some cases, fail to block cellular functions previously ascribed to PLD using primary alcohols. For example, exocytosis of insulin and degranulation of mast cells are blocked by primary alcohols, but not by the PLD inhibitor FIPI. In this study we show that 1-butanol reduces catecholamine secretion from adrenal chromaffin cells to a much greater extent than tert-butanol, and that the PLD inhibitor VU0155056 has no effect. Using fluorescent imaging we show the effect of these drugs on depolarization-evoked calcium entry parallel those on secretion. Patch-clamp electrophysiology confirmed the peak amplitude of voltage-gated calcium channel currents (I_{Ca}) is inhibited by 1-butanol, with little or no block by secondary or tert-butanol. Detailed comparison shows for the first time that the different butanol isomers exert distinct, and sometimes opposing, effects on the voltage-dependence and gating kinetics of I_{Ca}. We discuss these data with regard to PLD signaling in cellular physiology and the molecular targets of general anesthetics.

Editor: J. David Spafford, University of Waterloo, Canada

Funding: This work was supported in part by a pilot and feasibility grant from the Vanderbilt Diabetes Research and Training Center to KC [Grant P30 DK20593], and by the National Institutes of Health [Grant R01 NS052446] to KC. The funders had no role in study design, data collection and analysis, decision to publish, or preparation of the manuscript.

Competing Interests: Kevin Currie currently serves as an academic editor for PLOS ONE. This does not alter the authors' adherence to PLOS ONE policies on sharing data and materials.

* Email: kevin.currie@vanderbilt.edu

⁹ These authors contributed equally to this work.

Introduction

Butanol ($C_4H_{10}OH$) exists as multiple isomers; primary (1-butanol) and secondary butanol (2-butanol) have a straight carbon chain with the hydroxyl group located at the terminal or second carbon, respectively. The four-carbon chain can also be branched with the hydroxyl group located at a terminal carbon (isobutanol; also called 2-methyl-1-propanol) or at the internal carbon (tert-butanol; also called 2-methyl-2-propanol). Like other primary alcohols, 1-butanol serves as a substrate for phospholipase D (PLD) [1]. In the absence of alcohols, PLD catalyzes the hydrolysis of phosphatidylcholine to produce choline and phosphatidic acid, with the latter acting directly or indirectly through intracellular signaling cascades to control a diverse array of cellular functions [2–11]. However, in the presence of 1-butanol, PLD produces phosphatidylbutanol rather than phosphatidic acid [1]. Neither secondary nor tertiary butanols undergo this transphosphatidylation, so these alcohols are commonly used as controls for 1-butanol to implicate phosphatidic acid/PLD signaling. Recently, several selective pharmacological inhibitors of PLD have been developed [12–14], and some reports have noted a disparity between the effects of these and 1-butanol on cellular function. For example, 1-butanol inhibits insulin secretion, but the PLD inhibitor FIPI has no effect [12]. Similarly, 1-butanol inhibits membrane ruffling, blebbing, and degranulation (exocytosis) in mast cells, but FIPI does not [15]. The implication from these studies is that acute application of 1-butanol blocks exocytosis by a mechanism(s) distinct from PLD signaling.

This raises the question by which other target(s) might butanol inhibit exocytosis? It is known that primary alcohols induce anesthesia and act in a manner similar to inhalational anesthetics [16]. Potential molecular targets for alcohols/general anesthetics include ligand-gated, voltage-gated, and other ion channels [17–23]. Although much attention has focused on post-synaptic ligand-gated ion channels, there is also evidence for presynaptic effects of alcohols/anesthetics [23–25]. The critical roles of voltage-gated channels make them an attractive potential target for disruption of stimulus-secretion coupling by butanol (and other alcohols/

anesthetics). Voltage-gated sodium and potassium channels control electrical excitability, while calcium entry through voltage-gated calcium channels controls a multitude of cellular functions including vesicular trafficking and neurotransmitter/ hormone secretion. Indeed, primary alcohols have been shown to modulate voltage-gated channels: 1-butanol inhibits voltage-gated sodium channel currents [26], voltage-gated potassium channel currents [27–29], and voltage-gated calcium channel currents (I_{Ca}) [30–32]. However, it is not known if butanol isomers differ in their modulation of voltage-gated ion channel function.

In this study we investigated the effects of butanol isomers on catecholamine secretion and I_{Ca} in adrenal chromaffin cells, an important neuroendocrine component of the sympathetic nervous system and a well-characterized neurosecretory model [33]. Both PLD1 and PLD2 are expressed in chromaffin cells, and PLD1 has been implicated in controlling catecholamine secretion [11,34]. However, to our knowledge the effects of newer PLD inhibitors have not been reported prior to this study. We show that 1-butanol reduces catecholamine secretion to a much greater extent than tert-butanol, but VU0155056, a newly developed cell membrane permeable inhibitor of both PLD1 and PLD2 [13,14], has no effect. Fluorescent imaging approaches reveal parallel effects on depolarization-evoked calcium entry. With patch-clamp electrophysiology we demonstrate concentration-dependent inhibition of I_{Ca} by 1-butanol with little or no block by secondary or tert-butanol. Detailed comparison shows for the first time that different butanol isomers exert distinct, and sometimes opposing, effects on the gating and kinetics of I_{Ca}. We discuss these data with regard to PLD signaling in cellular physiology and the molecular targets of general anesthetics.

Materials and Methods

Cell culture

Bovine adrenal glands were obtained from a local slaughterhouse (C & F Meat Co. Inc., College Grove, TN), and chromaffin cells were prepared by digestion with collagenase followed by density gradient centrifugation as described previously [35]. The cells were plated onto coverslips coated with collagen (at a density of $0.3–0.4\times10^6$ cells/mL for $[Ca^{2+}]_i$ measurements or $\sim0.2\times10^6$ cell/mL for patch clamp recordings). For secretion studies, cells were plated in 24-well tissue culture plates at a density of $\sim0.3\times10^6$ cells per well. Fibroblasts were effectively suppressed with cytosine arabinoside (10 μM) (Sigma-Aldrich; St Louis MO), leaving relatively pure chromaffin cell cultures. The culture medium consisted of Dulbecco's modified Eagle medium \ F12 (1:1) supplemented with fetal bovine serum (10%), glutamine (2 mM), penicillin/streptomycin (100 unit mL^{-1}/100 μg mL^{-1}), cytosine arabinoside (10 μM) and 5-fluorodeoxyuridine (10 μM). Tissue culture reagents were from Life Technologies (Grand Island, NY). The culture medium was replaced the day after isolation and experiments were performed 2–5 days following cell isolation.

$[Ca^{2+}]_i$ Measurements

Free cytosolic Ca^{2+} concentration ($[Ca^{2+}]_i$) was measured using an InCyt IM2 fluorescence imaging system (Intracellular Imaging Inc., Cincinnati, OH) and a Nikon TE2000 fluorescence microscope (Nikon Instruments Inc., Melville, NY) [35]. Cells were washed twice with HEPES-buffered Hanks Balanced Salt Solution and incubated in the dark for 30–45 minutes with 3-5 μM FURA2-AM or FURA4F-AM at 37°C. Cells were then washed (in the dark) in FURA-free solution for 30–60 minutes before recording. The coverslip was transferred to a recording bath (volume ~300–400 μL) and continually perfused with fresh solution at a flow rate of ~4 ml/min from gravity-fed reservoirs. Cells were excited at 340 nm and 380 nm and emission at 510 nm detected using a Pixelfly digital camera. The ratio of fluorescence emission at 340 nm/380 nm excitation was collected every 1–2 s throughout the experiment and converted to $[Ca^{2+}]_i$ using an *in vitro* calibration curve. Data were transferred to OriginPro software (Originlab Corporation, Northampton, MA) for analyses.

Catecholamine secretion experiments

Cells in 24-well plates were washed twice with extracellular solution and equilibrated in this solution for 30 mins at ~37°C. This was next replaced with fresh solution to determine basal release or with solution containing 30 mM KCl to stimulate secretion. After a five-minute stimulation period at ~37°C the cells were placed on ice, and the solution was removed and added to an equal volume of ice-cold 0.4 M perchloric acid. The cells were lyzed by addition of perchloric acid and scraping to extract the non-secreted catecholamines. The catecholamine content of the samples was determined by a specific high performance liquid chromatography (HPLC) assay utilizing an Antec Decade (oxidation potential: 0.7 V) electrochemical detector in the Neurochemistry Core of the Vanderbilt Brain Institute as described previously [35]. The amount of catecholamine secreted during the 5-minute stimulation period was expressed as a percentage of the total catecholamine content for that dish of cells. For each experiment, duplicate wells for each condition (control and drug treated) were averaged (to yield n = 1). 1-butanol (0.4% v/v; ~44 mM), tert-butanol (0.4% v/v; ~42 mM), the PLD inhibitor VU0155056 (1 μM), or DMSO (0.01%) (vehicle for VU0155056) was added to the cells for 10 minutes during the preincubation period and throughout the stimulation with KCl. Statistical analyses were performed using Prism5 software (GraphPad Software Inc., La Jolla, CA).

Patch-clamp electrophysiology

Patch pipette electrodes were pulled from borosilicate glass capillary tubes (World Precision Instruments, Sarasota, FL) using a Sutter P-97 pipette puller (Sutter Intrument, Novato, CA), coated with dental wax (Electron Microscopy Sciences, Hatfield, PA) and fire-polished to a final resistance of ~2 MΩ when filled with a CsCl-based internal solution. Cells were voltage-clamped in the conventional whole-cell configuration using either an Axopatch 200B amplifier, Digidata 1400A interface, and PClamp10 (Clampex) acquisition software (Molecular Devices, Sunnyvale, CA) or a HEKA EPC10 amplifier and PatchMaster acquisition software (HEKA instruments). Analog data were filtered at 2–3 kHz and digitized at 50 kHz. Series resistance was partially compensated (~50–80%) and data for I_{Ca} were subjected to linear capacitance and leak subtraction using P/N protocols (P/-4 or P/-8) with the leak pulses applied following the test pulses. The recording bath (volume ~300 μL) was continually perfused with fresh solution at a flow rate of ~4 ml/min from gravity-fed reservoirs. The exception was when ω-conotoxin GVIA (CgTx) was used to block the N-type I_{Ca}. For these experiments the CgTx was added as a 50 μL bolus of 2 μM CgTx into a static bath. The estimated final concentration of CgTx was ~0.5–1 μM. Blockade of the channels by CgTx is irreversible over the time course of these experiments. Following plateau of the current inhibition by CgTx (approximately 4–5 minutes), the bath flow was restarted and butanol applied. Raw data were analyzed using PClamp10 (Clampfit) or HEKA FitMaster software. Graphing and statistical analyses were performed using Origin or Prism.

Solutions, drugs and reagents

The extracellular solution for calcium imaging and secretion studies comprised (in mM): 136 NaCl, 2 KCl, 1 MgCl, 10 glucose, 10 HEPES, 2 CaCl, pH 7.3 osmolarity ~305 mOsm. The extracellular solution for patch-clamp recording was (in mM): 136 NaCl, 2 KCl, 1 MgCl, 10 glucose, 10 HEPES, 5 CaCl, pH 7.3 osmolarity ~310 mOsm. Tetrodotoxin (TTX) (0.5–1 μM) was added to block voltage-gated sodium channels. The intracellular (patch pipette) solution consisted of (in mM): CsCl 110, $MgCl_2$ 4, HEPES 20, EGTA 10, GTP 0.35, adenosine triphosphate 4, creatine phosphate 14, pH 7.3, osmolarity ~310–315 mOsm.

The AM-ester of FURA was prepared as 1 mM stock in dimethyl sulfoxide (DMSO) and aliquots frozen until use. The pentapotassium salt used for in vitro calibration curves was prepared as an aqueous stock and stored at 4°C. Butanol was added to the extracellular solutions at the indicated concentrations on the day of each experiment. VU0155056 was kindly provided by Dr. Alex Brown (Vanderbilt University) (also available from Avanti Polar Lipids Inc., Alabaster, Alabama). Stock solutions were prepared in DMSO (10 mM) and diluted into extracellular solution (1 μM final concentration) on the day of use. Tetrodotoxin (R&D systems, Minneapolis, MN) was prepared as a 1 mM aqueous stock and aliquots frozen until use (final concentration when diluted into extracellular solution was ~0.5 μM). ω-conotoxin GVIA (R&D systems, Minneapolis, MN) was prepared as a 100–300 μM aqueous stock and stored as frozen aliquots until use. On the day of the use, the aliquot was diluted to 2 μM in extracellular solution and a 50 μL bolus of this solution was added to the static recording bath (300–400 μL).

Results

Differential inhibition of calcium entry and catecholamine secretion by butanol isomers and the PLD inhibitor VU0155056

Dishes of chromaffin cells were stimulated with 30 mM KCl for 5 minutes to evoke membrane depolarization, calcium entry through voltage-gated calcium channels, and thus catecholamine secretion. Pre-incubation of the cells with 1-butanol (0.4%; ~44 mM) dramatically reduced epinephrine secretion measured using HPLC (Fig 1A). Tert-butanol (0.4%; ~42 mM) also reduced catecholamine secretion but to a significantly lesser extent than 1-butanol (Fig 1A). In contrast, 1 μM VU0155056, a newly developed cell membrane permeable inhibitor of both PLD1 and PLD2 [13], had no effect on secretion compared to DMSO controls (Fig 1B). These results suggest that 1-butanol exerts the bulk of its inhibitory effect on exocytosis at a site(s) other than PLD.

Because calcium entry through voltage-gated calcium channels plays a pivotal role in catecholamine secretion [36–39], we used ratiometric imaging of FURA2-loaded cells to determine if 1-butanol altered KCl-evoked calcium entry. Cells were stimulated with three successive applications of 30 mM KCl (Fig 1C). 1-butanol (0.4%; ~44 mM) reversibly reduced the peak calcium transient by 52±3% (n = 51 cells: p<0.001, Tukey's post-test following repeated measures ANOVA). In contrast, only slight reductions in calcium entry were produced by tert-butanol (9±2%) or VU-155056 (12±3%), and these did not reverse upon washout of the drugs. In other experiments, we used longer preincubations with butanol or VU0155056 (10 - 15 minute preincubation) and measured the peak intracellular calcium transient evoked by a single application of KCl. The peak calcium transient in control cells was 1319±65 nM (n = 43) and was significantly smaller in cells treated with 0.4% 1-butanol

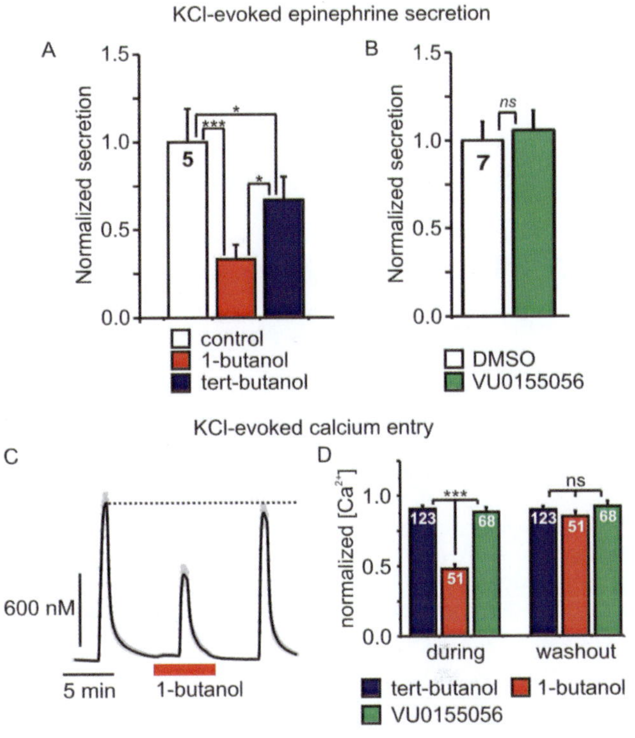

Figure 1. 1-butanol but not the phospholipase D inhibitor VU0155056 inhibits catecholamine secretion and calcium entry. A) Secretion was evoked by application of 30 mM KCl for five-minutes. Epinephrine secretion from cells treated with 1-butanol (0.4%; ~44 mM) or tert-butanol (0.4%; ~42 mM) was normalized to that from controls. Secretion was significantly inhibited by 1-butanol and to a lesser extent by tert-butanol (one-way ANOVA, F = 20.98, p = 0.0007: * p<0.05, *** p<0.001 for pairwise comparisons using Tukey's post-hoc test). **B**) KCl-evoked epinephrine secretion was not altered by the phospholipase D inhibitor VU0155056 (1 μM) (p = 0.49, paired t-test). **C**) A representative experiment showing the intracellular calcium transients evoked by 30 mM KCl (60 s applications) applied before, during, and after washout of 0.4% 1-butanol. **D**) Mean data from several experiments like that shown in panel C. The peak increase in intracellular $[Ca^{2+}]$ evoked by KCl in the presence (during) of 1-butanol (0.4%; ~42 mM), tert-butanol (0.4%; ~42 mM), or VU0155056 (1 μM) was normalized to the first control response in each cell. 1-butanol significantly inhibited Ca^{2+} entry compared to both tert-butanol and VU0155056 (one-way ANOVA, F = 54.8, p<0.0001: *** p<0.001 for pairwise comparisons using Tukey's post-hoc test). After washout of the drugs (washout) Ca^{2+} entry was not significantly different in any of the three treatment groups (one-way ANOVA, F = 1.03, p = 0.36).

(797±38 nM; n = 62; p<0.001 ANOVA with Tukey's post-test). In contrast, neither tert-butanol (1153±29 nM, n = 99) nor VU0155056 (1112±84 nM; n = 71) significantly reduced the peak calcium transient compared to controls (ANOVA followed by pair-wise comparison with Tukey's post-test).

Differential effects of butanol isomers on voltage-gated calcium channel currents (I_{Ca})

Based on the calcium imaging data (Fig 1), we compared the effects of butanol isomers on I_{Ca} using patch clamp electrophysiology. Cells were voltage-clamped in the standard whole-cell recording configuration and I_{Ca} activated by short (10–20 ms) steps from −80 mV to +10 mV every 20 s (Fig 2A). Acute application of 1-butanol (0.4%; ~44 mM) rapidly and reversibly inhibited the peak amplitude of I_{Ca}. The inhibition of I_{Ca} was concentration-dependent with an estimated EC_{50} of 52 mM (~0.48%) (Fig 2B). We then compared the ability of 1-butanol, 2-butanol, and tert-butanol (all at 0.4%) to inhibit the peak amplitude of I_{Ca}. 1-butanol inhibited I_{Ca} from 640±88 pA to 399±57 pA (n = 17, p<0.0001 paired t-test); 2-butanol inhibited I_{Ca} from 652±81 pA to 547±81 pA (n = 5; p<0.001 paired t-test); tert-butanol only slightly reduced the amplitude of I_{Ca} from 632±83 pA to 583±78 pA (n = 18, p = 0.06 paired t-test). The percent inhibition by 1-butanol was significantly greater than either 2-butanol or tert-butanol (Fig 2C).

1-butanol inhibits N-type and P/Q-type I_{Ca} to the same extent

The whole cell I_{Ca} in bovine chromaffin cells has been well characterized and is comprised of ~10% L-type current (blocked by dihydropyridine antagonists) with the remaining current carried by N-type and P/Q-type I_{Ca} in roughly equal proportions [37,40,41]. To determine if the N- and P/Q-type channels were differentially inhibited by 1-butanol, we pharmacologically isolated the two current components. Cells were voltage-clamped at −70 mV and nitrendipine (3 μM) was present throughout the experiment to block the L-type current. Cells were stimulated every 20 s with a 20 ms step to +10 mV. The inhibition of I_{Ca} produced by 1-butanol was determined twice, once before and once after application of ω-conotoxin GVIA (CgTx) to block the N-type channels (Fig 2D). Consistent with previous reports, CgTx blocked 48±7% (n = 5) of the current [37,42,43]. We have previously shown that the remaining CgTx resistant component of I_{Ca} is almost fully comprised of P/Q-type channels, as it is blocked by ω-Agatoxin IVA [42]. Calculating the "difference current" (i.e. subtracting the data recorded after CgTx from that recorded before CgTx) yields the CgTx-sensitive N-type I_{Ca}. Using this pharmacological dissection, we found that 1-butanol inhibited N-type I_{Ca} by 46±5% and P/Q-type I_{Ca} by 49±3.7% (n = 5) (Fig 2D).

Differential effects of primary and tert-butanol on channel activation

To assess the inhibition of I_{Ca} in more detail, current-voltage relationships were determined. 1-butanol inhibited the amplitude of I_{Ca} across a range of voltages with no obvious shift in the I-V curve (Fig 3A). In contrast, 2-butanol had much smaller effects (Fig 3B) and especially for tert-butanol there was an obvious hyperpolarizing shift in the I-V curve (Fig 3C). Indeed, the amplitude of I_{Ca} elicited by a step to −10 mV was significantly *increased* by tert-butanol (p<0.01, repeated measures ANOVA with pairwise comparison using Bonferroni post-test).

Given that tert-butanol produced a prominent shift in the I-V curve, we assessed the voltage-dependence of I_{Ca} activation by measuring the tail current amplitude following a series of depolarizing steps (Fig 4A). Figures 4B and 4C show the effects of 1-butanol and tert-butanol on the activation curves. The V_{50}

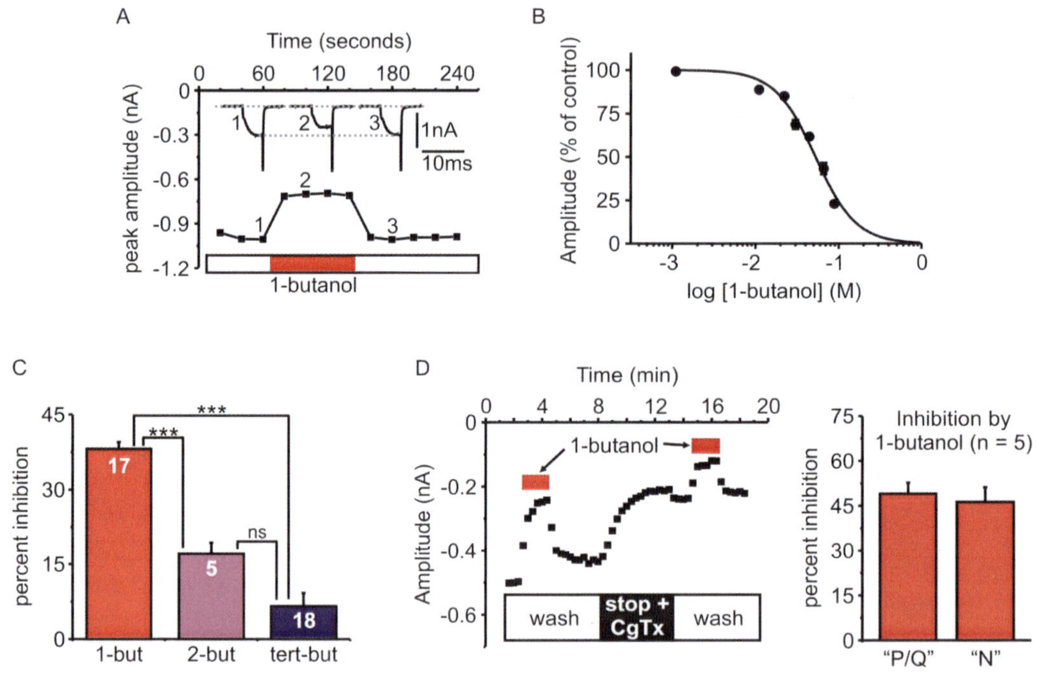

Figure 2. Concentration-dependent inhibition of I_{Ca} by 1-butanol. A) Representative time-course showing reversible inhibition of peak I_{Ca} amplitude by 1-butanol (0.4%; ~44 mM). Currents were evoked by 10 ms duration steps from −90 mV to +10 mV. **B**) Concentration-response curve showing the percent inhibition of I_{Ca} amplitude by 1-butanol. Points are mean ± s.e.m. of 4–17 cells (error bars are within the data points in some cases). The solid line shows the fit to a standard dose-response relationship which yielded an estimated EC_{50} of 52 mM and Hill slope of −1.73. **C**) Percent inhibition of peak I_{Ca} amplitude (elicited by a step from −90 mV to +10 mV) by 1-butanol (n = 17), 2-butanol (n = 5), or tert-butanol (n = 18) (all butanol isomers at 0.4%) (one-way ANOVA, F = 60.7, p<0.0001: *** p<0.001, ns = "not significant" for pairwise comparisons using Tukey's post-hoc test). **D**) *Left panel*: Representative experiment showing peak I_{Ca} amplitude plotted against time (elicited by a step from −70 mV to +10 mV). Nitrendipine (3 μM) was present throughout the experiment to block any L-type calcium channels. The bath was continually perfused with fresh solution (wash) and 1-butanol applied as indicated by the red bars. At the time indicated by the black bar, the solution flow was stopped and a bolus of ω-conotoxin GVIA was added to the bath (stop + CgTx) to irreversibly block N-type calcium channels. *Right panel*: The percent inhibition of pharmacologically isolated P/Q-type and N-type I_{Ca} by 1-butanol. "P/Q-type" I_{Ca} was defined as the CgTx resistant current (i.e. the current remaining after washout of CgTx). "N-type" I_{Ca} was defined as the CgTx sensitive component (i.e. the data after Cgtx subtracted from data before CgTx).

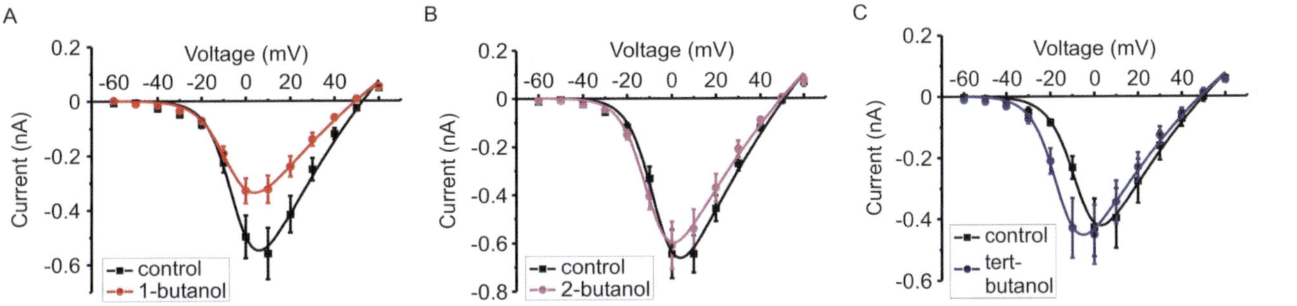

Figure 3. Differential effects of butanol isomers on the current-voltage relationship of I_{Ca}. Cells were stimulated by a series of steps, from a holding potential of −90 mV to test potentials ranging from −60 mV to +60 mV, first in control conditions and then in the presence of either 0.4% (~44 mM) 1-butanol (panel A, n = 6), 2-butanol (panel B, n = 5), or tert-butanol (panel C, n = 5). The mean current amplitude elicited by each step is plotted. Tert-butanol elicited a clear hyperpolarizing shift in the I-V relationship.

(potential at which half maximal activation is achieved) was determined by fitting a Boltzmann curve to the data. 1-butanol did not significantly shift the V_{50} for activation (0.6±0.4 mV in control conditions compared to −0.1±0.9 mV in the presence of 1-butanol, n = 6; p = 0.35, paired t-test). However, tert-butanol hyperpolarized the activation curve (Fig 4C) and significantly shifted the V_{50} from −2.7±1.4 mV to −11.4±0.8 (n = 6; p = 0.0018, paired t-test). The slope of the activation curve was significantly reduced by 1-butanol (Fig 4B) but not by tert-butanol (Fig 4C). Thus, the different butanol isomers exert distinct effects on channel activation which is opposed by 1-butanol but favored by tert-butanol.

Opposite effects of primary and tert-butanol on the deactivation kinetics of I_{Ca}

Figure 5A shows examples of tail currents following steps to + 40 mV to maximally activate I_{Ca}. The mean tail current amplitude was significantly reduced by 1-butanol (from 1.81±0.33 nA to 0.92±0.15 nA; n = 6; p = 0.006, paired t-test) but not by tert-butanol (1.17±0.22 nA to 1.01±0.15 nA; n = 6; p = 0.14, paired t-test). The decay of the tail currents reflects channel deactivation (i.e. the open to closed transition upon membrane hyperpolarization) and is well fit with a single exponential. 1-butanol significantly accelerated the decay (Fig 5B, C), decreasing the time constant of the exponential fit from 300±13 µS to 217±7 µS (n = 6, p = 0.004, paired t-test) (Fig 5C). In contrast, tert-butanol significantly slowed the decay of the tail currents, increasing the time constant of the exponential fit from 340±33 µS to 514±68 µS (n = 6, p = 0.03, paired t-test) (Fig 5B, C).

Primary and tert-butanol both promote voltage-dependent inactivation of I_{Ca}

The voltage-dependence of steady-state inactivation was determined by incrementally increasing the holding potential from − 90 mV to −20 mV for durations of 30 s (Fig 6A). Following recovery at −90 mV the cell was then exposed to either 1-butanol (0.4%; ~44 mM) or tert-butanol (0.4%; ~42 mM) and the

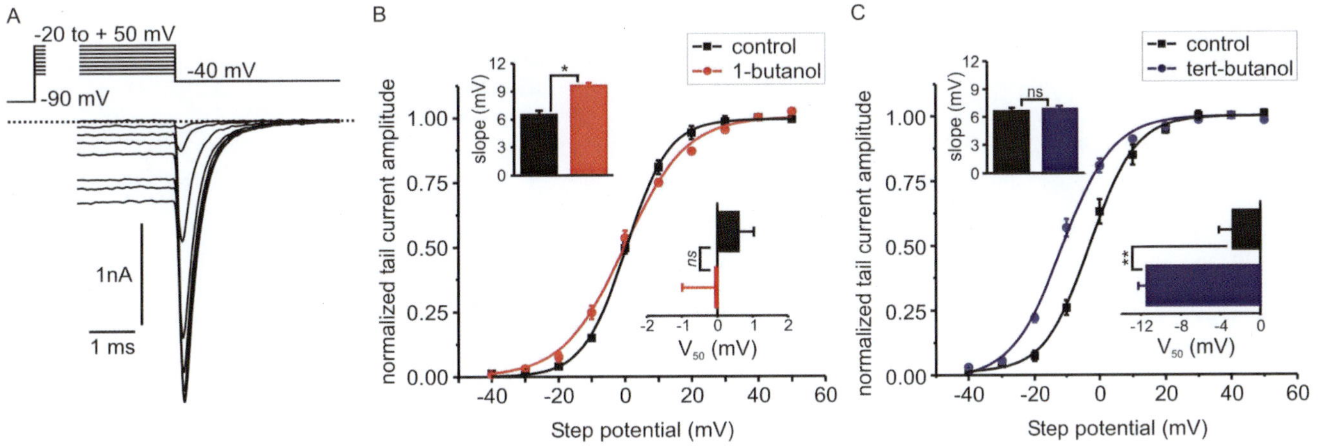

Figure 4. Butanol isomers differentially modulate the voltage-dependence of I_{Ca} activation. A) The upper panel shows the voltage command protocol and the lower panel shows a family of representative I_{Ca} tail current recordings. Cells were stimulated with depolarizing steps from a holding potential of −90 mV to test potentials ranging from −20 to +50 mV and tail currents were recorded upon repolarization to −40 mV. **B, C**) In each cell, tail currents were recorded first under control conditions and then in the presence of either 1-butanol (panel B, n = 6) or tert-butanol (panel C, n = 6). Tail current amplitude was normalized to that evoked by the +40 mV step and plotted against the potential of the step depolarization (mean ± s.e.m.). The solid line shows the fit with a Boltzmann curve. The inset bar graphs show the mean slope and V_{50} (potential at half maximal activation) derived from the Boltzmann fits to individual cells. 1-butanol had no effect on V_{50} but the slope of the curve was significantly shallower. In contrast, tert-butanol had no effect on the slope, but produced a strong hyperpolarizing shift in the V_{50} (* $p<0.05$; ** $P<0.01$; ns = not significant; paired t-test).

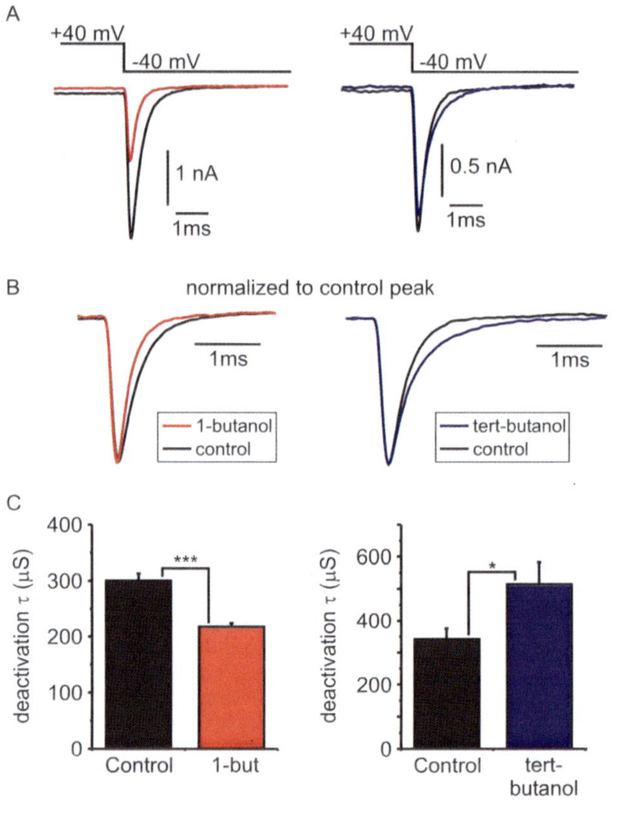

Figure 5. Differential effects of butanol isomers on the deactivation kinetics of I_{Ca}. A) Representative tail currents activated by a step depolarization from −90 mV to +40 mV. In each cell, tail currents were recorded first in control conditions and then in the presence of either 1-butanol (left) or tert-butanol (right). **B)** The same traces as in panel A, but the time-base was expanded and the currents in the presence of butanol were scaled to the same amplitude as control to more clearly illustrate changes in the decay kinetics. **C)** The decay of the tail currents was fit with a single exponential function. Bar charts plot the mean time constant of the fit (τ) in control conditions and in the presence of 1-butanol (n = 6) or tert-butanol (n = 6). (* $p < 0.05$; *** $p < 0.001$ compared to matched controls; paired t-test).

inactivation protocol was repeated. Both butanol isomers produced a similar hyperpolarizing shift in the inactivation curves (Fig 6B, C). 1-butanol significantly shifted the V_{50} (potential at half maximal inactivation) from −37.4±3.6 mV to -54.3±5.1 mV (n = 5, p = 0.0016, paired t-test). Similarly, tert-butanol shifted the V_{50} from -37.8±2.4 mV to −55.1±4.2 mV (n = 6, p = 0.0006, paired t-test).

The effect of butanol on voltage-dependent inactivation during a sustained depolarizing step was also determined (Fig 7A, B). EGTA (10 mM) was present in the patch-pipette solution to block Ca^{2+}-dependent inactivation. Cells were stimulated by a voltage step to +10 mV lasting 500 ms before and during application of either 1-butanol (0.4%; ~44 mM) or tert-butanol (0.4%; ~42 mM). Both butanol isomers significantly increased inactivation during the 500 ms step (Fig 7B). Accelerated inactivation will reduce calcium entry into cells during sustained or repetitive stimulation. To quantify this we calculated the charge (i.e. the integral) of I_{Ca} evoked by a 500 ms step depolarization. 1-butanol significantly inhibited the charge of I_{Ca} from 328±35 pC to 116±14 pC (n = 9; $p<0.0001$, paired t-test). Even though tert-butanol has little effect on the peak amplitude, it significantly reduced the charge of I_{Ca} from 297±48 pC to 184±40 pC (n = 7; $p<0.001$, paired t-test). Reflecting the dual actions of 1-butanol on both peak amplitude and inactivation, the integral of I_{Ca} was inhibited to a greater extent by 1-butanol (65±3%, n = 9) than by tert-butanol (41±4%, n = 7; $p<0.001$, independent t-test).

Discussion

In this study we investigated the effects of butanol isomers on calcium signaling and catecholamine secretion from adrenal chromaffin cells, an important component of the sympathetic nervous system and powerful model for investigating neurosecretory mechanisms. The rationale for the current investigation arose from two general uses of butanol in cellular physiology: implication of phosphatidic acid/PLD signaling in cellular functions, and investigating the molecular targets of general anesthetics. In spite of these two uses, there is little data comparing the effects of butanol isomers on pertinent cellular targets including voltage-gated ion channels.

Our data show that 1-butanol inhibited secretion to a much greater extent than tert-butanol, but the PLD inhibitor VU0155056 had no effect (Fig 1). We used VU0155056 at 1 µM, a concentration well above the reported cellular IC_{50} for PLD1 (20 nM) and PLD2 (380 nM) [13,14]. Our data parallel a previous report showing that 1-butanol inhibits insulin secretion but the PLD inhibitor FIPI has no effect [12]. Similarly, 1-butanol but not FIPI blocks degranulation (exocytosis) of mast cells [15]. Together, our data and these previous studies imply that acute application of 1-butanol blocks exocytosis by a PLD-independent mechanism(s). Our data demonstrate that disrupted calcium signaling is a likely mechanism by which 1-butanol acts. Using cellular imaging, we show that the calcium transient evoked by KCl-mediated depolarization was significantly reduced by 1-butanol, while tert-butanol and VU0155056 had negligible effects (Fig 1). Furthermore, we used patch clamp electrophysiology to confirm that 1-butanol rapidly and reversibly inhibited the peak amplitude of I_{Ca} while secondary and tert-butanol had minimal effects (Fig 2).

Ten genes encode for the pore-forming α_1 subunit of voltage-gated calcium channels, and these are sub-divided into three major families based on sequence homology (Ca_V1, Ca_V2, Ca_V3) [44,45]. Chromaffin cells from adult animals typically express Ca_V1 and Ca_V2 channels with the relative expression level depending on the species [37,39–41]. Low threshold T-type channels (Ca_V3) are typically not functionally expressed under normal conditions, but can be recruited by various signaling pathways or hypoxia [46–49]. In bovine cells, we have previously demonstrated that the whole cell I_{Ca} is comprised of ~10% L-type current and ~90% N + P/Q-type current in a roughly 1:1 ratio [42,50]. The concentration response relationship to 1-butanol (Fig 2B) shows that higher concentrations almost fully blocked I_{Ca}, suggesting that all the calcium channel subtypes present in these cells were targeted. To confirm this, we pharmacological dissected I_{Ca} using ω-conotoxin GVIA (a selective blocker of N-type channels) and found that the N-type and P/Q-type I_{Ca} were equally blocked by 1-butanol (Fig 2D). We speculate that L-type channels will be modulated in a similar manner, but due to the small amplitude of the L-type current in bovine chromaffin cells we did not determine this. In rodent chromaffin cells L-type channels ($Ca_V1.2$ and $Ca_V1.3$) comprise ~40% of the whole cell calcium current, and have been implicated in controlling action potential firing at rest or during sustained depolarization [51]. It is interesting to speculate that the butanol isomers will differentially modulate these aspects of rodent chromaffin cell function, but further experiments are needed to confirm this.

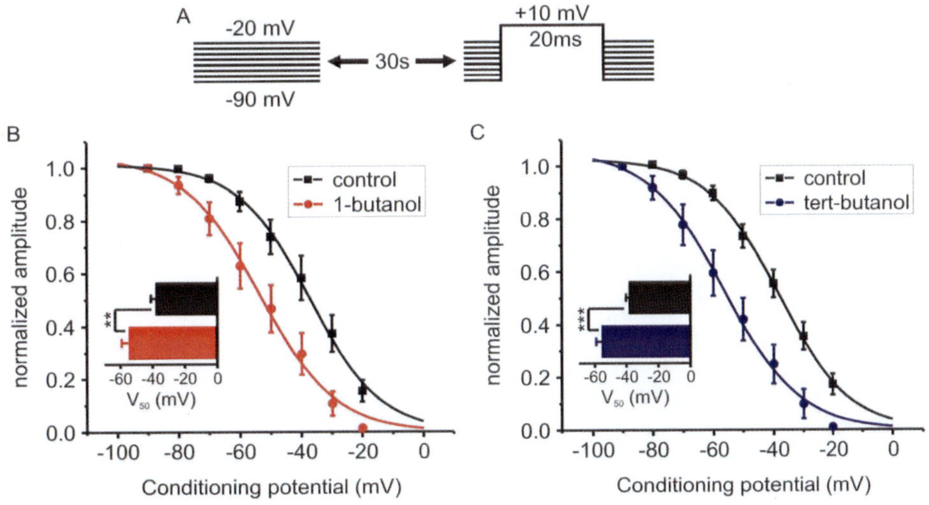

Figure 6. 1-butanol and tert-butanol produce a similar hyperpolarization of closed-state inactivation. A) Schematic depiction of the voltage-stimulus protocol. I_{Ca} were elicited by steps to +10 mV. The holding potential was increased in 10 mV increments from −90 mV to −20 mV and maintained at each potential for 30 s. In each cell this was done first in control conditions and then in the presence of either 1-butanol (panel B; n = 5) or tert-butanol (panel C; n = 6). **B, C)** I_{Ca} amplitude was normalized to that evoked from a holding potential of −90 mV and plotted against the holding potential. The graphs show the mean data fit using a Boltzmann function with three free parameters (upper plateau, slope, and V_{50}) and the lower plateau was constrained to ≥0. The inset bar graphs show the hyperpolarizing shift in mean V_{50} (voltage at half maximal inactivation) derived from the Boltzmann fits to individual cells (** $p<0.01$; *** $p<0.001$ compared to matched controls; paired t-test).

Our data showing isomer-specific block of I_{Ca} by butanol suggests the need to reassess at least some cellular functions previously attributed to PLD signaling using primary alcohols, especially those in which calcium signaling plays a prominent role. There is a body of work supporting a role for PLD in calcium-dependent exocytosis from chromaffin or PC12 cells [9,11,34],

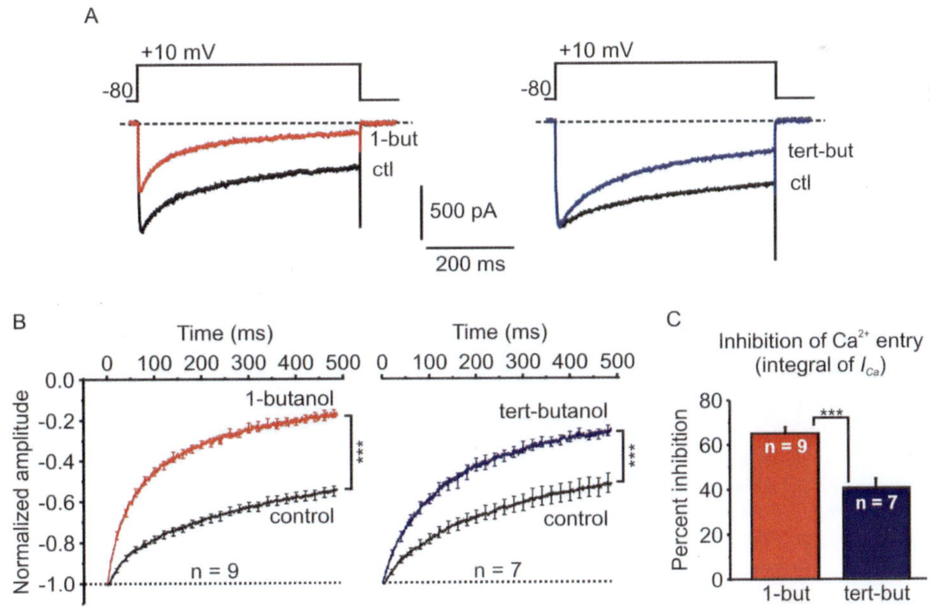

Figure 7. Butanol accelerates voltage-dependent inactivation and reduces total calcium entry during sustained depolarization. A) Representative recordings of I_{Ca} elicited by a 500 ms step depolarization under control conditions (ctl) and in the presence of either 0.4% (~44 mM) 1-butanol (1-but) or 0.4% (~42 mM) tert-butanol (tert-but). The patch pipette solution contained 10 mM EGTA to block calcium-dependent inactivation. Thus, the decay in I_{Ca} is due to voltage-dependent inactivation. 1-butanol inhibited the peak amplitude and accelerated the the inactivation of I_{Ca}. Tert-butanol also accelerated inactivation, but had minimal effects of the peak amplitude of I_{Ca}. **B)** Pooled data (mean ± sem) from multiple experiments like that shown in panel A. To facilitate comparison of inactivation, the amplitude of I_{Ca} in the presence of butanol was normalized to control conditions. For clarity, the displayed traces begin at the peak amplitude and error bars are only shown for some data points. 1-butanol and tert-butanol both significantly increased the extent of inactivation. (*** $p<0.001$ for the extent of inactivation at 490 ms in the presence of butanol compared to control conditions; paired t-test). **C)** The charge (integral) of I_{Ca} is directly proportional to the amount of calcium entry during the depolarizing step. 1-butanol produced a significantly greater inhibition than tert-butanol (*** $p<0.001$; paired t-test).

although some other studies have found no such link [52–54]. While the precise mechanism remains unclear, it has been proposed that generation of phosphatidic acid at vesicle release sites induces membrane curvature and thereby promotes the final stages of vesicle fusion with the plasma membrane [11]. Phosphatidic acid has also been shown to interact directly with SNARE proteins [55], or could lead to changes in other signaling lipids such as diacylglycerol or PiP2 [10]. Several approaches including RNAi-mediated knockdown of PLD and overexpression of wild-type or dominant negative mutants have been used to implicate PLD, and in particular PLD1, in exocytosis (for reviews see [9,11]). However, acute interventions have typically involved the use of primary alcohols, and to our knowledge the effects of newer PLD inhibitors have not been reported prior to this study. The main focus of the current investigation was not to dissect the role of PLD in catecholamine secretion *per se*, but our data suggest that acute block of PLD does not have a dramatic impact. Subtle effects on secretion are still possible as these would not be resolved in the assays used in this study, and we did not assess the impact of longer term block of PLD signaling. Further investigations will be required to address these issues and the precise role of PLD in neurotransmitter/hormone secretion.

This paper also provides the first detailed comparison of how butanol isomers modulate the function of voltage-gated channels. We used a concentration of 0.4% (~44 mM), typical for experiments probing PLD signaling and close to the EC_{50} for block of peak I_{Ca} amplitude by 1-butanol (Fig 2B). Although tert-butanol had minimal effects on peak I_{Ca} amplitude, it was not simply inert with respect to channel function. Tert-butanol accelerated inactivation of I_{Ca} during sustained depolarization and produced a pronounced (approximately −20 mV) shift in the steady state inactivation curve (Figs 6, 7). Distinct, even opposing effects of the butanol isomers were seen on other channel gating parameters, including the voltage-dependence of activation. 1-butanol produced no shift in the V_{50} and a modest reduction in the slope of the activation curve (Fig 4B). In contrast, tert-butanol hyperpolarized the V_{50} by ~−9 mV, with no change in the slope (Fig 4C). This likely will not increase the small "window current" (overlap of activation and inactivation curves (Figs 4 and 6)) because the much larger shift in steady-state inactivation will dominate. However, the hyperpolarizing shift in activation was apparent in the I-V relationship, and resulted in tert-butanol significantly *potentiating* the amplitude of I_{Ca} evoked by steps to −10 mV (Fig 3). The two isomers also had opposing effects on the kinetics of deactivation (tail current decay), which was accelerated by 1-butanol and slowed by tert-butanol (Fig 5). Again, as with the effects on activation gating, this would favor a potentiation of I_{Ca} by tert-butanol and inhibition by 1-butanol.

Perhaps the complex effects of butanol on I_{Ca} reflect multiple binding sites on the channel, some of which discern between the structurally distinct primary and tert-butanol isomers. 1-butanol has been used to map a binding site for general anesthetics/alcohols near the activation gate of Shaw-2 voltage-gated potassium channels [28,29]. The effects we observe on activation and deactivation gating are consistent with there being a similar binding site for butanol on the voltage-gated calcium channels, although this remains to be determined. Another recent study has reported multiple binding sites for general anesthetics on the bacterial sodium channel NaChBac [56]. It is also interesting to note that in virtually all cases reported to date, alcohols/general anesthetics *inhibit* voltage-gated channels. However, sevoflurane can potentiate voltage-gated potassium channels [57] and NaChBac [56]. It will be of interest in future to determine if sevoflurane also potentiates Ca_V channels, and conversely if tert-butanol potentiates potassium and sodium channels.

Although much progress has been made, the molecular targets and mechanisms of general anesthetics/alcohols are not completely understood. There is general consensus that post-synaptic ligand gated ion channels (e.g GABA, ACh) are important targets, but some evidence also points to presynaptic effects, perhaps on voltage-gated channels or the exocytotic machinery itself including SNARE proteins and munc18 [58–61]. In this study the estimated EC_{50} for 1-butanol block of peak I_{Ca} amplitude was ~52 mM (Fig 2B), which is somewhat higher than that producing anesthesia in vivo (10–20 mM) [62–64]. Moreover, even though secondary and tert-butanol also produce anesthesia, they had minimal effects on I_{Ca} amplitude (Fig 2,3). This would argue against Ca_V2 voltage-gated calcium channels being a primary target for the anesthetic actions. However, even relatively small changes in I_{Ca} can have a significant impact on neurotransmitter release, and as already discussed the effects of butanol are complex and extend well beyond the simple block of peak current amplitude. Further, investigations will be required to determine if these channels contribute to some of the anesthetic actions and/or side effects of alcohols/inhalational anesthetics.

In conclusion, we show for the first time that butanol isomers have distinct effects on the amplitude and gating properties of Ca_V2 voltage-gated calcium channel currents. This adds to existing literature demonstrating complex modulation of voltage-gated channels by alcohols and anesthetic agents. Our data also suggest the need to reassess at least some cellular functions previously attributed to PLD signaling by using primary alcohols as a tool, especially those in which calcium signaling plays a prominent role.

Supporting Information

Data S1 This file is provided as part of the PLOS ONE data availability policy. For figures in the manuscript that present averaged data (e.g. mean ± sem), the underlying raw data used to calculate those averages are provided. Refer to the main text of the manuscript or figure legends for further explanation of experimental design, protocols, etc.

Acknowledgments

We would like to thank: Ray Johnson, Manager of the Vanderbilt Brain Institute Neurochemistry Core, for assistance with high performance liquid chromatography analyses of catecholamines and Dr. Alex Brown, Dept. of Pharmacology, Vanderbilt University, for generously providing samples of the PLD inhibitor.

Author Contributions

Conceived and designed the experiments: KC. Performed the experiments: SM MB RB MJ. Analyzed the data: SM MB RB KC. Wrote the paper: SM MB RB MJ KC.

References

1. Brown HA, Henage LG, Preininger AM, Xiang Y, Exton JH (2007) Biochemical analysis of phospholipase D. Methods Enzymol 434: 49–87.
2. Cockcroft S (2001) Signalling roles of mammalian phospholipase D1 and D2. Cell Mol Life Sci 58: 1674–1687.
3. Exton JH (2000) Phospholipase D. Ann N Y Acad Sci 905: 61–68.

4. Selvy PE, Lavieri RR, Lindsley CW, Brown HA (2011) Phospholipase D: enzymology, functionality, and chemical modulation. Chem Rev 111: 6064–6119.
5. Peng X, Frohman MA (2012) Mammalian phospholipase D physiological and pathological roles. Acta Physiol (Oxf) 204: 219–226.
6. Rudge SA, Wakelam MJ (2009) Inter-regulatory dynamics of phospholipase D and the actin cytoskeleton. Biochim Biophys Acta 1791: 856–861.
7. Gomez-Cambronero J (2010) New concepts in phospholipase D signaling in inflammation and cancer. ScientificWorldJournal 10: 1356–1369.
8. Stace CL, Ktistakis NT (2006) Phosphatidic acid- and phosphatidylserine-binding proteins. Biochim Biophys Acta 1761: 913–926.
9. Bader MF, Vitale N (2009) Phospholipase D in calcium-regulated exocytosis: lessons from chromaffin cells. Biochim Biophys Acta 1791: 936–941.
10. Jenkins GM, Frohman MA (2005) Phospholipase D: a lipid centric review. Cell Mol Life Sci 62: 2305–2316.
11. Vitale N (2010) Synthesis of fusogenic lipids through activation of phospholipase D1 by GTPases and the kinase RSK2 is required for calcium-regulated exocytosis in neuroendocrine cells. Biochem Soc Trans 38: 167–171.
12. Su W, Yeku O, Olepu S, Genna A, Park JS, et al. (2009) 5-Fluoro-2-indolyl des-chlorohalopemide (FIPI), a phospholipase D pharmacological inhibitor that alters cell spreading and inhibits chemotaxis. Mol Pharmacol 75: 437–446.
13. Scott SA, Selvy PE, Buck JR, Cho HP, Criswell TL, et al. (2009) Design of isoform-selective phospholipase D inhibitors that modulate cancer cell invasiveness. Nat Chem Biol 5: 108–117.
14. Scott SA, Mathews TP, Ivanova PT, Lindsley CW, Brown HA (2014) Chemical modulation of glycerolipid signaling and metabolic pathways. Biochim Biophys Acta.
15. Yanase Y, Carvou N, Frohman MA, Cockcroft S (2010) Reversible bleb formation in mast cells stimulated with antigen is Ca2+/calmodulin-dependent and bleb size is regulated by ARF6. Biochem J 425: 179–193.
16. Fang Z, Ionescu P, Chortkoff BS, Kandel L, Sonner J, et al. (1997) Anesthetic potencies of n-alkanols: results of additivity and solubility studies suggest a mechanism of action similar to that for conventional inhaled anesthetics. Anesth Analg 84: 1042–1048.
17. Howard RJ, Trudell JR, Harris RA (2014) Seeking structural specificity: direct modulation of pentameric ligand-gated ion channels by alcohols and general anesthetics. Pharmacol Rev 66: 396–412.
18. Garcia PS, Kolesky SE, Jenkins A (2010) General anesthetic actions on GABA(A) receptors. Curr Neuropharmacol 8: 2–9.
19. Dopico AM, Lovinger DM (2009) Acute alcohol action and desensitization of ligand-gated ion channels. Pharmacol Rev 61: 98–114.
20. Franks NP (2006) Molecular targets underlying general anaesthesia. Br J Pharmacol 147 Suppl 1: S72–81.
21. Orestes P, Todorovic SM (2010) Are neuronal voltage-gated calcium channels valid cellular targets for general anesthetics? Channels (Austin) 4: 518–522.
22. Hemmings HC, Jr. (2009) Sodium channels and the synaptic mechanisms of inhaled anaesthetics. Br J Anaesth 103: 61–69.
23. Herold KF, Hemmings HC, Jr. (2012) Sodium channels as targets for volatile anesthetics. Front Pharmacol 3: 50.
24. Barclay JW, Graham ME, Edwards MR, Johnson JR, Morgan A, et al. (2010) Presynaptic targets for acute ethanol sensitivity. Biochem Soc Trans 38: 172–176.
25. Siggins GR, Roberto M, Nie Z (2005) The tipsy terminal: presynaptic effects of ethanol. Pharmacol Ther 107: 80–98.
26. Horishita T, Harris RA (2008) n-Alcohols inhibit voltage-gated Na+ channels expressed in Xenopus oocytes. J Pharmacol Exp Ther 326: 270–277.
27. Covarrubias M, Vyas TB, Escobar L, Wei A (1995) Alcohols inhibit a cloned potassium channel at a discrete saturable site. Insights into the molecular basis of general anesthesia. J Biol Chem 270: 19408–19416.
28. Bhattacharji A, Klett N, Go RC, Covarrubias M (2010) Inhalational anaesthetics and n-alcohols share a site of action in the neuronal Shaw2 Kv channel. Br J Pharmacol 159: 1475–1485.
29. Barber AF, Liang Q, Amaral C, Treptow W, Covarrubias M (2011) Molecular mapping of general anesthetic sites in a voltage-gated ion channel. Biophys J 101: 1613–1622.
30. Oyama Y, Akaike N, Nishi K (1986) Effects of n-alkanols on the calcium current of intracellularly perfused neurons of Helix aspersa. Brain Res 376: 280–284.
31. Hawthorn MH, Ferrante JN, Kwon YW, Rutledge A, Luchowski E, et al. (1992) Effect of an homologous series of aliphatic alcohols on neuronal and smooth muscle voltage-dependent Ca2+ channels. Eur J Pharmacol 229: 143–148.
32. Oz M, Tchugunova YB, Dunn SM (2001) Direct inhibition of voltage-dependent Ca(2+) fluxes by ethanol and higher alcohols in rabbit T-tubule membranes. Eur J Pharmacol 418: 169–176.
33. Jewell ML, Currie KPM (2013) Control of CaV2 calcium channels and neurosecretion by heterotrimeric G protein coupled receptors. In: Stephens GJ, Mochida S, editors. Modulation of presynaptic calcium channels: Springer Publishing. pp. 101–130.
34. Vitale N, Caumont AS, Chasserot-Golaz S, Du G, Wu S, et al. (2001) Phospholipase D1: a key factor for the exocytotic machinery in neuroendocrine cells. Embo J 20: 2424–2434.
35. Todd RD, McDavid SM, Brindley RL, Jewell ML, Currie KP (2012) Gabapentin inhibits catecholamine release from adrenal chromaffin cells. Anesthesiology 116: 1013–1024.
36. Douglas WW (1968) Stimulus-secretion coupling: the concept and clues from chromaffin and other cells. Br J Pharmacol 34: 451–469.
37. Garcia AG, Garcia-De-Diego AM, Gandia L, Borges R, Garcia-Sancho J (2006) Calcium signaling and exocytosis in adrenal chromaffin cells. Physiol Rev 86: 1093–1131.
38. Currie KP (2010) Inhibition of Ca2+ channels and adrenal catecholamine release by G protein coupled receptors. Cell Mol Neurobiol 30: 1201–1208.
39. Mahapatra S, Calorio C, Vandael DH, Marcantoni A, Carabelli V, et al. (2012) Calcium channel types contributing to chromaffin cell excitability, exocytosis and endocytosis. Cell Calcium 51: 321–330.
40. Marcantoni A, Carabelli V, Comunanza V, Hoddah H, Carbone E (2008) Calcium channels in chromaffin cells: focus on L and T types. Acta Physiol (Oxf) 192: 233–246.
41. Fox AP, Cahill AL, Currie KP, Grabner C, Harkins AB, et al. (2008) N- and P/Q-type Ca2+ channels in adrenal chromaffin cells. Acta Physiol (Oxf) 192: 247–261.
42. Currie KPM, Fox AP (1997) Comparison of N- and P/Q-type voltage-gated calcium channel current inhibition. J Neurosci 17: 4570–4579.
43. McDavid S, Currie KP (2006) G-proteins modulate cumulative inactivation of N-type (Cav2.2) calcium channels. J Neurosci 26: 13373–13383.
44. Ertel EA, Campbell KP, Harpold MM, Hofmann F, Mori Y, et al. (2000) Nomenclature of voltage-gated calcium channels. Neuron 25: 533–535.
45. Catterall WA, Perez-Reyes E, Snutch TP, Striessnig J (2005) International Union of Pharmacology. XLVIII. Nomenclature and structure-function relationships of voltage-gated calcium channels. Pharmacol Rev 57: 411–425.
46. Novara M, Baldelli P, Cavallari D, Carabelli V, Giancippoli A, et al. (2004) Exposure to cAMP and beta-adrenergic stimulation recruits Ca(V)3 T-type channels in rat chromaffin cells through Epac cAMP-receptor proteins. J Physiol 558: 433–449.
47. Carabelli V, Marcantoni A, Comunanza V, de Luca A, Diaz J, et al. (2007) Chronic hypoxia up-regulates alpha1H T-type channels and low-threshold catecholamine secretion in rat chromaffin cells. J Physiol 584: 149–165.
48. Souvannakitti D, Nanduri J, Yuan G, Kumar GK, Fox AP, et al. (2010) NADPH oxidase-dependent regulation of T-type Ca2+ channels and ryanodine receptors mediate the augmented exocytosis of catecholamines from intermittent hypoxia-treated neonatal rat chromaffin cells. J Neurosci 30: 10763–10772.
49. Hill J, Chan SA, Kuri B, Smith C (2011) Pituitary adenylate cyclase-activating peptide (PACAP) recruits low voltage-activated T-type calcium influx under acute sympathetic stimulation in mouse adrenal chromaffin cells. J Biol Chem 286: 42459–42469.
50. Currie KPM, Fox AP (1996) ATP serves as a negative feedback inhibitor of voltage-gated Ca2+ channel currents in cultured bovine adrenal chromaffin cells. Neuron 16: 1027–1036.
51. Marcantoni A, Vandael DH, Mahapatra S, Carabelli V, Sinnegger-Brauns MJ, et al. (2010) Loss of Cav1.3 channels reveals the critical role of L-type and BK channel coupling in pacemaking mouse adrenal chromaffin cells. J Neurosci 30: 491–504.
52. Glenn DE, Thomas GM, O'Sullivan AJ, Burgoyne RD (1998) Examination of the role of ADP-ribosylation factor and phospholipase D activation in regulated exocytosis in chromaffin and PC12 cells. J Neurochem 71: 2023–2033.
53. Purkiss J, Murrin RA, Owen PJ, Boarder MR (1991) Lack of phospholipase D activity in chromaffin cells: bradykinin-stimulated phosphatidic acid formation involves phospholipase C in chromaffin cells but phospholipase D in PC12 cells. J Neurochem 57: 1084–1087.
54. Coorssen JR (1996) Phospholipase activation and secretion: evidence that PLA2, PLC, and PLD are not essential to exocytosis. Am J Physiol 270: C1153–1163.
55. Lam AD, Tryoen-Toth P, Tsai B, Vitale N, Stuenkel EL (2008) SNARE-catalyzed fusion events are regulated by Syntaxin1A-lipid interactions. Mol Biol Cell 19: 485–497.
56. Barber AF, Carnevale V, Klein ML, Eckenhoff RG, Covarrubias M (2014) Modulation of a voltage-gated Na+ channel by sevoflurane involves multiple sites and distinct mechanisms. Proc Natl Acad Sci U S A 111: 6726–6731.
57. Barber AF, Liang Q, Covarrubias M (2012) Novel activation of voltage-gated K(+) channels by sevoflurane. J Biol Chem 287: 40425–40432.
58. Nagele P, Mendel JB, Placzek WJ, Scott BA, D'Avignon DA, et al. (2005) Volatile anesthetics bind rat synaptic snare proteins. Anesthesiology 103: 768–778.
59. Herring BE, Xie Z, Marks J, Fox AP (2009) Isoflurane inhibits the neurotransmitter release machinery. J Neurophysiol 102: 1265–1273.
60. Xie Z, McMillan K, Pike CM, Cahill AL, Herring BE, et al. (2013) Interaction of anesthetics with neurotransmitter release machinery proteins. J Neurophysiol 109: 758–767.
61. Graham ME, Edwards MR, Holden-Dye L, Morgan A, Burgoyne RD, et al. (2009) UNC-18 modulates ethanol sensitivity in Caenorhabditis elegans. Mol Biol Cell 20: 43–55.
62. Krasowski MD, Harrison NL (2000) The actions of ether, alcohol and alkane general anaesthetics on GABAA and glycine receptors and the effects of TM2 and TM3 mutations. Br J Pharmacol 129: 731–743.
63. Alifimoff JK, Firestone LL, Miller KW (1989) Anaesthetic potencies of primary alkanols: implications for the molecular dimensions of the anaesthetic site. Br J Pharmacol 96: 9–16.
64. Firestone S, Firestone LL (1995) Staurosporine, a protein kinase inhibitor, increases the intoxicating potencies of ethanol and other n-alkanols in Rana pipiens tadpoles. Alcohol Clin Exp Res 19: 416–419.

Nonspecific Adverse Events in Knee Osteoarthritis Clinical Trials

Yun Hyung Koog[1,2]*, **Jin Su Lee**[1,3], **Hyungsun Wi**[1]

1 Honam Research Center, Medifarm Hospital, Suncheon, Republic of Korea, **2** Department of Oriental Medicine, Medifarm Hospital, Suncheon, Republic of Korea, **3** Department of Rehabilitation, Medifarm Hospital, Suncheon, Republic of Korea

Abstract

Background: Adverse events (AEs) derived from nonspecific activity of treatments can impair the validity of trials, and even make it difficult to identify specific AEs associated with treatments. To better understand these nonspecific AEs, we investigated the AEs in placebo groups by using knee osteoarthritis clinical trials.

Methods: Randomized, placebo-controlled, knee osteoarthritis trials were identified by searching electronic databases. We determined the rate of patients with AEs and the rate of dropouts caused by AEs in the active and placebo groups. Furthermore, we calculated the rate of patients for individual AEs in the placebo groups. Finally, we performed secondary analyses to identify the factors associated with these rates.

Results: Overall, 272 papers reporting 281 trials were included in the analysis. The rates of patients with AEs were 31.8% in the active groups and 27.4% in the placebo groups. The rate of the placebo groups accounted for 86.2% of the rate of the active groups. The rates of dropouts caused by AEs were 5.2% in the active groups and 4.8% in the placebo groups. The rate of the placebo groups accounted for 92.3% of the rate of the active groups. AEs in the placebo groups included a number of clinical conditions, with elevated alanine aminotransferase (0.59%; 95% CI: 0.46 to 0.77) being the most common objective outcome and headache (4.48%; 95% CI: 4.20 to 4.79) being the most frequent subjective outcome. The rate of patients with AEs and the rate of dropouts caused by AEs were associated with the treatment type, delivery route, and study design.

Conclusions: The nonspecific AEs substantially accounted for the development of AEs in the active groups and included conditions involving the entire body.

Editor: Joel Joseph Gagnier, University of Michigan, United States of America

Funding: The authors have no support or funding to report.

Competing Interests: The authors declare that they have no competing interests.

* Email: samlungchim@hanmail.net (YHK)

Introduction

Osteoarthritis is one of the most prevalent musculoskeletal diseases affecting the elderly. Because it is characterized by the progressive degeneration of synovial joint structure [1], it causes pain, loss of motion, and physical disability, thus impairing quality of life. Current treatment strategies also aim to alleviate joint pain, reduce physical disability, and limit the progression of joint damage [2]. In line with this concept, basic efforts to establish treatment guidelines often focus on treatment efficacy [2,3].

Nonetheless, adverse events (AEs) are an essential aspect to be considered when evaluating treatments for clinical use [4]. Although AEs arise as direct results from the specific activity of the treatments, they can also be derived from nonspecific activity. Such nonspecific AEs can often hinder patients from adhering to their treatments, thus leading to attrition bias. Furthermore, if the nonspecific AEs are high, the specific AEs of the treatments can be difficult to identify.

To better understand nonspecific AEs, numerous reviews have investigated the AEs in placebo groups, linking them to the nocebo response [5–15]. When participants are informed about possible AEs caused by active treatments, and thus expect them during the trial, some participants may respond negatively to placebos. It was reported that osteoarthritic patients gained health benefits with placebos, indicating that the placebo response is significant in osteoarthritis [16]. Since the nocebo and placebo responses may occur simultaneously (e.g., acupuncture [17–20]), osteoarthritic patients may also experience a significant nocebo response.

On the basis of these considerations, we attempted to investigate nonspecific AEs using randomized osteoarthritis trials. This study focused on knee osteoarthritis, because the number of placebo-controlled trials focusing on the knee is almost 10 times higher than those focusing on any other site [16]. Moreover, the anatomy, physiology, risk factors, and responses to the same treatments may be different for each site [21,22].

Methods

Search strategy and study selection

The search strategy used in this study has been described previously [23,24]. Briefly, the final search was performed in PubMed, SCOPUS, and the Cochrane Central Register of Controlled Trials up to December 2011, using knee osteoarthritis-related terms with the limits set to trials. For example, in

PubMed, we used terms ["knee arthritis" OR "knee osteoarthritis" OR "gonarthritis" OR "gonarthrosis"], with limits to randomized controlled trials and humans. A search was also carried out in the Cochrane Review database to identify additional papers. The search was then expanded to all studies referenced in the papers. On the basis of a previous dataset of trials [23–28], two authors (HW and JSL) jointly selected randomized, placebo-controlled, clinical trials that investigated treatment efficacy or safety. Only trials written in English were included. We excluded trials investigating test treatments as an adjunct therapy (e.g., tramadol trial as an adjunct [29]), because nonspecific AEs may be affected by the addition of other treatments.

Data extraction

AEs were defined as "any untoward medical occurrences that may present during treatment ... but which do not necessarily have a causal relationship with this treatment" [30]. Specifically, any AEs occurring in placebo groups were defined as nonspecific AEs. First, we randomly selected 50 trials, and two authors (YHK and MG) independently extracted data, including the number of patients experiencing any AE and number of dropouts caused by AEs. After discussions, the two authors independently extracted data from the whole trials. In instances of multiple data found at more than one time point, the time point when both variables were reported together was preferred. If only one variable was reported, the time point that was considered primary was chosen. This time point was considered as trial duration. For crossover trials, only data acquired before the crossover were extracted. The inter-rater reliability was kappa = 0.905 for recording the number of patients with adverse events and kappa = 0.845 for recording the number of dropouts caused by adverse events. To determine the total number of patients in the two groups in each trial, initially randomized patients were considered. In addition, two authors independently extracted data for AEs and patient number corresponding to each AE. After referencing previous reviews [5–8], the final data were determined at team meetings. These data were rechecked by another author (HW).

Data analysis

First, the rate of patients with AEs and the rate of dropouts caused by AEs in the two groups were calculated using logit transformation. The proportions were then combined using a random effects model [31]. Summary rates were calculated by back-transforming the combined proportions, and presented as percentages with 95% confidence intervals. Heterogeneity was assessed using an I^2 test [32]. Small study effects were evaluated using a funnel plot and Egger's regression test [33].

Second, the frequencies in separate trials were summed to obtain the cumulative number of patients corresponding to each AE. If trials did not report relevant AEs, we assumed that there were no patients complaining of those AEs in the trials. Summary rates were then expressed as percentages with 95% confidence intervals. As large sample sizes were used for the calculations, the intervals were determined using the Agresti-Coull method [34]. We categorized these rates into objective and subjective rates.

Secondary analyses

We examined whether the rates of patients with AEs and dropouts caused by AEs in the placebo groups were affected by trial qualities (i.e., allocation concealment, provider blinding, patient blinding, and attrition rate). Allocation concealment was considered adequate if the researchers responsible for patient selection could not predict the next treatment for a patient. Provider or patient blinding was considered adequate if the provider or patient could not predict the treatment for a patient. Attrition rate was considered adequate if the attrition rate of all initially randomized patients was below 15% [26].

We further observed whether the rates were influenced by the following factors: treatment type; delivery route; trial duration; flare design (yes vs. no/unclear); prohibition of usual analgesics during the trial (yes vs. no/unclear); and allowance of escape medication (yes vs. no/unclear). A meta-regression analysis with a random effects model was performed [35]. To this end, individual treatments were categorized according to the treatment type (pharmacological, non-pharmacological, and mixed) and delivery route (oral, topical, injection/puncture, and surgical). Subsequently, both factors were coded in a descending order of rates. Statistical significance was defined as values of $P<0.05$. STATA 11.0 software (StataCorp LP, Texas, USA) was used for all analyses.

Results

We identified 36,691 records (PubMed, 1646; SCOPUS, 32,246; Cochrane Registered Trials, 2484; and other source, 315), of which 344 papers were identified as potentially eligible for our analyses (Figure 1). Of these, 72 papers were excluded because they lacked sufficient data (n = 42), were crossover studies not reporting enough data (n = 23), used test treatments as adjuncts (n = 5), included rheumatoid arthritis patients (n = 1), or reported data combined over the hip and knee joints (n = 1). Finally, a total of 272 papers reporting 281 trials were analyzed.

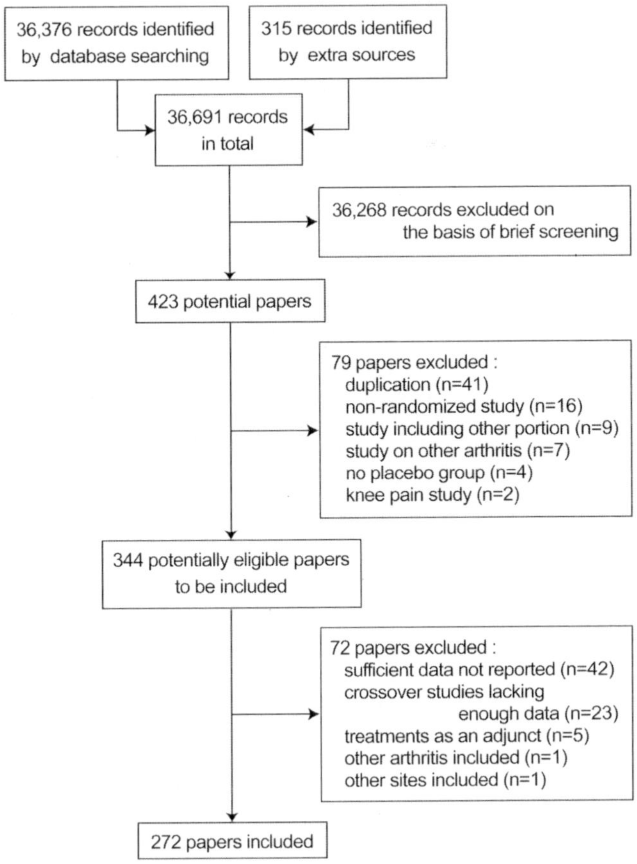

Figure 1. Study flow diagram.

Information regarding the trials included in our analysis is provided in Table 1. Diverse treatment strategies such as pharmacological, non-pharmacological, and surgical therapies were used. While these treatments were commonly investigated in trials without a flare design, they were evenly tested in trials with and without prohibition of usual analgesics or in trials with and without allowance of escape medication. The median trial duration was 12 weeks (interquartile range: 6 to 24) and the median time for provision of final placebo was 6 weeks (interquartile range: 3 to 12). In total, 44,976 patients were considered for the active groups and 22,284 for the placebo groups.

Primary analyses

The summary rates of patients with AEs were 31.8% (95% confidence interval: 29.1 to 34.7; $I^2 = 96\%$) in the active groups and 27.4% (24.7 to 30.3; $I^2 = 92\%$) in the placebo groups. The rate of the placebo groups accounted for 86.2% of the rate of the active groups. Using Egger's regression test, bias was detected in both groups ($P<0.001$ for each) (Figure 2). The summary rates of dropouts caused by AEs were 5.2% (4.6 to 5.9; $I^2 = 87\%$) in the active groups and 4.8% (4.3 to 5.4; $I^2 = 60\%$) in the placebo groups. The rate of the placebo groups accounted for 92.3% of the rate of the active groups. Using Egger's regression test, bias was found in both groups ($P<0.001$ for each) (Figure 2).

The profiles of nonspecific AEs are shown in Figure 3. Abnormalities in hemoglobin, creatinine, and liver enzymes were commonly identified objective AEs. Elevated alanine aminotransferase was the most commonly reported AE, with a rate of 0.59% (0.46 to 0.77). With regard to subjective AEs, a variety of symptoms pertaining to different parts of the body were reported. Headache was the most frequent AE, with a rate of 4.48% (4.20 to 4.79). For injection/puncture treatment-related nonspecific AEs, insertion pain was the most commonly reported, with a rate of 3.52% (2.98 to 4.15), followed by treated site swelling. When topical treatment-related nonspecific AEs were examined, dry skin was the most common symptom, with a rate of 3.39% (2.70 to 4.19), followed by rash.

Secondary analyses

When the analysis was separately restricted to studies with clearly concealed allocation (n = 109), explicit blinding of patients (n = 249) or providers (n = 73), or adequate dropout rate (n = 135), the significance of the rates of patients with AEs and dropouts caused by AEs remained unchanged. Furthermore, when the analysis was performed across trials that met all factors (n = 28), the respective rates were 24.9% (17.0 to 34.9; $I^2 = 85\%$) and 3.9% (2.8 to 5.3; $I^2 = 0\%$).

When the rate of patients with AEs was categorized by the treatment type, a linear trend was observed ($P<0.001$) (Figure 4). Pharmacological treatment had the largest impact on AEs, followed by non-pharmacological treatment. The rate decreased consistently for delivery route ($P<0.001$), with the highest number of AEs experienced for oral delivery, followed by injection/puncture, surgical, and topical routes.

When the rate of dropouts caused by AEs was categorized by the treatment type and delivery route, a linear trend was observed for both factors (Figure 4). The rate decreased ($P = 0.017$) in pharmacologic treatment studies, followed by non-pharmacological and mixed treatment studies. Likewise, a consistent decrease was observed ($P<0.001$) when the delivery routes were considered in the following order: oral, topical, injection/puncture, and surgical.

Table 1. Characteristics of the included trials.

	No. of paper (No. of trial)
Total study	272 (281)
Treatment type	
Pharmacological	203 (212)
Non-pharmacological	68 (68)
mixed	1 (1)
Delivery route*	
Oral	127 (135)
Topical	64 (64)
Percutaneous	71 (72)
Surgical	4 (4)
Flare design	
Yes	26 (26)
No/unclear	246 (255)
Prohibition of usual analgesics	
Yes	144 (152)
No/unclear	128 (129)
Allowance of escape medication	
Yes	135 (139)
No/unclear	137 (142)

No., number.
*Six studies administered treatments using mixed methods.

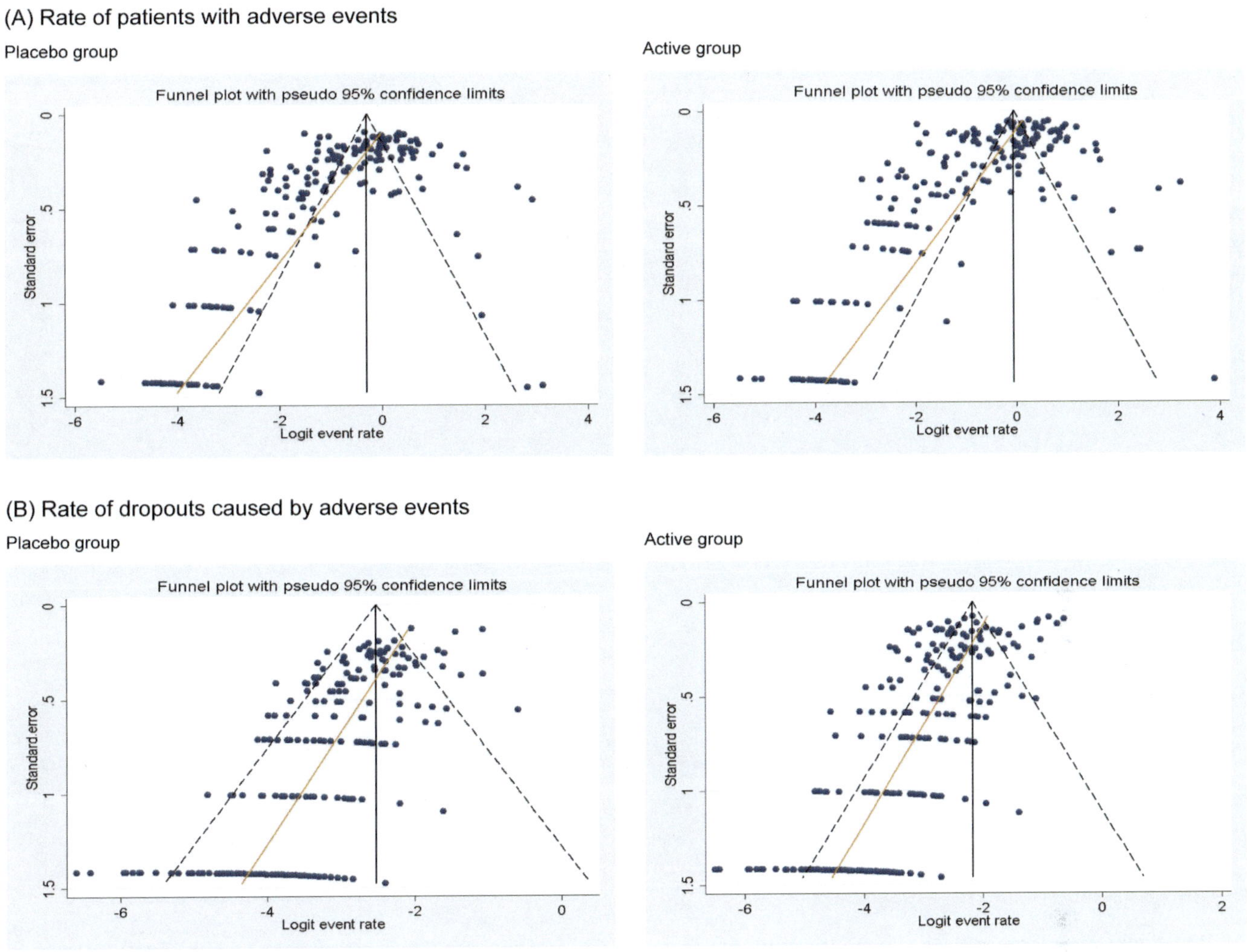

Figure 2. Funnel plots including an Egger's regression line.

The associations of two variables with the trial duration and study design are summarized in Table 2. The rate of patients with AEs was significantly associated with the trial duration (P = 0.021), flare design (P = 0.027), prohibition of usual analgesics (P = 0.003), and allowance of escape medication (P<0.001). In contrast, the rate of dropouts caused by AEs was only associated with the trial duration (P = 0.004).

Discussion

Previously, numerous reviews have reported that the rate of patients with AEs and the rate of dropouts caused by AEs in placebo groups were 10–50% and 2–6%, respectively [5–15,36]. When these rates were compared with those in the active groups, the rate of patients with AEs in the placebo groups was 72.8–81.7% of that in the active groups [8–12]. With respect to the rate of dropouts caused by AEs, the rate in the placebo groups was 43.9–99.6% of that in the active groups [6,11]. Our findings of 86.2% and 92.3% correspond with these other studies. All of these data imply that the nonspecific AEs may substantially account for the development of AEs in the active groups.

Previous reviews have also investigated the profiles of nonspecific AEs caused by the nocebo response [5–15]. According to these reviews, subjective nonspecific AEs included a number of conditions occurring throughout the body, and numerous events were significant. Our study also confirms these findings. Meanwhile, to our knowledge, none of the previous reviews investigated objective AEs. Our study found that the rates of some objective AEs were significant. Considering that these nonspecific AEs occurred in patients receiving inert placebos, the findings are surprising. Although these results may be explained by many factors (e.g., participation burden), previous studies have focused on the nocebo response linked to expectation and conditioning theories.

First, some reviews found that nonspecific AEs reflected the pattern of AEs caused by active treatments, suggesting that the nonspecific AEs may be triggered by expectation [5,7,8]. Expectation of AEs caused by active treatments may generate similar AEs in patients receiving placebos. To check whether the patterns of AEs were similar between the two groups in our study, we conducted correlation analyses with regard to the rates of patients with AEs, rates of dropouts caused by AEs, and rates of patients for some AEs. We found significant relationships for all factors (Table S1 and figure S1), which corresponds with the previous findings [5,7,8].

Second, some reviews indicated the possibility of conditioning-mediated nonspecific AEs [8]. Nonspecific AEs may occur in

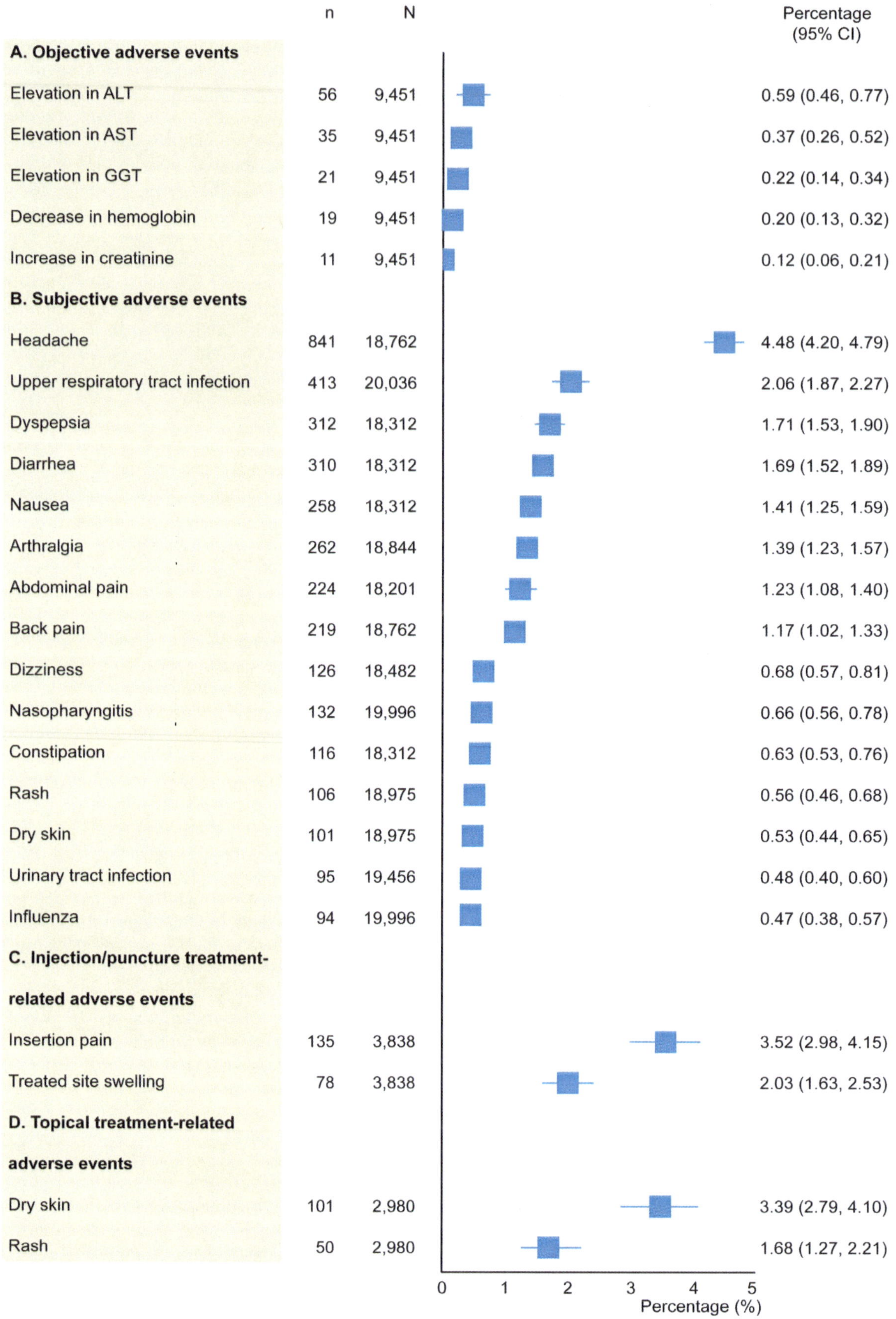

Figure 3. Rates of nonspecific adverse events. n, number of patients reporting adverse events; N, total sample size; ALT, alanine aminotransferase; AST, aspartate aminotransferase; GGT, gamma-glutamyltransferase.

	Paper No.	Patient No.	Percentage (95% CI)
A. Rate of patients with adverse events			
Treatment type			
Pharmacological	157	6,360	33.9 (30.8, 37.1)
Non-pharmacological	44	245	8.8 (6.6, 11.7)
Delivery route			
Oral	95	4,700	38.4 (34.8, 42.1)
Needle/puncture	58	1,312	19.1 (14.2, 25.3)
Surgical	3	9	9.1 (5.0, 16.2)
Topical	42	266	8.5 (5.6, 12.5)
B. Rate of dropouts caused by adverse events			
Treatment type			
Pharmacological	201	1,088	0.05 (0.05, 0.06)
Non-pharmacological	68	44	0.04 (0.03, 0.05)
Mixed	1	0	0.01 (0.00, 0.15)
Delivery route			
Oral	124	909	0.07 (0.06, 0.08)
Topical	64	65	0.04 (0.03, 0.05)
Needle/puncture	70	87	0.03 (0.02, 0.04)
Surgical	4	0	0.02 (0.00, 0.07)

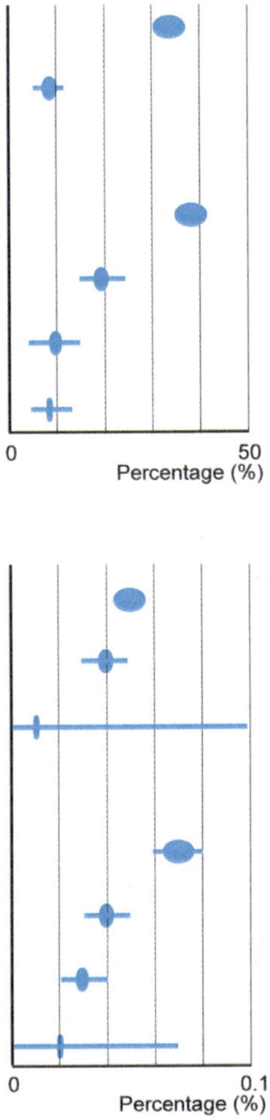

Figure 4. Rates for treatment type and delivery route.

patients who were previously exposed to similar treatments and thus experienced AEs. There is evidence that, when unconscious physiological functions such as hormonal secretion are involved, nocebo responses are mediated by conditioning [37]. However, verbally-induced expectations have no effect on unconscious physiological functions [37]. Therefore, our finding of significant objective nonspecific AEs may be explained by the conditioning theory, although we could not analyze how many patients were previously conditioned.

In our study, the magnitude of the nocebo response was found to be affected by the treatment type, delivery route, and study design. Specifically, the rate of patients with adverse events was closely related to the study design. Some trials described that, although escape medications were allowed for treating knee flare pain during trials, they were instead used to treat AEs [38,39]. This suggests that the nonspecific AEs may have been affected by strategies to deal with patients complaining of pain during the trials. We addressed this point, and found that a higher rate of patients with AEs was associated with longer trial duration, flare design, prohibition of usual analgesics, and allowance of escape medication. Hence, we think that escape medication may act as an alert, even when adverse events were minimal and could be ignored.

Although our study provides an excellent opportunity to study nonspecific AEs, the results should be interpreted with caution. First, we encountered different reporting styles across trials. Some trials enumerated AEs reported by >2% of patients in any group, and others by >5% of patients. In some cases, only generic AEs (e.g., gastrointestinal symptoms) were presented. We excluded data pertaining to generic AEs for practical reasons, while the remaining data were encoded as reported. Therefore, if all AEs were reported in trials, the rates of nonspecific AEs would have been greater.

Second, the data collection methods for subjective AEs were insufficiently detailed in trials. According to a study [40], patients who reported no side effects in an open questionnaire reported at least one side effect in a structured questionnaire. This suggests that the data collection methods can influence the rates of AEs.

Table 2. Results of the meta-regression analysis.

	Rate of patients with adverse events	Rate of dropouts caused by adverse events
	Coefficient (95% CI)	Coefficient (95% CI)
	P value	P value
Continuous outcome		
Trial duration (per week)	0.013 (0.002, 0.023)	0.006 (0.002, 0.010)
	P = 0.021	P = 0.004
Binary outcome*		
Flare design	0.784 (0.088, 1.480)	0.182 (−0.156, 0.521)
	P = 0.027	P = 0.291
Prohibition of usual analgesics	0.694 (0.240, 1.148)	0.038 (−0.208, 0.283)
	P = 0.003	P = 0.764
Allowance of escape medication	0.935 (0.500, 1.370)	0.003 (−0.238, 0.245)
	P<0.001	P = 0.979

CI, confidence interval.
The coefficients are values after logit transformation.
*For binary outcomes, "no/unclear" and "yes" were coded as 1 and 2, respectively.

However, most of the trials in our study either did not report the data collection methods or did not use a structured checklist. As our results may be confounded by these factors, it is necessary to clearly report the data collection methods in future trials.

The final major limitation includes the small study effects, in which smaller studies in a meta-analysis show larger treatment effects. Although the impact of such biases has been well demonstrated for efficacy outcomes [17], it has not yet been discussed for safety outcomes. Nonetheless, it is possible that smaller studies with greater AE rates may have a rare chance to be published in journals. For this reason, it is possible that our results may have been affected.

We believe that the present findings will have several useful implications for the design and conduct of clinical trials. First, substantial efforts have recently been directed toward reducing the magnitude of the nocebo response at the patient level, such as excluding patients with a higher risk of experiencing the nocebo response [36,41], and carefully explaining the possible AEs during a trial [36,42,43]. However, our findings imply that adopting an optimal study design (i.e., short trial duration, non-flare design, allowance of usual analgesics, and prohibition of escape medication) may be another option for reducing the nocebo response without intervening in patient-researcher interactions.

Second, in most trials, the patient recruitment strategies were based on a power calculation that aimed to demonstrate the efficacy of active treatments. Nonetheless, conclusions regarding the safety outcomes were presented on the basis of those sample sizes. However, such sample sizes may be insufficient to demonstrate the safety of active treatments, thereby leading to a type II error. For example, the continuous form of the odds ratio for patients with or without AEs between the two groups was 0.1 in our study. When compared with the effect sizes for the effectiveness of all treatments presented in a guideline study [3], this magnitude is very small. Therefore, caution should be observed when interpreting the safety outcomes in clinical trials.

Similarly, it can also be argued that most of the active treatments are safe, because most AEs seen in the treatment groups can be considered to be nonspecific. However, one study demonstrated that some AEs were frequently reported in the German population not taking any drugs [44]. Specifically, headache, back pain; and joint pain were experienced by >10% of the general population. When these data are compared with our data, the rates of AEs in our study are lower than those in the German population. As general clinical trials may report lower rates for AEs [6,8], the safety of active treatments should be determined on the basis of fully-powered clinical trials.

Conclusions

From the data based on 281 knee osteoarthritis trials, we found that nonspecific AEs substantially accounted for the development of AEs in the active groups. They accounted for 86.2% of the active groups for the rate of patients with AEs and 92.3% of the active groups for the rate of dropouts caused by AEs. In addition, nonspecific AEs included conditions involving the entire body, including musculoskeletal, gastrointestinal, respiratory, urogenital, cerebrovascular, psychiatric, and immune system manifestations. Upon further investigation, the rate of patients with AEs was associated with the treatment type, delivery route, and study design. We believe that our findings provide some clues toward reducing nonspecific AEs in the design and conduct of clinical trials.

Supporting Information

Figure S1 Plots of patient rates in the treatment groups against patient rates in the placebo groups.

Table S1 Correlation coefficients.

Checklist S1 PRISMA checklist.

Acknowledgments

We thank Min Sun Park, Eun-Ok Jeong, Munsoo Gil, and Seo Ryang We for searching electronic databases and Munsoo Gil for extracting data.

Author Contributions

Conceived and designed the experiments: YHK. Performed the experiments: YHK JSL HW. Analyzed the data: YHK JSL HW. Contributed reagents/materials/analysis tools: YHK JSL HW. Wrote the paper: YHK JSL HW.

References

1. Martel-Pelletier J, Pelletier JP (2010) Is osteoarthritis a disease involving only cartilage or other articular tissues? Eklem Hastalik Cerrahisi 21: 2–14.
2. Zhang W, Moskowitz RW, Nuki G, Abramson S, Altman RD, et al. (2008) OARSI recommendations for the management of hip and knee osteoarthritis, part II: OARSI evidence-based, expert consensus guidelines. Osteoarthritis Cartilage 16: 137–162.
3. Zhang W, Nuki G, Moskowitz RW, Abramson S, Altman RD, et al. (2010) OARSI recommendations for the management of hip and knee osteoarthritis: part III: changes in evidence following systematic cumulative update of research published through January 2009. Osteoarthritis Cartilage 18: 476–499.
4. Topol EJ (2004) Failing the public health—rofecoxib, Merck, and the FDA. N Engl J Med 351: 1707–1709.
5. Reuter U, Sanchez del Rio M, Carpay JA, Boes CJ, Silberstein SD, et al. (2003) Placebo adverse events in headache trials: headache as an adverse event of placebo. Cephalalgia 23: 496–503.
6. Rief W, Avorn J, Barsky AJ (2006) Medication-attributed adverse effects in placebo groups: implications for assessment of adverse effects. Arch Intern Med 166: 155–160.
7. Amanzio M, Corazzini LL, Vase L, Benedetti F (2009) A systematic review of adverse events in placebo groups of anti-migraine clinical trials. Pain 146: 261–269.
8. Rief W, Nestoriuc Y, von Lilienfeld-Toal A, Dogan I, Schreiber F, et al. (2009) Differences in adverse effect reporting in placebo groups in SSRI and tricyclic antidepressant trials: a systematic review and meta-analysis. Drug Saf 32: 1041–1056.
9. Papadopoulos D, Mitsikostas DD (2010) Nocebo effects in multiple sclerosis trials: a meta-analysis. Mult Scler 16: 816–828.
10. Mitsikostas DD, Mantonakis LI, Chalarakis NG (2011) Nocebo is the enemy, not placebo. A meta-analysis of reported side effects after placebo treatment in headaches. Cephalalgia 31: 550–561.
11. Häuser W, Bartram C, Bartram-Wunn E, Tölle T (2012) Systematic review: Adverse events attributable to nocebo in randomised controlled drug trials in fibromyalgia syndrome and painful diabetic peripheral neuropathy. Clin J Pain 28: 437–451.
12. Mitsikostas DD, Chalarakis NG, Mantonakis LI, Delicha EM, Sfikakis PP (2012) Nocebo in fibromyalgia. Meta-analysis of placebo-controlled clinical trials and implications for practice. Eur J Neurol 19: 672–680.
13. Papadopoulos D, Mitsikostas DD (2012) A meta-analytic approach to estimating nocebo effects in neuropathic pain trials. J Neurol 259: 436–447.
14. Stathis P, Smpiliris M, Konitsiotis S, Mitsikostas DD (2013) Nocebo as a potential confounding factor in clinical trials for Parkinson's disease treatment: a meta-analysis. Eur J Neurol 20: 527–533.
15. Mitsikostas DD, Mantonakis L, Chalarakis N (2014) Nocebo in clinical trials for depression: a meta-analysis. Psychiatry Res 215: 82–86.
16. Zhang W, Robertson J, Jones AC, Dieppe PA, Doherty M (2008) The placebo effect and its determinants in osteoarthritis: meta-analysis of randomised controlled trials. Ann Rheum Dis 67: 1716–1723.
17. Koog YH, We SR, Min BI (2011) Three-armed trials including placebo and no-treatment groups may be subject to publication bias: systematic review. PloS One 6: e20679.
18. We SR, Koog YH, Park MS, Min BI (2012) Placebo effect was influenced by publication year in three-armed acupuncture trials. Complement Ther Med 20: 83–92.
19. Koog YH, Jung WY (2013) Time course of placebo effect of acupuncture on pain: a systematic review. ISRN Pain 2013: 204108.
20. Koog YH, Lee JS, Wi H (2014) Clinically meaningful nocebo effect occurs in acupuncture treatment: a systematic review. J Clin Epidemiol 67: 858–869.
21. Zhang W, Doherty M (2006) EULAR recommendations for knee and hip osteoarthritis: a critique of the methodology. Br J Sports Med 40: 664–669.
22. Svensson O, Malmenäs M, Fajutrao L, Roos EM, Lohmander LS (2006) Greater reduction of knee than hip pain in osteoarthritis treated with naproxen, as evaluated by WOMAC and SF-36. Ann Rheum Dis 65: 781–784.
23. Koog YH, Wi H, Jung WY (2013) Eligibility criteria in knee osteoarthritis clinical trials: systematic review. Clin Rheumatol 32: 1569–1574.
24. Koog YH, Gil M, We SR, Wi H, Min BI (2013) Barriers to participant retention in knee osteoarthritis clinical trials: a systematic review. Semin Arthritis Rheum 42: 346–354.
25. Koog YH, Lee JS, Wi H (2014) External validity of knee osteoarthritis clinical trials: a systematic review. Arch Rehumatol (in press).
26. Koog YH (2013) Caution should be observed against the last observation carried forward analysis in opioid trials. Turk J Rheumatol 28: 282–283.
27. Ryang We S, Koog YH, Jeong KI, Wi H (2013) Effects of pulsed electromagnetic field on knee osteoarthritis: a systematic review. Rheumatology (Oxford) 52: 815–824.
28. We SR, Jeong EO, Koog YH, Min BI (2012) Effects of nutraceuticals on knee osteoarthritis: systematic review. Afr J Biotechnol 11: 2814–2821.
29. Schnitzer TJ, Kamin M, Olson WH (1999) Tramadol allows reduction of naproxen dose among patients with naproxen-responsive osteoarthritis pain: a randomized, double-blind, placebo-controlled study. Arthritis Rheum 42: 1370–1377.
30. Nebeker JR, Barach P, Samore MH (2004) Clarifying adverse drug events: a clinician's guide to terminology, documentation, and reporting. Ann Intern Med 140: 795–801.
31. DerSimonian R, Laird N (1986) Meta-analysis in clinical trials. Control Clin Trials 7: 177–188.
32. Higgins JP, Thompson SG, Deeks JJ, Altman DG (2003) Measuring inconsistency in meta-analyses. BMJ 327: 557–560.
33. Egger M, Davey Smith G, Schneider M, Minder C (1997) Bias in meta-analysis detected by a simple, graphical test. BMJ 315: 629–634.
34. Brown LD, Cai TT, DasGupta A (2001) Interval estimation for a binomial proportion. Stat Sci 16: 101–133.
35. Harbord RM, Higgins JP (2008) Meta-regression in Stata. Stata J 8: 493–529.
36. Häuser W, Hansen E, Enck P (2012) Nocebo phenomena in medicine: their relevance in everyday clinical practice. Dtsch Arztebl Int 109: 459–465.
37. Benedetti F, Pollo A, Lopiano L, Lanotte M, Vighetti S, et al. (2003) Conscious expectation and unconscious conditioning in analgesic, motor, and hormonal placebo/nocebo responses. J Neurosci 23: 4315–4323.
38. Ruff KJ, Winkler A, Jackson RW, DeVore DP, Ritz BW (2009) Eggshell membrane in the treatment of pain and stiffness from osteoarthritis of the knee: a randomized, multicenter, double-blind, placebo-controlled clinical study. Clin Rheumatol 28: 907–914.
39. Ergün H, Külcü D, Kutlay S, Bodur H, Tulunay FC (2007) Efficacy and safety of topical nimesulide in the treatment of knee osteoarthritis. J Clin Rheumatol 13: 251–255.
40. Sheftell FD, Feleppa M, Tepper SJ, Rapoport AM, Ciannella L, et al. (2004) Assessment of adverse events associated with triptans–methods of assessment influence the results. Headache 44: 978–982.
41. Barsky AJ, Saintfort R, Rogers MP, Borus JF (2002) Nonspecific medication side effects and the nocebo phenomenon. JAMA 287: 622–627.
42. Miller FG, Colloca L (2011) The placebo phenomenon and medical ethics: rethinking the relationship between informed consent and risk-benefit assessment. Theor Med Bioeth 32: 229–243.
43. Cohen S (2014) The nocebo effect of informed consent. Bioethics 28: 147–154.
44. Rief W, Barsky AJ, Glombiewski JA, Nestoriuc Y, Glaesmer H, et al. (2011) Assessing general side effects in clinical trials: reference data from the general population. Pharmacoepidemiol Drug Saf 20: 405–415.

22

Mutations at Beta N265 in γ-Aminobutyric Acid Type A Receptors Alter Both Binding Affinity and Efficacy of Potent Anesthetics

Deirde S. Stewart, David W. Pierce, Mayo Hotta[¤], Alex T. Stern, Stuart A. Forman*

Department of Anesthesia Critical Care and Pain Medicine, Massachusetts General Hospital, Boston, Massachusetts, United States of America

Abstract

Etomidate and propofol are potent general anesthetics that act via GABAA receptor allosteric co-agonist sites located at transmembrane β+/α− inter-subunit interfaces. Early experiments in heteromeric receptors identified βN265 (M2-15′) on β2 and β3 subunits as an important determinant of sensitivity to these drugs. Mechanistic analyses suggest that substitution with serine, the β1 residue at this position, primarily reduces etomidate efficacy, while mutation to methionine eliminates etomidate sensitivity and might prevent drug binding. However, the βN265 residue has not been photolabeled with analogs of either etomidate or propofol. Furthermore, substituted cysteine modification studies find no propofol protection at this locus, while etomidate protection has not been tested. Thus, evidence of contact between βN265 and potent anesthetics is lacking and it remains uncertain how mutations alter drug sensitivity. In the current study, we first applied heterologous α1β2N265Cγ2L receptor expression in Xenopus oocytes, thiol-specific aqueous probe modification, and voltage-clamp electrophysiology to test whether etomidate inhibits probe reactions at the β-265 sidechain. Using up to 300 μM etomidate, we found both an absence of etomidate effects on α1β2N265Cγ2L receptor activity and no inhibition of thiol modification. To gain further insight into anesthetic insensitive βN265M mutants, we applied indirect structure-function strategies, exploiting second mutations in α1β2/3γ2L GABAA receptors. Using α1M236C as a modifiable and anesthetic-protectable site occupancy reporter in β+/α− interfaces, we found that βN265M reduced apparent anesthetic affinity for receptors in both resting and GABA-activated states. βN265M also impaired the transduction of gating effects associated with α1M236W, a mutation that mimics β+/α− anesthetic site occupancy. Our results show that βN265M mutations dramatically reduce the efficacy/transduction of anesthetics bound in β+/α− sites, and also significantly reduce anesthetic affinity for resting state receptors. These findings are consistent with a role for βN265 in anesthetic binding within the β+/α− transmembrane sites.

Editor: Alexander G. Obukhov, Indiana University School of Medicine, United States of America

Funding: This work was supported by National Institutes of General Medical Sciences Grant R01GM089745 to SAF. The funders had no role in study design, data collection and analysis, decision to publish, or preparation of the manuscript.

Competing Interests: The authors have declared that no competing interests exist.

* Email: saforman@partners.org

¤ Current address: Keck School of Medicine of the University of Southern California, Los Angeles, California, United States of Amerca

Introduction

Etomidate and propofol are potent general anesthetics that act as positive allosteric modulators and agonists at $GABA_A$ receptors [1–3], the major inhibitory neurotransmitter receptors of the central nervous system and members of the pentameric ligand-gated ion channel (pLGIC) superfamily [4,5]. Typical synaptic $GABA_A$ receptors consist of α, β, and γ subunits, arranged β-α-β-α-γ counterclockwise viewed from the extracellular space [6]. Structural homology models of αβγ $GABA_A$ receptors, based on crystallography of distantly related pLGICs [5] and β3 homo-pentameric channels [7], are consistent with a large body of structure-function data. Each homologous subunit has a large extracellular domain, and four α-helices (M1 to M4) forming a transmembrane domain (Fig. 1A, B). The two GABA binding sites are located in the β+/α− interfaces of the extracellular domain. The transmembrane domains of each subunit form four-helix bundles with all five M2 domains around the central chloride channel (Fig. 1B). Surrounding the M2 domains is a second ring of M1 and M3 α-helices, with M4 domains outermost. Portions of M1, M3 and M4 contact membrane lipids.

Allosteric co-agonist sites for etomidate and propofol are located between the extracellular ends of α-M1 and β-M3 transmembrane helices; the transmembrane β+/α− interfaces (Fig. 1B, C). Combined, photolabeling with etomidate and propofol analogs [8–10], photolabel inhibition studies [10,11], and substituted cysteine accessibility method (SCAM) with protection experiments [12–14] have identified six residues near either etomidate or propofol: βM286 and βV290 on β-M3 as well as αL232, αM236, αT237, and αI239 on α-M1 (Fig. 1C). Tryptophan mutations at either αM236 or βM286, two photolabeled residues, mimic the channel gating effects of bound anesthetics and reduce sensitivity to both etomidate and propofol [15,16]. Disulfide bond formation

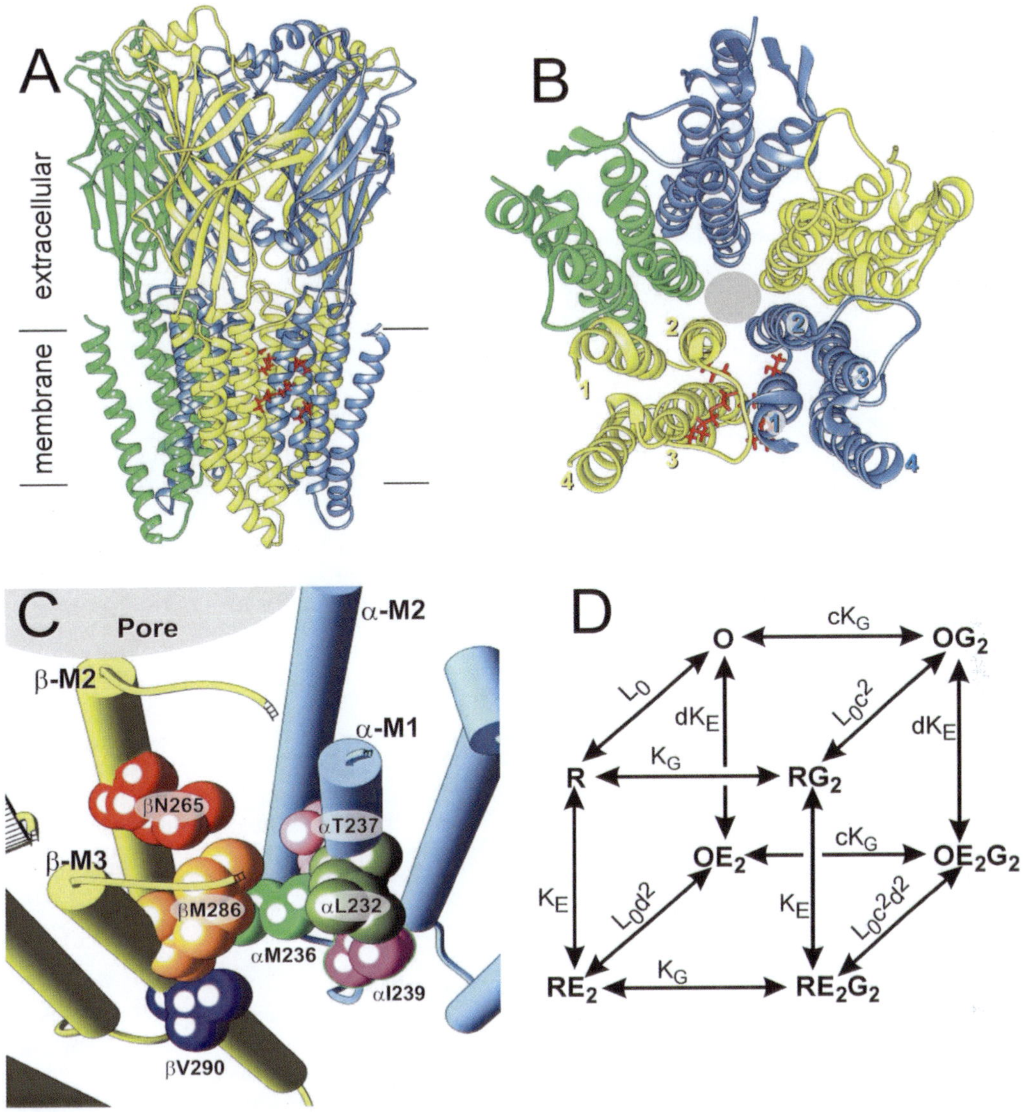

Figure 1. Functional and structural models of $GABA_A$ receptor interactions with etomidate. Panel A: A side-on ribbon depiction of a structural homology model for α1β3γ2L $GABA_A$ receptors based on the glutamate-gated chloride channel (GluCl) from *Caenorhabditis elegans* [20]. Both the extracellular domains and transmembrane domains are shown in relation to membrane lipids. Subunits are color-coded (α1 = blue; β3 = yellow; γ2L = green). βN265 and other residues involved in etomidate and propofol binding are depicted as red stick structures in one of two β+/α− transmembrane interfacial sites. **Panel B:** A view of the transmembrane domains from the extracellular space shows the structure of each subunit's four-helix bundle and the arrangement of subunits around the central chloride channel (grey circle). Residues in one interfacial anesthetic site are depicted as red stick structures. **Panel C:** A close-up view of one β+/α− transmembrane inter-subunit etomidate binding site in the homology model. Helix backbones are depicted as solid cylinders. The βN265 residue and six anesthetic contact residues identified by photolabeling or cysteine modification/protection are highlighted as labeled space-filling structures. **Panel D:** A Monod-Wyman-Changeux two-state (inactive = R; active = O) equilibrium co-agonist scheme with two equivalent orthosteric agonist (GABA; G) sites and two equivalent allosteric agonist (etomidate; E) sites is depicted [1]. For simplicity, states with only one occupied agonist site are omitted. The model is defined by five equilibrium parameters (see Eq. 3, methods): L_0 is a basal gating equilibrium (C/O); K_G and K_E are dissociation constants for respectively, GABA and etomidate binding to inactive receptors; c and d quantify the binding affinity ratios for respectively, GABA and etomidate to active vs. inactive receptors. Maximal agonist efficacies for GABA and etomidate are respectively, $(1+L_0c^2)^{-1}$ and $(1+L_0d^2)^{-1}$.

between engineered cysteines demonstrates that the photolabeled faces of α-M1 and β-M3 abut water-accessible transmembrane clefts [17,18]. Additionally, high resolution crystallography identifies homologous inter-subunit transmembrane pockets where ivermectin, an allosteric modulator/agonist of various pLGICs [19], binds to *Caenorhabditis elegans* glutamate-sensitive chloride channels (GluCl) [20].

In addition to the α-M1 and β-M3 residues identified above, M2 domain residues may contribute to the β+/α− transmembrane sites for propofol and etomidate. The focus of this study, β-M2 position 265 (M2-15′), is of particular and longstanding interest as one of the first sites where mutations were found to affect $GABA_A$ receptor sensitivity to alcohols and anesthetics [21,22]. This residue also plays a critical role in determining etomidate and propofol sensitivity in mammalian $GABA_A$

receptors. Interchanging the β-M2-15′ asparagine of β2 or β3 and the homologous serine of β1 accounts for the remarkable specificity of etomidate for receptors containing β2/3 subunits [22,23]. Methionine substitution at β2 or β3 N265 eliminates etomidate sensitivity and weakens propofol effects at the receptor level [24,25], and β3N265M transgenic mice show remarkable resistance to both anesthetics [26]. Quantitative mechanistic comparison of etomidate effects in voltage-clamped wild-type α1β2γ2L and α1βN265Sγ2L receptors expressed in *Xenopus* oocytes indicated that drug efficacy was reduced and that affinity for receptors might be weakened. Similar studies of α1βN265Mγ2L receptors were inconclusive due to the absence of anesthetic effects [27]. Homology models of αβγ $GABA_A$ receptors locate βN265 either near or within the β+/α− site (Fig. 1C), and *in silico* docking calculations suggest possible contact with anesthetics [9,12,28,29]. Moreover, contact with M2-15′ residues is evident in x-ray diffraction structures demonstrating allosteric modulators bound within inter-subunit sites of crystallized pLGIC homologs: ivermectin contacts M2-15′ of GluCl [20], while ethanol and the alkane anesthetic bromoform contact M2-15′ sidechains in positively modulated prokaryotic *Gloeobacter violaceus* ion channel (GLIC) mutants [30]. Nonetheless, no anesthetic photolabel incorporation at $GABA_A$ βN265 has been detected. One photoreactive propofol analog incorporates at β3H267 [31], which is predicted to be on the M2 helix face opposite the β+/α− interface. A SCAM protection study of α1βN265Cγ2L receptors reported no propofol protection [13], while another reported protection by n-octanol [32]. No studies have reported whether etomidate protects βN265C from modification. Thus, it remains uncertain whether βN265 mutations impair only the efficacy of etomidate and propofol, a result suggesting indirect interactions, or also the affinity of these drugs for $GABA_A$ receptors, consistent with a role in binding.

To discriminate between the effects of βN265 mutations on anesthetic binding *versus* efficacy, we applied both direct and indirect structure-function approaches. We first performed pharmacological sensitivity and thiol modification-protection studies of α1β2N265Cγ2L $GABA_A$ receptors expressed in *Xenopus* oocytes and monitored with voltage-clamp electrophysiology, using etomidate at concentrations up to 300 μM (intending to achieve high site occupancy). These experiments revealed that etomidate neither affects α1β2N265Cγ2L receptor function nor inhibits reaction with a water-soluble thiol modifier. We also explored βN265M effects in $GABA_A$ receptors containing previously characterized second point mutations: a modifiable and anesthetic-protectable cysteine (α1M236C), and a mutation that mimics bound anesthetic (α1M236W). Our results reveal that βN265M reduces both anesthetic binding affinity at β+/α− sites and transduction of gating effects associated with anesthetic binding.

Methods

Animal use

Adult female *Xenopus laevis* frogs were used as a source of oocytes for voltage-clamp electrophysiological experiments. Frogs were housed in a veterinarian-supervised facility and used in accordance with the NIH Guide for the Care and Use of Laboratory Animals. All animal procedures for this study were approved by the Massachusetts General Hospital Institutional Animal Care and Use Committee (Offices of Laboratory Animal Welfare assurance #A3596-01; MGH protocol 2005N000051). To ameliorate suffering, frogs were anesthetized by immersion in 0.2% tricaine prior to harvesting oocytes (Sigma-Aldrich, St. Louis, MO). Laparotomy wounds were minimized (<0.5 cm), and infiltrated with 0.25% bupivicaine to provide post-procedure analgesia. To reduce the number of frogs used, each frog was subjected to a maximum of six oocyte harvests with at least 8 weeks recovery between procedures.

Chemicals

R(+)-Etomidate (2 mg/ml in 35% propylene glycol:water) was from Bedford Laboratories (Bedford, OH). Propofol was purchased from Sigma-Aldrich (St. Louis, MO) and stored as stock solution in DMSO. Alphaxalone was purchased from MP Biomedical (Solon, OH) and prepared as a stock solution in DMSO. Drugs were diluted into electrophysiology solutions on the day of use. Maximal experimental concentrations of propylene glycol (<4%) and DMSO (≤0.1%) produced no functional effects on $GABA_A$ receptors [1]. Picrotoxin (PTX; from Sigma-Aldrich) was dissolved in electrophysiology buffer (2 mM). *p*-Chloromercuribenzenesulfonic acid sodium salt (pCMBS) was purchased from Toronto Research Chemicals (North York, Ontario, Canada). Salts and buffers were purchased from Sigma-Aldrich.

Molecular Biology

cDNAs for human $GABA_A$ receptor α1, β2, and γ2L subunits were cloned into pCDNA3.1 vectors (Invitrogen, Carlsbad, CA). Plasmids encoding concatenated dimer (β2-α1 and β3-α1) and trimer (γ2-β2-α1 and β3-α1-δ) subunit proteins were a generous gift from Professor Erwin Sigel (Institute for Biochemistry & Molecular Medicine, University of Bern, Switzerland) [6,33,34]. A β3-α1-γ2L trimer cDNA construct was created by excising δ and appending γ2L using overlap extension polymerase chain reaction. The β2-α1 (rat) constructs contain a 26 residue linker ($Q_5A_3PAQ_2A_3PA_2Q_5$) between the C-terminus of β2 and the N-terminus of the mature α1 (without its leader sequence). The γ2L-β2-α1 trimer also contains a 23 residue linker ($Q_5A_3PAQ_3AQA_3PA_2Q_5$) between γ2 and β2. In β3-α1 and β3-α1-γ2L constructs (rat β3, human α1 and γ2L), linkers between β3 and α1 were composed of 23 amino acids ($Q_5A_3PTGQA_3PA_2Q_5$), and that between α1 and γ2L subunits is 10 amino acids (Q_4TGQ_4). Mutations in cDNAs were created with oligonucleotide-directed mutagenesis using QuikChange kits (Agilent Technologies, Santa Clara, CA). Clones from each mutagenesis reaction were subjected to DNA sequencing through the entire cDNA region to confirm the presence of the mutation and absence of stray mutations.

Oocyte Electrophysiology

Messenger RNA synthesis and *Xenopus* oocyte expression were performed as previously described [16]. Electrophysiological experiments were done at 21 to 23°C. All drugs were delivered in ND96 electrophysiology buffer (in mM: 96 NaCl, 2 KCl, 0.8 $MgCl_2$, 1.8 $CaCl_2$, 5 HEPES, pH 7.5). Peak current responses to varying GABA concentrations (range 0.1 μM to 10 mM) alone or co-applied with anesthetics, were measured in *Xenopus* oocytes using two microelectrode voltage clamp electrophysiology, as previously described [12]. The duration of GABA application varied depending on the time to reach steady-state peak current. Responses to maximal GABA (1 to 10 mM), were recorded every 2nd or 3rd sweep for normalization. Picrotoxin-sensitive spontaneous channel activity was measured by applying 2 mM PTX, followed by >5 minute washout and a maximal GABA response test. Etomidate (10 μM) or alphaxalone (2 μM) were used as gating enhancers with high GABA concentrations to estimate maximal GABA efficacy. Oocyte currents were low-pass filtered at 1 kHz (Model OC-725B, Warner Instruments, Hamden, CT) digitized at 1–2 kHz (Digidata 1200, Molecular Devices, Sunnyvale, CA) and recorded digitally (pClamp 7, Molecular Devices).

Cysteine Modification with pCMBS and Etomidate Protection in Xenopus Oocytes

The pCMBS concentrations used for modification experiments were chosen so that initial modification rate conditions (less than 50% of maximal effect) were maintained at up to 40 s exposure. Oocytes were repetitively stimulated with GABA pulses every five minutes until at least three sequential current responses were constant (±5%). For modification and protection experiments, oocytes were exposed to pCMBS (alone, with GABA, with anesthetic, or with GABA+anesthetic) for 5 or 10 s, followed by 5–10 min wash in ND96. Responses to both low GABA (EC10) and high GABA (1 to 3 mM) were tested after each cycle of pCMBS exposure and wash. After up to ten cycles of modification and wash, maximal modification effect was checked using 10× higher pCMBS or 100 s pCMBS exposure. Modification rate analysis was performed on data from individual oocytes. For β2N265C receptor modification, spontaneous current after modification was plotted against [pCMBS] × time and fitted with single exponential functions. For α1M236C modification, the ratio of low GABA to high GABA responses were calculated, normalized to the pre-modification control, and plotted against [pCMBS] × time (mM×s). Linear least squares fits to the first three to five points were used to determine the initial modification rate in $M^{-1}s^{-1}$. A subset of oocytes were modified first in the absence of etomidate, then in the presence of etomidate. Modification rates in both conditions were independently fitted with linear least squares.

Electrophysiological Data Analysis

Analyses for agonist concentration-responses, etomidate-induced left shift, and allosteric co-agonist model fitting followed our approach described elsewhere [16,27]. Experimental peak currents were normalized to maximal GABA responses, and GABA concentration-response data for individual oocytes in the absence and presence of etomidate were fitted with logistic functions using non-linear least squares (Prism v.5, Graphpad Software):

$$I^{Agonist} = \frac{I_{\max} - I_{\min}}{1 + 10^{(\log EC50 - \log[Agonist]) \times nH}} + I_{\min} \quad (1)$$

where EC_{50} is the half-maximal activating concentration and nH is Hill slope. Etomidate-dependent direct activation of receptors was analyzed similarly.

EC_{50} shift ratios were calculated from the difference in log(GABA EC_{50}) values ($\Delta\log(EC_{50})$) measured in the presence of 3.2 μM etomidate versus control.

PTX-sensitive leak currents (I_{PTX}) normalized to $I_{\max GABA}$ ($\frac{I_{PTX}}{I_{\max GABA}}$) provided estimates of basal open probability. GABA efficacy was estimated based on enhancement of maximal GABA responses by etomidate or alphaxalone [27].

The estimated fraction of activated receptors, P^{est}_{open} corrected for both basal activity and maximal GABA efficacy, was calculated as previously described [35]:

$$P^{est}_{open} = \frac{\frac{I}{I^{GABA}_{\max}} + \frac{I_{PTX}}{I^{GABA}_{\max}}}{\frac{I^{GABA+Enhancer}}{I^{GABA}_{\max}} + \frac{I_{PTX}}{I^{GABA}_{\max}}} \quad (2)$$

A Monod-Wyman-Changeux (MWC) co-agonist mechanism with two equivalent sites each for GABA and etomidate (Fig. 1D; Eq. 3) was fitted by non-linear least squares to P^{est}_{open} values derived from GABA concentration-responses with and without etomidate as well as etomidate direct activation. Both [GABA] and [ETO] were independent variables:

$$P_{open} = \frac{1}{1 + L_0\left(\frac{1+[GABA]/K_G}{1+[GABA]/cK_G}\right)^2\left(\frac{1+[ETO]/K_E}{1+[ETO]/dK_E}\right)^2} \quad (3)$$

In Eq. 3, L_0 is a dimensionless basal closed:open gating equilibrium variable, K_G and K_E are dissociation constants for respectively, GABA and etomidate binding to inactive receptors, and c and d are the respective (dimensionless) ratios of dissociation constants in activated versus inactive receptors. The maximal agonist efficacies of GABA and etomidate are inversely related to, respectively, L_0c^2 and L_0d^2.

Estimation of etomidate binding affinity from cysteine protection

Because α1M236C is fully protectable by etomidate [12] or propofol, anesthetic-dependent inhibition of the α1M236C modification rate reflects anesthetic site occupancy, as we reported for β2M286C [14]. We therefore plotted α1M236C modification rate results as a function of etomidate concentration and fitted logistic functions (Eq. 1) to the data using non-linear least squares with a Hill slope of 1.0. The 50% protection concentration (PC_{50}) is assumed to be the anesthetic dissociation constant (K_E).

Structural Homology Modeling

A model of the human α1β3γ2 $GABA_A$ receptor was constructed using the Prime module in Schrödinger Maestro 9.7 (release 2014-1, run on the SBGrid Consortium cluster housed at Harvard Medical School, Boston, MA). The structure was based on the GluCl structure template PDB 3RHW [20] after removal of co-crystallized ivermectin and antibody fragments. Separate amino acid sequence alignments of each $GABA_A$ subunit to GluCl were performed using the ClustalW algorithm. Alignments were gap-free in all M1 through M3 domains. The intracellular ends of $GABA_A$ subunit M3 and M4 were established by the strong alignment of homologous sequences in the middle of these domains and the length of the helices in the GluCl crystal structure. Intervening M3–M4 loops of $GABA_A$ subunit sequences were then truncated and replaced with that of the modified GluCl used for crystallography. Alignment introduced a modest number of gaps into extracellular domains and M4 sequences. Some of these were edited out or moved to preserve local GluCl secondary structure. The final sequence alignments (Figure S1) are similar to those of Bertaccini et al [28]. Subunit monomer models were built using the "knowledge-based methods" option in Prime, and the heteropentamer model was assembled from five subunit monomer models in the established pentameric arrangement [6]. Model refinement used VSGB solvation [36] and a simulated membrane forcefield (dielectric = 80) bracketing the transmembrane helices. Stepwise structural energy minimization proceeded first with non-template loops, then non-conserved sidechain rotamers, and finally full all-atom minimization. Molecular graphics images were produced using UCSF Chimera software version 1.8.1.

Statistical Analysis

Results are reported as mean ± standard deviation unless otherwise noted. Statistical comparisons of results for three or more groups were performed using ANOVA with Tukey's *post-hoc* test. Pairwise comparisons were performed using Students t-tests. Statistical significance was inferred at $p<0.05$.

Results

Structural Homology Modeling

A homology model for α1β3γ2L $GABA_A$ receptors based on GluCl is depicted in Fig. 1, panels A through C. This model is similar to other $GABA_A$ receptor homology models based on both GLIC and GluCl [9,12,28,37]. The transmembrane structure of β3 subunits in our model closely matches that of crystallized β3 homomeric $GABA_A$ (PDB 4COF) [7]. Residues thought to contribute to etomidate or propofol binding (αL232, αM236, αT237, αI239, βM286, and βV290) all appear in or near the β+/α− transmembrane interfacial pockets of the model structure. In addition, βN265 (M2-15′) is also adjacent to the β+/α− interface of the model.

Functional characteristics of α1β2N265Cγ2L $GABA_A$ receptors

Our initial approach to testing steric interactions between βN265 and etomidate followed the substituted cysteine modification and protection strategy that we and others have used to test anesthetic interactions with $GABA_A$ receptor transmembrane domains [12–14,32]. We electrophysiologically characterized α1β2N265Cγ2L $GABA_A$ receptors for spontaneous activity, GABA EC_{50} and efficacy, and sensitivity to both etomidate modulation and direct activation (Fig. 2). Oocytes expressing α1β2N265Cγ2L receptors produced GABA-activated chloride currents with GABA EC_{50} similar to α1β2γ2L receptors (Fig. 2A, solid symbols, Table 1). However, etomidate at a concentration that produces general anesthesia in tadpoles (3.2 μM) did not significantly enhance GABA-activated α1β2N265Cγ2L currents and did not alter GABA EC_{50} (Fig. 2A, open symbols). High concentrations of etomidate (>30 μM) elicited very small currents with maximal amplitudes around 1 to 2% of maximal GABA responses (Fig. 2B), consistent with a prior report by McCracken et al [32]. Picrotoxin-sensitive spontaneous chloride leak in α1β2N265Cγ2L receptors was not detectable (Fig. 2C) and, thus less than experimental noise (~0.2% of maximal GABA-elicited currents), indicating a very low spontaneous opening probability. In contrast to etomidate, alphaxalone (2 μM) strongly modulated low GABA responses in α1β2N265Cγ2L receptors, and enhanced maximal GABA currents by 5 to 10% (Fig. 2D). This indicates that over 90% of α1β2N265Cγ2L receptors are activated at GABA concentrations of 1 to 10 mM, which is slightly higher than GABA efficacy estimates for α1β2γ2L (Table 1). Thus, α1β2N265Cγ2L receptors, like α1β2N265Mγ2L [27], display a functional phenotype with basal activity and GABA sensitivity similar to wild-type receptors, but extremely low sensitivity to etomidate. These functional data do not indicate whether insensitivity to etomidate is due to low drug affinity, low drug efficacy, or both.

Etomidate does not protect β2N265C from pCMBS modification

Exposing α1β2N265Cγ2L $GABA_A$ receptors to a water soluble thiol-reactive probe, para-chloromercuribenzene sulfonate (pCMBS), produced currents that did not fully reverse with pCMBS washout (Fig. 3A). These currents were blocked by picrotoxin (not shown), indicating that covalent modification of β2N265C with pCMBS irreversibly activated α1β2N265Cγ2L channels. Plotting the post-wash current against cumulative pCMBS exposure resulted in an average apparent modification

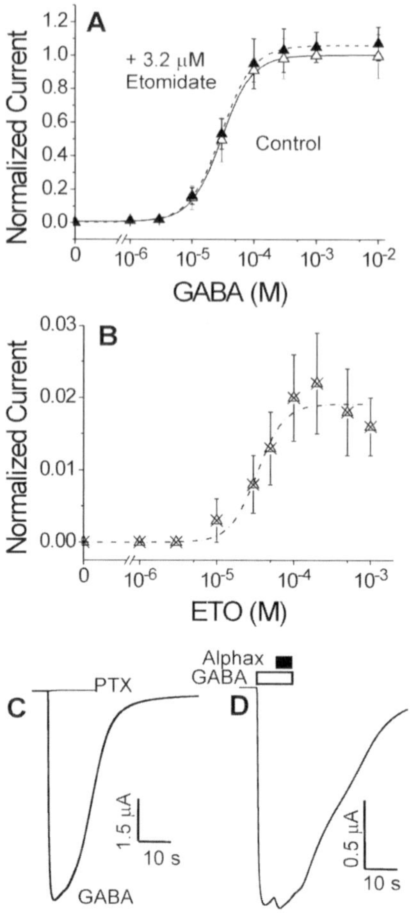

Figure 2. Electrophysiological characterization of α1β2N265Cγ2L $GABA_A$ receptors. Panel A: GABA concentration response in oocytes. Data points are mean ± sd (n ≥4) peak currents normalized to maximal GABA (1 mM) responses. Lines through data represent fits to logistic equations (Eq. 1, Methods). Open symbols: GABA alone; $EC_{50} = 31 \pm 4.7$ μM; nH = 1.75±0.088. Filled symbols: GABA plus 3.2 μM etomidate; $EC_{50} = 30 \pm 3.2$; nH = 1.67±0.068; maximum response = 1.06±0.01. **Panel B:** Etomidate agonism concentration response in oocytes. Data points are mean ± sd (n ≥4) peak currents normalized to maximal GABA (1 mM) responses. The line represents a logistic fit. $EC_{50} = 35 \pm 5.7$ μM; nH = 2.5±1.1; maximum response = 0.020±0.007. **Panel C:** Spontaneous channel gating activity in an oocyte, assessed using picrotoxin (PTX). No outward current during PTX application was observed. Current elicited with 1 mM GABA in the same cell is also displayed. **Panel D:** Estimation of maximal GABA efficacy in oocytes. GABA (3 mM; white bar) alone elicits a current that is enhanced about 5% with co-application of alphaxalone (2 μM; black bar). Average results for GABA efficacy are reported in Table 1.

rate of 950±155 $M^{-1}s^{-1}$ (n = 6). Addition of GABA increased the apparent rate of modification to 3800±600 $M^{-1}s^{-1}$, (n = 3). In contrast, control experiments in wild-type α1β2γ2L receptors revealed no functional effects of 2 mM pCMBS exposures up to 60 s (120 mM×s; n = 5; data not shown).

Absent any data to guide estimation of etomidate affinity in α1β2N265Cγ2L receptors, we tested protection using a range of concentrations up to 300 μM, which fully protected β2M286C from modification in both the absence and presence of GABA [14]. However, in α1β2N265Cγ2L receptors, co-administration of pCMBS with etomidate at up to 300 μM, with or without GABA,

Table 1. Wild-type and Mutant $GABA_A$ receptor functional characteristics in *Xenopus* oocytes.

Receptor	GABA EC_{50} (μM)	Max. GABA Efficacy [a]	ETO EC_{50} (μM)	Max. ETO Efficacy [a]	Spontaneous Activity [b]	EC_{50} Ratio (Ctl/3.2 ETO) [c]
α1β2γ2L	34±7	0.85±0.04	30±9.2	0.35±0.06	<0.002	17±3.5
	(n = 4)	(n = 4)	(n = 4)	(n = 6)	(n = 4)	(n = 4)
α1β2N265Cγ2L	31±5	0.91±0.05	35+5.7	0.02±0.006 **	<0.002 **	1.0±0.16 **
	(n = 4)	(n = 4)	(n = 3)	(n = 3)	(n = 5)	(n = 4)
β3-α1M236C/β3-α1M236C-γ2L	58±4.6*	0.63±0.08	40+3.9	0.60±0.10	<0.002	18±2.3
	(n = 4)	(n = 4)	(n = 3)	(n = 3)	(n = 3)	(n = 3)
β3N265M-α1M236C/β3N265M-α1M236C-γ2L	110±15**	0.60±0.12	n.a.	<0.002 **	<0.002	1.0±0.16 **
	(n = 3)	(n = 3)	(n = 3)	(n = 3)	(n = 3)	(n = 3)

[a]Efficacy is the estimated fraction of activatable receptors that open in the presence of an agonist (either GABA or etomidate). The detection limit for etomidate agonist efficacy is about 0.2% of maximal GABA response.
[b]Spontaneous activity is the estimated fraction of active receptors in the absence of either GABA or etomidate. The detection limit for spontaneous activity is about 0.2% of maximal GABA response.
[c]EC_{50} ratio is the ratio of control GABA EC_{50} to GABA EC_{50} measured in the presence of 3.2 μM etomidate. Large ratios indicate sensitivity to etomidate modulation.
*Differs from wild-type value at $p<0.05$. **Differs from wild-type value at $p<0.01$.

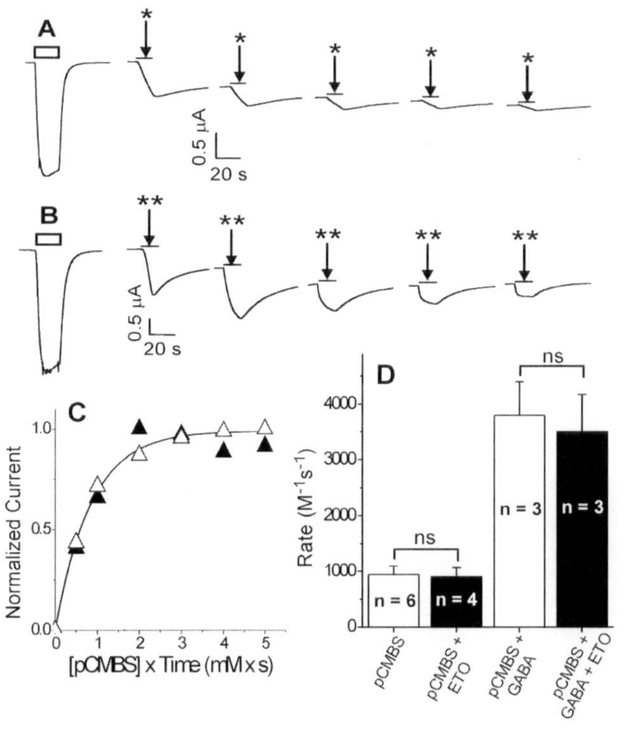

Figure 3. pCMBS modification and lack of etomidate protection in oocyte-expressed α1β2N265Cγ2L $GABA_A$ receptors. **Panel A:** The first trace is elicited with EC_{10} GABA (10 μM; white bar) and subsequent traces were recorded during sequential 10 s exposures to 0.1 mM *p*-chloromercuribenzenesulfonate (pCMBS; arrows; *), followed by wash. Basal currents increase with incremental exposure to pCMBS. **Panel B:** Traces are from another oocyte. Arrows (**) indicate 10 s exposures to 0.1 mM pCMBS plus 300 μM etomidate, followed by wash. **Panel C:** Rate analysis of current data from panels A (open symbols) and B (solid symbols) is shown, plotted against cumulative pCMBS exposure time. The line represents a nonlinear least squares single exponential fit to control data (no etomidate). The fitted rate constant is 1200±50 $M^{-1}s^{-1}$. The fitted rate for protection data (+ etomidate) is 1300±270 $M^{-1}s^{-1}$. **Panel D:** Average ± sd pCMBS modification rates in the absence and presence of 1 mM GABA and/or 300 μM etomidate.

did not alter the rate or extent of the pCMBS-receptor reaction (Fig. 3, B–D).

There are several hypotheses for this lack of etomidate protection at βN265C: 1) etomidate may bind normally, but not near the βN265 residue, implying that the βN265C mutation eliminates drug transduction/efficacy; 2) the βN265C mutation may reduce affinity for etomidate so that site occupancy remains low at concentrations up to 300 μM; and 3) etomidate may bind near βN265, but without obstructing pCMBS access. To address some of these possibilities, we assessed the effects of combining βN265M with previously characterized second mutations in the etomidate site. In order to reduce potential receptor assembly variations caused by subunit-subunit interfacial mutations, we also used concatenated dimer and trimer subunit assemblies for these double-mutant experiments.

A β+/α− site occupancy reporter reveals that βN265M mutations reduce etomidate affinity

We previously reported that $GABA_A$ receptors with cysteine substitutions at α1M236 are modified by pCMBS and that bound etomidate blocks α1M236C modification [12]. Thus, as we showed for βM286C [14], anesthetic-dependent reduction in the α1M236C modification rate reflects β+/α− site occupation. For the experiments described here, we preferred α1M236C as a site occupancy reporter because, unlike βM286C, it maintains etomidate sensitivity [12]. We first demonstrated that, in $GABA_A$ receptors assembled from concatenated subunit dimers and trimers, α1M236C is both pCMBS modifiable and protected by both etomidate and propofol (Fig. 4). We then examined anesthetic protection at α1M236C in receptors assembled from concatenated dimers and trimers with βN265M mutations, for comparison (Fig. 5).

Voltage-clamped oocytes expressing β3-α1M236C dimers and β3-α1M236C-γ2L trimers produced GABA-activatable receptor-channels that were both modulated and directly activated by etomidate (Fig. 4A, B; Table 1). Etomidate efficacy as an agonist was similar to that of GABA (Fig. 4B, which was 63±4.4% (n = 3) based on enhancement of maximal currents at high GABA (Fig. 4A, C). These pharmacological responses were quantitatively consistent with an MWC allosteric co-agonist model (Fig. 4D). Exposing β3-α1M236C/β3-α1M236C-γ2L receptors to pCMBS

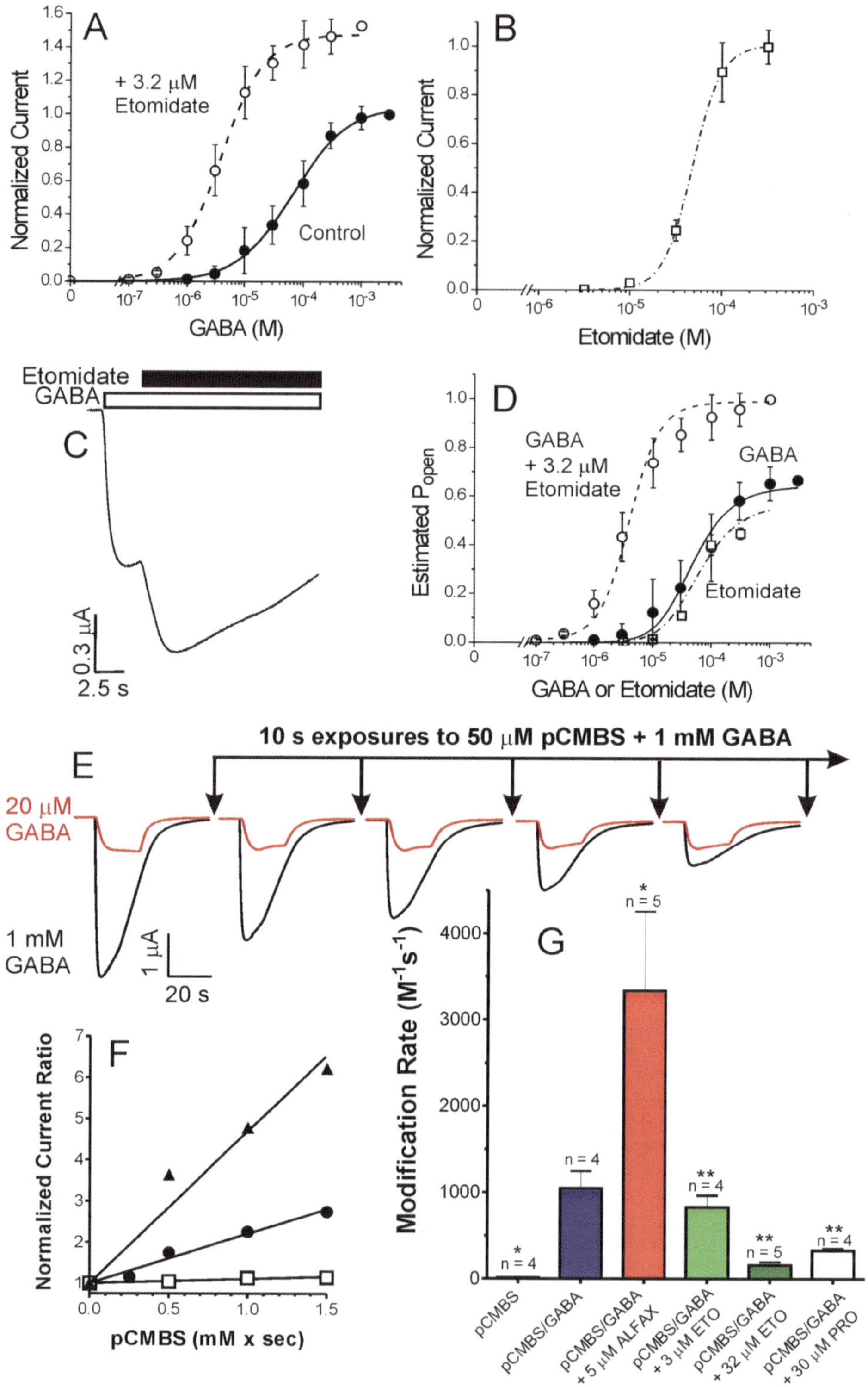

Figure 4. Modification and protection at α1M236C reflects anesthetic site occupancy. Panel A) Data represent mean ± SD peak current responses to GABA from oocytes (n = 4) expressing β3-α1M236C/β3-α1M236C-γ2L $GABA_A$ receptors, normalized to maximal GABA responses. Lines represent logistic fits to responses using GABA alone (solid circles; EC_{50} = 58 μM) and GABA with 3.2 μM etomidate (open circles; EC_{50} = 3.2 μM). **Panel B)** Data represent mean ± SD peak current responses to etomidate from oocytes (n = 3) expressing β3-α1M236C/β3-α1M236C-γ2L $GABA_A$ receptors, normalized to maximal GABA responses. The line represents a logistic fit with etomidate EC_{50} = 47 μM. **Panel C)** A single voltage-clamp current trace illustrating maximal GABA (3 mM; white bar above trace) efficacy in oocyte-expressed β3-α1M236C/β3-α1M236C-γ2L $GABA_A$ receptors, enhanced with addition of 10 μM etomidate (black bar). **Panel D)** Data from panels A and B were renormalized to maximal GABA efficacy (methods; Eq. 2) and fitted with a global MWC equilibrium co-agonist equation (methods; Eq. 3). Lines through data points represents the fitted MWC model: L_0 = 10,000; K_G = 42 ± 8.7 μM; c = 0.0075 ± 0.00048; K_E = 50 ± 12 μM; d = 0.0089 ± 0.00096. **Panel E)** Traces are from a single oocyte expressing β3-α1M236C/β3-α1M236C-γ2L $GABA_A$ receptors, demonstrating the effects of repeated pCMBS applications on the relative responses to low versus high

GABA stimulation. **Panel F)** Points represent response ratios to low (EC10) vs. high GABA, normalized to pre-modification control values. Lines through data represent linear fits used to determine relative bimolecular modification rates: GABA+pCMBS (circles; 1200±57 $M^{-1}s^{-1}$); GABA+pCMBS +5 μM alphaxalone (triangles; 3700±270 $M^{-1}s^{-1}$); and GABA+pCMBS +32 μM etomidate (squares; 106±8.4 $M^{-1}s^{-1}$). **Panel G)** Summary of modification rate results (mean ± se) for all oocytes expressing β3-α1M236C/β3-α1M236C-γ2L $GABA_A$ receptors under different conditions. The rate with pCMBS alone is significantly accelerated with addition of GABA and GABA/alphaxalone. Relative to GABA+alphaxalone, modification in the presence of GABA is slowed 65% by 3 μM etomidate, 95% by 32 μM etomidate, and 91% by 30 μM propofol. * $p<0.05$; ** $p<0.01$.

irreversibly increased their sensitivity to low GABA (20 μM ≈ EC10–20) relative to high GABA, indicating enhanced channel gating (Fig. 4E). The apparent rate of α1M236C modification increased about 3-fold when pCMBS was co-applied with GABA, and was further accelerated by addition of alphaxalone, a positive allosteric modulator that does not interact with etomidate or propofol sites (Fig. 4F, G). Because etomidate directly activates β3-α1M236C/β3-α1M236C-γ2L receptors, we did not test etomidate protection in the absence of GABA. Etomidate at 3 μM did not significantly alter the apparent rate of α1M236C modification in GABA-activated receptors (Fig. 4G). We hypothesized that this result reflected two opposing effects of etomidate, as we have previously reported [12,14]: etomidate both increased the fraction of activated channels relative to GABA alone (see Figs. 4A, C), while also blocking pCMBS access. Therefore, we used the GABA+alphaxalone modification rate as a control for analysis of etomidate-dependent protection results, because the fraction of activated receptors was maximized when GABA was co-applied with either alphaxalone or etomidate. Relative to the rate observed with GABA plus alphaxalone, 3.2 μM etomidate slowed modification about three-fold, and 32 μM etomidate reduced the modification rate over twenty-fold (Fig. 4G). Logistic analysis of these modification rate data indicated 50% protection at 1.07 μM etomidate (PC_{50}; 95% CI = 0.24 to 4.7 μM).

Double-mutant β3N265M-α1M236C/β3N265M-α1M236C-γ2L $GABA_A$ receptors produced GABA-activated currents that were insensitive to both etomidate modulation and direct etomidate activation (Table 1). Currents mediated by β3N265M-α1M236C/β3N265M-α1M236C-γ2L double-mutant receptors also demonstrated cumulative irreversible gating changes following repeated exposures to pCMBS (Fig. 5A). Modification by pCMBS was accelerated over 10-fold in the presence of GABA. Because β3N265M-α1M236C/β3N265M-α1M236C-γ2L receptors were etomidate insensitive, we were able to study etomidate protection at α1M236C in both the absence and presence of GABA (i.e. inactive vs. mostly activated channels). Insensitivity to etomidate also enabled sequential measurement in the same oocytes of modification rates in the absence vs. presence of etomidate, (e.g. Fig. 5B). Etomidate at 32 μM did not significantly alter the apparent rate of α1M236C modification in either the absence (Fig. 5C) or presence of GABA (Fig. 5D). Using 300 μM etomidate, rates of modification were reduced by about two-fold from control in both conditions (Fig. 5B–D). Logistic fits to these data estimated that in the absence of GABA etomidate PC_{50} ≈ 300 μM (95% CI = 215 to 423 μM) and is similar in the presence of GABA (PC_{50} ≈ 290 μM; 95% CI = 206 to 412 μM). Assuming that the PC_{50} estimates reflect etomidate occupancy, we infer that etomidate binds very weakly (dissociation constant ≈ 300 μM) to

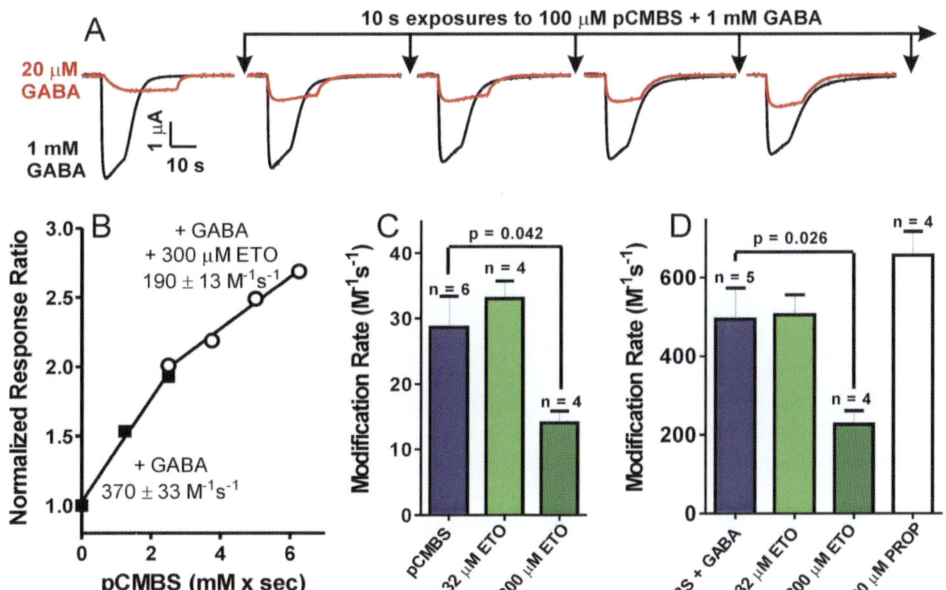

Figure 5. The βN265M mutation reduces anesthetic-dependent site occupancy. Panel A) Voltage-clamp current traces are from a single oocyte expressing β3N265M-α1M236C/β3N265M-α1M236C-γ2L $GABA_A$ receptors, showing the effects of repeated pCMBS+GABA applications on responses to low versus high GABA. **Panel B)** Points represent response ratios to low (EC10) vs. high GABA, normalized to pre-modification control values, for one oocytes exposed to: GABA+pCMBS (solid squares) followed by GABA+pCMBS +300 μM etomidate (open circles). Lines through data represent linear fits; labels are the apparent bimolecular modification rates (slopes). **Panel C)** Summary of modification rate results for all oocytes expressing β3N265M-α1M236C/β3N265M-α1M236C-γ2L $GABA_A$ receptors modified with pCMBS, in the absence vs. presence of etomidate. Etomidate (300 μM) reduced the apparent modification rate by 51%. **Panel D)** Summary of modification rate results for GABA-activated receptors (modified in the presence of 1 mM GABA). Modification is inhibited 54% by 300 μM etomidate. Propofol (30 μM) does not significantly inhibit modification.

both inactive and GABA-activated β3N265M-α1M236C/β3N265M-α1M236C-γ2L receptors, in comparison to activated β3-α1M236C/β3-α1M236C-γ2L receptors (dissociation constant ≈ 1 μM).

Propofol occupancy of β+/α− sites is also reduced by βN265M mutations

We also demonstrated that propofol at 30 μM, like etomidate, reduced the rate of pCMBS modification at α1M236C by about 90% in activated free subunit α1M236Cβ3γ2L receptors (not shown) and in concatenated β3-α1M236C/β3-α1M236C-γ2L receptors (Fig. 4G). In comparison, 30 μM propofol did not reduce the rate of pCMBS modification in GABA-activated β3N265M-α1M236C/β3N265M-α1M236C-γ2L receptors (Fig. 5D), indicating very low β+/α− site occupancy.

A β+/α− site mutation that mimics bound anesthetic reveals that βN265M impairs transduction

To study the effect of βN265M mutations on β+/α− site transduction, without the need to establish drug site occupancy, we used another mutation. The azi-etomidate photolabeled α1M236 sidechain abuts the β+/α− cleft where etomidate binds, and α1M236W mutation mimics the positive allosteric effects of anesthetic binding while reducing etomidate modulation [16]. Thus, the tryptophan substituted sidechain at α1M236 likely occupies the same space as bound etomidate, and shares transduction mechanisms that enhance channel gating.

In α1β2γ2L receptors formed from free subunits, α1M236W produced a 20-fold reduction in GABA EC_{50} [16]. In receptors where pentameric subunit assembly is constrained by co-expression of concatenated β2-α1 dimers and γ2L-β2-α1 trimers, α1M236W mutations in both subunit assemblies produced a 36-fold reduction in GABA EC_{50} (Fig. 6A) [38]. We introduced β2N265M mutations into both dimer and trimer concatenated subunit assemblies, and then added α1M236W mutations to both constructs. GABA concentration response data from β2N265M-α1/γ2L-β2N265M-α1 receptors resulted in GABA EC_{50} = 76 μM; n = 4 oocytes; Fig. 6B). This represents about a two-fold increase in GABA EC_{50} relative to β2-α1/γ2L-β2-α1 receptors, consistent with previous studies of βN265M [25,27,39]. Etomidate neither modulated nor directly activated β2N265M-α1/γ2L-β2N265M-α1 receptors (4 cells tested for each effect, not shown). GABA concentration-responses for β2N265M-α1M236W/γ2L-β2N265M-α1M236W (n = 4 oocytes) were characterized by GABA EC_{50} = 25 μM, three-fold lower than the β2N265M-α1/γ2L-β2N265M-α1 value (Fig. 6B). Thus, α1M236W produced a small but significant channel gating effect when βN265M mutations were present. The GABA EC_{50} shift produced by α1M236W when βN265M was present was about 10-fold smaller than the shift in the wild-type receptor background. In other words, βN265M mutations dramatically reduced, but did not eliminate β+/α− site transduction.

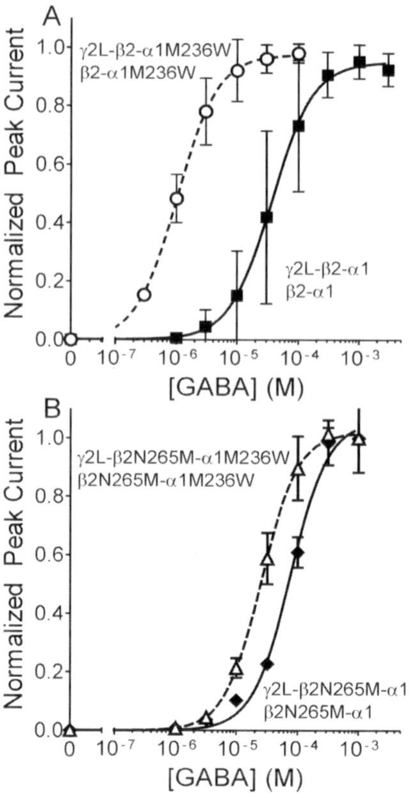

Figure 6. The βN265M mutation reduces the channel gating effects of a α1M236W mutation that mimics etomidate. Panel A) Data are reproduced from Guitchounts et al [38] showing mean ± SD GABA concentration-response, normalized to maximal currents, from oocytes expressing concatenated receptor dimer and trimer constructs. Lines through data points represent non-linear least squares logistic fits (Eq. 1, methods). Solid squares represent β2-α1/γ2L-β2-α1 receptors (GABA EC_{50} = 36 μM) and open circles represent β2-α1M236W/γ2L-β2-α1M236W receptors (EC_{50} = 1.0 μM). **Panel B)** Data points are mean ± SD current responses to GABA, normalized to maximal currents. Solid diamonds represent β2N265M-α1/γ2L-β2N265M-α1 receptors (GABA EC_{50} = 76 μM; 95% CI = 63 to 92 μM) and open triangles represent β2N265M-α1M236W/γ2L-β2N265M-α1M236W- receptors (EC_{50} = 25 μM; 95% CI = 22 to 29 μM).

Discussion

Major findings

We used both direct and indirect structure-function strategies to investigate the role of the $GABA_A$ receptor βN265 (M2-15′) residue in the binding and efficacy of etomidate and propofol within their established β+/α− interfacial sites. Cysteine substitution at βN265 produced receptors that were profoundly insensitive to etomidate (Fig. 2). Moreover, etomidate at concentrations up to 300 μM did not protect βN265C from covalent thiol modification (Fig. 3). The absence of etomidate effects obscures whether βN265C alters anesthetic binding vs. efficacy. However, the impact of βN265M mutations was revealed in studies of receptors containing second "reporter" mutations within the β+/α− anesthetic sites. These indirect experiments show that βN265M mutations both weaken anesthetic binding and impair β+/α− site transduction (efficacy).

Anesthetic binding versus efficacy in $GABA_A$ receptors

The challenge of distinguishing whether ligand-gated ion channel mutations affect agonist binding, efficacy, or both, is well-known [40]. Both etomidate and propofol are allosteric agonists at $GABA_A$ receptors [1,2]. Within the MWC mechanistic framework, mutations can affect apparent sensitivity to anesthetics in three ways [41]: 1) altering the basal inactive-active equilibrium (L_0 in Eq. 3), 2) altering anesthetic binding to inactive receptors (K_E), and 3) altering anesthetic efficacy (d), which is equivalent to selectively altering binding to activated receptor states (dK_E).

The βN265M mutation reduces both etomidate efficacy and binding affinity

Both current and previous [25,27,32] functional studies reveal that βN265C and βN265M mutations eliminate etomidate sensitivity, providing no information regarding changes in drug binding or efficacy. To investigate drug occupancy (binding) of β+/α− anesthetic sites independent of drug effects, we used a modifiable and protectable reporter cysteine, α1M236C. Concatenated β3-α1M236C/β3-α1M236C-γ2L receptors, like free subunit α1M236Cβ2γ2L receptors [12], retained sensitivity to both etomidate modulation and direct activation. MWC model analysis indicated that the respective dissociation constants for etomidate in inactive (K_E) and active (dK_E) receptors are approximately 50 μM and 0.5 μM (Figs. 4D, 7A). Thus, etomidate allosteric efficacy (d) in this receptor is approximately 0.01 (Figs. 4D, 7A), comparable to estimates for both wild-type receptors [1] and free subunit α1M236Cβ2γ2L receptors [12]. Etomidate occupation of its two sites per β3-α1M236C/β3-α1M236C-γ2L receptor is thus predicted to shift the closed:open equilibrium by $d^{-2} \approx 10{,}000$-fold toward open states (Fig. 7A). This accounts for the robust etomidate agonism observed in these channels (Fig. 4B). The MWC estimate for etomidate affinity in activated β3-α1M236C/β3-α1M236C-γ2L receptors ($dK_E \approx 0.5$ μM) is also in good agreement with that for free-subunit α1M236Cβ2γ2L receptors($dK_E \approx 1$ μM) [12] and our current etomidate protection results ($PC_{50} \approx 1$ μM; Fig. 5).

In comparison, protection experiments in double-mutant concatenated β3N265M-α1M236C/β3N265M-α1M236C-γ2L receptors indicated only ~50% occupancy at 300 μM etomidate, implying extremely low-affinity binding to both inactive ($K_E \approx$ 300 μM) and GABA-activated ($dK_E \approx$ 300 μM) receptors (Fig. 7B). Etomidate's similar affinity for both inactive and active receptors in the double mutant receptors implies an allosteric efficacy near 1.0 (Fig. 7B). This means that etomidate binding to receptors with βN265M mutations doesn't shift the closed:open state distribution, consistent with the observed absence of drug effects on channel activity. This estimated effect of βN265M on etomidate efficacy (10,000-fold reduction for two sites) is much larger than the efficacy effect (25-fold reduction for two sites) that was previously estimated for β2N265S mutations [27]. Comparing results for α1M236Cβ3γ2L and α1M236Cβ3N265Mγ2L receptors (Fig. 7) suggests that methionine substitution reduces etomidate affinity for inactive receptors about 6-fold ($K_E \approx$ 50 μM vs. 300 μM), while efficacy (d) is weakened about 100-fold per site. Together, reductions of both drug affinity and efficacy account for the approximately 600-fold reduction in apparent etomidate binding affinity for GABA-activated receptors ($dK_E \approx$ 0.5 μM vs. 300 μM).

Our evidence demonstrating reduced etomidate affinity in both inactive and GABA-activated receptors is consistent with a direct role for βN265 in drug binding. This interaction is also suggested by *in silico* docking calculations [12]. Additional indirect support for this hypothesis comes from studies of M2-15′ residues on other pLGICs that contact alcohols and anesthetics [30,39,42]. In addition, other outer M2 domain residues may also contribute to anesthetic sites in $GABA_A$ receptors [31] and related pLGICs [30,43,44]. However, the indirect nature of our evidence cannot rule out the possibility that βN265 mutations indirectly influence etomidate binding.

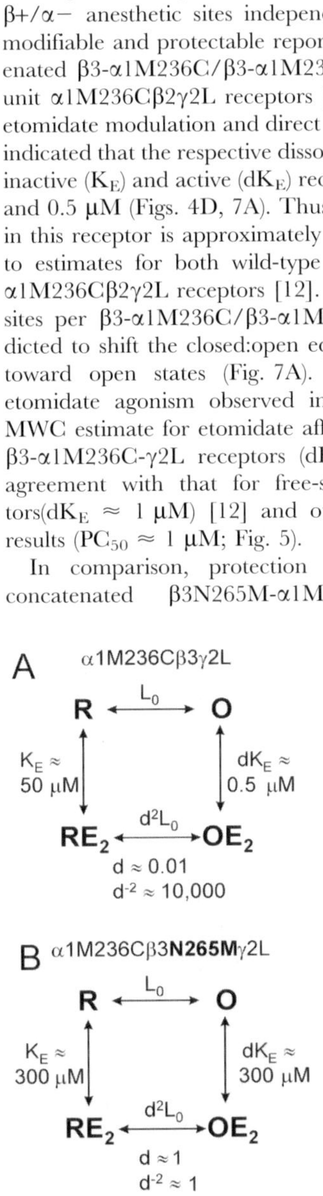

Figure 7. Effects of βN265M mutation on etomidate in inactive versus active $GABA_A$ receptors. Monod-Wyman-Changeux equilibrium allosteric models are diagrammed for both α1M236Cβ2γ2L (A) and α1M236Cβ2N265Mγ2L (B) receptors, each with two equivalent etomidate sites. Etomidate dissociation constants for both inactive (R; K_E) and GABA-activated (O; dK_E) receptors are rounded estimates based on both functional analysis and modification/protection results (Figs. 6 and 7). Etomidate-sensitive α1M236Cβ2γ2L receptors bind etomidate 100-fold more avidly in the active vs. inactive state, resulting in a 10,000-fold shift in the open-closed equilibrium constant (d^2L_0 vs. L_0) when both sites are occupied. In contrast, etomidate-insensitive α1M236Cβ2N265Mγ2L receptors display low affinity ($K_E \approx dK_E \approx$ 300 μM) for etomidate in both resting and GABA-activated states. Thus, high etomidate concentrations result in only partial site occupancy and weak modulatory effects.

The propofol sites in β+/α− interfaces overlap with the etomidate sites

Recently, both αM236 and βM286 in α1β3 receptors were identified as incorporation sites for a propofol photo-label analog [10]. Our protection studies at α1M236C confirm this locus as a propofol contact residue. Propofol also protects βM286C from thiol modification [13]. Azi-etomidate photolabeling [8] and SCAM protection [12] identify both α1M236 and βM286 as etomidate contact points, and propofol inhibits azi-etomidate photolabeling at these residues [45]. Thus, both αM236 and βM286 are common contact points for both etomidate and propofol. Our results (Figs. 4, 5) also show that βN265M reduces β+/α− site affinity for propofol. Bali & Akabas [13] noted that propofol modulates α1β2N265Cγ2 receptors, and we also observed propofol effects in receptors with βN265M mutations. This likely reflects propofol modulation *via* at least two other transmembrane interfacial sites: β-/α+ and β-/γ+ [45], that also bind a potent barbiturate photolabel [46] but not etomidate. The presence of at least four propofol sites per αβγ $GABA_A$ receptor present challenges for interpretation of its effects in mutant channels.

The βN265M mutation impairs transduction between β+/α− anesthetic sites and channel gating

We further assessed the effect of βN265M on β+/α− anesthetic site transduction by testing the gating effects of α1M236W, a mutation that mimics bound anesthetic [16,38]. The β2N265M mutation reduced the gating effects of α1M236W mutations about ten-fold, but did not eliminate them (Fig. 6). Extending this conclusion to bound etomidate suggests that reduced efficacy/transduction alone may not fully account for the profound etomidate-insensitivity of receptors containing βN265M mutations. This is consistent with our result from α1M236C protection studies that also show profound effects on anesthetic efficacy combined with more modest, but significant reductions in etomidate affinity for resting state receptors.

The impact of βN265 mutations also appears to be highly selective for β+/α− anesthetic site ligands, further supporting its involvement through local steric interactions. Both GABA EC_{50} and basal channel gating are weakly altered by β2N265S or βN265M mutations [27], and our current results indicate that the same is true for βN265C mutations. Based on our data and others [32], receptors with βN265 mutations also retain modulation by alphaxalone, pentobarbital, and benzodiazepines. Evidence indicates that all of these drugs act primarily *via* allosteric sites that do not overlap with the β+/α− interfacial sites where both etomidate and propofol bind.

Anesthetics and βN265C protection

In contrast to negative βN265C protection results with etomidate (this study) and propofol [13], McCracken et al [32] reported that n-octanol blocks thiol modification at β2N265C. If all of these anesthetics bind in the β+/α− sites, why don't they all protect βN265C? One explanation consistent with our results is that βN265C reduces anesthetic affinity more than βN265M; thus β+/α− site occupancy may have been very low during our etomidate protection experiments. Secondly, the possibility that 300 μM etomidate occupies α1β2N265Cγ2L sites without obstructing pCMBS modification cannot be excluded. βN265C forms disulfide bonds with other cysteine substitutions on α-M1, β-M3, and β-M1 [18], revealing potential βN265 interactions with both β+/α− *inter-subunit* anesthetic sites and β *intra-subunit* helix bundles. Structural homology models (e.g. Fig. 1) also show βN265 oriented toward β-M3, lying between intra- and inter-subunit pockets. Other pLGIC subunit helix bundles are known to form sites that anesthetics occupy [47] and the $GABA_A$ β helix bundles could be access pathways for pCMBS to reach the thiol of βN265C without interference from propofol or etomidate. If octanol, a small flexible molecule, binds in both β helix bundles and β+/α− sites, this could explain its unique protection at βN265C. Thirdly, the small size and flexibility of n-octanol relative to propofol and etomidate may allow it to bind closer to βN265 within the β+/α− sites. Intriguingly, high-resolution structures of GLIC mutants suggest that the relative size and occupancy of inter-subunit and intra-subunit transmembrane pockets influences whether small alcohols and anesthetics act as gating enhancers *versus* inhibitors [30]. Moreover, the positive modulating anesthetic sites on GLIC are formed between M2 domains on adjacent subunits, rather than between M1 and M3 domains. Thus, examination of anesthetic interactions with both intra-subunit helix bundle pockets and various parts of the inter-subunit pockets of $GABA_A$ receptor may reveal distinct sites where small versus large drugs bind and act.

βN265 and etomidate photolabels

If βN265 sidechains contact anesthetics, how also to explain the absence of anesthetic photolabeling at this residue? The large effects of βN265 mutations on etomidate sensitivity are fully consistent with complementary structure-function data on etomidate derivatives, if we assume limitations on their binding orientation. Modification at the ester leaving group of etomidate, including appending large photoreactive groups, preserves anesthetic activity and $GABA_A$ receptor modulating efficacy [48,49]. Photolabels of this type label residues on α–M1 and β-M3, near the lipid-protein interface. In contrast, based on inhibition of azietomidate labeling, p-trifluorodiaziryl (TFD) substitution on the phenyl ring of etomidate reduces affinity for etomidate sites ~50-fold relative to a similar p-TFD-benzyl substitution at the ester position [45]. Other bulky additions to the phenylethyl group or reorientation around the chiral carbon adjacent to the phenyl group of etomidate also dramatically reduce anesthetic activity in animals and/or modulatory efficacy in $GABA_A$ receptors [49–53]. Together, these results suggest that the phenylethyl end of bound etomidate is oriented toward the transmembrane pore and M2 domains (i.e. βN265), in a sterically constrained posture that likely contributes to etomidate stereoselectivity.

Finally, $GABA_A$ receptors form other transmembrane anesthetic sites, including other inter-subunit pockets, intra-subunit helical bundles, and the ion channel [54,55]. Different anesthetics display distinctive specificities for these various sites [10,45]. Defining the pLGIC structural elements involved in site-selective anesthetic binding will be essential to understanding the mechanisms of these important drugs, while also informing development of more receptor sub-type selective modulators.

Supporting Information

Figure S1 Alignment of $GABA_A$ receptor subunit amino acid sequences with GluCl. Each subunit sequence was independently aligned as described in methods. Predicted secondary structure domains are indicated by blue bars for beta sheet and red bars for alpha-helix.

Acknowledgments

We thank Youssef Jounaidi (Massachusetts General Hospital, Boston, MA) for technical help with subunit expression constructs. Some concatenated subunit cDNA constructs were gifts from Prof. Erwin Sigel (Institute for Biochemistry & Molecular Medicine, University of Bern, Switzerland). Prof. Keith W. Miller (Massachusetts General Hospital, Boston MA), provided guidance on sequence alignments for homology modeling and comments on the manuscript. Prof. Jonathan B. Cohen (Harvard Medical School, Boston, MA) also provided helpful comments on the manuscript. Molecular graphics images were produced using the University of California, San Francisco, Chimera version 1.8.1 from the Resource for Biocomputing, Visualization, and Informatics at the University of California, San Francisco (supported by NIH P41 RR-01081).

Author Contributions

Conceived and designed the experiments: DSS SAF. Performed the experiments: DSS DWP MH ATS. Analyzed the data: DSS DWP MH SAF. Contributed reagents/materials/analysis tools: SAF. Contributed to the writing of the manuscript: DSS ATS SAF.

References

1. Rüsch D, Zhong H, Forman SA (2004) Gating allosterism at a single class of etomidate sites on alpha1beta2gamma2L GABA-A receptors accounts for both direct activation and agonist modulation. J Biol Chem 279: 20982–20992.
2. Rüsch D, Neumann E, Wulf H, Forman SA (2012) An Allosteric Coagonist Model for Propofol Effects on alpha1beta2gamma2L gamma-Aminobutyric Acid Type A Receptors. Anesthesiology 116: 47–55.
3. Zeller A, Arras M, Jurd R, Rudolph U (2007) Mapping the contribution of beta3-containing GABAA receptors to volatile and intravenous general anesthetic actions. BMC Pharmacol 7: 2.
4. Olsen RW, Sieghart W (2008) International Union of Pharmacology. LXX. Subtypes of gamma-aminobutyric acid(A) receptors: Classification on the basis of subunit composition, pharmacology, and function. Pharmacol Rev 60: 243–260.

5. Corringer PJ, Poitevin F, Prevost MS, Sauguet L, Delarue M, et al. (2012) Structure and pharmacology of pentameric receptor channels: from bacteria to brain. Structure 20: 941–956.
6. Baumann SW, Baur R, Sigel E (2002) Forced subunit assembly in alpha1beta2gamma2 GABAA receptors. Insight into the absolute arrangement. J Biol Chem 277: 46020–46025.
7. Miller PS, Aricescu AR (2014) Crystal structure of a human GABAA receptor. Nature doi:10.1038/nature13293: 1–8.
8. Li GD, Chiara DC, Sawyer GW, Husain SS, Olsen RW, et al. (2006) Identification of a $GABA_A$ receptor anesthetic binding site at subunit interfaces by photolabeling with an etomidate analog. J Neurosci 26: 11599–11605.
9. Chiara DC, Dostalova Z, Jayakar SS, Zhou X, Miller KW, et al. (2012) Mapping general anesthetic binding site(s) in human alpha1beta3 gamma-aminobutyric acid type A receptors with [(3)H]TDBzl-etomidate, a photoreactive etomidate analogue. Biochemistry 51: 836–847.
10. Jayakar SS, Zhou X, Chiara DC, Dostalova Z, Savechenkov PY, et al. (2014) Multiple Propofol Binding Sites in a gamma-Aminobutyric Acid Type A Receptor (GABAAR) Identified Using a Photoreactive Propofol Analog. J Biol Chem 289: 456–468.
11. Li GD, Chiara DC, Cohen JB, Olsen RW (2010) Numerous classes of general anesthetics inhibit etomidate binding to gamma-aminobutyric acid type A (GABAA) receptors. J Biol Chem 285: 8615–8620.
12. Stewart DS, Hotta M, Li GD, Desai R, Chiara DC, et al. (2013) Cysteine Substitutions Define Etomidate Binding and Gating Linkages in the alpha-M1 Domain of gamma-Aminobutyric Acid Type A (GABAA) Receptors. J Biol Chem 288: 30373–30386.
13. Bali M, Akabas MH (2004) Defining the propofol binding site location on the GABAA receptor. Mol Pharmacol 65: 68–76.
14. Stewart DS, Hotta M, Desai R, Forman SA (2013) State-Dependent Etomidate Occupancy of Its Allosteric Agonist Sites Measured in a Cysteine-Substituted GABAA Receptor. Mol Pharmacol 83: 1200–1208.
15. Krasowski MD, Nishikawa K, Nikolaeva N, Lin A, Harrison NL (2001) Methionine 286 in transmembrane domain 3 of the GABAA receptor beta subunit controls a binding cavity for propofol and other alkylphenol general anesthetics. Neuropharmacology 41: 952–964.
16. Stewart DS, Desai R, Cheng Q, Liu A, Forman SA (2008) Tryptophan mutations at azi-etomidate photo-incorporation sites on alpha-1 or beta-2 subunits enhance GABAA receptor gating and reduce etomidate modulation Mol Pharmacol 74: 1687–1695.
17. Bali M, Jansen M, Akabas MH (2009) GABA-induced intersubunit conformational movement in the GABAA receptor alpha1M1-beta2M3 transmembrane subunit interface: Experimental basis for homology modeling of an intravenous anesthetic binding site. J Neurosci 29: 3083–3092.
18. Borghese CM, Hicks JA, Lapid DJ, Trudell JR, Harris RA (2014) GABA(A) receptor transmembrane amino acids are critical for alcohol action: disulfide cross-linking and alkyl methanethiosulfonate labeling reveal relative location of binding sites. J Neurochem 128: 363–375.
19. Lynagh T, Lynch JW (2012) Ivermectin binding sites in human and invertebrate Cys-loop receptors. Trends Pharmacol Sci 33: 432–441.
20. Hibbs RE, Gouaux E (2011) Principles of activation and permeation in an anion-selective Cys-loop receptor. Nature 474: 54–60.
21. Mihic SJ, Ye Q, Wick MJ, Koltchine VV, Krasowski MD, et al. (1997) Sites of alcohol and volatile anaesthetic action on GABA(A) and glycine receptors. Nature 389: 385–389.
22. Belelli D, Lambert JJ, Peters JA, Wafford K, Whiting PJ (1997) The interaction of the general anesthetic etomidate with the gamma-aminobutyric acid type A receptor is influenced by a single amino acid. Proc Natl Acad Sci U S A 94: 11031–11036.
23. Hill-Venning C, Belelli D, Peters JA, Lambert JJ (1997) Subunit-dependent interaction of the general anaesthetic etomidate with the gamma-aminobutyric acid type A receptor. Br J Pharmacol 120: 749–756.
24. Siegwart R, Jurd R, Rudolph U (2002) Molecular determinants for the action of general anesthetics at recombinant alpha(2)beta(3)gamma(2)gamma-aminobutyric acid(A) receptors. J Neurochem 80: 140–148.
25. Siegwart R, Krahenbuhl K, Lambert S, Rudolph U (2003) Mutational analysis of molecular requirements for the actions of general anaesthetics at the gamma-aminobutyric acidA receptor subtype, alpha1beta2gamma2. BMC Pharmacol 3: 13.
26. Jurd R, Arras M, Lambert S, Drexler B, Siegwart R, et al. (2003) General anesthetic actions in vivo strongly attenuated by a point mutation in the GABA(A) receptor beta3 subunit. FASEB J 17: 250–252.
27. Desai R, Rüsch D, Forman SA (2009) Gamma-amino butyric acid type A receptor mutations at beta2N265 alter etomidate efficacy while preserving basal and agonist-dependent activity. Anesthesiology 111: 774–784.
28. Bertaccini EJ, Yoluk O, Lindahl ER, Trudell JR (2014) Assessment of homology templates and an anesthetic binding site within the gamma-aminobutyric acid receptor. Anesthesiology 119: 1087–1095.
29. Jansen M, Akabas MH (2006) State-dependent cross-linking of the M2 and M3 segments: Functional basis for the alignment of GABAA and acetylcholine receptor M3 segments. J Neurosci 26: 4492–4499.
30. Sauguet L, Howard RJ, Malherbe L, Lee US, Corringer PJ, et al. (2013) Structural basis for potentiation by alcohols and anaesthetics in a ligand-gated ion channel. Nature Comm 4: 1697.
31. Yip GM, Chen ZW, Edge CJ, Smith EH, Dickinson R, et al. (2013) A propofol binding site on mammalian GABA receptors identified by photolabeling. Nature Chem Biol 9: 715–720.
32. McCracken ML, Borghese CM, Trudell JR, Harris RA (2010) A transmembrane amino acid in the GABAA receptor beta2 subunit critical for the actions of alcohols and anesthetics. J Pharmacol Exp Ther 335: 600–606.
33. Baumann SW, Baur R, Sigel E (2001) Subunit arrangement of gamma-aminobutyric acid type A receptors. J Biol Chem 276: 36275–36280.
34. Kaur KH, Baur R, Sigel E (2009) Unanticipated structural and functional properties of delta subunit containing GABAA receptors. J Biol Chem 284: 7889–7896.
35. Forman SA, Stewart D (2011) Mutations in the GABAA receptor that mimic the allosteric ligand etomidate. Meth Mol Biol 796: 317–333.
36. Li J, Abel R, Zhu K, Cao Y, Zhao S, et al. (2011) The VSGB 2.0 model: a next generation energy model for high resolution protein structure modeling. Proteins 79: 2794–2812.
37. Bali M, Akabas MH (2012) Gating-induced Conformational Rearrangement of the gamma-Aminobutyric Acid Type A Receptor beta-alpha Subunit Interface in the Membrane-spanning Domain. J Biol Chem 287: 27762–27770.
38. Guitchounts G, Stewart DS, Forman SA (2012) The Two Etomidate Sites in alpha1beta2gamma2 gamma-Aminobutyric Acid Type A Receptors Contribute Equally and Noncooperatively to Modulation of Channel Gating. Anesthesiology 116: 1235–1244.
39. Nishikawa K, Jenkins A, Paraskevakis I Harrison NL (2002) Volatile anesthetic actions on the GABAA receptors: Contrasting effects of alpha 1(S270) and beta 2(N265) point mutations. Neuropharmacology 42: 337–345.
40. Colquhoun D (1998) Binding, gating, affinity and efficacy: the interpretation of structure-activity relationships for agonists and of the effects of mutating receptors. Br J Pharmacol 125: 924–947.
41. Galzi JL, Edelstein SJ, Changeux J (1996) The multiple phenotypes of allosteric receptor mutants. Proc Natl Acad Sci U S A 93: 1853–1858.
42. Foadi N, Leuwer M, Demir R, Dengler R, Buchholz V, et al. (2010) Lack of positive allosteric modulation of mutated alpha(1)S267I glycine receptors by cannabinoids. Naunyn-Schmiedeberg's Arch Pharmacol 381: 477–482.
43. Borghese CM, Xiong W, Oh SI, Ho A, Mihic SJ, et al. (2012) Mutations M287L and Q266I in the glycine receptor alpha1 subunit change sensitivity to volatile anesthetics in oocytes and neurons, but not the minimal alveolar concentration in knockin mice. Anesthesiology 117: 765–771.
44. Lynagh T, Laube B (2014) Opposing effects of the anesthetic propofol at pentameric ligand-gated ion channels mediated by a common site. J Neurosci 34: 2155–2159.
45. Chiara DC, Jayakar SS, Zhou X, Zhang X, Savechenkov PY, et al. (2013) Specificity of intersubunit general anesthetic binding sites in the transmembrane domain of the human alpha1beta3gamma2 GABAA receptor. J Biol Chem 288: 19343–19357.
46. Savechenkov PY, Zhang X, Chiara DC, Stewart DS, Ge R, et al. (2012) Allyl m-Trifluoromethyldiazirine Mephobarbital: An Unusually Potent Enantioselective and Photoreactive Barbiturate General Anesthetic. J Med Chem 55: 6554–6565.
47. Nury H, Van Renterghem C, Weng Y, Tran A, Baaden M, et al. (2011) X-ray structures of general anaesthetics bound to a pentameric ligand-gated ion channel. Nature 469: 428–431.
48. Husain SS, Ziebell MR, Ruesch D, Hong F, Arevalo E, et al. (2003) 2-(3-Methyl-3H-diaziren-3-yl)ethyl 1-(1-phenylethyl)-1H-imidazole-5-carboxylate: A derivative of the stereoselective general anesthetic etomidate for photolabeling ligand-gated ion channels. J Med Chem 46: 1257–1265.
49. Husain SS, Nirthanan S, Ruesch D, Solt K, Cheng Q, et al. (2006) Synthesis of trifluoromethylaryl diazirine and benzophenone derivatives of etomidate that are potent general anesthetics and effective photolabels for probing sites on ligand-gated ion channels. J Med Chem 49: 4818–4825.
50. Husain SS, Stewart D, Desai R, Hamouda AK, Li SG, et al. (2010) p-Trifluoromethyldiazirinyl-etomidate: a potent photoreactive general anesthetic derivative of etomidate that is selective for ligand-gated cationic ion channels. J Med Chem 53: 6432–6444.
51. Godefroi EF, Janssen PAJ, Van der Eycken CAM, Van Heertum AHMT, Niemegeers CJE (1965) DL-(1-arylalkyl)imidazole-5-carboxylate esters. A novel type of hypnotic agents. J Med Chem 56: 220–223.
52. Atucha E, Hammerschmidt F, Zolle I, Sieghart W, Berger ML (2009) Structure-activity relationship of etomidate derivatives at the GABA(A) receptor: Comparison with binding to 11beta-hydroxylase. Bioorg Med Chem Lett 19: 4284–4287.
53. Pejo E, Santer P, Jeffrey S, Gallin H, Husain SS, et al. (2014) Analogues of Etomidate: Modifications around Etomidate's Chiral Carbon and the Impact on In Vitro and In Vivo Pharmacology. Anesthesiology 121: 290–301.
54. Forman SA, Miller KW (2011) Anesthetic sites and allosteric mechanisms of action on Cys-loop ligand-gated ion channels. Can J Anaesth 58: 191–205.
55. Spurny R, Billen B, Howard RJ, Brams M, Debaveye S, et al. (2013) Multisite binding of a general anesthetic to the prokaryotic pentameric Erwinia chrysanthemi ligand-gated ion channel (ELIC). J Biol Chem 288: 8355–8364.

Inflammation and MiR-21 Pathways Functionally Interact to Downregulate PDCD4 in Colorectal Cancer

Oliver Peacock, Andrew C. Lee, Fraser Cameron, Rebecca Tarbox, Natasha Vafadar-Isfahani, Cristina Tufarelli*, Jonathan N. Lund

Surgery Group, Division of Medical Sciences and Graduate Entry Medicine, School of Medicine, University of Nottingham, Royal Derby Hospital, Derby, United Kingdom

Abstract

Inflammation plays a direct role in colorectal cancer (CRC) progression; however the molecular mechanisms responsible for this effect are unclear. The inflammation induced cyclooxygenase 2 (COX-2) enzyme required for the production of Prostaglandin E2 (PGE_2), can promote colorectal cancer by decreasing expression of the tumour suppressor gene Programmed Cell Death 4 (PDCD4). As PDCD4 is also a direct target of the oncogene microRNA-21 (miR-21) we investigated the relationship between the COX-2 and miR-21 pathways in colorectal cancer progression. Gene expression profile in tumour and paired normal mucosa from 45 CRC patients demonstrated that up-regulation of COX-2 and miR-21 in tumour tissue correlates with worse Dukes' stage. In vitro studies in colonic adenocarcinoma cells revealed that treatment with the selective COX-2 inhibitor NS398 significantly decreased miR-21 levels ($p = 0.0067$) and increased PDCD4 protein levels ($p < 0.001$), whilst treatment with PGE_2 up-regulated miR-21 expression ($p = 0.019$) and down-regulated PDCD4 protein ($p < 0.05$). These findings indicate that miR-21 is a component of the COX-2 inflammation pathway and that this pathway promotes worsening of disease stage in colorectal cancer by inducing accumulation of PGE_2 and increasing expression of miR-21 with consequent downregulation of the tumour suppressor gene PDCD4.

Editor: Kalpana Ghoshal, The Ohio State University, United States of America

Funding: The work was supported by a donation from the Derby Colorectal Cancer Fund. The funders had no role in study design, data collection and analysis, decision to publish, or preparation of the manuscript.

Competing Interests: The authors have declared that no competing interests exist.

* Email: cristina.tufarelli@nottingham.ac.uk

Introduction

Colorectal cancer is the third most common cause of cancer related deaths worldwide [1]. Approximately half of all patients diagnosed with colorectal cancer ultimately die of the condition [2]. The five year survival rate has increased to approximately 50–55%, which is attributed mainly to an earlier diagnosis and better tailoring of treatments [3]. Death from colorectal cancer can be prevented by early stage disease detection, but unfortunately it is often detected at an advanced stage when prognosis is worse [4]. The prognosis in colorectal cancer patients is associated with disease stage at the time of diagnosis.

The exact "trigger" for the development of colorectal cancer is still unknown. In 1990, a series of morphological steps known as the normal mucosa-adenoma-adenocarcinoma sequence in colorectal cancer due to genetic alterations was proposed [5]. However, many genetic events lead to the development of sporadic colorectal cancer; no single event occurs in all cancers and therefore no single pattern is applicable to every tumour [6]. Therefore, understanding specific genetic events that occur in colorectal carcinogenesis may have significant implications for diagnosis, prognosis and potentially gene therapy in the future.

There has been a recent resurgence in interest into the causal link between inflammation and cancer. Epidemiological studies have shown that chronic inflammation predisposes individuals to various types of cancer [7]. It is estimated that 15% to 20% of all cancer deaths worldwide are linked with underlying chronic infections and inflammatory responses within such individuals [7]. There is evidence from animal studies and observations in humans that a daily aspirin might be effective in preventing several common cancers [8,9]. This has been confirmed recently in follow-up studies of patients recruited originally for randomised trials of daily aspirin versus control in the prevention of vascular events [10–12]. In these trials, allocation to aspirin resulted in a 40% reduction in cancer deaths from 5 years onwards [11] and a sustained reduction in cancer-related death at 20 year follow-up [10,12]. Observational studies have also shown that aspirin use is associated with reduced distant metastasis and recurrence in common adenocarcinomas [13–15], suggesting that inflammation could play a role in progression as well as in development of cancer.

One of the possible reasons for the observed chemo preventive effects of aspirin in colorectal cancer is its ability to reduce tumour development by inhibition of cyclooxygenase 2 (COX-2) [16]. There is increasing evidence linking the pro-inflammatory enzyme COX-2 with the development and progression of colorectal cancer. COX-2 is induced in colonic epithelium in active inflammatory bowel disease (IBD) [17] and its up-regulation results in elevated levels of prostaglandin (PG), in particular PGE_2 that is a downstream mediator of COX-2 and promotes many carcinogenic pathways including cellular proliferation, inhibition of apoptosis and angiogenesis [18]. This contributes to the chronic inflammatory process orchestrating a tumour-supporting micro-environment, further linking inflammation with carcinogenesis.

The mechanistic linkage between inflammation and cancer is still not completely clear. Increasing evidence suggests that micro-RNAs (miRNAs) are involved in the regulation of inflammatory processes and are dysregulated in inflammatory conditions [19], including ulcerative colitis [20]. Therefore miRNAs dysregulation represents a potential molecular mechanism for inflammatory pathways to mediate cancer development and progression [21]. In particular, expression levels of miR-21 are increased in active inflammation in ulcerative colitis, which may be associated with the increased risk of cancer development with this condition [22]. Up-regulation of miR-21 has also been reported in other inflamed states including allergic airway inflammation [23], inflammatory skin conditions [19] and *Helicobacter pylori* associated gastric cancer [24]. miR-21 has been recently demonstrated to be a genuine oncogene in pre-B-cell lymphoma [25] and found to be over-expressed in most tumour types [26]. miR-21 is a potent stimulator of tissue and vascular invasion in colorectal cancer and these effects appear in part mediated by its ability to prevent translation of one of the miR-21 target genes, Programmed Cell Death 4 (PDCD4) [27]. More recently, a study has also shown significant down-regulation of PDCD4 in active IBD compared with inactive IBD, which also correlated with up-regulation of miR-21 [28], further supporting the link between inflammation, miR-21 and carcinogenesis.

Our aim was to investigate whether a functional interaction exist between the COX-2 (pro-inflammatory enzyme with increased expression in CRC) and miR-21 (oncogenic miR overexpressed in CRC) pathways leading to downregulation of the tumour suppressor PDCD4 in colorectal cancer not associated with previous chronic inflammatory disease.

Materials and Methods

Human tissues

This study received ethical approval from the Derbyshire Research Ethics Committee for collection of colorectal cancer tissue and matched normal mucosa from patients who underwent surgical resection for colorectal cancer between August and December 2010 at the Royal Derby Hospital, Derby, UK.

All patients diagnosed with colorectal cancer were discussed at the Royal Derby Hospital colorectal Multidisciplinary Team Meeting after radiological staging, and those deemed suitable for resection with curative intent were eligible for inclusion. Written informed consent was taken and patients unable or not willing to provide informed consent were excluded from the study, as were those withdrawing consent at any stage.

Cell Culture

The HCA-7 cell line was obtained from the Health Protection Agency Culture Collection (HPACC, Porton Down, UK). Cells were cultured in Dulbecco's Modified Eagle Media (DMEM) (GIBCO, Paisley, UK) supplemented with 10% foetal bovine serum (Fisher Scientific, Loughborough, UK), 2mM L-Glutamine (Sigma-Aldrich, Poole, UK), penicillin (50 units/ml) and streptomycin (50 μg/ml) (Sigma-Aldrich). Cells were cultured in 75cm^3 vented flasks (TSZ Scientific, Framingham, MA, USA) in humidified incubators at 37°C with 5% CO_2 (Sanyo, Osaka, Japan).

Cell Line Transfections and treatments

Cells were seeded at 500,000 cells/well into a 6 well plate and incubated at 37°C with 5% CO_2 until they reached 70% confluence.

For miR-21 inhibition studies, cells were transfected with miR-21 inhibitor (100nM) or a negative scrambled control (100nM) (miRIDIAN, Dharmacon Lafayette, CO, USA), using Dharmafect 2 lipid transfection reagent (Dharmacon Lafayette, CO, USA) according to the manufacturer's instructions.

For COX-2 inhibition, cells were treated with serum free medium containing the control (0.1% DMSO) or 100 μM NS398 (selective COX-2 inhibitor, Cayman Chemical, Michigan, USA) for 72 hours. For Prostaglandin E_2 (PGE_2) treatment, cells were grown 24 hours with serum free medium containing DMSO vehicle alone or 1 μM PGE_2 so that the final concentration of DMSO in both conditions was the same (0.1%). For combined miR-21 inhibition and PGE_2 treatment, PGE_2 was added to the culture 48 hours after miR-21 inhibitor transfection and cells were cultured for a further 24 hours.

RNA analyses

Total RNA extraction was performed using TRI Reagent following the manufacturer's protocol (Sigma-Aldrich) and quantified using a Nanodrop spectrophotometer (Thermo Fisher Scientific, Wilmington, DE, USA).

For the miR-21 studies, a total of 6 ng of total RNA was used to reverse transcribe miR-21 and RNU44 control into cDNA following the TaqMan miRNA protocol (Applied Biosystems, Foster City, CA, USA), using hairpin primers directed to miR-21 and RNU44 as a control in a thermocycler (GeneAmp PCR System 9700, Applied Biosystems) for 30min at 16°C, 30 min at 42°C, 5min at 85°C. Real-time quantitative polymerase chain reaction was then performed using miRNAs specific TaqMan probe assays (miR-21, ID 000397; RNU44, ID 001094; Applied Biosystems) in a Chromo4 thermal cycler (Bio-Rad Laboratories LTD, Hemel Hempstead, UK). miR-21 expression levels were normalised to RNU44 and calculated using the $2^{-\Delta\Delta Ct}$ method [29] using commercially available normal colon RNA as a calibrator.

For *COX-2* and *PDCD4* analyses, 30ng of total RNA was converted to cDNA with random hexamers using the TaqMan high capacity cDNA reverse transcription protocol (Applied Biosystems, Foster City, CA, USA). Real time PCRs were performed according to the manufacturer instructions in a Chromo4 real time cycler (Bio-Rad Laboratories Ltd) using commercially available 20x TaqMan assays (Applied Biosystems) for *PDCD4* (Hs00377253_m1) and *COX-2* (PTGS2 - Hs00153133_m1), alongside the control genes *GAPDH* (Hs02258991_g1), *PGK1* (Hs00943178_g1) and *HPRT* (Hs01003267_m1). For the experiments in cell lines, quantification was performed in accordance to MIQE (Minimum Information for Publication of Quantitative Real-Time PCR Experiments) guidelines [30] relatively to the geometric mean of the reference genes *GAPDH*, *PGK1*, *HPRT* using the GenEX software (MultiD Analysis; Göteborg, Sweden). Due to limited sample's amounts, in human tissues expression was quantified relatively to *GAPDH* alone as described above for miR-21 analyses.

Protein analyses

Protein extractions and quantification were performed as previously described [31]. Western blotting was performed using the loading control anti-beta actin antibody (1:1000 dilution; Abcam, Cambridge, UK) in combination with anti-PDCD4 antibody (1:500 dilution; Sigma-Aldrich) or anti-COX-2 (1:1000

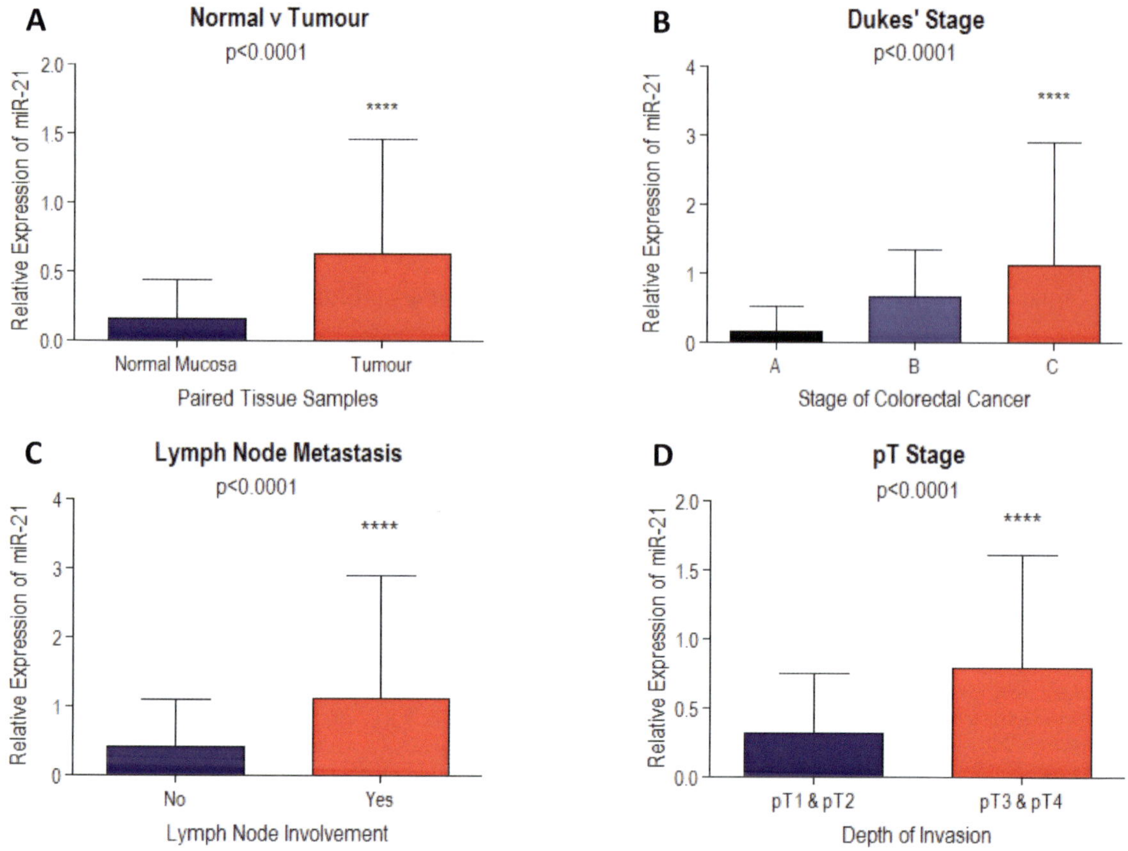

Figure 1. miR-21 expression in primary colorectal tissue samples, calculated relatively to that of the control miRNA RNU44, was studied in primary tumour and matched adjacent normal mucosa (n = 45; A); in Dukes' A (n = 9), B (n = 23) and C (n = 13) stages (B); in lymph node negative (No; n = 32) versus lymph node positive (Yes, n = 13) cases (C); and in tumours displaying lower (pT1 & pT2; n = 11) versus higher (pT3 & pT4; n = 34) depth of invasion (D). Column bar graphs indicate the median and whiskers demonstrate the IQR of miR-21 expression. Note that significant increase in miR-21 expression is observed in tumours, and this increases further with worsening stage, lymphnode involvement and depth of invasion. Statistical significance was calculated using the Wilcoxon signed-rank test in A, the Kruskall-Wallis test in B, and the Mann-Whitney U test in C and D.

dilution; Abcam). Anti-rabbit IgG antibody conjugated to alkaline phosphatase was used as secondary antibody (1:30,000 dilution; DAKO, Ely, UK) for detection of primary antibody binding. Immunocomplexes were visualised by enhanced chemiluminescence using the ECL kit (Bio-Rad) according to the manufacturer's protocol. The chemidoc system was used to capture images and Quantity One (Bio-Rad) software was used for quantification of bands' intensities.

Elisa Analysis

PGE_2 levels were measured in the media of HCA-7 treated and untreated cells using the PGE_2 elisa detection kit (Cayman Chemical, Ann Arbor, Michigan USA) according to the manufacturer's instructions. Plates were read with a plate photocytometer at 450 nm (Wallac 1420 Victor; Perkin-Elmer, Waltham, MA, USA).

Statistical Analysis

Statistical analysis was performed using GraphPad Prism Version 5.03 (GraphPad Software, La Jolla, CA, USA). The Kolmogorov-Smirnov test demonstrated all the tissue sample data to be non-parametric and all the cell line data to be parametric. Therefore patient's data is expressed as medians and range, whilst cell line data is expressed as mean and standard error of the mean. The Wilcoxon signed-rank test (paired data); the Mann-Whitney U test (unpaired) and the Kruskall-Wallis test were used for comparative analysis of patient's data. The paired t-test (paired data); the t-test (unpaired) and the ANOVA test were used for comparative analysis of cell line's data.

Statistical significance was determined at $p \leq 0.05$ for both patient's and cell line's data.

Results

Increase in miR-21 directly relates to increase in COX-2 mRNA levels in CRC patients

We performed our study on primary colorectal cancer tissue and paired normal mucosa collected between August and December 2010 from 45 elective patients with sporadic cases of CRC. A prospectively maintained database was populated with patient demographics, neoadjuvant therapies and tumour characteristics. The tumour histopathology was classified according to the national minimum data set for colorectal cancer designed by the Royal College of Pathologists, UK [32]. No patients were excluded or had withdrawn from the study and none had benign disease. The median age was 69 (range 51–88) years and the majority were male patients. Four patients with rectal cancer who received neo-adjuvant chemo-radiotherapy were also included based on previous studies demonstrating that expression of miR-21 is equivalent between radiated and non-radiated tissue [33]. All patients had a complete resection and histology confirmed all tumours were adenocarcinomas. (Table S1 and S2 in File S1)

Using by real time RT-PCR we studied expression of *COX-2* and miR-21 in tumour tissues as compared to normal mucosa in our cohort of CRC patients. Relative expression of miR-21 was significantly up-regulated in the CRC tissue compared with the matched normal mucosa ($p<0.0001$, Wilcoxon matched-pairs signed rank test; Fig. 1A). Moreover, expression levels of miR-21 were correlated with the commonly used clinical-pathological features for CRC (Table 1). Higher expression of miR-21 in tumour tissues significantly correlated with a worse Dukes' stage ($p<0.0001$, Kruskall-Wallis test; Fig. 1B), lymph node metastasis ($p<0.0001$, Mann-Whitney U test; Fig. 1C), and depth of tumour invasion (pT stage; $p<0.0001$, Mann-Whitney U test; Fig. 1D). These findings are in agreement with previous reports [34,35], and confirm that miR-21 is up-regulated in CRC with increasing expression levels correlating with increased severity of the disease.

Relative expression of *PDCD4* was significantly down-regulated in CRC tissues compared with matched normal mucosa ($p<0.0001$, Wilcoxon matched-pairs signed rank test; Fig. 2A). However, there was no correlation between *PDCD4* expression in tumour tissues and the Dukes' stage, with expression in Dukes'A stage being already significantly decreased as compared to normal tissue and no further decrease seen in more advanced stages (Fig. 2B). It is unlikely that the observed downregulation of *PDCD4* at the RNA level is caused by miR-21 given that this micro-RNA acts to prevent PDCD4 mRNA translation rather than induce its degradation or transcriptional repression [27]. Given that all the patients studied carried malignant tumours with an assigned Dukes' stage, the data suggest that during progression of malignancy increasing amounts of miR-21 lead to inhibition of translation of the already decreased levels of *PDCD4* mRNA. Ethics constraints prevented us from analysing PDCD4 protein levels in these patients to confirm this hypothesis and we recurred to *in vitro* studies to gain mechanistic insights (see next section).

Interestingly, relative expression of *COX-2* mRNA was significantly up-regulated in tumour tissues compared with their matched normal mucosa ($p<0.0001$, Wilcoxon matched-pairs signed rank test; Fig. 2C). Moreover, similarly to what was observed with miR-21, relative expression of *COX-2* mRNA in tumour tissues significantly correlated with a worse Dukes' stage ($p<0.0001$, Kruskall-Wallis test; Fig. 2D). Given that miR-21 and inflammation have both been shown to decrease PDCD4 protein levels [27,36], a possible interpretation of these findings is that increase in miR-21 and *COX-2* may be functionally related and that they could lead to downregulation of PDCD4 through a common pathway.

HCA-7 cells are a suitable system for analysing the relationship between miR-21 and COX-2 overexpression in CRC

To further investigate the potential of a functional relationship between COX-2 and miR-21 in the down-regulation of PDCD4 in CRC we recurred to an *in vitro* cell culture system. We chose the human colonic adenocarcinoma cell line HCA-7 isolated from a Dukes' B tumour [37] because it has high endogenous levels of COX-2 [38] and following treatment with the COX-2 inhibitor NS398 increases expression of *PDCD4* [39]. In order to determine whether HCA-7 cells are a good system in which to study the functional relationship between the miR-21 and COX-2 pathways, we first needed to determine whether miR-21 is expressed and is responsible for *PDCD4* downregulation in these cells. To achieve these we used RT-PCR to study the levels of miR-21 in untreated HCA-7 cells or in cells treated with 100nM of a miR-21 inhibitor or scramble control based on published work showing that this concentration is non-cytotoxic and effective in inhibitory studies [40].

We found that miR-21 is expressed at high levels in HCA-7 cells and these levels are not affected by treatment with scramble small RNAs but are significantly decreased ($p<0.0001$, unpaired t-test) following 72 hours treatment with a specific miR-21 small RNA inhibitor (Fig. 3A). No significant differences in PDCD4 mRNA

Table 1. Relative expression of miR-21 with common clinical-pathological features of colorectal cancer.

Variables	Patients	p-Value
Histological Type:		
Well Differentiated	4	
Moderate & Poorly Differentiated	41	p = 0.0002
Depth of Invasion:		
pT1 & pT2	11	p<0.0001
pT3 & pT4	34	
Dukes' Stage:		
A	9	
B	23	p<0.0001
C	13	
Lymph Node Metastasis:		
Positive	13	p<0.0001
Negative	32	
Vascular Invasion		
Positive	13	p = 0.01
Negative	32	

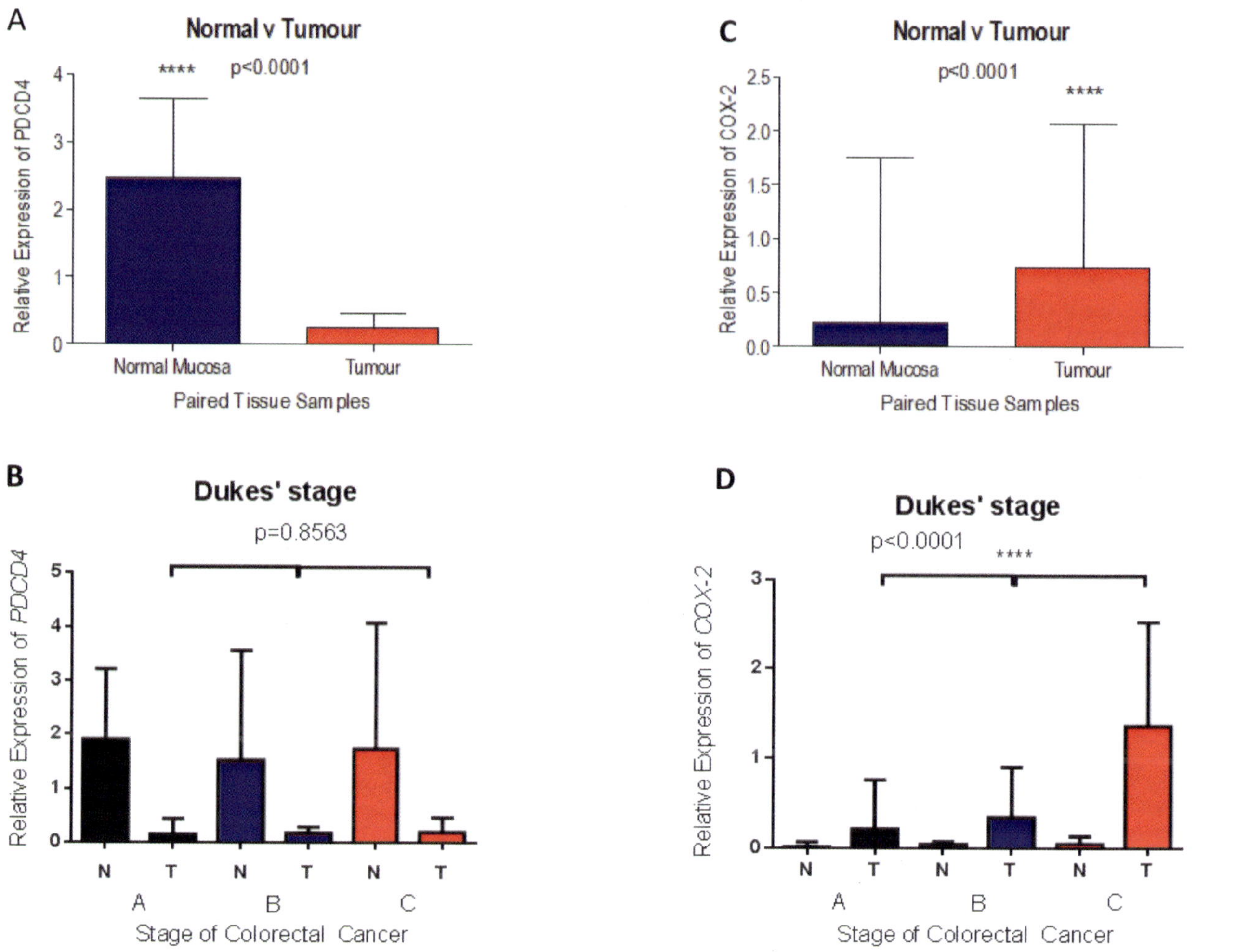

Figure 2. Expression of *PDCD4* and *COX-2* mRNA in primary colorectal tissue samples calculated relatively to that of the control gene *GAPDH*. Combined relative expression of PDCD4 and COX-2 was analysed in primary tumour versus matched adjacent normal mucosa (n = 45; A and C respectively), and in normal (N) and tumour (T) tissues from Dukes' A (n = 9), B (n = 23) and C (n = 13) stages (B and D respectively). The column bar graph indicates the median and the whiskers demonstrate the IQR of mRNA expression. Statistical significance was calculated using the Wilcoxon signed-rank test in A and C; the Kruskall-Wallis test in B and D. Note that *PDCD4* is downregulated in tumour versus normal, but no differences are seen in the remaining expression in tumours of different Dukes' stages. By contrast *COX-2* levels increase in tumour and with disease stage.

levels were observed by quantitative RT-PCR in any of the treatment conditions (Fig. 3B); by contrast, a significant increase ($p = 0.002$, unpaired t-test) in PDCD4 was observed at the protein level by western blot in the miR-21 inhibitor treated cells compared to untreated or scramble control treated cells. These findings are consistent with miR-21 acting to inhibit translation of PDCD4 mRNA rather than directing its degradation and confirm that miR-21 plays a role in PDCD4 downregulation in HCA-7 cells. Therefore both the COX-2 and miR-21 pathways contribute to downregulation of PDCD4 in HCA-7 cells, making them a suitable system in which to study whether a functional relationship exists between the two pathways.

Relation between miR-21 and COX-2 in the downregulation of PDCD4 in HCA-7 cells

To further investigate the functional interaction between the miR-21 and COX-2 pathways, we first analysed COX-2 mRNA and protein levels in HCA-7 cells after 72 hours treatment with the miR-21 inhibitor compared to scramble control and untreated cells. No difference in COX-2 expression was observed neither at the mRNA nor at the protein levels ($p = 0.62$ and $p = 0.83$ respectively, unpaired t test), showing that COX-2 is not a target of miR-21 (Fig. S1 in File S1).

We next treated HCA-7 cells with 100 μM NS398, a specific COX-2 inhibitor reported to be non-cytotoxic and effective at this concentration in cell culture [41], or with vehicle alone (0.1% DMSO). COX-2 plays a critical role during inflammation in the initial steps of the conversion of arachidonic acid to prostaglandins including prostaglandin E (PGE_2) and up-regulation of COX-2 in colorectal cancer has been shown to associate with marked increase in the production of PGE_2 [42]. Using Elisa to measure levels of PGE_2 we found a significant decrease ($p = 0.006$, unpaired t test) in the media of cells treated with NS398 compared to untreated cells or cells treated with vehicle alone, consistent with inhibition of COX-2 catalytic activity (Fig. S2 in File S1).

Having established effectiveness of the treatment we then measured the relative expression of miR-21 and we could detect a significant decrease in miR-21 following NS398 treatment for 72 hours ($p < 0.01$, unpaired t test; Fig. 4A). By contrast, treatment of HCA-7 cells with NS398 did not alter expression of PDCD4

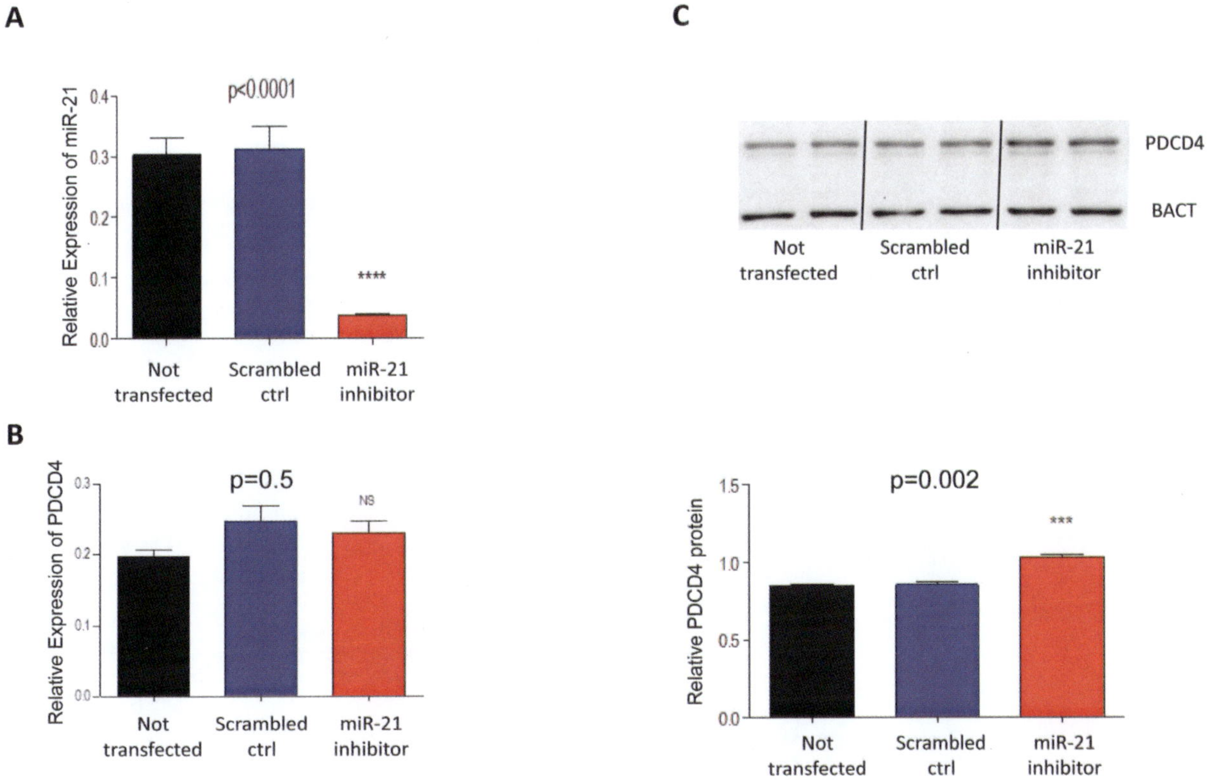

Figure 3. miR-21 and *PDCD4* expression in HCA-7 cells treated with miR-21 inhibitor. Following 72 hours from transfection significant decrease in miR-21 levels are seen only in cells transfected with miR-21 inhibitor (**A**). *PDCD4* mRNA levels were not affected by inhibition of miR-21 (**B**). Western blot analysis of PDCD4 (**C** top panel for a representative blot) reveals a significant increase in protein levels in cells transfected with the inhibitor as compared to untreated or scramble control treated cells, when quantified relatively to beta actin protein (BACT) as a loading control (**C** bottom panel). The column bar graph indicates the mean and the whiskers demonstrate the standard error of the mean (SEM). Statistical significance was calculated using the unpaired t-test. Experiments were repeated three times and analysed in duplicate. Untreated = cells culture in media; scramble = cells transfected with scramble RNA inhibitors; miR-21 inhibitor = cells treated with the miR-21 RNA inhibitor.

mRNA ($p = 0.74$, unpaired t test) (Fig. 4B), an observation that is in contrast to the previously reported 1.5 fold upregulation of PDCD4 mRNA following treatment of HCA-7 cells with NS398 [39]. The difference might be due to the methods used: the latter study analysed PDCD4 mRNA expression by northern blot and quantified it relatively to GAPDH, whilst in our study we have measured mRNA levels using quantitative RT-PCR and normalised the data using the geometric mean of three reference genes (GAPDH, PGK and HPRT) in accordance to the MIQE guidelines [30] (see methods). Our real time PCR data suggests that NS398 treatment leads to a decrease in GAPDH levels (Fig. S3 in File S1) and this change would result in an apparent increase in PDCD4 levels if GAPDH was used as the sole reference gene. Therefore we conclude that NS398 treatment does not alter PDCD4 transcription rate or mRNA stability; however, consistent with the observed decrease in miR-21, significant up-regulation in PDCD4 protein expression ($p<0.001$, unpaired t test) was observed in NS398 treated cells as compared to untreated or vehicle alone cells (Fig. 4C). These data indicate that downregulation of PDCD4 by COX-2 is not a consequence of decreased PDCD4 mRNA synthesis or stability, but rather that COX-2 may act by promoting an increase in miR-21 which in turn inhibits translation of PDCD4 mRNA.

COX-2 activation of miR-21 in HCA-7 cells is mediated by PGE_2

Given the role of COX-2 in the production of prostaglandins, to investigate the mechanism underlying activation of miR-21 by COX-2 we treated HCA-7 cells with 1 μM PGE_2 for 24 hours as this concentration was shown to work effectively on these cells [38]. We found that miR-21 expression was significantly upregulated ($p = 0.019$, unpaired t test) in PGE_2 treated cells as compared to vehicle (0.1% DMSO) treated or untreated cells (Fig. 5A). No changes in PDCD4 mRNA levels were observed in PGE_2 treated cells (Fig. 5B); however a significant decrease ($p< 0.05$, unpaired t test) in PDCD4 protein levels was observed which paralleled the increase in miR-21 (Fig. 5C). Combined treatment with PGE_2 and miR-21 inhibitor brought the levels of miR-21 down to levels comparable with those in untreated cells (Fig. S4 in File S1), and treatment with aspirin also led to a decrease in miR-21 levels (Fig. S5 in File S1). These data suggest that COX-2 driven downregulation of PDCD4 in this model system is mainly due to PGE_2 induced upregulation of miR-21.

Discussion

Dysregulation of miRNAs is a recognised step in the pathogenesis of many cancer types, including CRC. miR-21 is a miRNA frequently upregulated in CRC, whose increased expression levels are associated with poorer therapeutic outcomes in CRC [34]. We

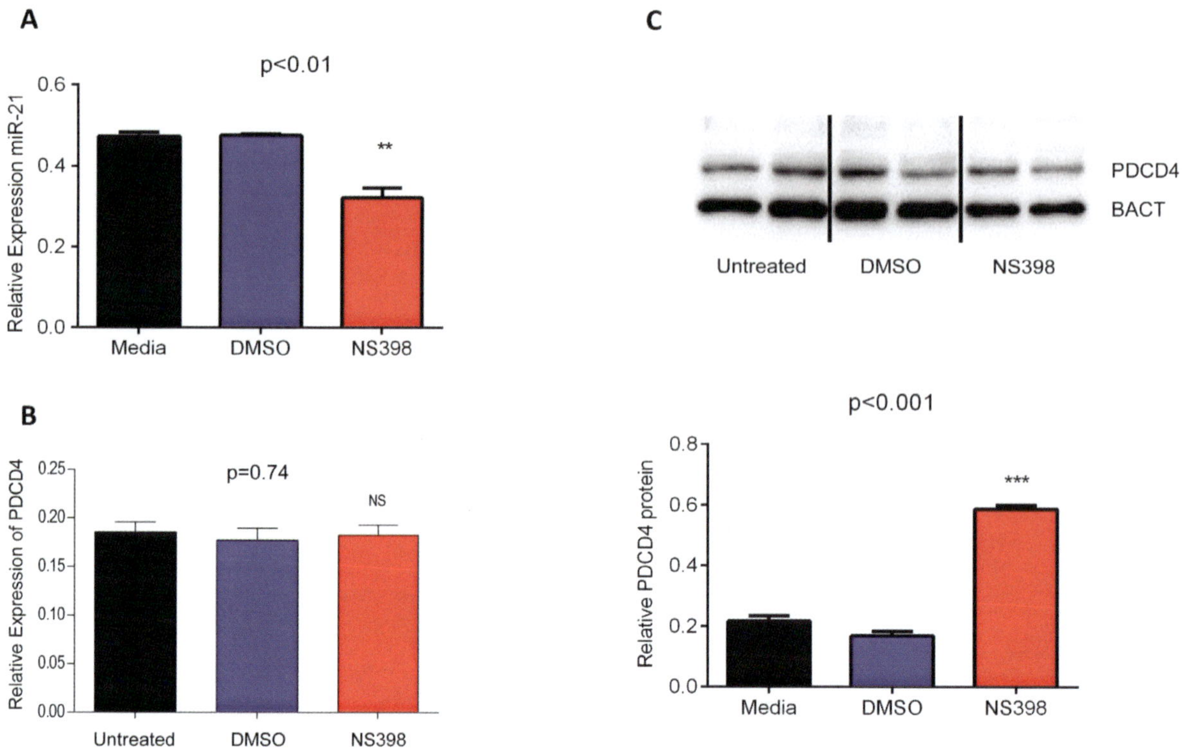

Figure 4. miR-21 and *PDCD4* expression in HCA-7 cells treated with the COX-2 inhibitor NS398. Following 72 hours treatment significant decrease in miR-21 levels is seen in NS398 treated cells (**A**). *PDCD4* mRNA levels are not affected by NS398 treatment (**B**). Western blot analysis of PDCD4 (**C** top panel for a representative blot) reveals a significant increase in protein levels in NS398 treated cells as compared to untreated or vehicle alone (DMSO) treated cells, when quantified relatively to beta actin protein (BACT) as a loading control (**C** bottom panel). The column bar graph indicates the mean and the whiskers demonstrate the standard error of the mean (SEM). Statistical significance was calculated using the unpaired t-test. Experiments were repeated three times and analysed in triplicate. Untreated = cells cultured in media; DMSO = cells cultured in media supplemented with 0.1% DMSO vehicle; NS398 = cells cultured in media supplemented with NS398 prepared in DMSO to a final concentration of 100 μM NS398 and 0.1% DMSO.

have confirmed that over-expression of miR-21 correlates significantly with worse pathological staging in our CRC patient's cohort (Fig. 1), comprised of patients who presented with tumours of an assigned Dukes' stage, suggesting an important role of miR-21 in cancer invasion and dissemination.

Few of the potential downstream targets regulated by miR-21 have been confirmed, and these include the programmed cell death 4 (PDCD4) tumour suppressor gene that inhibits neoplastic transformation [43]. Recent studies have shown a progressive reduction in PDCD4 expression from normal mucosa, to polyp, to colorectal tumour [33]. Interestingly a significant increase in miR-21 was seen in CRC compared to normal, but not between adenomatous polyps and normal, although a decrease in PDCD4 expression was evident at this transition [33]. In our cohort we observed a decrease in PDCD4 mRNA levels in the tumours relative to the normal tissues, but no changes as disease progressed by Dukes' stage (Fig. 2A). Taken together these observations suggest that at the transition from normal to hyperproliferation downregulation of PDCD4 might be due to regulation at the level of transcription and/or RNA and protein stability. However, in the transition to malignancy miR-21 mediated inhibition of translation of PDCD4 protein levels of the already decreased levels of *PDCD4* mRNA becomes predominant, thus promoting further progression of malignancy. Therefore determining the upstream factors that influence miR-21 expression is instrumental in establishing whether and how miR-21 contributes to malignancy progression and to provide potential therapeutic targets.

Given that in our cohort of CRC patients upregulation of miR-21 is positively related to that of COX-2 mRNA and with worse pathological staging (Fig. 1 and 2B), we hypothesised that miR-21 upregulation in CRC might be linked to an inflammatory response. Circumstantial evidence supporting this hypothesis includes the observations that inflammation can lead to down-regulation of PDCD4 in colorectal tissue [36] and that miR-21 upregulation in gastric cancer is due to PGE_2 induced activation of NF-kB [44]. Using an *in vitro* culture system we have shown that in HCA-7 cells PDCD4 downregulation is mediated by miR-21 at the post-transcriptional level as no change in PDCD4 mRNA levels were seen (Fig. 3). This confirms the work of a previous group who identified a conserved target site for miR-21 within the 3′-UTR of PDCD4 [27]. We found that whilst down-regulation of miR-21 by transfection of a miR-21 inhibitor had no effect on the expression of COX-2 (Fig. S1 in File S1), inhibition of COX-2 by the specific COX-2 inhibitor NS398 or use of the anti-inflammatory aspirin led to decrease in miR-21 levels (Fig. 3 and Fig. S5 in File S1). In NS398 treated cells, miR-21 downregulation correlates with an increase in PDCD4 protein without changes in PDCD4 mRNA levels (Fig. 4), further supporting a role of miR-21 in the downregulation of PDCD4. Previous studies have demonstrated that NS398 exerts several anti-carcinogenic effects in colon cancer by inducing apoptosis [45], whilst also inhibiting cell cycle progression [39], angiogenesis [46] and metastasis [47]. Our novel finding of a significant up-regulation in PDCD4 protein levels following NS398 treatment

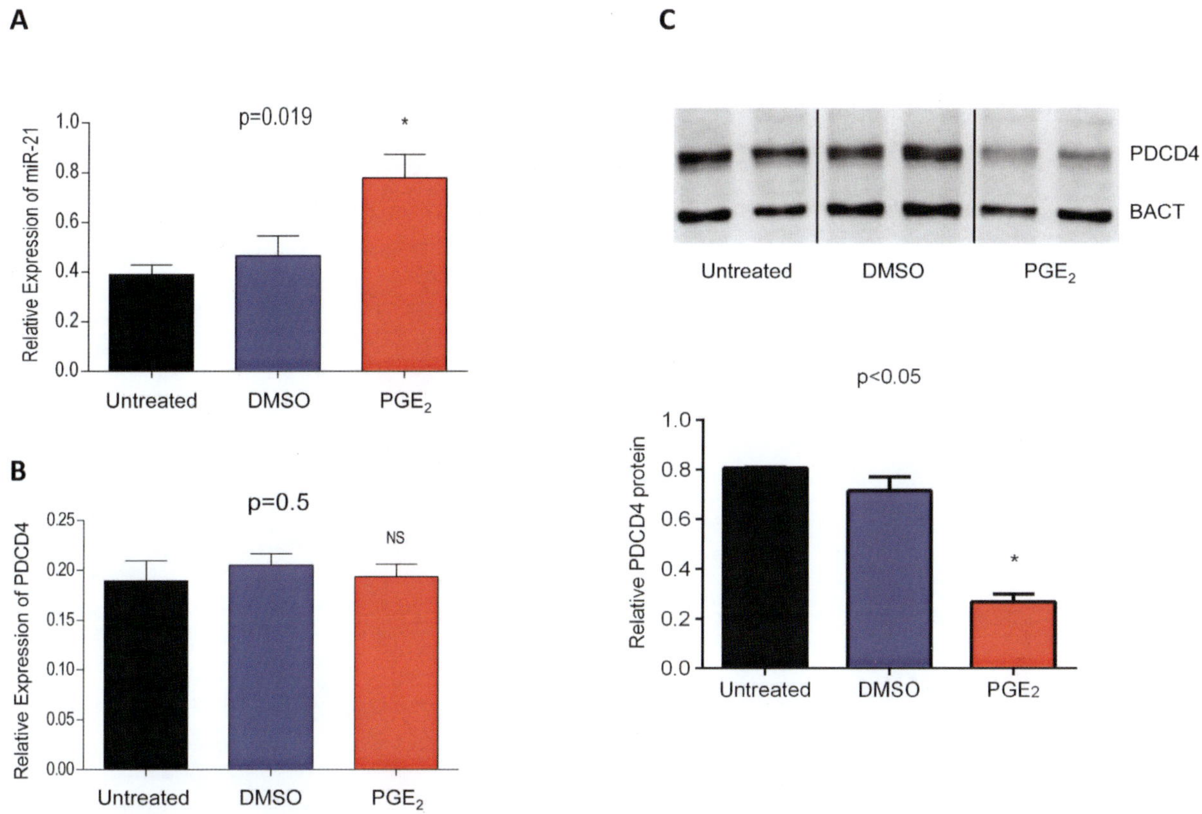

Figure 5. miR-21 and *PDCD4* expression in HCA-7 cells treated with PGE_2. After 24 hours treatment significant increase in miR-21 levels is seen in PGE_2 treated cells (**A**). *PDCD4* mRNA levels are not affected by PGE_2 treatment (**B**). Western blot analysis of PDCD4 (**C** top panel for a representative blot) reveals a significant decrease in protein levels in PGE_2 treated cells as compared to untreated or vehicle alone (DMSO) treated cells, when quantified relatively to beta actin protein (BACT) as a loading control (**C** bottom panel). The column bar graph indicates the mean and the whiskers demonstrate the standard error of the mean (SEM). Statistical significance was calculated using the unpaired t-test. Experiments were repeated three times and analysed in duplicate. Untreated = cells cultured in media; DMSO = cells cultured in media supplemented with 0.1% DMSO vehicle; PGE_2 = cells cultured in media supplemented with PGE_2 prepared in DMSO to a final concentration of 1 µM PGE_2 and 0.1% DMSO.

suggests that the chemo preventive effects of NS398 may in part be attributed to its action on PDCD4. Moreover, the relationship between COX-2 and miR-21 is unidirectional, whereby increase in COX-2 activity drives overexpression of miR-21; therefore miR-21 is a component of the COX-2 pathway, downstream of COX-2. Indeed we found that miR-21 upregulation is a consequence of COX-2 mediated PGE_2 production as treatment of cells with PGE_2 led to increase in miR-21 and decrease in PDCD4 protein, which was reversed by combining PGE_2 and miR-21 inhibitor treatments (Fig. 5 and Fig. S2 in File S1). These findings are in agreement with work by other groups indicating that COX-2 inhibitors induce apoptosis and inhibit angiogenesis *in vitro*, [48,49] whilst also attenuating invasion, angiogenesis and metastasis *in vivo* [50,51].

Our study provides mechanistic insights into the link between inflammation, miR-21 and PDCD4 expression and colorectal cancer progression. Based on our findings it is feasible to propose a model of one of the ways in which persistent inflammation at a site of invasive early stage colorectal tumour can induce progression to more malignant states (Fig. 6). According to our model, continued inflammation at the tumour site leads to progressive increase in COX-2 expression and consequent PGE_2 accumulation which can be blocked by the use of NS398 COX-2 inhibitor (Fig. 6, left side). PGE_2 induces increase in miR-21 expression causing further downregulation of PDCD4 protein levels (and potentially other miR-21 targets) thus facilitating further progression of the tumour to more malignant stages and these effects can be reversed using miR-21 inhibitors (Fig. 6, right side). Interestingly, it has just been reported that the 15-hydroxyprostaglandin dehydrogenase (15-PGDH) mRNA which codes for a key enzyme required for PGE_2 degradation, is a direct target of miR-21 in cholangiocarcinoma cells [52]. Although the presence of this miR-21 mediated effect remains to be proven in CRC, the observation suggests that a reinforcing positive feedback may exists whereby increase in miR-21 induced by PGE_2 favours further accumulation of PGE_2 by preventing its degradation.

Conclusions

In conclusion, we have highlighted the potential benefits of analysing COX-2 and miR-21 expression levels for tumour staging and of correlating these levels to therapeutic response or disease outcome. Moreover, this study has contributed to an improved understanding of the role of miR-21, PDCD4 and COX-2 in colorectal cancer progression. We have demonstrated a functional link between COX-2, miR-21 and PDCD4, which provides further understanding into the beneficial effects of COX-2 inhibitors in colorectal cancer control. Further investigation of the pathway linking inflammation to miR-21 will reveal key intermediate players and their potential to be targeted therapeutically, with the final goal to determine the feasibility of combining

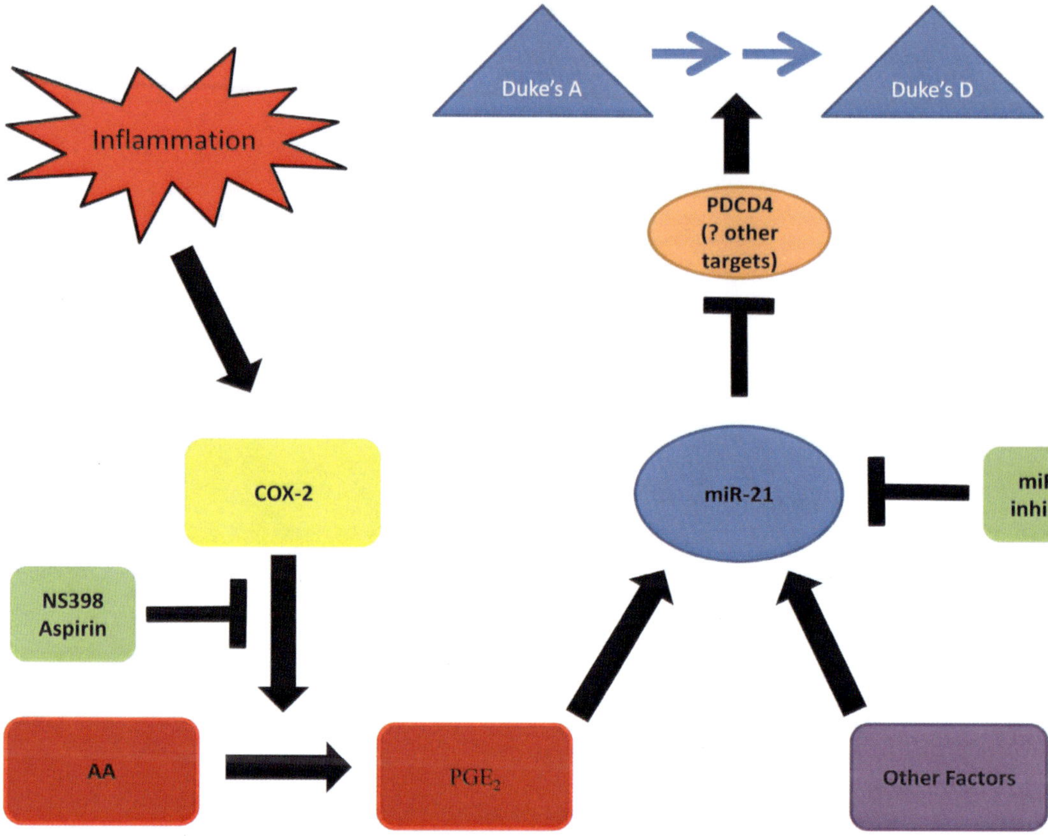

Figure 6. Proposed model of how the inflammation pathway can promote colorectal cancer progression by linking inflammation to downregulation of PDCD4 via miR-21 induction mediated by COX-2 driven accumulation of PGE_2. Persistent inflammation at the tumour site drives increase in COX-2 expression leading to accumulation of PGE_2. This in turn leads to the increase in expression of miR-21 and subsequent downregulation of PDCD4 protein levels facilitating progressive increase to more invasive and metastatic forms of colorectal cancer (from Dukes' A to B, C and D). Our experiments indicate that this pathway can be blocked by COX-2 inhibitors (NS398 and Aspirin) by preventing accumulation of PGE_2 as well as by miR-21 inhibitors. ↑ Activation, ⊤ Inhibition. See text for further details.

the use of anti-inflammatory drugs, with miR-21 inhibitors and strategies targeting intermediate components in the treatment of CRC. These findings therefore provide a basis for identification of potential therapeutic targets in the future management of colorectal cancer.

Supporting Information

File S1 Table of Contents: Method S1. Aspirin treatment of HCA-7 cells (page 1). **Figure S1.** *COX-2* mRNA expression in HCA-7 cells treated with miR-21 inhibitor (page 2). **Figure S2.** PGE2 levels in the media of cells treated with the COX-2 inhibitor NS398 (page 3). **Figure S3.** Expression of *GAPDH* in cells treated with NS398 (page 4). **Figure S4.** miR-21 expression in cells treated with PGE2 and miR-21 inhibitor (page 5). **Figure S5.** miR-21 expression in cells treated with Aspirin (page 6). **Table S1.** Demographics for the cohort of colorectal cancer patients (page 7). **Table S2.** Clinical-pathological staging (page 8).

Acknowledgments

We are grateful to Dr Raheela Khan for support and constructive discussions throughout the course of the project.

Author Contributions

Conceived and designed the experiments: OP CT JNL. Performed the experiments: OP ACL FC RT NV-I CT. Analyzed the data: OP ACL NV-I CT. Contributed reagents/materials/analysis tools: OP CT JNL. Wrote the paper: OP CT JNL. Study supervision: CT JNL.

References

1. Jemal A, Bray F, Center MM, Ferlay J, Ward E, et al. (2011) Global cancer statistics. CA Cancer J Clin 61: 69–90.
2. Figueredo A, Coombes ME, Mukherjee S (2008) Adjuvant therapy for completely resected stage II colon cancer. Cochrane Database Syst Rev: CD005390.
3. UK CR (2011) Bowel Cancer Survival Statistics.
4. Walsh JM, Terdiman JP (2003) Colorectal cancer screening: scientific review. JAMA 289: 1288–1296.
5. Fearon ER, Vogelstein B (1990) A genetic model for colorectal tumorigenesis. Cell 61: 759–767.
6. Smith G, Carey FA, Beattie J, Wilkie MJ, Lightfoot TJ, et al. (2002) Mutations in APC, Kirsten-ras, and p53–alternative genetic pathways to colorectal cancer. Proc Natl Acad Sci U S A 99: 9433–9438.
7. Pisani P, Parkin DM, Munoz N, Ferlay J (1997) Cancer and infection: estimates of the attributable fraction in 1990. Cancer Epidemiol Biomarkers Prev 6: 387–400.
8. Elwood PC, Gallagher AM, Duthie GG, Mur LA, Morgan G (2009) Aspirin, salicylates, and cancer. Lancet 373: 1301–1309.
9. Flossmann E, Rothwell PM (2007) Effect of aspirin on long-term risk of colorectal cancer: consistent evidence from randomised and observational studies. Lancet 369: 1603–1613.

10. Rothwell PM, Wilson M, Elwin CE, Norrving B, Algra A, et al. (2010) Long-term effect of aspirin on colorectal cancer incidence and mortality: 20-year follow-up of five randomised trials. Lancet 376: 1741–1750.
11. Rothwell PM, Price JF, Fowkes FG, Zanchetti A, Roncaglioni MC, et al. (2012) Short-term effects of daily aspirin on cancer incidence, mortality, and non-vascular death: analysis of the time course of risks and benefits in 51 randomised controlled trials. Lancet 379: 1602–1612.
12. Rothwell PM, Fowkes FG, Belch JF, Ogawa H, Warlow CP, et al. (2011) Effect of daily aspirin on long-term risk of death due to cancer: analysis of individual patient data from randomised trials. Lancet 377: 31–41.
13. Chan AT, Ogino S, Fuchs CS (2009) Aspirin use and survival after diagnosis of colorectal cancer. JAMA 302: 649–658.
14. Holmes MD, Chen WY, Li L, Hertzmark E, Spiegelman D, et al. (2010) Aspirin intake and survival after breast cancer. J Clin Oncol 28: 1467–1472.
15. Leitzmann MF, Stampfer MJ, Ma J, Chan JM, Colditz GA, et al. (2002) Aspirin use in relation to risk of prostate cancer. Cancer Epidemiol Biomarkers Prev 11: 1108–1111.
16. Chan AT, Ogino S, Fuchs CS (2007) Aspirin and the risk of colorectal cancer in relation to the expression of COX-2. N Engl J Med 356: 2131–2142.
17. Singer, II, Kawka DW, Schloemann S, Tessner T, Riehl T, et al. (1998) Cyclooxygenase 2 is induced in colonic epithelial cells in inflammatory bowel disease. Gastroenterology 115: 297–306.
18. Greenhough A, Smartt HJ, Moore AE, Roberts HR, Williams AC, et al. (2009) The COX-2/PGE2 pathway: key roles in the hallmarks of cancer and adaptation to the tumour microenvironment. Carcinogenesis 30: 377–386.
19. Sonkoly E, Stahle M, Pivarcsi A (2008) MicroRNAs: novel regulators in skin inflammation. Clin Exp Dermatol 33: 312–315.
20. Wu F, Zikusoka M, Trindade A, Dassopoulos T, Harris ML, et al. (2008) MicroRNAs are differentially expressed in ulcerative colitis and alter expression of macrophage inflammatory peptide-2 alpha. Gastroenterology 135: 1624-1635 e1624.
21. Schetter AJ, Heegaard NH, Harris CC (2010) Inflammation and cancer: interweaving microRNA, free radical, cytokine and p53 pathways. Carcinogenesis 31: 37–49.
22. Lin CJ, Gong HY, Tseng HC, Wang WL, Wu JL (2008) miR-122 targets an anti-apoptotic gene, Bcl-w, in human hepatocellular carcinoma cell lines. Biochem Biophys Res Commun 375: 315–320.
23. Lu TX, Munitz A, Rothenberg ME (2009) MicroRNA-21 is up-regulated in allergic airway inflammation and regulates IL-12p35 expression. J Immunol 182: 4994–5002.
24. Zhang Z, Li Z, Gao C, Chen P, Chen J, et al. (2008) miR-21 plays a pivotal role in gastric cancer pathogenesis and progression. Lab Invest 88: 1358–1366.
25. Medina PP, Nolde M, Slack FJ (2010) OncomiR addiction in an in vivo model of microRNA-21-induced pre-B-cell lymphoma. Nature 467: 86–90.
26. Volinia S, Calin GA, Liu CG, Ambs S, Cimmino A, et al. (2006) A microRNA expression signature of human solid tumors defines cancer gene targets. Proc Natl Acad Sci U S A 103: 2257–2261.
27. Asangani IA, Rasheed SA, Nikolova DA, Leupold JH, Colburn NH, et al. (2008) MicroRNA-21 (miR-21) post-transcriptionally downregulates tumor suppressor Pdcd4 and stimulates invasion, intravasation and metastasis in colorectal cancer. Oncogene 27: 2128–2136.
28. Ludwig K, Fassan M, Mescoli C, Pizzi M, Balistreri M, et al. (2013) PDCD4/miR-21 dysregulation in inflammatory bowel disease-associated carcinogenesis. Virchows Arch 462: 57–63.
29. Pfaffl MW (2001) A new mathematical model for relative quantification in real-time RT-PCR. Nucleic Acids Res 29: e45.
30. Bustin SA, Benes V, Garson JA, Hellemans J, Huggett J, et al. (2009) The MIQE guidelines: minimum information for publication of quantitative real-time PCR experiments. Clin Chem 55: 611–622.
31. Bhatti I, Lee A, James V, Hall RI, Lund JN, et al. (2011) Knockdown of microRNA-21 inhibits proliferation and increases cell death by targeting programmed cell death 4 (PDCD4) in pancreatic ductal adenocarcinoma. J Gastrointest Surg 15: 199–208.
32. The Royal College of Pathologists U (2007) Dataset for colorectal cancer (2nd edition).
33. Chang KH, Miller N, Kheirelseid EA, Ingoldsby H, Hennessy E, et al. (2011) MicroRNA-21 and PDCD4 expression in colorectal cancer. Eur J Surg Oncol.
34. Schetter AJ, Leung SY, Sohn JJ, Zanetti KA, Bowman ED, et al. (2008) MicroRNA expression profiles associated with prognosis and therapeutic outcome in colon adenocarcinoma. JAMA 299: 425–436.
35. Slaby O, Svoboda M, Fabian P, Smerdova T, Knoflickova D, et al. (2007) Altered expression of miR-21, miR-31, miR-143 and miR-145 is related to clinicopathologic features of colorectal cancer. Oncology 72: 397–402.
36. Schmid T, Bajer MM, Blees JS, Eifler LK, Milke L, et al. (2011) Inflammation-induced loss of Pdcd4 is mediated by phosphorylation-dependent degradation. Carcinogenesis 32: 1427–1433.
37. Kirkland SC (1985) Dome formation by a human colonic adenocarcinoma cell line (HCA-7). Cancer Res 45: 3790–3795.
38. O'Callaghan G, Kelly J, Shanahan F, Houston A (2008) Prostaglandin E2 stimulates Fas ligand expression via the EP1 receptor in colon cancer cells. Br J Cancer 99: 502–512.
39. Zhang Z, DuBois RN (2001) Detection of differentially expressed genes in human colon carcinoma cells treated with a selective COX-2 inhibitor. Oncogene 20: 4450–4456.
40. Wang P, Zou F, Zhang X, Li H, Dulak A, et al. (2009) microRNA-21 negatively regulates Cdc25A and cell cycle progression in colon cancer cells. Cancer Res 69: 8157–8165.
41. Foreman JE, Sorg JM, McGinnis KS, Rigas B, Williams JL, et al. (2009) Regulation of peroxisome proliferator-activated receptor-beta/delta by the APC/beta-CATENIN pathway and nonsteroidal antiinflammatory drugs. Mol Carcinog 48: 942–952.
42. Kutchera W, Jones DA, Matsunami N, Groden J, McIntyre TM, et al. (1996) Prostaglandin H synthase 2 is expressed abnormally in human colon cancer: evidence for a transcriptional effect. Proc Natl Acad Sci U S A 93: 4816–4820.
43. Cmarik JL, Min H, Hegamyer G, Zhan S, Kulesz-Martin M, et al. (1999) Differentially expressed protein Pdcd4 inhibits tumor promoter-induced neoplastic transformation. Proc Natl Acad Sci U S A 96: 14037–14042.
44. Shin VY, Jin H, Ng EK, Cheng AS, Chong WW, et al. (2011) NF-{kappa}B targets miR-16 and miR-21 in gastric cancer: involvement of prostaglandin E receptors. Carcinogenesis 32: 240–245.
45. Li M, Wu X, Xu XC (2001) Induction of apoptosis in colon cancer cells by cyclooxygenase-2 inhibitor NS398 through a cytochrome c-dependent pathway. Clin Cancer Res 7: 1010–1016.
46. Abdelrahim M, Safe S (2005) Cyclooxygenase-2 inhibitors decrease vascular endothelial growth factor expression in colon cancer cells by enhanced degradation of Sp1 and Sp4 proteins. Mol Pharmacol 68: 317–329.
47. Yao M, Lam EC, Kelly CR, Zhou W, Wolfe MM (2004) Cyclooxygenase-2 selective inhibition with NS-398 suppresses proliferation and invasiveness and delays liver metastasis in colorectal cancer. Br J Cancer 90: 712–719.
48. Nagatsuka I, Yamada N, Shimizu S, Ohira M, Nishino H, et al. (2002) Inhibitory effect of a selective cyclooxygenase-2 inhibitor on liver metastasis of colon cancer. Int J Cancer 100: 515–519.
49. Sheng H, Shao J, Kirkland SC, Isakson P, Coffey RJ, et al. (1997) Inhibition of human colon cancer cell growth by selective inhibition of cyclooxygenase-2. J Clin Invest 99: 2254–2259.
50. Leahy KM, Ornberg RL, Wang Y, Zweifel BS, Koki AT, et al. (2002) Cyclooxygenase-2 inhibition by celecoxib reduces proliferation and induces apoptosis in angiogenic endothelial cells in vivo. Cancer Res 62: 625–631.
51. Masferrer JL, Leahy KM, Koki AT, Zweifel BS, Settle SL, et al. (2000) Antiangiogenic and antitumor activities of cyclooxygenase-2 inhibitors. Cancer Res 60: 1306–1311.
52. Lu L, Byrnes K, Han C, Wang Y, Wu T (2014) MiR-21 Targets 15-PGDH and Promotes Cholangiocarcinoma Growth. Mol Cancer Res.

Permissions

All chapters in this book were first published in PLOS ONE, by The Public Library of Science; hereby published with permission under the Creative Commons Attribution License or equivalent. Every chapter published in this book has been scrutinized by our experts. Their significance has been extensively debated. The topics covered herein carry significant findings which will fuel the growth of the discipline. They may even be implemented as practical applications or may be referred to as a beginning point for another development.

The contributors of this book come from diverse backgrounds, making this book a truly international effort. This book will bring forth new frontiers with its revolutionizing research information and detailed analysis of the nascent developments around the world.

We would like to thank all the contributing authors for lending their expertise to make the book truly unique. They have played a crucial role in the development of this book. Without their invaluable contributions this book wouldn't have been possible. They have made vital efforts to compile up to date information on the varied aspects of this subject to make this book a valuable addition to the collection of many professionals and students.

This book was conceptualized with the vision of imparting up-to-date information and advanced data in this field. To ensure the same, a matchless editorial board was set up. Every individual on the board went through rigorous rounds of assessment to prove their worth. After which they invested a large part of their time researching and compiling the most relevant data for our readers.

The editorial board has been involved in producing this book since its inception. They have spent rigorous hours researching and exploring the diverse topics which have resulted in the successful publishing of this book. They have passed on their knowledge of decades through this book. To expedite this challenging task, the publisher supported the team at every step. A small team of assistant editors was also appointed to further simplify the editing procedure and attain best results for the readers.

Apart from the editorial board, the designing team has also invested a significant amount of their time in understanding the subject and creating the most relevant covers. They scrutinized every image to scout for the most suitable representation of the subject and create an appropriate cover for the book.

The publishing team has been an ardent support to the editorial, designing and production team. Their endless efforts to recruit the best for this project, has resulted in the accomplishment of this book. They are a veteran in the field of academics and their pool of knowledge is as vast as their experience in printing. Their expertise and guidance has proved useful at every step. Their uncompromising quality standards have made this book an exceptional effort. Their encouragement from time to time has been an inspiration for everyone.

The publisher and the editorial board hope that this book will prove to be a valuable piece of knowledge for researchers, students, practitioners and scholars across the globe.

List of Contributors

Xin Luo, Wai Lydia Tai, Liting Sun and Qiu Qiu
Department of Anaesthesiology, The University of Hong Kong, HKSAR, China,
Laboratory and Clinical Research Institute for Pain, The University of Hong Kong, HKSAR, China

Zhengyuan Xia
Department of Anaesthesiology, The University of Hong Kong, HKSAR, China
Research Center of Heart, Brain, Hormone and Healthy Aging, The University of Hong Kong, HKSAR, China

Sookja Kim Chung
Department of Anatomy, The University of Hong Kong, HKSAR, China
Research Center of Heart, Brain, Hormone and Healthy Aging, The University of Hong Kong, HKSAR, China
Laboratory and Clinical Research Institute for Pain, The University of Hong Kong, HKSAR, China

Chi Wai Cheung
Department of Anaesthesiology, The University of Hong Kong, HKSAR, China
Research Center of Heart, Brain, Hormone and Healthy Aging, The University of Hong Kong, HKSAR, China
Laboratory and Clinical Research Institute for Pain, The University of Hong Kong, HKSAR, China

Carlos A. Valdez, Roald N. Leif and Brian P. Mayer
Physical and Life Sciences Directorate, Lawrence Livermore National Laboratory, Livermore, California, United States of America
Forensic Science Center, Lawrence Livermore National Laboratory, Livermore, California, United States of America

Chenlong Liao, Wenchuan Zhang, Min Yang, Qiufeng Ma, Guowei Li and Wenxiang Zhong
Department of Neurosurgery, XinHua Hospital, affiliated to Shanghai JiaoTong University School of Medicine, Shanghai, P. R. China

Andrée Aubin
Centre ostéopathique du Québec, Montréal, Québec, Canada

Chantal Morin
Centre ostéopathique du Québec, Montréal, Québec, Canada
School of Rehabilitation, Faculty of Medicine and Health Sciences, University of Sherbrooke, Sherbrooke Québec, Canada

Jin Xu, Zhigang Lu, Mingming Xu, Gavril W. Pasternak and Ying-Xian Pan
Department of Neurology and Molecular Pharmacology and Chemistry Program, Memorial Sloan Kettering Cancer Center, New York, New York, United States of America

Grace C. Rossi
Department of Psychology, Long Island University, Post Campus, Brookville, New York, United States of America

Benjamin Kest and Amanda R. Waxman
Department of Psychology and Center for Developmental Neuroscience, City University of New York, Staten Island, New York, United States of America

Michael E. Herce
Department of Medicine, Division of Infectious Diseases, University of North Carolina School of Medicine, Chapel Hill, North Carolina, United States of America,
Abwenzi Pa Za Umoyo, Neno, Malawi
Partners in Health, Boston, Massachusetts, United States of America

Shekinah N. Elmore
Department of Global Health and Social Medicine, Harvard Medical School, Boston, Massachusetts, United States of America

Noel Kalanga, Atupere Phiri, James W. Keck, Junior Bazile, Jason A. Beste and Jonas Rigodon
Abwenzi Pa Za Umoyo, Neno, Malawi, 3 Partners in Health, Boston, Massachusetts, United States of America

Emily B. Wroe
Abwenzi Pa Za Umoyo, Neno, Malawi, 3 Partners in Health, Boston, Massachusetts, United States of America
Partners in Health, Boston, Massachusetts, United States of America
Department of Medicine, Brigham and Women's Hospital, Boston, Massachusetts, United States of America

Alishya Mayfield
Department of Medicine, Brigham and Women's Hospital, Boston, Massachusetts, United States of America

Felix Chingoli and Listern Tengatenga
Neno District Health Office, Neno District Hospital, Ministry of Health, Government of the Republic of Malawi, Neno, Malawi

Eric L. Krakauer
Partners in Health, Boston, Massachusetts, United States of America
Department of Global Health and Social Medicine, Harvard Medical School, Boston, Massachusetts, United States of America
Department of Medicine, Division of Palliative Care, Massachusetts General Hospital, Boston, Massachusetts, United States of America

Mingzhu Zhuang and Lianzhu Lin
College of Light Industry and Food Sciences, South China University of Technology, Guangzhou, China

Mouming Zhao
College of Light Industry and Food Sciences, South China University of Technology, Guangzhou, China
State Key Laboratory of Pulp and Paper Engineering, South China University of Technology, Guangzhou, China

Huijuan Qiu, Dingbo Shi, Jingshu Wang, Yun Tian and Wuguo Deng
State Key Laboratory of Oncology in South China, Sun Yat-Sen University Cancer Center, Guangzhou, China

Laura S. Stone
Alan Edwards Centre for Research on Pain, McGill University, Montreal, Quebec, Canada
Faculty of Dentistry, McGill University, Montreal, Quebec, Canada,
Department of Anesthesiology, Faculty of Medicine, McGill University, Montreal, Quebec, Canada
Department of Pharmacology and Therapeutics, Faculty of Medicine,
McGill University, Montreal, Quebec, Canada
Department of Neurology and Neurosurgery, Faculty of Medicine, McGill University, Montreal, Quebec, Canada

Jonathan P. German and Kelly F. Kitto
Department of Neuroscience, Medical School, University of Minnesota, Minneapolis, Minnesota, United States of America

Carolyn A. Fairbanks and George L. Wilcox
Department of Pharmaceutics, College of Pharmacy, University of Minnesota, Minneapolis, Minnesota, United States of America
Department of Neuroscience, Medical School, University of Minnesota, Minneapolis, Minnesota, United States of America
Department of Pharmacology, Medical School, University of Minnesota, Minneapolis, Minnesota, United States of America
Department of Dermatology, Medical School, University of Minnesota, Minneapolis, Minnesota, United States of America

Anuradha Venugopalan, Ravi P. Ghorpade and Arvind Chopra
Center for Rheumatic Diseases, Pune, India

Eivind Aadland
Sogn og Fjordane University College, Faculty of Health Studies, Førde, Norway

Torkil Terum
Sogn og Fjordane University College, Faculty of Teacher Education and Sports, Sogndal, Norway

Asgeir Mamen
Sogn og Fjordane University College, Faculty of Teacher Education and Sports, Sogndal, Norway
University College of Health Sciences - Campus Kristiania, Oslo, Norway

Geir Kåre Resaland
Sogn og Fjordane University College, Faculty of Teacher Education and Sports, Sogndal, Norway
Sogn og Fjordane Center for Health Research, Førde Central Hospital, Førde, Norway

Lars Bo Andersen
Department of Sports Medicine, Norwegian School of Sport Sciences, Oslo, Norway
Department of Sport Sciences and Clinical

Biomechanics, University of Southern Denmark, Odense, Denmark

Zhenhong Zou and Yuming Jiang
Department of General Surgery, Nanfang Hospital, Southern Medical University, Guangzhou City, Guangdong Province, China

Mingjia Xiao
Department of Hepatobiliary Surgery, Wuxi People's Hospital of Nanjing Medical University, Wuxi, Jiangsu Province, China

Ruiyao Zhou
Department of General Surgery, The Third Affiliated Hospital of Wenzhou Medical University, Ruian City, Zhejiang Province, China

Diana Amorim, Ana David-Pereira, Patrícia Marques, Sónia Puga, Patrícia Rebelo, Patrício Costa, Armando Almeida and Filipa Pinto-Ribeiro
Life and Health Sciences Research Institute (ICVS), School of Health Sciences (ECS), University of Minho, Braga, Portugal
ICVS/3B's - PT Government Associate Laboratory, Braga/Guimarães, Portugal

Antti Pertovaara
Institute of Biomedicine/Physiology, University of Helsinki, Helsinki, Finland

Svend Erik Mathiassen, David M. Hallman and Eugene Lyskov
Centre for Musculoskeletal Research, Department of Occupational and Public Health Sciences, University of Gävle, Gävle, Sweden

Staffan Hygge
Department of Building, Energy and Environmental Engineering, University of Gävle, Gävle, Sweden

Ahmed M. Al-Abd
Department of Pharmacology and Toxicology, Faculty of Pharmacy, King Abdulaziz University, Jeddah, Saudi Arabia

Fahad A. Al-Abbasi
Department of Biochemistry, Faculty of Science, King Abdulaziz University, Jeddah, Saudi Arabia

Salwa M. Nofal and Wafaa I. El-Eraky
Department of Pharmacology, Medical Division, National Research Centre, Giza, Egypt

Amani E. Khalifa and Ashraf B. Abdel-Naim
Department of Pharmacology and Toxicology, Faculty of Pharmacy, Ain Shams University, Cairo, Egypt

Richard O. Williams
Kennedy Institute of Rheumatology, University of Oxford, Oxford, United Kingdom

Ayman A. Nagy
Department of Forensic Medicine and Clinical Toxicology, Faculty of Medicine, Tanta University, Egypt

Patrizia Maria Carrieri, Caroline Lions, Julien Cohen, Marion Mora, Fabienne Marcellin, Bruno Spire and Perrine Roux
INSERM UMR912 (SESSTIM), Marseille, France
Aix Marseille Université , UMR_S912, Marseille, France
ORS PACA, Observatoire Régional de la Santé Provence Alpes Côte d'Azur, Marseille, France

Laurent Michel
INSERM, Research Unit 669, Paris, France, 5 Univ Paris-Sud and Univ Paris Descartes, UMR-S0669, Paris, France, 6 Centre Pierre Nicole, Paris, France

Muriel Vray
Unité de Recherche et d'Expertise en Epidémiologie des Maladies Emergentes, Institut Pasteur, Paris, France, 8 Institut National de la Santé et de la Recherche
Médicale (INSERM), Paris, France

Alain Morel
Oppelia, Paris, France

Hyun Jung Jho, Jin Young Choi and Eun Jung Park
Hospice & Palliative Care Branch, National Cancer Control Institute, National Cancer Center, Goyang, Republic of Korea

Yeol Kim
Division of Cancer Management & Policy, National Cancer Control Institute, National Cancer Center, Goyang, Republic of Korea

Kyung Ae Kong
Clinical Trial Center, Ewha Womans University Medical Center, Seoul, Republic of Korea

Dae Hyun Kim
Department of Pain and Anesthesiology, Hospital, National Cancer Center, Goyang, Republic of Korea

Eun Jeong Nam and Jin Young Choi
Department of Nursing, Hospital, National Cancer Center, Goyang, Republic of Korea

Sujin Koh
Department of Hematology and Oncology, Ulsan University Hospital, Ulsan, Republic of Korea

Kwan Ok Hwang
Korean Hospice & Palliative Nurse Association, Daejeon, Republic of Korea

Sun Kyung Baek
Department of Medical Oncology and Hematology, Kyung Hee University Medical Center, Seoul, Republic of Korea

Joakim M. Bischoff, Thomas K. Ringsted, Marian Petersen and Mads U. Werner
Multidisciplinary Pain Center 7612, Neuroscience Center, Rigshospitalet, Copenhagen University, Copenhagen, Denmark

Claudia Sommer and Nurcan Üçeyler
Department of Neurology, University Hospital of Würzburg, Würzburg, Germany

Charles N. Rudick, Aisha K. Taylor, Ryan E. Yaggie and Anthony J. Schaeffer
Department of Urology, Feinberg School of Medicine, Northwestern University, Chicago, Illinois, United States of America

David J. Klumpp
Department of Urology, Feinberg School of Medicine, Northwestern University, Chicago, Illinois, United States of America
Microbiology-Immunology, Feinberg School of Medicine, Northwestern University, Chicago, Illinois, United States of America

Laura Anselmi
CURE Digestive Diseases Research Center, Division of Digestive Diseases and Department of Medicine, David Geffen School of Medicine, University of California Los Angeles, Los Angeles, California, United States of America

Celine Duraffourd and Erica Kumala
CURE Digestive Diseases Research Center, Division of Digestive Diseases and Department of Medicine, David Geffen School of Medicine, University of California Los Angeles, Los Angeles, California, United States of America
CURE Digestive Diseases Research Center, Division of Digestive Diseases and Department of Neurobiology, David Geffen School of Medicine, University of California Los Angeles, Los Angeles, California, United States of America

Nicholas C. Brecha Catia Sternini
Veteran Administration Greater Los Angeles Healthcare System, Los Angeles, California, United States of America

Sarah McDavid, Mary Beth Bauer and Rebecca L. Brindley
Department of Anesthesiology, Vanderbilt University School of Medicine, Nashville, Tennessee, United States of America

Mark L. Jewell
Department of Pharmacology, Vanderbilt University School of Medicine, Nashville, Tennessee, United States of America

Kevin P. M. Currie
Department of Anesthesiology, Department of Pharmacology, and Vanderbilt Brain
Institute, Vanderbilt University School of Medicine, Nashville, Tennessee, United States of America

Yun Hyung Koog
Honam Research Center, Medifarm Hospital, Suncheon, Republic of Korea
Department of Oriental Medicine, Medifarm Hospital, Suncheon, Republic of Korea

Jin Su Lee
Honam Research Center, Medifarm Hospital, Suncheon, Republic of Korea
Department of Rehabilitation, Medifarm Hospital, Suncheon, Republic of Kore

Hyungsun Wi
Honam Research Center, Medifarm Hospital, Suncheon, Republic of Korea

Deirdre S. Stewart, David W. Pierce, Mayo Hotta¤, Alex T. Stern and Stuart A. Forman
Department of Anesthesia Critical Care and Pain Medicine, Massachusetts General Hospital, Boston, Massachusetts, United States of America

Oliver Peacock, Andrew C. Lee, Fraser Cameron, Rebecca Tarbox, Natasha Vafadar-Isfahani, Cristina Tufarelli and Jonathan N. Lund
Surgery Group, Division of Medical Sciences and Graduate Entry Medicine, School of Medicine, University of Nottingham, Royal Derby Hospital, Derby, United Kingdom

Index